ALLOGENEIC STEM CELL TRANSPLANTATION

CURRENT CLINICAL ONCOLOGY

Maurie Markman, MD, SERIES EDITOR

ALLOGENEIC STEM CELL TRANSPLANTATION

Clinical Research and Practice

Edited by

MARY J. LAUGHLIN, MD

*Ireland Cancer Center,
Case Western Reserve University, Cleveland, OH*
and

HILLARD M. LAZARUS, MD

*Ireland Cancer Center,
Case Western Reserve University, Cleveland, OH*

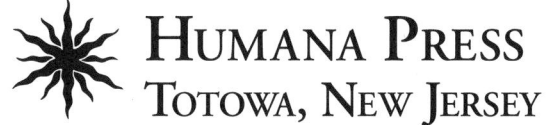 HUMANA PRESS
TOTOWA, NEW JERSEY

To Robert O'Connor and our twins Robert and Margaret for their continued love and patience.
— M. J. L.

To my loving wife Joan and my sons Jeffrey and Adam, for all their support.
— H. M. L.

Production Editor: Tracy Catanese
Cover design by Patricia F. Cleary.

For additional copies, pricing for bulk purchases, and/or information about other Humana titles, contact Humana at the above address or at any of the following numbers: Tel: 973-256-1699; Fax: 973-256-8341; E-mail: humana@humanapr.com or visit our website at www.humanapress.com

This publication is printed on acid-free paper. ∞
ANSI Z39.48-1984 (American National Standards Institute)
Permanence of Paper for Printed Library Materials.

Printed in the United States of America.   10 9 8 7 6 5 4 3 2 1

Library of Congress Cataloging-in-Publication Data

Allogeneic stem cell transplantation : clinical research and practice / edited by Mary J. Laughlin and Hillard M. Lazarus
          p. ; cm. -- (Current clinical oncology)
       Includes bibliographical references and index.
       ISBN 0-89603-979-X (alk. paper); 1-59259-333-X (e-book)
          1. Blood--Diseases. 2. Hematopoietic stem cells--Transplantation. I. Laughlin, Mary J. II. Lazarus, Hillard M. III. Current clinical oncology (Totowa N.J.)
          [DNLM: 1. Hematopoietic Stem Cell Transplantation. 2. Transplantation, Homologous--methods. WH 380 A441 2003]
       RC636 .A45 2003
       617.4'4--dc21

                                                                                                                    200268939

PREFACE

Hematopoietic stem cell transplantation for patients with hematologic disorders is undergoing fast-paced changes, owing to evolving paradigms of stem cell plasticity and improved understanding of mechanisms underlying immunologic tolerance. In *Allogeneic Stem Cell Transplantation*, the editors have focused on assigning topics relevant to evolving knowledge in the field in order to guide clinicians in decision-making and management of their patients. The leaders in this discipline have responded by providing state-of-the-art discussions addressing these topics.

Important advances in patient management include the use of tyrosine kinase inhibitors in the treatment of chronic myelogenous leukemia that has abruptly changed previous standard care paths for these patients in tracking toward allografting as consolidative therapy. Moreover, the results of randomized trials in breast cancer over the past few years have guided clinicians away from use of autologous transplantation to focus now on newer perspectives of potential graft-vs-tumor effects after allogeneic transplantation. The administration of nonmyeloablative conditioning has also brought forth new concepts in the management of hematologic malignancies, thought to be of particular importance in patients with multiple myeloma and low grade non-Hodgkin's lymphomas. The reduced toxicity of these novel conditioning regimens has also raised new possibilities in the application of allogeneic stem cell transplantation for patients with non-malignant hematologic disorders and selected solid tumors such as renal cell carcinoma.

Further examples of innovation in allogeneic transplantation outlined in this text include the results of phase I trials of umbilical cord blood as a new stem cell source, confirming its safety and thereby alleviating previous restrictions for patients for whom an HLA-matched graft from an adult donor is not available. The previous focus of stem cell transplant physicians on measurement and characterization of CD34-expressing hematopoietic stem cells has broadened recently to examine the role of marrow mesenchymal stem cells and graft accessory cells in facilitating engraftment and immune reconstitution. These issues of graft engineering play an important role as the field has transitioned from the routine use of bone marrow to mobilized peripheral blood stem cell grafting. Finally, the ongoing attempts to discern lymphocyte populations critical in mediating graft-vs-leukemia/lymphoma effects and immune tolerance are anticipated to benefit clinicians and patients, as well to reduce graft-vs-host disease incidence and severity while preserving antitumor effects in patients undergoing allogeneic transplantation.

The editors hope that this new information, well-summarized by the authors in *Allogeneic Stem Cell Transplantation*, will prove of significant benefit to clinicians in the approach to and care of their patients.

Mary J. Laughlin, MD
Hillard M. Lazarus, MD

CONTENTS

PART V. PREVENTION AND MANAGEMENT OF RELAPSE AFTER ALLOGENEIC TRANSPLANTATION

PART VI. PRECLINICAL STUDIES IN ALLOGENEIC TRANSPLANTATION

PART VII. EPILOGUE

CONTRIBUTORS

DANIEL ANDERSON, MD, *Adult Blood and Marrow Transplant Program, Department of Medicine, University of Minnesota, Minneapolis, MN*

FREDERICK R. APPELBAUM, MD, *Clinical Research Division, Fred Hutchinson Cancer Research Center, Seattle, WA*

DAVID AVIGAN, MD, *Bone Marrow Transplantation, Beth Israel-Deaconess Medical Center, Boston, MA*

JULIET BARKER, MBBS (HONS), *Blood and Marrow Transplant Program, Department of Medicine, University of Minnesota, MN*

ERNEST BEUTLER, MD, *Molecular and Experimental Medicine, The Scripps Research Institute, La Jolla, CA*

PHILIP J. BIERMAN, MD, *Oncology/Hematology, University of Nebraska Medical Center, Omaha, NE*

RANDY BROWN, MD, *Section of Bone Marrow Transplant and Leukemia, Division of Medical Oncology, Washington University School of Medicine, St. Louis, MO*

NELSON J. CHAO, MD, *Division of Oncology and Bone Marrow Transplantation, Duke University Medical Center, Durham, NC*

ROBERT H. COLLINS, JR., MD, *Bone Marrow Transplantation Program, University of Texas Southwestern Medical Center at Dallas, Dallas, TX*

EDWARD COPELAN, MD, *BMT Program, The Ohio State University Hospital, Columbus, OH*

STEVEN M. DEVINE, MD, *Section of Bone Marrow Transplantation and Leukemia, Division of Medical Oncology, Washington University School of Medicine, St. Louis, MO*

JOHN F. DIPERSIO, MD, PhD, *Section of Bone Marrow Transplantation and Leukemia, Division of Medical Oncology, Washington University School of Medicine, St. Louis, MO*

IGOR ESPINOZA-DELGADO, MD, *National Institute on Aging, National Institutes of Health, Baltimore, MD*

STEPHEN J. FORMAN, MD, *Division of Hematology and Bone Marrow Transplantation, City of Hope National Medical Center, Duarte, CA*

HENRY C. FUNG, MD, *Division of Hematology and Bone Marrow Transplantation, City of Hope National Medical Center, Duarte, CA*

STANTON L. GERSON, MD, *Ireland Cancer Center, University Hospitals of Cleveland, Case Western Reserve University, Cleveland, OH*

ANDREAS H. GROLL, MD, *Center for Bone Marrow Transplantation, Wilhelms-University Medical Center, Muenster, Germany*

THOMAS G. GROSS, MD, PhD, *BMT Program, Department of Medicine, Children's Hospital Medical Center, Cincinnati, OH*

RONALD HOFFMAN, MD, *Chief, Section of Hematology and Oncology, and Director, UIC Cancer Center, College of Medicine, University of Illinois at Chicago, Chicago, IL*

CARL H. JUNE, *Abramson Family Cancer Research Institute and the Department of Pathology and Laboratory Medicine, University of Pennsylvania, Philadelphia, PA*

PARTOW KEBRIAEI, MD, *Section of Hematology/Oncology, Department of Medicine, University of Chicago Medical Center, Chicago, IL*

OMER N. KOÇ, MD, *Ireland Cancer Center, University Hospitals of Cleveland, Case Western Reserve University, Cleveland, OH*

GINNA G. LAPORT, *Division of Bone Marrow Transplantation, Stanford University Medical Center, Stanford, CA*

MARY J. LAUGHLIN, MD, *Allogeneic Transplant Program, Ireland Cancer Center, University Hospitals of Cleveland, Case Western Reserve University, Cleveland, OH*

HILLARD M. LAZARUS, MD, *Blood and Marrow Transplant Program, Ireland Cancer Center, University Hospitals of Cleveland, Case Western Reserve University, Cleveland, OH*

BRETT J. LOECHELT, MD, *Division of Hematology/Oncology, Children's Hospital Medical Center, Cincinnati, OH*

DAN L. LONGO, MD, *National Institute on Aging, National Institutes of Health, Baltimore, MD*

MASSIMO F. MARTELLI, MD, PhD, *Chair of Hematology, University of Perugia, Perugia, Italy*

JAMES R. MASON, MD, *Blood and Marrow Transplantation Program, Scripps Clinic, La Jolla, CA*

WILLIAM J. MURPHY, PhD, *Department of Microbiology, University of Nevada Reno, Reno, NV*

ROBERT S. NEGRIN, MD, *Bone Marrow Transplantation, Stanford University School of Medicine, Stanford, CA*

DONNA PRZEPIORKA, MD, PhD, *Malignant Hematology and Transplantation, University of Tennessee, Memphis, TN*

JERALD P. RADICH, MD, *Clinical Research Division, Fred Hutchinson Cancer Research Center, Seattle, WA*

YAIR REISNER, PhD, *Immunology, Weizmann Institute of Science, Rehovot, Israel*

DAVID A. RIZZIERI, MD, *Department of Medicine, Duke University Medical Center, Durham, NC*

JACOB M. ROWE, MD, *Department of Hematology, Rambam Medical Center, Technion, Haifa, Israel*

ABBY B. SIEGEL, MD, *Division of Medical Oncology, Department of Medicine, Herbert Irving Comprehensive Cancer Center, Columbia University College of Physicians and Surgeons, New York, NY*

WENDY STOCK, MD, *Section of Hematology/Oncology, Department of Medicine, University of Chicago Medical Center, Chicago, IL*

KAI SUN, MD, PhD, *Department of Microbiology, University of Nevada Reno, Reno, NV*

JAMES E. TALMADGE, PhD, *Departments of Pathology and Microbiology, University of Nebraska Medical Center, Omaha, NE*

STEFANO TARANTOLO, MD, *Oncology/Hematology, University of Nebraska Medical Center, Omaha, NE*

LINDA T. VAHDAT, MD, *Medical Oncology Department, Milstein Hospital, Columbia University, New York, NY*

MICHAEL R. VERNERIS, MD, *Division of Pediatric Hematology, Oncology, and Bone Marrow Transplantation, Stanford University, Stanford, CA*

RAVI VIJ, MD, *Section of Bone Marrow Transplantation and Leukemia, Division of Medical Oncology, Washington University School of Medicine, St. Louis, MO*

JOHN E. WAGNER, MD, *Department of Pediatrics, Blood and Marrow Transplant Program of the University of Minnesota School of Medicine, Minneapolis, MN*

THOMAS J. WALSH, *Immunocompromised Host Section, Pediatric Oncology Branch, National Cancer Institute, National Institutes of Health, Bethesda, MD*

DANIEL WEISDORF, MD, *Adult Blood and Marrow Transplant Program, Department of Medicine, University of Minnesota, Minneapolis, MN*

LISBETH A. WELNIAK, PhD, *Department of Microbiology, University of Nevada Reno, Reno, NV*

STEVEN N. WOLFF, MD, *Stem Cell Transplantation Program, Department of Medicine, Vanderbilt University, Nashville, TN, and Aastrom Biosciences, Ann Arbor, MI*

I   HISTORICAL PERSPECTIVE

1

Hematopoietic Stem Cell Transplantation
A Historical Perspective

Frederick R. Appelbaum, MD

1. INTRODUCTION

Over the last half-century, hematopoietic cell transplantation has evolved from an idea to a well-established therapy used in the treatment of tens of thousands of individuals annually. This evolution is the product of laboratory-based investigations, studies using animal models, and especially clinical trials involving human subjects. The following brief account highlights some of the more outstanding contributions, with particular emphasis on those made during the earlier development of the procedure (Table 1). In this brief recounting it is possible to include only a small fraction of the valuable contributions, and apologies are prospectively offered to all of those whose important work is not mentioned. For a more complete retelling of the story, with more extensive bibliographies, the reader is referred to a number of other excellent papers (1–4).

2. EARLY STUDIES LEADING TO THE FIRST HUMAN TRIALS

While earlier references to oral or intravenous administration of bone marrow exist, the story of hematopoietic cell transplantation really begins shortly after World War II and the first (and only) use of nuclear weapons. The realization that bone marrow failure was a predictable and fatal consequence of exposure to relatively low levels of radiation spurred considerable interest in the biology of radiation exposure. A landmark study was published in 1949 by Jacobson et al., who showed that mice exposed to an otherwise lethal dose of radiation would survive if their spleens were protected by lead foil (5). Lorenz et al. showed that this protective

From: *Current Clinical Oncology: Allogeneic Stem Cell Transplantation*
Edited by: Mary S. Laughlin and Hillard M. Lazarus © Humana Press Inc., Totowa, NJ

Table 1
Milestones in the Development of Hematopoietic Cell Transplantation

1949	Spleen shielding experiment of Jacobson.
1957	First human twin transplants for leukemia.
1962	Successful allogeneic transplants in dogs.
1968	First successful allogeneic transplants in humans.
1977	Successful application of autologous marrow transplantation.
1990	Dr. Thomas awarded Nobel Prize.

effect could be transferred between animals when they demonstrated that infusion of marrow or spleen cells from a healthy animal to an irradiated one reversed the otherwise lethal effects of radiation (6). At the time, it was unclear whether this protective effect was due to humoral factors produced by the nonirradiated cells or due to the cells themselves. Two experiments proved the cellular nature of radiation protection. Main and Prehn in 1955 reported that radiated mice given marrow grafts from nonsyngeneic donors not only recovered, but could no longer reject donor skin grafts. This demonstration of active tolerance strongly implied that the radiation protection effect was not simply the result of a humoral factor stimulating recovery of host hematopoiesis (7). The following year, Ford et al. provided definitive evidence of the cellular nature of radiation protection when they used cytogenetic markers to demonstrate the donor identity of marrow in irradiated hosts post-transplant (8). Finally, in 1956, Barnes et al. published their classic paper describing the use of supralethal radiation followed by marrow grafting as treatment for murine leukemia (9). In these studies, they noted eradication of leukemia in irradiated mice receiving allogeneic marrow, but not syngeneic marrow, thus demonstrating for the first time the possibility of a graft-vs-leukemia effect.

3. INITIAL TRIALS IN HUMANS

The demonstration that systemic irradiation could eradicate a normal marrow and that marrow function could be restored by infusion of syngeneic marrow, at least in mice, led Thomas et al. to attempt a similar approach in humans (10). In 1957, he reported the results of treating two patients suffering from advanced leukemia using supralethal radiation followed by an infusion of marrow from their identical twins (11). Both patients engrafted promptly, demonstrating the feasibility of the approach, but subsequently their leukemia recurred. Further attempts at marrow transplants using donors other than identical twins were made over the next decade. The first patient engrafted using allogeneic marrow was reported by Mathe in 1965, but the patient died of complications probably related to graft-vs-host disease (12). In 1970, Bortin et al. published a report summarizing the results of approx 200 allogeneic transplants performed during the 1950s and 1960s and concluded that none had resulted in long-term survival (13). The problems that limited the success of transplantation during this era were the limited understanding of details of human histocompatibility, lack of experience with the use of immunosuppressive drugs, and shortcomings in supportive care techniques.

4. LABORATORY STUDIES LEADING TO THE FIRST SUCCESSES IN PATIENTS

A number of critical laboratory studies were performed during the 1950s and 1960s, which led to the first successful allogeneic transplants in humans. In the late 1950s, Dausset (14) and van Rood et al. (15) described a number of antigens expressed on human leukocytes (human leukocyte antigens or HLA) that influenced the success of skin grafts and, thus, were thought to be generally involved in histocompatibility. The ability to select HLA-compatible siblings as marrow donors was one of the major advances leading to the ultimate success of allogeneic transplantation in humans. A series of experiments conducted in dogs defined many additional principles necessary for the ultimate success of transplantation in humans. Dogs, unlike mice, are an outbred species, and the relative importance of histocompatibility or incompatibility turns out to reasonably parallel their importance in humans. Studies in dogs, conducted primarily by Thomas and his colleagues, demonstrated the dose of radiation necessary to achieve engraftment, the requirement for histocompatibility matching to prevent graft rejection or lethal graft-versus-host disease, and the ability of postgrafting methotrexate to adequately suppress acute graft-vs-host disease to allow for the majority of animals to become long-term healthy survivors after receiving marrow grafts from histocompatible donors (16–19). The increased understanding of human histocompatibility, coupled with advances in the techniques of transplantation and improvements in supportive care, set the stage for the first successes in human marrow transplantation.

5. INITIAL SUCCESSES IN HUMAN MARROW TRANSPLANTATION

The first therapeutically successful human marrow transplants were reported in 1968 and 1969, when three infants with severe combined immunodeficiency disease were successfully transplanted from their HLA-matched siblings (20–22). According to recent reports, these patients continue to survive more than three decades after transplantation. Transplantation for severe combined immunodeficiency from HLA-identical siblings does not require a preparative regimen to prevent graft rejection or eliminate disease. The first successful transplants requiring a preparative regimen were reported three years later, in 1972, when the Seattle group reported success in transplanting patients for aplastic anemia from HLA-identical siblings using a preparative regimen of high-dose cyclophosphamide and posttransplant methotrexate (23). At approximately the same time, the first successful transplants for acute leukemia were being performed. In 1975, Thomas et al. published a review article describing the state of the art at that time, and noting that successful engraftment could be achieved in most patients with aplastic anemia and acute leukemia and that some of these patients appeared to be surviving without evidence of their disease for at least several years posttransplant (24). Two years later the same group published a follow-up of the first 100 patients transplanted for advanced leukemia and provided convincing evidence that transplantation could, in fact, cure at least a portion of such patients (25).

Over the next several years, a number of other notable hematopoietic cell transplant "firsts" were reported. These firsts involved the use of alternate sources of stem cells, the use of transplantation to treat additional diseases, and the use of transplantation earlier in the disease course. Prior to 1977, there had been several attempts to use autologous marrow to support the administration of high-dose curative therapy. While these reports suggested that autologous transplants might lead to engraftment, lack of genetic markers or control groups prohibited definitive conclusions, and the clinical situations studied were so advanced that no clinical benefit was obvious (26,27). In 1977, the group at the National Institute of Health (NIH) published a controlled trial demonstrating that previously cryopreserved autologous marrow was capable of establishing hematopoietic function in humans (28). These same studies demonstrated that the high-dose therapy made possible by transplantation could cure selected patients of recurrent non-Hodgkin's lymphoma (29).

The demonstration that transplantation could be effective therapy for patients with endstage disease led a number of investigators to study the role of transplantation earlier in the disease course. In 1979, the first reports emerged showing encouraging results in patients with acute myeloid leukemia transplanted in first remission *(30,31)* and for patients with chronic myeloid leukemia transplanted while in chronic phase *(32)*. Several years later, the first successful transplants for patients with hemoglobinopathies, including β-thalassemia and sickle cell anemia, were reported *(33,34)*. It was also during the early 1980s that the first reports of successful transplants using marrow from HLA-matched unrelated donors began to emerge.

6. SUBSEQUENT ADVANCES IN THE APPLICATION OF HEMATOPOIETIC CELL TRANSPLANTATION

Since the early 1980s, there have been a large number of notable advances, a few of which are mentioned here. These advances, and many others that are not discussed here for lack of space, have substantially improved the outcome of hematopoietic cell transplantation and are the subject of this textbook.

6.1. Source of Stem Cells

The use of growth-factor-mobilized hematopoietic stem cells harvested from peripheral blood was shown to dramatically hasten engraftment and has replaced marrow as the preferred source of stem cells for autologous, and in some cases allogeneic, engraftment *(35,36)*. Placental cord blood has become a useful source of stem cells, especially for pediatric patients *(37)*. Large donor registries have been created, making matched unrelated donor transplantation available for the majority of patients *(38,39)*. Advances in HLA-typing technology have allowed for continued improvements in selection of appropriate donors *(40)*.

6.2. Preparative Regimens

Preparative regimens based on busulfan and cyclophosphamide were developed and have become the most frequently used for treating myeloid malignancies *(41)*. The development of nonablative preparative regimens provides a method for capturing a graft-vs-tumor effect without exposing patients to the toxicities of high-dose therapy *(42–44)*. The demonstration that infusion of viable donor lymphocytes can result in complete disappearance of leukemia after posttransplant recurrence, not only provides physicians with another therapeutic tool, but has generally fueled efforts in the field of clinical tumor immunology *(45)*.

6.3. Graft-vs-Host Disease

The combination of methotrexate plus cyclosporin was shown to provide better prophylaxis of acute graft-vs-host disease than either agent alone and became the standard of care *(46,47)*. Techniques involving the removal of T-cells from the stem cell inoculum were shown to offer an alterative method to prevent graft-vs-host disease *(48,49)*.

6.4. Supportive Care Techniques

The use of hematopoietic growth factors was shown to accelerate hematopoietic recovery after autologous stem cell transplantation *(50)*. Methods to prevent cytomegalovirus (CMV) disease, by the use of CMV seronegative blood products in CMV seronegative patients or by the use of ganciclovir, dramatically reduced the death rate from CMV *(51,52)*. The prophylactic use of fluconazole likewise improved overall survival following allogeneic transplantation *(53)*.

The advances noted above, as well as many others, have led to the widespread application of hematopoietic cell transplantation as an effective treatment for selected patients with essentially all hematologic diseases, both malignant and nonmalignant. Important experiments are underway determining whether approaches requiring hematopoietic cell transplantation have a role in the treatment of autoimmune disorders and nonhematopoietic malignancies.

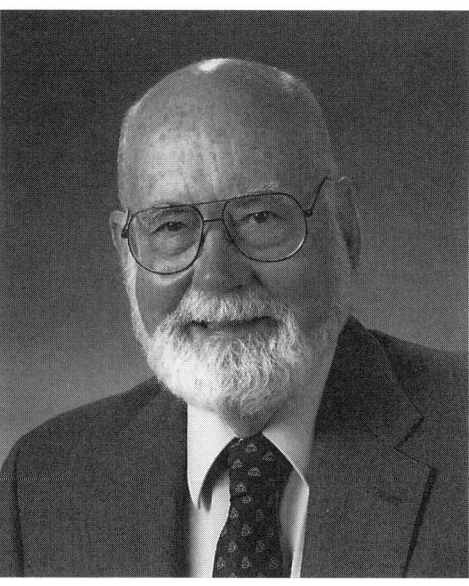

Fig. 1. Dr. E. Donnall Thomas, recipient of the 1990 Nobel Prize for Physiology and Medicine (along with Dr. Joseph Murray), recognizing the field of organ transplantation.

7. A TRIBUTE TO E. DONNALL THOMAS

While many individuals, including Robert Good, George Santos, and Rainer Storb, have made enormous contributions to the field of hematopoietic cell transplantation, the role of E. Donnall Thomas stands out (Fig. 1). In the mid-1950s, Thomas became aware of the studies of Leon Jacobson and others and became convinced of the clinical potential of marrow transplantation. In 1955, Thomas moved to the Mary Imogene Bassett Hospital in Cooperstown, New York, where he began working with Dr. Joe Ferrebee on marrow transplantation, both in dogs and in humans. It was there that Thomas published the first report of successful transplantation in identical twins, but became aware of failures of the procedure in the nontwin setting. Thomas moved to the University of Washington in Seattle in 1963, and there he and his colleagues developed techniques for histocompatibility typing in dogs and demonstrated that by selecting matched donors and using posttransplant methotrexate, it was possible to successfully transplant marrow between matched litter mates in virtually every case. These experiments set the stage for renewed attempts to apply transplantation to the treatment of human disease. In the late 1960s, Thomas wrote a program project grant that was funded by the National Cancer Institute and began to assemble a team of physicians, nurses, and support staff that remains largely intact to this day. During the early 1970s, Thomas and his group developed many of the clinical techniques that established hematopoietic cell transplantation as a lifesaving treatment for large numbers of patients. For his pioneering work Thomas has received almost every possible prize, including, of course, the 1990 Nobel Prize in Medicine, which he shared with Dr. Joseph Murray. On receipt of every award, Thomas is quick to point out the contributions of other scientists to the field of transplantation. He never fails to credit the nursing and support staff workers who have been so much a part of this effort, and he always acknowledges the patients and their families who have been partners in his work. While hematopoietic cell transplantation might have developed as a therapeutic tool without Thomas' contribution, it would not have happened nearly as quickly or become as effective as it is without his leadership.

REFERENCES

1. Brent L. A *History of Transplantation Immunology*. Academic Press, San Diego, CA, 1997.
2. Thomas ED, Blume KG. Historical markers in the development of allogeneic hematopoietic cell transplantation [review]. *Biol Blood Marrow Transplantation* 1999;5:341-346.
3. Blume KG, Thomas ED. A review of autologous hematopoietic cell transplantation [review]. *Biol Blood Marrow Transplantation* 2000;6:1–12.
4. Good RA, Verjee T. Historical and current perspectives on bone marrow transplantation for prevention and treatment of immunodeficiencies and autoimmunities [review]. *Biol Blood Marrow Transplantation* 2001;7:123–135.
5. Jacobson LO, Marks EK, Robson MJ, Gaston EO, Zirkle RE. Effect of spleen protection on mortality following x-irradiation. *J Lab Clin Med* 1949;34:1538–1543.
6. Lorenz E, Uphoff D, Reid TR, Shelton E. Modification of irradiation injury in mice and guinea pigs by bone marrow injections. *J Natl Cancer Inst* 1951;12:197–201.
7. Main JM, Prehn RT. Successful skin homografts after the administration of high dosage X radiation and homologous bone marrow. *J Natl Cancer Inst* 1955;15:1023–1029.
8. Ford CE, Hamerton JL, Barnes DWH, Loutit JF. Cytological identification of radiation-chimaeras. *Nature* 1956;177:452–454.
9. Barnes DWH, Corp MJ, Loutit JF, Neal FE. Treatment of murine leukaemia with x-rays and homologous bone marrow. Preliminary communication. *Br Med J* 1956;2:626–627.
10. Thomas ED, Lochte HL, Jr., Lu WC, Ferrebee JW. Intravenous infusion of bone marrow in patients receiving radiation and chemotherapy. *N Engl J Med* 1957;257:491–496.
11. Thomas ED, Lochte HL, Jr., Cannon JH, Sahler OD, Ferrebee JW. Supralethal whole body irradiation and isologous marrow transplantation in man. *J Clin Invest* 1959;38:1709–1716.
12. Mathe G, Amiel JL, Schwarzenberg L, Catton A, Schneider M. Adoptive immunotherapy of acute leukemia: experimental and clinical results. *Cancer Res* 1965;25:1525–1531.
13. Bortin MM. A compendium of reported human bone marrow transplants. *Transplantation* 1970;9:571–587.
14. Dausset J. Iso-leuco-anticorps. *Acta Haematol* 1958;20:156–166.
15. van Rood JJ, Eernisse JG, van Leeuwen A. Leukocyte antibodies in sera from pregnant women. *Nature* 1958;181:1735,1736.
16. Thomas ED, Collins JA, Herman EC, Jr., Ferrebee JW. Marrow transplants in lethally irradiated dogs given methotrexate. *Blood* 1962;19:217–228.
17. Epstein RB, Storb R, Ragde H, Thomas ED. Cytotoxic typing antisera for marrow grafting in littermate dogs. *Transplantation* 1968;6:45–58.
18. Storb R, Epstein RB, Graham TC, Thomas ED. Methotrexate regimens for control of graft-versus-host disease in dogs with allogeneic marrow grafts. *Transplantation* 1970;9:240–246.
19. Storb R, Rudolph RH, Thomas ED. Marrow grafts between canine siblings matched by serotyping and mixed leukocyte culture. *J Clin Invest* 1971;50:1272–1275.
20. Gatti RA, Meuwissen HJ, Allen HD, Hong R, Good RA. Immunological reconstitution of sex-linked lymphopenic immunological deficiency. *Lancet* 1968;ii:1366–1369.
21. Bach FH, Albertini RJ, Joo P, Anderson JL, Bortin MM. Bone-marrow transplantation in a patient with the Wiskott-Aldrich syndrome. *Lancet* 1968;2:1364–1366.
22. deKoning J, van Bekkum DW, Dicke KA, Dooren LJ, Radl J, van Rood JJ. Transplantation of bone-marrow cells and fetal thymus in an infant with lymphopenic immunological deficiency. *Lancet* 1969;i:1223–1227.
23. Thomas ED, Buckner CD, Storb R, et al. Aplastic anaemia treated by marrow transplantation. *Lancet* 1972;i:284–289.
24. Thomas ED, Buckner CD, Banaji M, et al. One hundred patients with acute leukemia treated by chemotherapy, total body irradiation, and allogeneic marrow transplantation. *Blood* 1977;49:511–533.
25. Thomas ED, Buckner CD, Clift RA, et al. Marrow transplantation for acute nonlymphoblastic leukemia in first remission. *N Engl J Med* 1979;301:597–599.
26. Kurnick NB, Montano A, Gerdes JC, Feder BH. Preliminary observations on the treatment of postirradiation hematopoietic depression in man by the infusion of stored autogenous bone marrow. *Ann Intern Med* 1958;49:973–986.
27. McGovern JJ, Jr., Russel PS, Atkins L, Webster EW. Treatment of terminal leukemic relapse by total-body irradiation and intravenous infusion of stored autologous bone marrow obtained during remission. *N Engl J Med* 1959;260:675–683.
28. Appelbaum FR, Herzig GP, Ziegler JL, Graw RG, Levine AS, Deisseroth AB. Successful engraftment of cryopreserved autologous bone marrow in patients with malignant lymphoma. *Blood* 1978;52:85–95.
29. Appelbaum FR, Deisseroth AB, Graw RG, et al. Prolonged complete remission following high dose chemotherapy of Burkitt's lymphoma in relapse. *Cancer* 1978;41:1059–1063.

30. Thomas ED. Marrow transplant for acute nonlymphoblastic leukemia in first remission: a follow-up [letter]. *N Engl J Med* 1983;308:1539,1540.
31. Beutler E, Blume KG, Bross KJ, et al. Bone marrow transplantation as the treatment of choice for "good risk" adult patients with acute leukemia. *Trans Assoc Am Physicians* 1979;92:189–195.
32. Fefer A, Cheever MA, Thomas ED, et al. Disappearance of Ph1-positive cells in four patients with chronic granulocytic leukemia after chemotherapy, irradiation and marrow transplantation from an identical twin. *N Engl J Med* 1979;300:333–337.
33. Thomas ED, Buckner CD, Sanders JE, et al. Marrow transplantation for thalassaemia. *Lancet* 1982;ii:227–229.
34. Johnson FL, Look AT, Gockerman J, Ruggiero MR, Dalla-Pozza L, Billings FT, III. Bone-marrow transplantation in a patient with sickle-cell anemia. *N Engl J Med* 1984;311:780–783.
35. Gianni AM, Siena S, Bregni M, et al. Granulocyte-macrophage colony-stimulating factor to harvest circulating haemopoietic stem cells for autotransplantation. *Lancet* 1989;ii:580–585.
36. Bensinger WI, Martin PJ, Storer B, et al. Transplantation of bone marrow as compared with peripheral-blood cells from HLA-identical relatives in patients with hematologic cancers. *N Engl J Med* 2001;344:175–181.
37. Gluckman E, Broxmeyer HE, Auerbach AD, et al. Hematopoietic reconstitution in a patient with Fanconi's anemia by means of umbilical-cord blood from an HLA-identical sibling. *N Engl J Med* 1989;321:1174–1178.
38. Kernan NA, Bartsch G, Ash RC, et al. Analysis of 462 transplantations from unrelated donors facilitated by The National Marrow Donor Program. *N Engl J Med* 1993;328:593–602.
39. Hansen JA, Gooley TA, Martin PJ, et al. Bone marrow transplants from unrelated donors for patients with chronic myeloid leukemia. *N Engl J Med* 1998;338:962–968.
40. Petersdorf EW, Hansen JA, Martin PJ, et al. Major-histocompatibility-complex class I alleles and antigens in hematopoietic-cell transplantation. *N Engl J Med* 2001;345:1794–1800.
41. Santos GW. Busulfan (Bu) and cyclophosphamide (Cy) for marrow transplantation. *Bone Marrow Transplant* 1989;4:236–239.
42. Slavin S, Nagler A, Naparstek E, et al. Nonmyeloablative stem cell transplantation and cell therapy as an alternative to conventional bone marrow transplantation with lethal cytoreduction for the treatment of malignant and nonmalignant hematologic diseases. *Blood* 1998;91:756–763.
43. Giralt S, Estey E, Albitar M, et al. Engraftment of allogeneic hematopoietic progenitor cells with purine analog-containing chemotherapy: harnessing graft-versus-leukemia without myeloablative therapy. *Blood* 1997;89:4531–4536.
44. McSweeney PA, Niederwieser D, Shizuru JA, et al. Hematopoietic cell transplantation in older patients with hematologic malignancies: replacing high-dose cytotoxic therapy with graft-versus-tumor effects. *Blood* 2001;97:3390–3400.
45. Kolb HJ, Mittermüller J, Clemm Ch, et al. Donor leukocyte transfusions for treatment of recurrent chronic myelogenous leukemia in marrow transplant patients. *Blood* 1990;76:2462–2465.
46. Deeg HJ, Storb R, Weiden PL, et al. Cyclosporin A and methotrexate in canine marrow transplantation: engraftment, graft-versus-host disease, and induction of tolerance. *Transplantation* 1982;34:30–35.
47. Storb R, Deeg HJ, Whitehead J, et al. Methotrexate and cyclosporine compared with cyclosporine alone for prophylaxis of acute graft versus host disease after marrow transplantation for leukemia. *N Engl J Med* 1986;314:729–735.
48. Reisner Y, Kapoor N, Kirkpatrick D, et al. Transplantation for acute leukaemia with HLA-A and B nonidentical parental marrow cells fractionated with soybean agglutinin and sheep red blood cells. *Lancet.* 1981;ii:327–331.
49. Prentice HG, Blacklock HA, Janossy G, et al. Depletion of T lymphocytes in donor marrow prevents significant graft-versus-host disease in matched allogeneic leukaemic marrow transplant recipients. *Lancet* 1984;1:472–476.
50. Nemunaitis J, Rabinowe SN, Singer JW, et al. Recombinant granulocyte-macrophage colony-stimulating factor after autologous bone marrow transplantation for lymphoid cancer. *N Engl J Med* 1991;324:1773–1778.
51. Bowden RA, Slichter SJ, Sayers MH, Mori M, Cays MJ, Meyers JD. Use of leukocyte-depleted platelets and cytomegalovirus-seronegative red blood cells for prevention of primary cytomegalovirus infection after marrow transplant. *Blood* 1991;78:246–250.
52. Goodrich JM, Mori M, Gleaves CA, et al. Early treatment with ganciclovir to prevent cytomegalovirus disease after allogeneic bone marrow transplantation. *N Engl J Med* 1991;325:1601–1607.
53. Marr KA, Seidel K, Slavin M, et al. Prolonged fluconazole prophylaxis is associated with persistent protection against cadidiasis-related death in allogeneic marrow transplant recipients: long-term follow-up of a randomized, placebo-controlled trial. *Blood* 2000;96:2055–2061.

II DISEASE INDICATIONS: ALLOGENEIC TRANSPLANTATION

2

Allogeneic Hematopoietic Cell Transplantation for Adult Patients with Acute Myelogenous Leukemia

Henry C. Fung, MD *and Stephen J. Forman,* MD

CONTENTS

1. INTRODUCTION

The role of allogeneic marrow transplantation in the management of acute leukemia has grown considerably since the initial reports many years ago describing the safe infusion of marrow cells into humans with acute myelogenous leukemia (AML). A landmark report by Thomas describing 100 patients with acute leukemia beyond first remission, including 54 cases of AML treated with a total body irradiation (TBI) containing regimen and an allogeneic transplant, showed the curative potential of the therapy (1). The use of bone marrow transplantation (BMT) for AML has expanded in the past three decades and has moved from an experi-

From: *Current Clinical Oncology: Allogeneic Stem Cell Transplantation*
Edited by: Mary S. Laughlin and Hillard M. Lazarus © Humana Press Inc., Totowa, NJ

mental treatment used only for patients with refractory disease to a first line of treatment for patients with AML in their first remission, depending on biological characteristics and response to initial therapy, as described here *(2–6)*. This chapter summarizes the data on the results of allogeneic transplantation for AML, interpreted within the context of the evolving understanding of the molecular biology and cytogenetics of AML, and the implications of these disease-related factors in the treatment and long-term survival in patients with this disease.

Historically, the classification of treatment of AML has been based completely on morphologic and clinical observations; however, the identification of the molecular events involved in the pathogenesis of human tumors has refined their classification and understanding, including the acute leukemias *(7)*. In AML, a large number of leukemia-specific cytogenetic abnormalities have been identified, and the involved genes cloned. These studies have helped elucidate the molecular pathways that may be involved in cellular transformation, provided methods for monitoring of patients after chemotherapy, and helped evaluate the response to therapy correlated with various clinical and phenotypic characteristics *(8)*. Although the leukemia cells in many patients do not have detectable structural chromosome abnormalities at diagnosis, some may show molecular changes at diagnosis, such as involvement of the MLL gene *(9)*. Taken together, these observations have led to the concept that AML is a heterogeneous disease with its variants best defined by molecular defects and cytogenetic changes, some of which are more common in different age groups. In previous treatment trials with standard therapy, allogeneic and autologous transplantation, patients were often treated as a homogeneous group. As described here, recent studies have refined the way patients are allocated to various treatments, as well as in the analysis of the data, and provide the basis for now making a biologically and response-based treatment decision, rather than a global one, for patients with AML.

2. CYTOGENETIC CHARACTERIZATION OF AML

Cytogenetic risk groups form the backbone of a decision tree for postremission consolidation at the present time *(10–12)*. Other disease-related factors ,which influence the risk of relapse after induction chemotherapy, include high leukocyte count at diagnosis or extramedullary disease and residual leukemia in marrow examinations 7–10 d after completion of induction therapy. The availability of a sibling or unrelated donor also affects the risk assessment for consolidation treatment. Human leukocyte antigen (HLA) typing is now part of the National Cancer Comprehensive Network (NCCN) guideline recommendations for initial evaluation of patients with newly diagnosed AML who do not have co-morbid medical conditions, which would be a contraindication to transplantation.

Patients with acute promyelocytic leukemia (APL) enjoy an excellent disease-free survival (DFS) (80–90%) with current conventional dose chemotherapy combined with All-transretinoic acid (ATRA) in induction and maintenance *(13,14)*. Remission status can be monitored by following the level of the fusion protein promyelocytic leukemia/retinoic receptor alpha (PML/RARα) produced by the t(15;17) translocation using polymerase chain reaction (PCR) techniques *(14)*. Patients who either fail to achieve molecular remission by completion of consolidation or who show re-emergence and a rising level of the fusion protein are likely to relapse. Transplantation, using either an allogeneic donor or a molecular negative autologous stem cell product, is reserved for patients with APL who show evidence of relapse.

Patients with good risk cytogenetics [t(8;21), inv(16), t(16;16)] may achieve long-term remission with multiple cycles of high dose 1-β-D-arabinofuranosylcytosine (ARA-C) in 50–60% of patients with relapse as the major cause of treatment failure *(15)*. Autologous transplant following one or more dose intensive chemotherapy consolidations have shown somewhat better DFS of 70–85% in cooperative groups and single institution studies *(16)*. Although molecular probes exist for these translocations, their use in monitoring minimal residual disease is not as clinically useful as the probes for chronic myeloid leukemia (CML) or APL *(17,18)*. Many patients with t(8;21) in clinical remission remain PCR positive for 10–20 yr without relapse. Thus, the treatment approach for consolidation therapy of this subgroup of patients would include either: (i) multiple cycles of high dose ARA-C (HDAC) with allogeneic transplant reserved for treatment of relapse in patients having a sibling donor; (ii) one or two cycles of high dose ARA-C (HDAC) followed by autologous peripheral blood stem cell transplantation (PBSCT) in complete remission (CR); or (iii) multiple cycles of HDAC with autologous stem cells collected in remission and reserved for salvage in patients without a sibling donor.

The majority of adults with de novo AML are in the intermediate risk group. Unfortunately, the DFS for this group declines to 30–35% when HDAC alone is used for consolidation. In this group of patients, both autologous and allogeneic (sibling) transplant in CR offer an improved DFS of 50–60% *(19–21)*. Factors that might influence the type of transplant are patient age, tumor burden at diagnosis and infectious complications during induction. In younger patients (≤30 yr) in whom the risk of graft-vs-host disease (GVHD) is relatively low, allogeneic transplantation may be more attractive due to a low (15–20%) relapse rate. In an older patient (50–60 yr), the higher treatment-related mortality (20–40%) and long-term morbidity associated with allogeneic marrow transplant suggests that autologous PBSCT offers at least an equivalent chance of relapse-free survival with less long-term toxicity. Recent studies using PBSCs rather than marrow in the allogeneic setting have shown a significant decrease in the toxicity profile of dose-intensive regimen, which may make these treatments safer in older patients but longer follow-up is needed *(22)*. In addition, the development of nonmyeloablative allogeneic transplant approaches may allow for the use of allogeneic BMT in older patients with AML as described in more detail later in this chapter.

3. PATIENTS WITH POOR RISK CYTOGENETICS

Patients with loss of chromosomes 5 or 7 or complex karyotypic abnormalities, as well as those patients with antecedent myelodysplasia or therapy-related leukemia have a very poor outcome when treated with conventional HDAC (10–12% 5-yr DFS). Autologous transplants have failed to improve on these results in most series. Allogeneic transplants can cure approx 40% of patients in this group *(1,23)*. In patients with any of these poor risk features who lack a sibling donor, an unrelated donor search should be initiated early while the patient is still undergoing induction.

4. MYELODYSPLASTIC SYNDROMES

The myelodysplastic syndromes (MDSs) encompass a spectrum of marrow disorders with variable degrees of ineffective hematopoiesis and predisposition to leukemic transformation with survival ranging from months to decades after diagnosis *(24)*. Factors influencing the outcome are the number of significant cytopenias, cytogenetic abnormalities, and presence of increasing marrow blasts, which have recently been codified into a prognostic index that reflects both the survival and leukemic transformation as described below *(25)*. While the majority of patients with MDS are above 60 yr of age and, therefore, above the usual age for transplant, there are an increasing number of younger patients developing MDS as a sequelae of chemotherapy or radiation for lymphomas, germ cell tumors, and breast cancer *(26,27)*. These secondary MDS patients tend to be at high risk for early transformation to AML and often have poor risk cytogenetics.

Decisions to utilize transplantation to replace the defective stem cells are influenced by the patient's age, prognostic index score, and co-morbid conditions *(28)*. Patients with low risk disease are usually not recommended for transplant until they progress, unless they have treatment-related MDS. For patients with intermediate risk disease allogeneic transplant from a sibling or volunteer unrelated donor should be considered as primary therapy for patients under 55; such procedures successfully restore normal hematopoiesis in 40–50% of patients. For patients with high risk disease (with 15% blasts in the marrow) or secondary AML, there is controversy as to whether induction chemotherapy to reduce the "leukemic" burden is beneficial. Whereas the relapse rate is less in patients who respond to induction treatment, there are also many who fail to respond and who become too debilitated to receive a transplant. In patients who do not have a sibling donor, induction chemotherapy may be necessary as a temporizing measure while a donor is sought.

As described below, there is also interest in exploring nonmyeloablative transplant for older patients with AML and for those patients with intermediate risk MDS. While the early morbidity of this approach is low, much longer follow-up will be needed to learn whether the allogeneic graft-vs-leukemia (GVL) effect can be utilized to improve the outcome for these patients.

5. TRANSPLANT STRATEGY FOR ADULT PATIENTS WITH AML

Anthracycline containing primary induction therapy for newly diagnosed AML will lead to CR in 65–80% of patients treated *(7)*. The likelihood of remaining in CR is, however, highly dependent on prognostic factors found at the time of diagnosis, including cytogenetic analysis as well as response to treatment. Patients who require more than one cycle of chemotherapy to achieve remission have a poor prognosis regardless of cytogenetic subgroup *(29)*. Subsequent treatment options for patients who successfully enter first CR (CR1) after primary induction therapy include: (i) repeated courses of intensive consolidation chemotherapy; (ii) autologous bone marrow transplantation; or (iii) allogeneic bone marrow transplantation.

Currently, the decision on which of the above options to choose should take into account the predicted benefit in terms of DFS and quality of life vs risk of morbidity and mortality. An important component of this decision depends on identification of an available matched sibling donor. In most series, allogeneic transplantation results in a lower rate of relapse for patients undergoing BMT for AML in first remission *(2)*. These results, however, do not always factor in the new information on the biology of AML and the impact of various treatment modalities on the outcome.

Compared to autologous transplantation or consolidation chemotherapy, allogeneic BMT carries with it a higher potential for complications, with particular difficulty arising from regimen-related toxicity, infection, and GVHD, but offers the therapeutic potential of GVL effect (Table 1). Decision making should also take into account the knowledge that AML treated by allogeneic transplantation at the time of relapse is less likely to induce a lasting remission than transplantation at the time of first remission, because the disease may become treatment-resistant, accompanied by the development of additional somatic mutations and drug resistance. Patients who relapse and who are then treated with chemotherapy may develop organ dysfunction, as a result of chemotherapy or treatment for fungal or bacterial infections and become less able to withstand subsequent chemotherapy or a BMT preparative regimen.

The decision to proceed to allogeneic transplantation thus becomes less controversial as patients move from lesser to greater risk of relapse (and risk of death from leukemia), i.e., beyond CR1, and toward first relapse (R1) , second complete remission (CR2), or for primary refractory disease. Much research has, therefore, centered on the determination of which patients are the most likely to benefit from allogeneic BMT early on in their treatment course.

Table 1
Comparison of Allogeneic vs Autologous Stem Cell Transplant

Allogeneic	*Autologous*
Advantages	Advantages
1. No tumor contamination of graft and no prior marrow injury from chemotherapy (less risk of late MDS).	1. No need to identify donor if peripheral blood and/or marrow uninvolved by tumor at time of collection.
2. Graft-vs-tumor effect.	2. No immunosuppression equals less risk of infections.
3. Can be used for patients with marrow involvement by tumor or with bone marrow dysfunction such as aplastic anemia, hemoglobinopathies, or prior pelvic radiation.	3. No GVHD.
	4. Dose-intensive therapy can be used for older patients (usually up to age 70).
	5. Low early treatment related mortality (2–5%).
Disadvantages	Disadvantages
1. Dose-intensive regimen limited by toxicity (usually to patients <55).	1. Not feasible if PBSC/marrow involved.
2. Time to identify donor if no sibling donor available and/or limited availability of donor for some ethnic groups.	2. Possible marrow injury leading to late MDS (either from prior chemotherapy or transplant regimen).
3. Higher early treatment-related mortality from GVHD and infectious complications (20–40% depending on age and donor source).	3. No graft-vs-tumor effect.
	4. Not all patients can be mobilized to give adequate cell doses for reconstitution

6. WHEN TO BEGIN CONSIDERATION FOR BMT

Because AML carries with it a high risk of relapse after achievement of remission, patients under the age of 60 who have no obvious contraindications for allogeneic blood or BMT (ALLOBMT) should be evaluated regarding the number, health, and availability of siblings or other close relatives who are potential candidates for bone marrow donation. HLA typing can be performed at any time, but should be performed early so that all treatment options can be defined, particularly if the patient does not achieve a remission. This applies particularly to patients with poor risk cytogenetics or other poor prognostic features who are at very high risk for early relapse. This approach provides for minimal delay for transplantation in the possible event of primary refractory disease, early disease relapse after primary therapy, or persistent cytogenetic abnormalities in the marrow after CR is attained. In addition, there is currently no evidence that consolidation therapy used before proceeding to allogeneic transplant has any benefit in reducing relapse after allogeneic transplant *(30)*. Thus, for patients in a first morphologic and cytogenetic remission who are candidates for allogeneic BMT, consolidation therapy is not necessary and may lead to complications that either delay or increase the risk of transplantation.

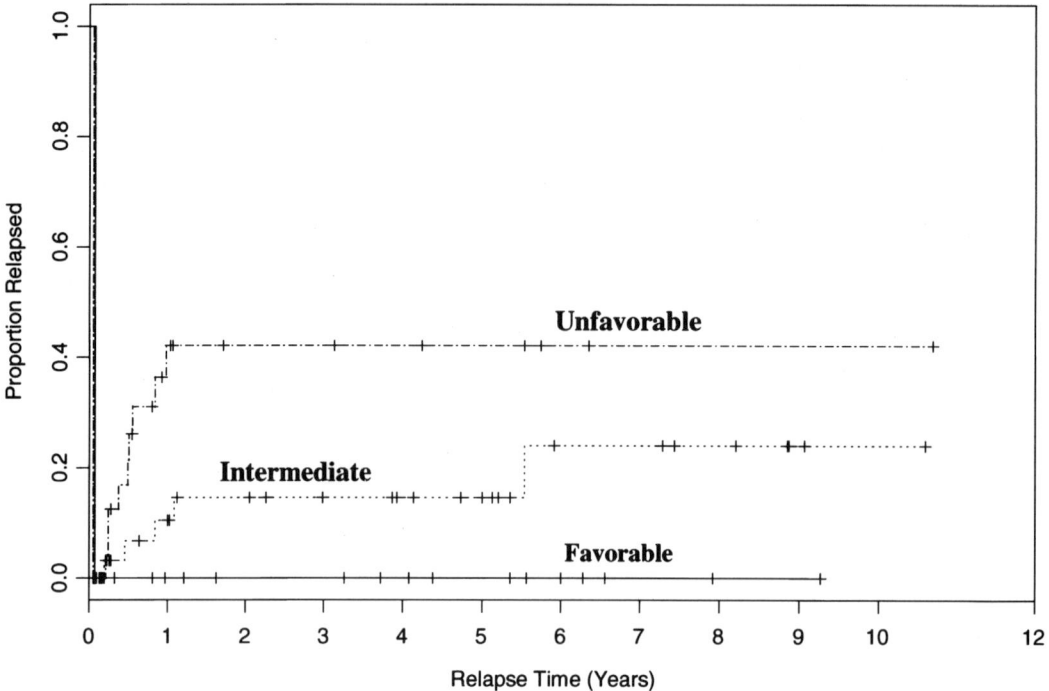

Fig. 1. Actuarial relapse rate for patients undergoing allogeneic transplantation for AML in first remission with a regimen of fractionated TBI and VP-16. Based on pretransplant cytogenetics, those patients with poor risk cytogenetics showed a higher rate of relapse compared to those with more favorable cytogenetic findings.

7. OUTCOME AFTER BMT FOR AML

Studies demonstrate a 5-yr DFS of 46–62% for patients treated with allogeneic BMT in CR1 *(31–35)*. In a representative study from City of Hope National Medical Center and Stanford University, 61 consecutive patients with AML in CR1 under age 50 with a histocompatible sibling donor received, an allogeneic BMT, after conditioning with fractionated TBI (1,320 cGy) and high-dose etoposide (60 mg/kg) *(36)*. The patients with AML demonstrated a 3-yr DFS of 61% with a relapse rate of 12%. By stepwise Cox regression analysis, significant prognostic variables for patients with AML were the presence of acute GVHD, increasing age and the cytogenetic risk category of the AML at the time of diagnosis *(36,37)*. Relapse was 0% in patients with good risk cytogenetics and approached 40% in those patients with poor risk cytogenetics *(37)* (Fig. 1). Complications related to GVHD and relapse of leukemia were the major causes of death. Additional studies from multiple institutions support a DFS ranging from 46 to 62% after 5 yr of observation *(38–43)*.

In order to reduce the limitations of GVHD on survival, Papadopoulos and colleagues at Memorial Sloan-Kettering Cancer Center studied the use of T-cell-depleted allografts in 31 patients with AML in CR1 or CR2. Patients treated in CR1, attained a DFS of 77% at 56 mo, while those treated in CR2 had a DFS of 50% at 48 mo. All patients were treated with a conditioning regimen of TBI, thiotepa, and cytoxan. Probability of relapse in patients treated in CR1 was 3.2%. Nonleukemic mortality in this group was 19.4%. There were no cases of grade II–IV acute GVHD *(44)*.

8. EFFECT OF CONDITIONING REGIMEN ON SURVIVAL OR RELAPSE RATE

Several studies have been published comparing outcome after different conditioning regimens. Although the use of higher doses of TBI results in a lower rate of relapse, patients suffered a higher incidence of GVHD and transplant-related mortality *(45)*. Other studies have found no significant differences between conditioning regimens using cyclophosphamide (CY)/single-dose TBI vs CY/fractionated-dose TBI (FTBI), chemotherapy (CT)/TBI vs melphalan/TBI *(28)*. There are conflicting data as to whether busulfan (BU)/CY results in a higher relapse rate than CY/TBI, but recent data suggest that optimal use of BU (intravenous or targeted therapy) may have an impact on both toxicity and relapse *(46)*. Recent studies utilizing radioimmunotherapy designed to target hematopoietic tissue have shown promising results with a low relapse rate and no increase in transplant-related toxicity *(47)*. Presently, there are no data to determine whether one regimen is more or less effective for each of the cytogenetic subtypes of AML.

9. ALLOGENEIC BMT FOR AML IN FIRST RELAPSE OR CR2

For patients in relapse after failure of standard therapy for AML, allogeneic transplantation offers the only chance for cure for those patients who have a sibling donor. For those patients who are able to achieve a second remission, particularly after a long first remission and a lack of a sibling donor, an autologous transplant is a potentially curative therapy *(48,49)*. A common dilemma is the question of whether to proceed directly to allogeneic transplantation at the time of relapse (if a suitable donor has been identified) or whether to proceed to reinduction chemotherapy first, in an attempt to reach a second CR (required for autologous BMT). Although no randomized data are available, one study demonstrates statistically nonsignificant survival rate differences of 29% in patients transplanted in untreated first relapse vs 22% in second remission and in 10% with refractory relapse *(2,50,51)*. Another study retrospectively evaluated outcomes in patients transplanted at various stages of disease. DFS was significantly better in patients transplanted in first remission, but no statistical difference was found between the various groups transplanted beyond first CR. Thus, the decision concerning reinduction is often based on the age, condition, duration of first remission, and cytogenetic category of the patient with relapsed AML *(2)*.

10. RECOMMENDATIONS FOR ALLOGENEIC BMT FOR AML

Information on cytogenetics at the time of diagnosis is vital to identify patients who might have a good prognosis after standard chemotherapy, as opposed to those who should have allogeneic transplant during first complete remission. Those who should be considered for standard consolidation therapy or autologous transplantation include those with t(8;21) or inv(16), in the absence of any other poor prognostic indicators for these subtypes. Other patients should be strongly considered for allogeneic BMT during first CR.

For those patients with poor prognosis and who lack a matched family donor, alternative donors (matched unrelated donors, cord blood transplants) should be pursued *(52,53)*.

Figure 2 shows an approach to the timing and use of BMT based on prognostic features found at diagnosis and response to treatment *(2)*.

11. ALLOGENEIC TRANSPLANTATION AND MDS

Because MDS is not curable with conventional treatment, feasibility studies of allogeneic transplantation began in the 1980s. Reports from several groups showed that the disease could be cured by allogeneic BMT *(54,55)*.

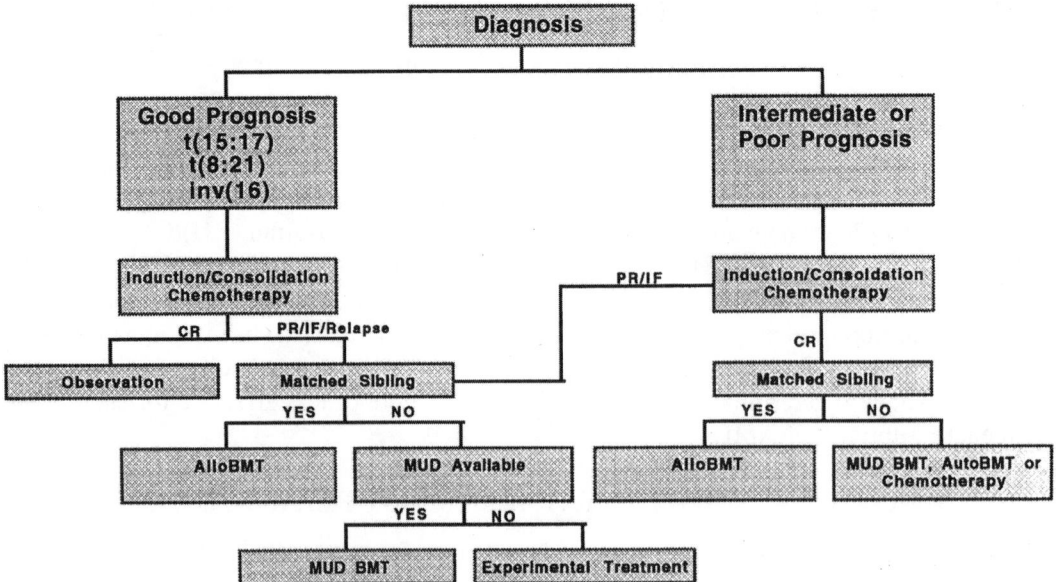

Fig. 2. Proposed algorithm for treatment of adults diagnosed with AML based primarily on cytogenetic analysis of the patients' leukemia at the time of diagnosis. CR, complete remission; PR, partial remission; IF, induction failure; ALLOBMT, allogeneic bone marrow transplantation; AUTOBMT, autologous bone marrow transplantation; MUD, matched unrelated donor.

A large retrospective survey of the European Group for Blood and Marrow Transplantation (EBMT) Leukaemia Working Party describes 78 patients with myelodysplasia (MDS) or secondary acute myelogenous leukemia (sAML) that received an allogeneic BMT *(56)*. The status of underlying disease at the time of transplantation was prognostic for the 2-yr DFS. Thirty-four patients received intensive chemotherapy prior to the conditioning for BMT. The 2-yr DFS was 60% for the 16 patients transplanted in CR. The results were significantly less favorable for those with more advanced disease who only partially responded prior to intensive chemotherapy (2-yr DFS: 18%), while none of those who either relapsed or were resistant to chemotherapy became long-term survivors after BMT. Forty-four patients had not received any prior intensive chemotherapy. The DFS at 2 yr after BMT was 58 ± 19% when a patient was transplanted for refractory anemia with ringed sideroblasts (RARS), 74 ± 14% for refractory anemia with excess blasts (RAEB), 50 ± 16% for RAEB in transformation (RAEB-T), and 18 ± 11% for secondary AML. Allogeneic BMT can, therefore, be considered as a potential curative treatment for patients with MDS.

12. FACTORS INFLUENCING OUTCOME

Initial studies involving allogeneic transplant for MDS focused mainly on the feasibility of the procedure, but lacked the statistical power to evaluate the effect of factors such as timing of transplantation, cytogenetics, or disease status on outcome. Addressing the question of which pretransplant factors are most predictive of favorable posttransplant outcome, the Chronic Leukemia Working Party of the EBMT retrospectively analyzed 131 patients who underwent BMT for MDS from HLA-identical siblings *(57)*. No patient received prior remission induction chemotherapy. The 5-yr DFS and overall survival (OS) for the entire group of patients was 34 and 41%, respectively. DFS and OS were dependent on pretransplant bone marrow blast counts. Patients with RA/RARS, RAEB, RAEB-T, and sAML had a 5-yr DFS of 52, 34, 19, and 26%, respectively, while the 5-yr OS for the respective patient groups was 57, 42, 24, and 28%, respectively. In a multivariate analysis, younger age, shorter disease duration, and absence of excess of blasts were associated with improved outcome.

13. IPSS SCORE AND RESULTS OF BMT FOR MDS

Several classification systems have been used for evaluating prognosis in patients with MDS, including the French–American–British (FAB) system. The International MDS Risk Analysis Workshop performed a global analysis on clinical data from seven large previously reported risk-based studies that had generated prognostic systems. The International Prognostic Scoring System (IPSS) was developed by evaluating critical prognostic variables and, in particular, by using a more refined bone marrow cytogenetic classification. A multivariate analysis combined these cytogenetic subgroups with percentage of bone marrow blasts and number of cytopenias to generate a prognostic model. Weighting these variables by their statistical power separated patients into four distinctive subgroups of risk. Patients receive a separate score based on percentage of marrow blasts, karyotype, and information on cytopenias. These scores are then combined into a total score which is then used to predict progression to AML, as well as for median survival *(58)*.

Appelbaum et al., analyzed data for all MDS patients transplanted in Seattle from 1981 to 1996, using multivariate analysis to determine factors predictive for nonrelapse mortality, relapse, and DFS. A total of 251 MDS patients were transplanted *(59)*. The IPSS score correlated significantly with relapse and DFS. The 5-yr DFS was 60, 36, and 28% for low- and intermediate-1 risk, intermediate-2 risk, and high-risk patients, respectively, leading to the conclusion that patients with intermediate-1, intermediate-2, or high-risk MDS are most likely to benefit from early transplantation.

14. EVIDENCE FOR GVL EFFECT

It has been recognized for some that the therapeutic benefit and potential cure achieved by allogeneic transplant is contributed by the dose-intensive regimen of either high-dose chemotherapy or high-dose chemotherapy and radiation combined with a graft-vs-tumor effect *(60)*. Over time, the potency of the graft-vs-tumor effect has been further understood and represents a significant immune-mediated effect to prevent relapse after the high dose chemotherapy and allogeneic stem cell transplant. Data that support the presence of GVL effect after allogeneic transplant include:

1. Reduced risk of relapse in patients with acute and chronic GVHD.
2. Detection of minimal residual disease early after transplantation, which clears over time.
3. Increased risk of relapse after syngeneic transplant.
4. Increased risk of relapse after T-cell-depleted transplants.
5. Induction of remission by donor lymphocyte infusions in patients relapsing after BMT.

Among hematologic malignancies, there are major differences in their susceptibility to the graft-vs-tumor effect, with CML being the most potent target; however, for patients with AML undergoing allogeneic transplantation, compared to syngeneic transplant, the relapse rate is lower following allogeneic transplant, suggesting that the allogeneic effect on AML is contributing to the long-term benefit *(61)*. This observation provides the basis for the exploration of nonmyeloablative transplants in patients with AML, particularly those older persons with AML in whom the disease is more common, but in whom allogeneic transplantation has not been commonly utilized.

15. NONMYELOABLATIVE ALLOGENEIC BMT (MINI-BMT)

The high-dose chemotherapy and radiation typically used in the conditioning regimens for BMT produces considerable morbidity and mortality and limits the use of this modality to those patients who are young and have medical conditions that would preclude its use. With regard to AML, although allogeneic transplantation has been an effective therapy in younger patients, it has not been utilized in older patients where the disease is not only more common, but the biology of the disease is different. Older patients with AML often have worse cytogenetics and phenotypes, such as expression of multidrug resistance that correlate with a decreased response to therapy and poor OS and DFS (62). Given the role of the GVL effect in curing some hematologic malignancies, an alternative strategy has evolved to utilize low dose nonmyeloablative conditioning regimens designed to provide sufficient immune suppression to achieve engraftment of an allogeneic blood cell or marrow graft, thus facilitating the development of a graft-vs-malignancy effect. The generation of a GVL effect requires engraftment and ultimate in vivo expansion of donor immunocompetent cells that can recognize allogeneic target antigens including both the normal and abnormal marrow of the recipient. The overall goal of this approach is to facilitate less intensive conditioning regimen treatment that would be associated with decreased regimen-related toxicity and to allow a graft-vs-tumor effect (63). This approach has been utilized by a number of investigators with varying regimens from a pure nonmyeloablative regimen utilizing TBI and fludarabine followed by posttransplant mycophenolate mofetil (MMF) and cyclosporin, to more intensive ones utilizing busulfan, fludarabine, and antithymocyte globulin with encouraging results (64). A study from a consortium of centers exploring a purely nonmyeloablative regimen has shown that the overall mortality in a group of patients whose median age was 60 at d 100 was 10%, half of which is contributed by disease progression (65). Thus, this approach is being explored for patients with AML, particularly those who are older and have poor risk features, such as high white count, more than two cycles of therapy to go into remission, multidrug resistance (MDR) phenotype, or poor risk cytogenetics.

16. APPROACH TO THE PATIENT WITH PRIMARY REFRACTORY AML

The survival of patients with AML who do not achieve a remission with primary therapy is very poor and, in general, is independent of all other cellular characteristics. The lack of achievement of remission is the clearest demonstration of the resistance of the disease to chemotherapy. Some studies have been performed which indicate that the use of allogeneic transplantation in patients who have not achieved a remission may result in long-term DFS in approx 15–30% of patients (66–68). In a recent analysis of 71 patients with primary refractory AML who underwent an allogeneic BMT, an analysis was performed to determine whether there are pretransplant features of this unique patient population that predict treatment outcome (69). Although relapse and regimen-related toxicity was high in this high-risk patient population, the probability of DFS and relapse at 3 yr was 29 and 54%, respectively. Remarkably, unfavorable cytogenetics before stem cell transplantation was significantly associated with decreased DFS and a TBI-based regimen appeared to convey a better outcome. The actuarial probability of DFS and relapse at 3 yr was 44 and 38% for patients with intermediate cytogenetics and 18 and 68% for those patients with unfavorable cytogenetics. Figure 3 shows the DFS for a group of patients who failed to achieve a remission and were then treated with an allogeneic BMT.

The data suggest that allogeneic transplantation can cure some patients with primary refractory AML and that cytogenetic analysis before stem cell transplantation correlates with trans-

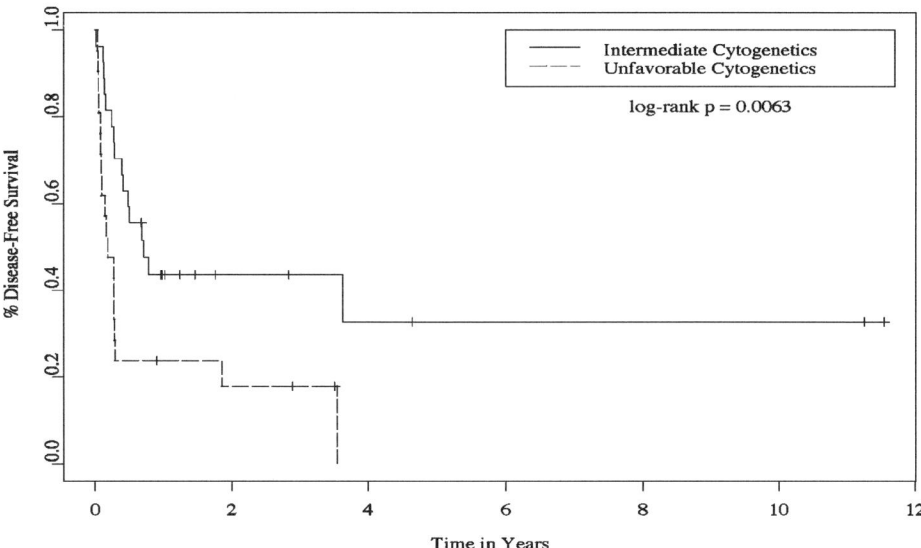

Fig. 3. DFS for a group of patients with AML undergoing allogeneic transplantation after having failed to achieve a remission with either conventional dose of ARA-C or high-dose ARA-C and an anthracycline. Patients with intermediate cytogenetics had a better DFS than those with unfavorable cytogenetics. Overall, the actual probability of DFS at 3 yr was 44% for patients with intermediate cytogenetics and 18% for those with unfavorable cytogenetics.

plant outcome as well as relapse. Thus, for patients who do not achieve remission with either one or two cycles of induction therapy, particularly with a high-dose ARA-C-based regimen, proceeding to allogeneic transplantation when a sibling donor is identified appears to be the optimal strategy rather than utilizing repeated courses of chemotherapy, which are unlikely to result in remission. Patients who require more than one cycle of chemotherapy to achieve a remission should also be considered at high risk for relapse and should be considered for early BMT *(8)*.

17. INNOVATIONS IN ALLOGENEIC TRANSPLANTATION FOR AML

Although the most common regimens, namely, FTBI and CY, BU and CY, and FTBI and etoposie (VP-16) have a long and stable track record, studies are being conducted to improve both the toxicity profile and efficacy of the regimens utilized in the treatment of AML. In general, TBI-based regimens have been more effective than non-TBI regimens, but have more toxicity to gastrointestinal (GI) mucosa and may be more associated with increased risk of second malignancies over time. Studies are being performed with the use of radio-immunoconjugates utilizing anti-CD45 or anti-CD33 antibodies conjugated to a variety of radioisotopes including iodine and yttrium. Early studies suggest the addition of radio-immunoconjugates to a regimen of BU and CY is an effective approach without, as yet, increasing toxicity *(70)*. Phase II studies are ongoing in AML with this approach, but the early data would suggest that incorporation of the radioimmunoconjugate into the preparative regimen is tolerable and will require further studies to determine the impact on preventing relapse in the various subgroups of AML.

In addition, the optimal use of chemotherapy as part of the preparative regimen is receiving increasing attention based on observations concerning the different pharmacokinetic and pharmacogenetic disposition of these agents in individual patients undergoing transplantation. Most recently, studies utilizing the intravenous form of BU have shown a better toxicity profile and less individual variation in the area under the plasma concentration vs time curve (AUC) achieved by the drugs *(71)*. Studies performed in CML and myelodysplasia suggest that targeting the dose of BU, either orally or intravenous, not only improves the toxicity profile and facilitates the use of these regimens in patients with myelodysplasia who are older, but has an impact on the risk of relapse *(72)*.

Nonmyeloablative transplantation, as noted above, which utilizes the immunotherapeutic effect of allogeneic T-cells, is being explored in older patients with AML and, depending upon the results, could be applied in younger patients with AML, particularly those for whom retaining fertility is an important consideration. In addition, the use of a nonmyeloablative approach may be utilized as immunotherapy following an autologous transplant for AML to help combine the benefits of the high-dose regimen utilized with autologous transplantation with the immunotherapeutic contribution of the allograft.

The stem cell source also may contribute to the overall benefit of allogeneic transplantation. Studies have been performed, comparing peripheral blood to marrow, that demonstrate the improved hematopoietic recovery and decreased toxicity without an obvious increase in acute or chronic graft-vs-host reaction *(22)*. Further studies are being performed to determine the incidence and extent of chronic GVHD in patients receiving PBSCT and the use of this cellular product is now being explored in patients with AML undergoing transplant in first remission.

ACKNOWLEDGMENT

This work was supported in part by United States Public Service Grants NCI PPG CA 30206 and NCI CA 33572.

REFERENCES

1. Thomas ED, Buckner CD, Banaji M, et al. One hundred patients with acute leukemia treated by chemotherapy, total body irradiation, and allogeneic marrow transplantation. *Blood* 1977;49:511–533.
2. Stockerl-Goldstein KE, Blume KG. Allogeneic hematopoietic cell transplantation for adult patients with acute myeloid leukemia. In: Thomas ED, Blume KG, Forman SJ, eds. *Hematopoietic Cell Transplantation*, 2nd ed. Blackwell Science, London, 1999, pp. 823–834.
3. Forman SJ, Krance RA, O'Donnell MR, et al. Bone marrow transplantation for acute nonlymphoblastic leukemia during first complete remission. An analysis of prognostic factors. *Transplantation* 1987;43:650–653.
4. Mehta J, Powles R, Treleaven J, et al. Long-term follow-up of patients undergoing allogeneic bone marrow transplantation for acute myeloid leukemia in first complete remission after cyclophosphamide-total body irradiation and cyclosporine. *Bone Marrow Transplant* 1996;18:741–746.
5. Snyder DS, Chao NJ, Amylon MD, et al. Fractionated total body irradiation high-dose etoposide as a preparatory regimen for bone marrow transplantation for 99 patients with acute leukemia in first complete remission. *Blood* 1993;82:2920–2928.
6. Keating S, Suciu S, de Witte T, et al. Prognostic factors of patients with acute myeloid leukemia (AML) allografted in first complete remission: an analysis of the EORTC-GIMEMA AML 8A trial. The European Organization for Research and Treatment of Cancer (EORTC) and the Gruppo Italiano Malattie Ematologiche Maligne dell' Adulto (GIMEMA) Leukemia Cooperative Groups. *Bone Marrow Transplant* 1996;17:993–1001.
7. Löwenberg B, Downing J, Burnett A. Acute myeloid leukemia. *N Engl J Med* 1999;341:1051–1062.
8. Golub TR, Slonim DK, Tamayo P, et al. Molecular classification of cancer: class discovery and class pr gene expression monitoring. *Science* 1999;286:531–537.
9. Caligiuri MA, Strout MP, Lawrence D, et al. Rearrangement of ALL1 (MLL) in acute myeloid leukemia with normal cytogenetics. *Cancer Res* 1998;58:55–59.
10. Yunis JJ, Brunning RD, Howe RB, Lobell M. High-resolution chromosomes as an independent prognostic indicator in adult acute nonlymphocytic leukemia. *N Engl J Med* 1984;311:812–818.
11. Keating MJ, Smith TL, Kantarjian H, et al. Cytogenetic pattern in acute myelogenous leukemia: a major reproducible determinant of outcome. *Leukemia* 1988;2:403–412.

12. Mrozek K, Heinonen K, de la Chapelle A, Bloomfield CD. Clinical significance of cytogenetics in acute myeloid leukemia. *Semin Oncol* 1997;24:17–31.

13. Fenaux P, Chastang C, Chevret S, et al. A randomized comparison of all-transretinoic acid (ATRA) followed by chemotherapy and ATRA plus chemotherapy and the role of maintenance therapy in newly diagnosed acute promyelocytic leukemia. *Blood* 1999;94:1192–1200.

14. Niu C, Yam H, Yu T, et al. Studies on treatment of acute promyelocytic leukemia with arsenic trioxide: remission induction, follow-up, and molecular monitoring in 11 newly diagnosed and 47 relapsed acute promyelocytic leukemia patients. *Blood* 1999;94:3315–3324.

15. Bloomfield CD, Lawrence D, Byrd JC, et al. Frequency of prolonged remission duration after high-dose cytarabine intensification in acute myeloid leukemia varies by cytogenetic subtype. *Cancer Res* 1998;58:4173–4179.

16. Stein AS, Slovak ML, Sniecinski I, et al. Immunotherapy with IL-2 after autologous stem cell transplant for acute myelogenous leukemia in first remission. *Proceedings of the Ninth International Symposium on Autologous Blood and Marrow Transplantation* 1999;1:46–53.

17. Saunders MJ, Tobal K, Liu Yin JA. Detection of t(8;21) by reverse transcriptase polymerase chain reaction in patients in remission of acute myeloid leukaemia type M2 after chemotherapy or bone marrow transplantation. *Leuk Res* 1994;18:891–895.

18. Nucifora G, Larson RA, Rowley RD. Persistence of the 8;21 translocation in patients with acute myeloid leukemia type M2 in long term remission. *Blood* 1993;82:712–715.

19. Burnett AK, Goldstone AH, Stevens RMF, et al. Randomised comparison of addition of autologous bone-marrow transplantation to intensive chemotherapy for acute myeloid leukemia in first remission. Results of MRC AML 10 trial. *Lancet* 1998;351:700–708.

20. Zittoun RA, Mandelli F, Willemze R, et al. Autologous or allogeneic bone marrow transplantation compared with intensive chemotherapy in acute myelogenous leukemia. *N Engl J Med* 1995;332:217–223.

21. Cassileth PA, Harrington DP, Appelbaum FR, et al. Chemotherapy compared with autologous or allogeneic bone marrow transplantation in the management of acute myeloid leukemia in first remission. *N Engl J Med* 1998;339:1649–1656.

22. Bensinger W, Martin P, Storer B, et al. Transplantation of bone marrow as compared with peripheral blood cells from HLA-identical relatives in patients with hematologic malignancies. *N Engl J Med* 2001;344:175–181.

23. Slovak ML, Kopecky KJ, Cassileth PA, et al. Karyotypic analysis predicts outcome of preremission and postremission therapy in adult acute myeloid leukemia: a Southwest Oncology Group/Eastern Cooperative Oncology Group study. *Blood* 2000;96:4075–4083.

24. Greenberg PL. Myelodysplastic syndrome. In: Hoffman R, Benz Jr. EJ, Shattil SJ, Furie B, Cohen HJ, Silberstein LE, McGlave P, eds. *Hematology. Basic Principles and Practice*, 3rd ed. Churchill Livingstone, New York, 2000, pp. 1106–1129.

25. Bennett JM, Catovsky D, Daniel MT, et al. Proposals for the classification of the myelodysplastic syndromes. *Br J Haematol* 1982;51:189–199.

26. Pedersen-Bjergaard J. Radiotherapy-and-chemotherapy-induced myelodysplasia and acute myeloid leukemia: a review. *Leuk Res* 1992;16:61–65.

27. Tucker MA, Coleman CN, Cox RS, et al. Risk of second cancers after treatment for Hodgkin's disease. *N Engl J Med* 1988;318:76–81.

28. Popplewell L, Forman SJ. Allogeneic hematopoietic stem cell transplantation for acute leukemia, chronic leukemia, and myelodysplasia. *Hematol/Oncol Clin North Am* 1999;13:987–1015.

29. Estey EH, Shen Y, Thall PF. Effect of time to complete remission on subsequent survival and disease-free survival time in AML, RAEB-t, and RAEB. *Blood* 2000;95:72–77.

30. Tallman MS, Rowlings PA, Milone G, et al. Effect of postremission chemotherapy before human leukocyte antigen-identical sibling transplantation for acute myelogenous leukemia in first complete remission. *Blood* 2000;96:1254–1258.

31. Blaise D, Maraninchi D, Archimbaud E, et al. Allogeneic bone marrow transplantation for acute myeloid leukemia in first remission: a randomized trial of a busulfan-cytoxan versus cytoxan-total body irradiation as preparative regimen: a report from the Group d'Etudes de la Greffe de Moelle Osseuse. *Blood* 1992;79:2578–2582.

32. Soiffer RJ, Fairclough D, Robertson M, et al. CD6-depleted allogeneic bone marrow transplantation for acute leukemia in first complete remission. *Blood* 1997;89:3039–3047.

33. Thomas ED, Buckner CD, Clift RA, et al. Marrow transplantation for acute nonlymphoblastic leukemia in first remission. *N Engl J Med* 1979;301:597–599.

34. Appelbaum FR, Dahlberg S, Thomas ED, et al. Bone marrow transplantation or chemotherapy after remission induction for adults with acute nonlymphoblastic leukemia: a prospective comparison. *Ann Intern Med* 1984;101:581–588.

35. Champlin RE, Ho WG, Gale RP, et al. Treatment of acute myelogenous leukemia: a prospective controlled trial of bone marrow transplantation versus consolidation chemotherapy. *Ann Intern Med* 1985;102:285–291.

36. Snyder DS, Chao NJ, Amylon MD, et al. Fractionated total body irradiation and high-dose etoposide as a preparatory regimen for bone marrow transplantation for 99 patients with acute leukemia in first complete remission. *Blood* 1993;82:2920–2928.

37. Fung H, Jamieson C, Snyder D, et al. Allogeneic bone marrow transplantation (BMT) for AML in first remission (1CR) utilizing fractionated total body irradiation (FTBI) and allogeneic bone marrow transplantation for bcr-abl positive acute lymphoblastic leukemia. VP-16: Analysis of risk factors for relapse and disease-free survival. *Blood* 1999;94:167a.

38. Bostrom B, Brunning RD, McGlave P, et al. Bone marrow transplantation for acute nonlymphoblastic leukemia in first remission: Analysis of prognostic factors. *Blood* 1985;65:1191–1196.

39. Clift RA, Buckner CD, Thomas ED, et al. The treatment of acute nonlymphoblastic leukemia by allogeneic transplantation. *Bone Marrow Transplant* 1987;2:243–258.

40. Forman SJ, Spruce WE, Farbstein MJ, et al. Bone marrow ablation followed by allogeneic marrow grafting during first complete remission of acute nonlymphocytic leukemia. *Blood* 1983;61:439–442.

41. Helenglass G, Powles RL, McElwain, TJ, et al. Melphalan and total body irradiation (TBI) versus cyclophosphamide and TBI as conditioning for allogeneic matched sibling bone marrow transplants for acute myeloblastic leukemia in first remission. *Bone Marrow Transplant* 1988;3:21–29.

42. Kim TH, McGlave PB, Ramsay N, et al. Comparison of two total body irradiation regimens in allogeneic bone marrow transplantation for acute nonlymphoblastic leukemia in first remission. *Int J Radiat Oncol Biol Phys* 1990;19:889–897.

43. McGlave PB, Haake RJ, Bostrom BC, et al. Allogeneic bone marrow transplantation for acute nonlymphocytic leukemia in first remission. *Blood* 1988;72:1512–1517.

44. Papadopoulos EB, Carabasi MH, Castro-Malaspina H, et al. T-cell-depleted allogeneic bone marrow transplantation as postremission therapy for acute myelogenous leukemia: freedom from relapse in the absence of graft-versus-host disease. *Blood* 1998;91:1083–1090.

45. Mehta J, Powles R, Singhal S, et al. Clinical and hematologic response of chronic lymphocytic and prolymphocytic leukemia persisting after allogeneic bone marrow transplantation with the onset of acute graft-versus-host disease: possible role of graft-versus-leukemia effect. *Bone Marrow Transplant* 1996;18:371-375.

46. Andersson BS, Gajewski J, Donato M, et al. Allogeneic stem cell transplantation (BMT) for AML and MDS following IV busulfan and cyclophosphamide (i.v. BuCy). *Bone Marrow Transplantation* 2000;25:S35–S38.

47. Appelbaum FR. Radioimmunotherapy and hematopoietic cell transplantation. In: Thomas ED, Blume KG, Forman SJ, eds. *Hematopoietic Cell Transplantation*, 2nd ed. Blackwell Science, London, 1999, pp. 168–175.

48. Stein AS, Forman SJ. Autologous hematopoietic cell transplantation for acute myeloid leukemia. In: Thomas ED, Blume KG, Forman SJ, eds. *Hematopoietic Cell Transplantation*, 2nd ed. Blackwell Science, London, 1999, pp. 287–295.

49. Miller CB, Rowlings PA, Zhang MJ, et al. The effect of graft purging with 4-hydroperoxycyclophosphamide in autologous bone marrow transplantation for acute myelogenous leukemia. *Exp Hematol* 2001;29:1336–1346.

50. Appelbaum FR, Clift RA, Buckner CD, et al. Allogeneic marrow transplantation for acute nonlymphoblastic leukemia after first complete relapse. *Blood* 1983;61:949–953.

51. Buckner CD, Clift RA, Thomas ED, et al. Allogeneic marrow transplantation for patients with acute non-lymphoblastic leukemia in second remission. *Leuk Res* 1982;6:395–399.

52. Broxmeyer HE, Smith FO. Cord blood stem cell transplantation. In: Thomas ED, Blume KG, Forman SJ, eds. *Hematopoietic Cell Transplantation*, 2nd ed. Blackwell Science, London, 1999, pp. 431–443.

53. Hansen JA, Petersdorf, EW. Unrelated donor hematopoietic cell transplantation. In: Thomas ED, Blume KG, Forman SJ, eds. *Hematopoietic Cell Transplantation*, 2nd ed. Blackwell Science, London, 1999, pp. 915–928.

54. Anderson JE, Appelbaum FR, Schoch G, et al. Allogeneic marrow transplantation for refractory anemia: a comparison of two preparative regimens and analysis of prognostic factors. *Blood* 1996;87:51–58.

55. O'Donnell MR, Long GD, Parker PM, et al. Busulfan/cyclophosphamide as conditioning regimen for allogeneic bone marrow transplantation for myelodysplasia. *J Clin Oncol* 1995;13:2973–2979.

56. De Witte T, Zwaan F, Hermans J, et al. Allogeneic bone marrow transplantation for secondary leukaemia and myelodysplastic syndrome: a survey by the Leukaemia Working Party of the European Bone Marrow Transplantation Group. *Br J Haematol* 1990;74:151–155.

57. Runde V, de Witte T, Arnold R, et al. Bone marrow transplantation from HLA-identical siblings as first-line treatment in patients with myelodysplastic syndromes: early transplantation is associated with improved outcome. Chronic Leukemia Working Party of the European Group for Blood and Marrow Transplantation. *Bone Marrow Transplant* 1998;21:255–261.

58. Greenberg P, Cox C, LeBeau MM, et al. International scoring system for evaluating prognosis in myelodysplastic syndromes. *Blood* 1997;89:2079–2088.

59. Appelbaum FR, Anderson J. Allogeneic bone marrow transplantation for myelodysplastic syndrome: outcomes analysis according to IPSS score. *Leukemia* 1998;12 (suppl. 1):S25–S29.

60. Fefer A. Graft-versus-tumor responses. In: Thomas ED, Blume KG, Forman SJ, eds. *Hematopoietic Cell Transplantation*, 2nd ed. Blackwell Science, London, 1999, pp. 316–326.

61. Fefer A, Sullivan K, Weiden P, et al. Graft versus leukemia effect in man: the relapse rate of acute leukemia is lower after allogeneic than after syngeneic marrow transplantation. In: Truitt R, Gale RP, Bortin MM, eds. *Cellular Immunotherapy of Cancer*. Alan R Liss, New York, 1987, pp. 401–408.

62. Leith CP, Kopecky KJ, Godwin JE, et al. Acute myeloid leukemia in the elderly: assessment of multidrug resistance (MDRI) and cytogenetics distinguishes biologic subgroups with remarkably distinct responses to standard chemotherapy. A Southwest Oncology Group study. *Blood* 1997;89:3323–3329.

63. Storb R, Yu C, McSweeney P. Mixed chimerism after transplantation of allogeneic hematopoietic cells. In: Thomas ED, Blume KG, Forman SJ, eds. *Hematopoietic Cell Transplantation*, 2nd ed. Blackwell Science, London, 1999, pp. 287–295.

64. Champlin R, Khouri I, Kornblau S, et al. Allogeneic hematopoietic transplantation as adoptive immunotherapy. In: Schiller GJ, guest ed. *Hematology/Oncology Clinics of North America*. W.B. Saunders, Phialdelphia, 1999, pp. 1041–1057.

65. McSweeney PA, Niederwieser D, Shizuru JA, et al. Hematopoietic cell transplantation in older patients with hematologic malignancies: replacing high-dose cytotoxic therapy with graft-versus-tumor effects. *Blood* 2001;97:3390–3400.

66. Forman SJ, Schmidt GM, Nademanee AP, et al. Allogeneic bone marrow transplantation as therapy for primary induction failure for patients with acute leukemia. *J Clin Oncol* 1991;9:1570–1574.

67. Mehta J, Powles R, Horton C, et al. Bone marrow transplantation for primary refractory acute leukemia. *Bone Marrow Transplant* 1994;14:415–418.

68. Biggs JC, Horowitz MM, Gale RP, et al. Bone marrow transplants may cure patients with acute leukemia never achieving remission with chemotherapy. *Blood* 1992;80:1090–1093.

69. Fung HC, O'Donnell M, Popplewell L, et al. Allogeneic stem cell transplantation (SCT) for patients with primary refractory acute myelogenous leukemia (AML): impact of cytogenetic risk group on the transplant outcome. In press.

70. Matthews DC, Appelbaum FR, Eary JF, et al. ¹³¹I-anti-CD45 antibody plus busulfan/cyclophosphamide in matched related transplants for AML in first remission. *Blood* 1996;88:142a.

71. Andersson BS, Kashyap A, Gian V, et al. Conditioning therapy with intravenous busulfan and cyclophosphamide (IV BuCy2) for hematologic malignancies prior to allogeneic stem cell transplantation: a phase II study. *Biol Blood Marrow Transplant* 2002;3:145–154.

72. Deeg HJ, Shulman HM, Anderson JE, et al. Allogeneic and syngeneic marrow transplantation for myelodysplastic syndrome in patients 55 to 66 years of age. *Blood* 2000;95:1188–1194.

3

Allogeneic Stem Cell Transplantation for Adult Acute Lymphoblastic Leukemia

Partow Kebriaei, MD and Wendy Stock, MD

CONTENTS

1. INTRODUCTION

Current treatment strategies for adult acute lymphoblastic leukemia (ALL) have resulted in the achievement of complete remission (CR) rates of 70–95%. Approximately 25–50% of these patients may enjoy long-term disease-free survival (DFS), and current research efforts are focused on innovative postremission strategies with the goal of improving the overall survival for adults with ALL. The identification of different prognostic groups based on the biology of the malignant clone and clinical patterns of disease presentation has begun to alter our therapeutic approach to this biologically heterogeneous disease. Treatment strategies tailored to specific prognostic groups have already resulted in dramatic improvements in the outcome for children with ALL *(1)*, and similar risk-adapted strategies based on the biologic heterogeneity of the disease are now being applied to adults with ALL to improve survival. Allogeneic stem cell transplantation (SCT) is one strategy that has been demonstrated to improve the outcome of high-risk adults with ALL. In this chapter, we will define this high-risk group, discuss indications for transplantation based on biologic risk group, and review current strategies and clinical outcome for allogeneic SCT in adults with ALL.

2. PROGNOSTIC FACTORS IN ADULT ALL

Several biologic features and specific clinical characteristics have been consistently noted to influence the outcome of adult ALL and impact on risk stratification (Fig. 1). Age greater

From: *Current Clinical Oncology: Allogeneic Stem Cell Transplantation*
Edited by: Mary S. Laughlin and Hillard M. Lazarus © Humana Press Inc., Totowa, NJ

- Age >60 yr
- WBC count >30,000/uL
- Cytogenetics: t(9;22)(q34;q11), trisomy 8, t(4;11)(q21;q23), monosomy 7, hypodiploid karyotype, t(1;19)(q23;p13)
- Delayed time to CR, >4 wk

Fig. 1. Adverse prognostic features in adult ALL.

than 60 yr, a high white blood cell count (WBC) at presentation, and failure to achieve a clinical remission within the first 4 wk of treatment are all considered adverse clinical features. The detection of specific recurring cytogenetic abnormalities has emerged as the most important prognostic factor for risk stratification of adults with ALL. Clonal chromosomal aberrations can be detected in cells from 62 to 85% of adult ALL patients, and several studies have shown their significance as predictors of outcome *(2,3)*. In a multivariate analysis of risk factors in adult ALL, karyotype was identified as the most important factor for DFS *(4)*. In general, patients with a normal karyotype have improved survival compared with those harboring a cytogenetic abnormality. In a recent review of this literature, six abnormalities were noted to result in unfavorable outcome, defined as having a 0.25 or less probability of continuous CR at 5 yr. These include in decreasing frequency, patients with t(9;22) (q34;q11), trisomy 8, t(4;11) (q21;q23), monosomy 7, a hypodiploid karyotype, and t(1;19) *(5,6)*.

The most common and clinically relevant cytogenetic abnormalities in adults with ALL include the t(9;22) (q34;q11) resulting in the *BCR/ABL* fusion gene that is present in as many as 30% of adult ALL patients, the t(4;11) (q21;q23) involving the *MLL* gene on chromosome 11q23 that results in the *MLL/AF4* fusion gene, and the t(8;14) (q24;q32) chromosomal translocation seen in mature B lineage ALL (Burkitt's type) that results in overexpression of the c-*MYC* proto-oncogene. With each of these abnormalities, patients have improved outcome if they are treated with an approach other than standard induction, consolidation, and maintenance regimens. For example, treatment insights from the pediatric groups have resulted in the successful implementation of fractionated high doses of alkylating agents in combination with high dose methotrexate and intensive central nervous system prophylaxis to improve significantly the outcome for adults with mature B-CR to use B-cell ALL *(7–10)*. Using this intensive but short-duration chemotherapeutic approach, these high-risk patients now achieve CR in 70–80% of cases and have DFS approaching 50%. As described above, and discussed in detail below, ALL patients with a t(9;22) (q34;q11) have fared very poorly with standard ALL chemotherapy, but can achieve prolonged DFS when allogeneic SCT approaches are used.

A number of investigators have combined these prognostic factors to predict the efficacy of the planned chemotherapy and to assess the potential use of allogeneic transplantation for patients with ALL. Hoelzer et al. initially proposed a risk classification of adult ALL focusing on age, WBC count, immunophenotype, and time to achievement of CR *(4)*. This classification scheme identified patients who had either good long-term DFS or poor outcome with a high risk of relapse. Similarly, Table 1 shows the impact of four adverse features and the outcome of treatment of ALL in two studies of intensive combination chemotherapy from the Cancer and Leukemia Group B (CALGB studies 8811 and 9111) *(10,11)*. This analysis demonstrates that a large number of adults with ALL have disease features at diagnosis that put them into a high-risk group with a DFS of less than 30%. These types of analyses, combined with advances in cytogenetic and molecular monitoring techniques to detect minimal residual disease (MRD) (discussed below), are useful for the identification of patients who might benefit from early hematopoietic SCT while in first remission.

Table 1
Impact of Adverse Features on the Outcome of Treatment

No. of adverse features	No. of patients	Age <60 yr	WBC <30,000/μL	No medstinal mass	Laboratory features[a]	Estimated survival at 3 yr
0	22	0	0	0	0	91% (66–98%)
1	83	1	16	63	3	64% (51–75%)
2	146	12	25	145	110	49% (36–61%)
3	89	25	68	89	85	21% (12–35%)
4	13	13	13	13	13	0

[a]Adverse laboratory features include the presence of the Ph or *BCR/ABL*+ PCR analysis, L3 morphology, or precursor B lineage disease.

2.1. Prognostic Role of MRD Monitoring

In addition to the adverse prognostic factors listed in Table 1, the detection of MRD using qualitative or semiquantitative polymerase chain reaction (PCR) or flow cytometric techniques is also beginning to provide important prognostic information. A number of large prospective studies in pediatric ALL have demonstrated the independent prognostic significance of MRD detection. Using semiquantitative PCR for the detection of the leukemia "clone-specific" immunoglobulin heavy chain or T cell receptor gene rearrangement, these studies have shown that persistent MRD detection at various time points following achievement of morphologic and cytogenetic remission is a highly significant and independent prognosticator of relapse *(12,13)*. Less is known about the significance of MRD detection in adult ALL. Brisco et al. studied 27 adults with B lineage ALL for MRD in CR1. Eight of nine patients with higher levels of disease (levels >10^{-3}) detected using semiquantitative PCR relapsed, compared to 6 of 13 patients with lower MRD levels (levels <10^{-3}) *(14)*. Larger, prospective studies are currently underway using more precise quantitative PCR (real time PCR) to determine the significance of MRD detection in predicting relapse in adult ALL *(15)*. These data may provide critical new prognostic information about "low risk" patients in CR1 who are actually at high risk for relapse and identify a new group of patients who might benefit from allogeneic SCT while still in first remission.

3. ALLOGENEIC TRANSPLANTATION FOR HIGH RISK ALL DURING FIRST CR

Several studies have investigated allogeneic SCT approaches in high-risk ALL patients following achievement of first CR (Table 2). These studies are difficult to compare directly with results of trials utilizing postremission chemotherapy, since the transplant series are usually small phase II studies that tend to include only healthy, younger patients who are already in remission. Nevertheless, a number of these trials provide some interesting insights into the potential efficacy of allogeneic SCT in CR1. To better clarify the relative roles of chemotherapy and SCT in adults with high-risk ALL, Horowitz et al. analyzed International Bone Marrow Transplant Registry (IBMTR) data for 484 patients who had received intensive postremission chemotherapy, and 251 recipients of HLA-identical allogeneic SCT for ALL in CR1. Patients ranged from 15 to 45 yr of age and were treated between 1980 and 1987. Similar prognostic factors, including non-T lineage phenotype, high leukocyte count at presentation, and greater than 8 wk to achieve CR, predicted treatment failure in both treatment groups. After statistical adjustments were made for differences in disease characteristics, 5-yr leukemia-free survival (LFS) was similar in the chemotherapy (38%) and allogeneic SCT (44%) cohorts;

Table 1
Comparative Trials of Transplantation vs Chemotherapy for ALL in CR1

Study	No. of patients	Median age (yr)	Prep. regimen	GVHD proph.	II–IV GVHD	5-yr DFS(%)
Horowitz, 1991 (16)						
ASCT	234	15–45	CY/TBI	MR	NR	44
Chemotherapy	484	15–45	MR			38
Rowe, 1999 (17)						
ASCT	173	14–60	VP-16/TBI	NR	NR	58 (3 yr)
Chemotherapy/ aSCT	426	14–60				39 (3 yr)
Sebban, 1994 (LALA 87) (17)						
ASCT	116	26	CY/TBI	CSA/MTX	NR	45
Chemotherapy/ aSCT	141	24	CY/TBI for SCT L10 regimen			31
Thiebaut, 2000 (LALA 87 f/u) (18)						
ASCT	116	15–40	CY/TBI	CSA/MTX	NR	46
High risk	41					44
Standard risk	75					49
Chemotherapy	141	≤50	L10 regimen			31
High risk	55					11
Standard risk	86					43
Oh, 1998 (19)						
ASCT	87	>30	CY ± Ara-C/TBI	CSA/MTX	NR	30
Chemotherapy	38	>30	MR			26
ASCT	127	<30	CY ± Ara-C/TBI	CSA/MTX	NR	53
Chemotherapy	38	<30	MR			30

ASCT, allogeneic SCT; aSCT, autologous SCT; CY, cytoxan; TBI, total body irradiation; MR, multiple regimens; NR, not reported; VP-16, etoposide; CSA, cyclosporine; MTX, methotrexate.

however, causes of treatment failure differed between the two groups. In the chemotherapy group, 96% of failures were due to relapse and 4% were treatment-related, while in the SCT group, 32% were due to relapse and 68% were treatment-related (16). Thus, while there was no difference in overall survival, this retrospective analysis suggests a decreased risk of relapse for high-risk patients treated with allogeneic SCT in CR1.

The MRC UKALL XII/ECOG E2993 is an international effort to prospectively define the role of allogeneic SCT, autologous SCT, and chemotherapy in adult patients with ALL in CR1. Initiated in 1993, over 1100 patients have been enrolled to date (HM Lazarus, personal communication, May 2001). All patients received two phases of induction therapy, and continued to allogeneic SCT if they achieved CR and had a histocompatible donor. The remaining patients were randomized to standard consolidation/maintenance therapy for 2.5 yr vs a single autologous SCT. The conditioning regimen for both allogeneic and autologous transplants was fractionated TBI (1320 cGy) and VP-16 (60 mg/kg). Available date on the first 800 patients revealed a CR rate of 91% for Philadelphia (Ph) patients and 83% for Ph+ patients; these results are corroborated by earlier, smaller trials. Details regarding the reponse of Ph+ patients to standard therapy vs allogeneic SCT will be discussed in the section on Ph+ patients. Based on the data presented in an abstract published in 1999 (17), 173 patients received an allogeneic SCT and 426 patients received chemotherapy or autologous SCT. The overall event free survival (EFS) for the allogeneic SCT group was 58 vs 39% for the chemotherapy or autologous BMT group. When patients (excluding Ph+ patients) were stratified into high or standard risk, the difference in EFS becomes more dramatic in the high risk subset (allogeneic BMT 57% vs chemotherapy/autologous BMT 32%), illustrating the advantage of allogeneic BMT in high risk patients. Standard risk was defined as Ph–, age <35, time to CR <4 wk, and WBC count <30,000/μL for B lineage and <50,000/μL for T lineage leukemia.

The French (Leucemie Aigue Lymphoblastique de l'Adulte [LALA]) group is another cooperative study which defined the role of chemotherapy and SCT for adult ALL patients. This was a prospective randomized study, initiated in November 1986 and completed in July 1991, which enrolled 634 patients in the LALA 87 protocol to assess the role of allogeneic SCT and autologous SCT in adult ALL. After exclusions, 572 patients were analyzed, and 10-yr follow-up results have recently been published. The median age of patients entered onto this trial was 33 yr. Patients received induction chemotherapy with cyclophosphamide, vincristine, prednisone, and one of two anthracyclines. Central nervous system (CNS) prophylaxis was administered. Four hundred and thirty-six patients (76%) achieved CR. After CR was achieved, patients older than 50 yr received postremission chemotherapy. Patients between 15 and 40 yr of age were assigned to the allogeneic SCT trial if they had an HLA-matched sibling donor. Patients between ages 40 and 50, and those under the age of 40 without a matched sibling donor, were further randomized to consolidation chemotherapy or autologous SCT using bone marrow purged with antibodies or mafosfamide. Consolidation chemotherapy consisted of three monthly courses of daunorubicin or zorubicin, Ara-C, and asparaginase followed by long-term maintenance therapy. The transplant preparative regimen consisted of total body irradiation (TBI) and cyclophosphamide. The 10-yr overall survival rate of patients greater than 50 yr treated with chemotherapy only was 27%. There was no statistically significant difference in outcome between patients who received autologous SCT vs consolidation chemotherapy (34% SCT, 29% chemotherapy, $p = 0.6$). After stratification into high and standard risk, there was still no statistical difference between these two groups. High risk was defined as having one or more of the following factors: presence of the Ph chromosome, null ALL, age > 35 yr, WBC count > 30×10^9/L, time to CR >4 wk. Importantly, this study showed that survival at 10 yr was significantly greater for the allogeneic SCT group compared to consolidation chemotherapy (46% SCT, 31% chemotherapy, $p = 0.04$). Furthermore, when these groups were stratified into high and standard risk, there was a highly significant benefit for allogeneic SCT in the high-risk subset, but no statistically significant benefit seen for the standard-risk subset (high risk: 44% SCT, 11% chemotherapy, $p = 0.009$; standard risk: 49% SCT, 43% chemotherapy, $p = 0.6$) (18,19). Thus, both the large IBMTR retrospective review and the LALA study suggest a clear role for allogeneic SCT over consolidation chemotherapy in younger adults with high-risk features in CR1. Another study by Oh et al. reinforces the observation that a significant survival advantage is gained in high-risk younger patients undergoing allogeneic SCT (20). Presumably, the lower mortality and morbidity sustained by younger patients undergoing SCT highlights the advantage of this method over chemotherapy.

In addition, review of a number of smaller phase II trials in high-risk adult ALL who have undergone ASCT in CR1 suggest a higher DFS when compared with conventional chemotherapy (21–27). High risk in these studies was defined as patients having at least one or more of the following: age greater than 30 yr, WBC greater than 30×10^9/L at presentation, extramedullary disease, unfavorable cytogenetic abnormalities, and requiring more than 4 wk to achieve a CR. As shown in Table 3, these phase II trials demonstrate a DFS ranging broadly from 21–71% during a 3- to 8-yr follow-up. The DFS for patients treated with conventional chemotherapy ranges from 30 to 40%. The large difference in outcome of patients entered onto these small phase II studies is influenced by multiple variables, including differences in patient

Table 3
Allogeneic Transplantation for ALL in CR1

Study	No. of patients	Median age (yr)	Prep. regimen	GVHD proph.	II–IV GVHD	3-yr DFS(%)
Wingard, 1990 (20)	18	24 (5–36)	CY/TBI	CSA ± MP	8	42
Blaise, 1990 (21)	25	22 (4–36)	CY/fTBI, ML/fTBI CY/ML/fTBI	MR	7	71
Chao, 1991 (22)	53	28 (1–45)	Ara-C/CY/TBI CY/TBI	CSA ± MP MTX ± MP	6	61
Doney, 1991 (23)	41	22 (18–50)	Cy/fTBI or single dose	MR	7	21 (5 yr)
Sutton, 1993 (24) (retrospective review)	184	25 (15–44)	CY/TBI (majority)	MR	15 deaths	49.5 (6 yr)
Vey, 1994 (25)	29	24 (16–41)	CY/TBI	CSA/MTX	7	62 (8 yr)
DeWitte, 1994 (26)	22	15–51	CY/TBI	CSA	NR	58

CY, cytoxan; fTBI, fractionated total body irradiation; MR, multiple regimens; NR, not reported; CSA, cyclosporine; MTX, methotrexate; MP, methylprednisolone.

selection, choice of preparative regimen, type of graft-vs-host disease (GVHD) prophylaxis, and different supportive care regimens.

4. ALLOGENEIC TRANSPLANTATION BEYOND CR1 USING HLA-IDENTICAL SIBLING DONORS

There are no data suggesting that durable remissions can be achieved with standard chemotherapy for adults with ALL in/or beyond CR2. Similar to the transplant literature in pediatric ALL beyond first remission, it appears that allogeneic SCT for adults in/beyond CR2 is superior to chemotherapy in achieving LFS. Adult ALL patients who undergo an allogeneic SCT in CR2 achieve long-term LFS rates of 14–43%, as illustrated in Table 4. The primary cause of failure is relapse (>50%).

5. PRIMARY REFRACTORY ALL

With current induction regimens, only 5–10% of adults with newly diagnosed ALL fail to achieve remission with initial induction chemotherapy. These patients often have one or more poor prognostic factors at presentation, and additional attempts at induction chemotherapy may be unsuccessful. Several studies suggest that patients with an HLA-identical sibling can benefit if they proceed directly to allogeneic transplantation without undergoing a second attempt at induction therapy (32–34). In the largest of these studies, 38 patients with ALL, failing to achieve remission, received HLA-identical sibling transplants. Approximately 35% of these patients with refractory disease had long-term DFS. A second study with 22 patients (five patients with ALL) with refractory disease had a similar survival of 38% following HLA-matched sibling transplants. Other studies suggest lower survival rates of 20% or less for these refractory patients (32,34); nevertheless, allogeneic transplant should be considered for these patients with an otherwise dismal chance of long-term survival.

6. PHILADELPHIA CHROMOSOME-POSITIVE ALL

The presence of the Philadelphia chromosome (Ph) represents an independent adverse risk factor, and carries an exceptionally poor prognosis. Although many patients can achieve a CR,

Table 4
Allogeneic Transplantation for ALL in CR2

Study	No. of patients	LFS (%)	Risk of relapse (%)
IBMTR, 1989 *(28)*			
High risk	208	22 (4 yr)	56
Standard risk	97	36 (4 yr)	49
Barrett et al., 1989 *(29)*	391	26 (5 yr)	52
Wingard et al., 1990 *(21)*	36	43 (5 yr)	26
Doney et al., 1991 *(24)*	48	15 (5 yr)	64
Greinex et al., 1998 *(30)*	27	14 (3 yr)	78
Michallet et al., 2000 *(31)*	47	30 ± 8 (5 yr)	44 ± 12

the median duration of remission is less than 1 yr with chemotherapy. Using intensive conventional chemotherapy, the CALGB observed similar CR rates between Ph+ and Ph- ALL patients (76% Ph+, 86% Ph-); however, only 17% of the Ph+ patients were reported to be in CR at 3 yr vs 48% of the Ph- patients *(5)*. Data from the MRC UKALL XII/ECOG E2993 study described earlier reveals similar poor results for Ph+ patients treated with chemotherapy only. In this ongoing, prospective, randomized study, 43 Ph+ patients were treated with chemotherapy only. They had a 3 yr overall survival (OS) of 19%, which was significantly worse than the Ph− group (47%, $p = 0.002$). The EFS at 3 yr was 0% for the Ph+ group vs. 38% for the Ph− ($p = $ <0.001) *(35)*. Therefore, studies have been conducted to test the efficacy of allogeneic SCT as a consolidative treatment after achievement of first remission in these patients.

In the MRC UKALL XII/ECOG E2993 study, 35 patients have undergone a matched, related allogeneic SCT and had a 38% EFS at 3 yr compared to an EFS of only 5% for those PH+ patients who received chemotherapy or autologous SCT. In another study, 23 patients with Ph+ ALL in CR1 underwent allogeneic SCT from a matched sibling between 1984 and 1997 at the City of Hope National Medical Center and Stanford University. The median age of the patients transplanted was 30 yr. The preparative regimen involved fractionated TBI and etoposide (VP-16). At 3 yr, the probability of DFS was reported at 65%. For patients transplanted after 1992, the probability of DFS increased to 81%, presumably due to improvements in GVHD prophylaxis and supportive care *(36)*. Of note, the DFS rate reported in this study is much higher than others reported for Ph+ patients undergoing allogeneic SCT. In a retrospective review of 67 Ph+ patients reported to the IBMTR between 1978 and 1990, with a median age of 28 yr, the 2-yr DFS rate was 31%, and was similar for patients in CR1, in CR2, or in relapse *(28)*. In a small study by Dunlop et al. *(37)*, 11 patients underwent an allogeneic transplant between 1986 and 1995. The estimated 3-yr probability of DFS was 21.8%. Of note, this small study included patients in CR1, in CR2, or in relapse. In another small study of 14 Ph+ patients undergoing transplantation (4 autologous SCT in CR1 or CR2 and 10 allogeneic SCT in CR1, CR2, or relapse), the overall DFS was 46% for all patients; however, of those patients who received an allogeneic SCT, 60% (6 of 10 patients) of patients undergoing allogeneic SCT were in remission during a median follow-up of 503 d *(38)*.

It is difficult to draw conclusions from these small series that vary considerably with respect to type of patient (CR1 or beyond), type of preparative regimen, GVHD prophylaxis, and supportive care; however, some general observations can be made. Taken together, the DFS rate for Ph+ adult patients in CR1 undergoing allogeneic transplant appears to be somewhere between 30 and 60%. Although the retrospective IBMTR review indicated that patients in CR1, CR2, or relapse have similar outcomes following allogeneic transplant, data from most of these series suggest that Ph+ patients fare best when transplanted in first remission. It is difficult to determine if a particular preparative regimen contributes to better outcome. Of note, fractionated TBI and VP-16 was used exclusively in the City of Hope trial. However, very similar regimens were used in some of the other series reported above.

In summary, survival for Ph+ patients following an allogeneic SCT is superior to what is achieved with standard chemotherapy. Although in most transplant series, Ph+ patients still have a more adverse outcome than other ALL subsets. Thus, much work remains to develop more effective treatment for these extremely high-risk patients. Novel transplant preparative regimens are currently being examined. Deane et al. *(39)* used fludarabine, cytarabine, idarubicin, and granulocyte colony stimulating factor (G-CSF) (FLAG-idarubicin) followed by allogeneic transplant in 8 Ph+ patients with advanced stage disease. The median age was 25 yr; 7 of 8 patients had other cytogenetic abnormalities in addition to the t(9;22) (q34;q11). One patient underwent a sibling bone marrow transplantation (BMT), 3 underwent matched unrelated donor (MUD) BMTs, and 4 underwent sibling peripheral blood SCT (PBSCT). All six patients with bone marrow involvement had a response following a single course of FLAG-idarubucin (5 CR, 1 partial remission [PR]). The DFS beyond 2 yr was 47.6%. This is comparable to other studies, but is intriguing because this study included patients with very advanced/refractory Ph+ disease.

The efficacy of HLA-MUD transplants for Ph+ ALL has also been investigated in a limited fashion to allow more Ph+ patients to undergo transplantation. At the Fred Hutchinson Cancer Research Center, MUD transplantation was investigated in 18 patients with Ph+ ALL between 1988 and 1995. The study included children and adults, with the median age being only 25 yr. Of 18 patients who underwent transplant, 6 who were transplanted in CR1, 1 in CR2, and 2 in first relapse remained leukemia free. The preparative regimen involved TBI and cyclophosphamide. Of 6 who were transplanted in CR1, 1 patient was in CR1, and 2 patients, while in second remission, remained leukemia-free at a median follow-up of 17 mo. The probability of LFS at 2 yr was 49%, which is similar to rates reported for matched-sibling SCT *(39)*. These data appear very promising; however, it must be emphasized that this was a highly selected population of extremely young Ph+ patients.

The role of donor lymphocyte infusion (DLI) has also been investigated in these patients. Interestingly, one theory for DLI's tremendous efficacy in chronic myelogenous leukemia (CML) postallotransplant is based on the inherent immunogenicity of the *BCR/ABL* protein. Yet, DLI has had very limited efficacy in Ph+ ALL *(41,42)*. It is not known whether the differences in DLI efficacy in Ph+ ALL compared to CML results from differences in immunogenicicty of the p190 *BCR/ABL* (most Ph+ ALL) vs the p210 *BCR/ABL* (most CML), differences in growth kinetics of Ph+ ALL relapse (high tumor burden) vs those in CML (lower tumor burden), or other disease specific factors. Interestingly, in a study of 11 patients, including one with Ph+ ALL, allogeneic PBSC from the original donor were administered following transplant relapse. All patients achieved CR, although responses were not durable. This suggests that cells, in addition to lymphocytes present in the PBSC, may have an important "anti-leukemia" role. Experiences using PBSC infusions, rather than DLI, are described in greater detail in a later section. The patient with Ph+ ALL achieved a complete clinical and molecular response, but died at 12 wk due to CNS relapse. This was the only site of disease at time of death *(43)*.

The most exciting recent development in the treatment of Ph+ ALL has been the intriguing early results observed with STI-571, a molecule specifically targeted to the *BCR/ABL* tyrosine kinase that is overexpressed as a result of the t(9;22) in CML and Ph+ ALL. STI-571 is a specific inhibitor of the *abl* protein tyrosine kinase that has demonstrated remarkable targeted therapeutic efficacy in patients with CML and ALL with increased *bcr/abl* activity. In a phase I pilot study of 58 patients treated with STI-571, including 38 patients with myeloid blast crisis and 20 patients with Ph+ ALL or lymphoid blast crisis, 55% of patients with myeloid blast crisis and 70% of patients with ALL achieved a response. A reduction of peripheral blasts was observed within 1 wk of treatment initiation. Four patients (20%) with ALL had a complete response, but 12 of 14 patients relapsed a median of 58 d after initiation of treatment (range 42–123 d); 1 patient underwent SCT and 1 patient was not evaluable due to short length of follow-up *(44)*. The mechanism(s) of resistance is currently under study; however, the rapid initial response to therapy and minimal side effects make STI-571 an ideal candidate for clinical trials to test efficacy in the treatment of newly diagnosed Ph+ ALL. CALGB, in combination with the Southwest Oncology Group (SWOG), are initiating a phase II trial of sequential chemotherapy, STI-571, and allogeneic or auto-SCT for adults with newly diagnosed Ph+ ALL. The primary objectives of this study will be to determine the ability of STI-571 to produce a complete molecular response (achieve *BCR/ABL* status by reverse transcription PCR [RT-PCR]) following sequential chemotherapy, STI-571, and transplantation, and to determine the ability of STI-571 to prolong DFS and overall survival in this high-risk group of patients.

6.1. Predicting Outcome: Role of Monitoring MRD in Ph+ ALL Following Transplantation

Several studies of MRD status following allogeneic transplantation provide intriguing information about the risk of relapse in Ph+ ALL and may help to identify patients who are likely to relapse *(45–49)*. All of these studies found that patients who are consistently *BCR/ABL–* following transplantation are unlikely to relapse and may become long-term survivors. Conversely, patients who are *BCR/ABL+* following transplantation seem to be at high risk for subsequent relapse. In the largest published series (28 patients), Radich and coworkers found that the relative risk (RR) for relapse was significantly higher for patients with a detectable *BCR/ABL* transcript following transplantation than for those without detectable *BCR/ABL* (RR = 5.7; $p = 0.025$) *(48)*. The prognostic significance of the PCR assay remained after controlling for other variables that could influence relapse risk. The risk of relapse was greater for patients with a p190 fusion transcript than for those with p210 *BCR/ABL*. The median time from detection of a positive PCR result to relapse was 94 d. Additional insights into the kinetics of disappearance of *BCR/ABL* will be obtained from current studies using *real-time* PCR techniques to quantify transcript number reproducibly *(49,50)*. Using rigorous monitoring techniques, it may be possible to introduce DLI prior to overt clinical relapse, when it may be more effective *(48)*, or other novel therapies (e.g., STI 571) that could eliminate subclinical disease and avoid the dire consequences of a clinical relapse in these patients.

7. FACTORS INFLUENCING TRANSPLANT OUTCOME

7.1. Preparative Regimens

Several different preparative regimens for allogeneic SCT have been described in attempts to decrease transplanted-related mortality (TRM) and improve DFS. The most widely used regimen is the combination of TBI and cyclophosphamide developed by Thomas and colleagues in the 1970s *(51)*. The TBI can be administered as single dose or fractionated over 3–5 d. A comparative analysis of fractionated-dose vs single-dose TBI in adult ALL patients showed a significantly higher TRM in the single dose group ($p = 0.017$), but an increase in the relapse rate of the fractionated-dose group; consequently, there were no differences in the overall LFS between the two groups *(25)*. The Minnesota Group compared TBI/cyclophosphamide with TBI/cytarabine (Ara-C) in a study including both adults and children and found no difference in regards to toxicity or outcome *(51)*. The City of Hope group studied fractionated TBI with etoposide followed by SCT in patients with advanced leukemia. A phase I/II trial indicated that etoposide at 60 mg/kg is the maximum tolerated dose when compared with TBI. In that study,

36 ALL patients were treated; 20 patients had relapsed disease. The DFS was 57%, with a 32% relapse rate suggesting that the regimen has significant activity in advanced ALL *(52)*. The fractionated TBI/etoposide regimen has also demonstrated activity in patients with high-risk Ph+ ALL, as discussed in more detail below.

Novel methods to allow selective delivery of radiation to sites of leukemia without increasing systemic toxicity are currently under investigation. A phase I transplant trial using ^{131}I-labeled anti-CD45 antibody combined with cyclophosphamide at 120 mg/kg and 12-gy TBI was recently published *(53)*. All patients had advanced hematologic malignancies. The dose limiting toxicity was grade III/IV mucositis. Nine patients with ALL (5 patients with relapsed/refractory ALL; 4 patients in CR2 or CR3) received allogeneic (6 patients) or autologous (t3 patients) transplants using this preparative regimen; 3 patients were disease-free 19, 54, and 66 mo posttransplant. The ultimate benefits of this approach, with respect to safety and improvements in survival, will be defined by phase II studies for patients with ALL.

Nonradiation-containing regimens, most commonly busulfan and cyclophosphamide, have been investigated in hopes of decreasing radiation-related complications. Fractionated TBI (FTBI)/etoposide was tested against busulfan/cyclophosphamide in a prospective randomized study conducted by SWOG (8612). One hundred twenty-two patients with leukemia beyond CR1 received either FTBI/etoposide or busulfan/cyclophosphamide in preparation for SCT. One hundred fourteen patients (93%) proceeded to SCT. All patients received cyclosporine and prednisone for posttransplant immunosuppression. There was no significant difference with respect to toxicity, incidence of acute GVHD, overall survival, or DFS between the two groups. The leading cause for treatment failure was leukemic relapse (39%) *(54)*. Furthermore, retrospective analysis of registry data from the IBMTR shows similar rates for LFS and relapse when busulfan/cyclophosphamide is compared to TBI/cyclophosphamide *(55)*. Careful comparisons of the incidence of second malignancies with each of these regimens have not been made but may have importance. Thus, a variety of preparative regimens can be used, but leukemic relapse remains the most significant factor affecting DFS.

7.2. Source of Stem Cells

Bensinger et al. *(56)* recently published a prospective, randomized trial comparing bone marrow to peripheral blood as the source of stem cells. Between March 1996 and July 1999, 172 patients, including 22 with ALL with a median age of 42 yr, were randomly assigned to receive bone marrow or filgrastim-mobilized PBSC from HLA-identical relatives for hematopoietic rescue after dose-intensive chemotherapy. After randomization, patients were stratified according to age (<30 or >30 yr), and stage of cancer (for ALL, CR1 was defined as less advanced; for all others, it was defined as advanced), with roughly equal numbers in the two groups. It was concluded from this study that allogeneic peripheral blood cells used for hematopoietic rescue restore blood counts faster than bone marrow without increasing the risk of GVHD. It was also observed that patients who received peripheral blood cells had a lower incidence of relapse at 2 yr, and a higher overall survival and DFS *(56)*. The authors did not analyze individual hematologic malignancies due to the small numbers; however, based on the faster count recovery and the overall lower relapse rate, it appears that the use of mobilized PBSC rather than the bone marrow may be advantageous for all patients with acute leukemias. Little data currently exist on the outcome of patients receiving umbilical cord stem cell transplants for adults with ALL.

7.3. Source of Donor Cells: Partially Matched Related or MUD

The majority of studies indicate that the best chance for cure for refractory or high-risk ALL is allogeneic SCT with matched related donor. Unfortunately, <30% of these patients have a matched sibling donor. Thus, much work continues to be done in making partially matched related donor (haplotype transplants) and MUD transplantation safe and more feasible as curative therapy. Typically, these transplants are associated with a higher risk of graft rejection, GVHD, and infection. The experience with these transplants for adults with ALL is still small. A recent study from the IBMTR compared MUD and haplo-identical transplantation with HLA-identical sibling transplants *(57)*. TRM was higher (>50%) and LFS was lower for patients receiving MUD transplants. Among the challenges to improving outcomes of patients receiving MUD transplants include more effective HLA matching of donor and recipient. Current innovations in molecular typing of HLA loci using high resolution allele-based typing for class I and II HLA molecules appears to decrease the incidence of severe GVHD and improves survival of patients undergoing MUD transplantation *(58)*.

Godder et al. evaluated the efficacy of partially matched allo-SCT in 43 pediatric ALL patients. Grafts were partially T cell depleted, and patients received posttransplant immunosuppression with cyclosporine, corticosteroids, and antithymocyte globulin (ATG). The study illustrated that the rate of engraftment and DFS was comparable to HLA identical grafts. Of note, the blast count at the start of transplantation and the donor's age were the two most influential variables. Improved rates of DFS and decreased risk of relapse were seen with younger donors. In addition, the estimated probability of grade II–IV acute GVHD was 0.24 and was not affected by recipient antigen mismatch *(59)*. Given the current data from series that include many young patients and patients with advanced leukemia beyond CR1, it is not yet clear whether SCT should be recommended over chemotherapy for the high-risk adult ALL patient in CR1 who does not have a matched sibling.

7.4. Partially Matched Related/MUD vs Autologous SCT

The theoretical advantage of MUD over autologous SCT in high-risk patients is a decreased risk of relapse, presumably due to the graft-vs-leukemia (GVL) effect. Weisdorf et al. *(60)* reported the results of 337 ALL patients (121 adults; 216 children) who received MUD-SCT and compared them to 214 patients (54 adults; 160 children) who underwent autologous SCT during 1987 to 1993. For those transplanted in CR1, autologous SCT yielded a significantly higher DFS (42% autologous SCT vs 32% MUD, $p = 0.03$). In contrast, for those transplanted in CR2, MUD-SCT yielded a better DFS (20% autologous SCT vs 42% MUD, $p = 0.02$). The worse outcome with autologous SCT in CR2 likely reflects the increased relapse hazard in the advanced leukemia group. When the data were analyzed separately for children and adults in CR2, MUD-SCT still yielded a higher DFS when compared to autologous SCT (adults, MUD 42% ± 22% vs autologous SCT 0%, $p = 0.006$) *(60)*. The Acute Leukemia Working Party of the European Cooperative Group for Blood and Marrow Transplantation (EBMT) analyzed data from ALL patients undergoing SCT between January 1987 and December 1994 *(61)*. One hundred eighteen patients with a median age of 14 yr received MUD-SCT; 236 patients with a median age of 16 yr received autologous SCT. Disease status ranged from CR1 to CR3. There were no significant differences in the 2-yr LFS for MUD-SCT vs autologous SCT (39% MUD-SCT, 32% autologous SCT) in this retrospective analysis of ALL patients matched for diagnosis, age, stage of disease, and year of transplantation. However, relapse was significantly lower in the MUD-SCT group (MUD-SCT 32% vs autologous SCT 61%, $p = <0.0001$), while TRM was significantly higher in this group (MUD 42% vs auto 17%, $p = <0.0001$). As expected, GVHD and graft failure were major sources of TRM in the MUD-SCT group. Interpretation of the results of retrospective analyses is always difficult. Nevertheless, both of these studies suggest an advantage for MUD-SCT with respect to decreased rates of relapse. Owing to the significant morbidity involved with this procedure and the low overall survival, the decision to proceed with MUD or autologous transplantation or to proceed with other "phase I" approaches for these high-risk patients currently remains very complex and is based on the specific situation of each individual patient.

7.5. The Role of T Cell Depletion

The role of T cell-depleted SCT remains controversial. T cell-depleted SCT have been shown to be better tolerated with less TRM, due to the lower incidence of GVHD, and present an appealing option for both older patients with a matched sibling and HLA-mismatched transplants. As described previously, T cell-purged SCT have higher relapse rates. Recently, several groups have reported a decreased risk of relapse with T cell-depleted SCT by manipulating the preparative regimen to compensate for potential lack of a GVL effect. Aversa et al. evaluated 54 consecutive acute leukemia patients with a median age 30 yr (30 acute myelogenous leukemia [AML], 24 ALL) undergoing ex vivo, T cell-depleted BMT using bone marrow from HLA identical or D-DR-mismatched (two patients) sibling donors (62). ATG and thiotepa were added to standard TBI/cyclophosphamide conditioning. The risk of relapse was 12% for AML patients and 28% for ALL patients. At median follow-up of 6.9 yr, the event-free survival (EFS) for AML was 74%, and 59% for ALL. Schattenberg et al. compared the outcome of HLA identical, T cell-depleted BMT in patients less than 50-yr-old vs those greater than 50-yr-old (63). The standard conditioning regimen of TBI/cyclophosphamide was intensified with the addition of idarubicin at 42 mg/m^2. The study evaluated 131 patients, which included 32 patients with ALL less than 50-yr-old, and two patients greater than 50-yr-old. Outcome did not differ significantly between the two age groups. The 2-yr LFS for the ALL patients in this small study was 64%, which compares very favorably with HLA identical transplants that are not T cell-depleted.

7.6. Immunomodulation: GVHD and GVL Effect

The presence of a GVL effect is based on observations of higher relapse rates following autologous or syngeneic SCT vs allogeneic SCT, lower relapse rates in patients who develop GVHD, and higher relapse rates in patients receiving T cell-depleted SCT. Table 5 summarizes results obtained from both single institution and registry data and demonstrates a consistent decrease in relapse rates for patients who develop GVHD vs those who do not. A GVL effect that is associated with the presence of GVHD has been described in ALL, AML, and CML; interestingly, this effect appears most potent in ALL and is reflected by the data in Table 5 (66). In distinct contrast to these consistent observations of the benefit of GVHD in reducing relapse rate following ALL allogeneic SCT is the marked absence of a significant GVL effect in ALL following DLI. In contrast to CML and AML, where DLI often results in complete remissions in patients with relapsed disease following allogeneic transplant, DLI does not appear to be effective for ALL relapses in this setting. The European Group for Blood and Marrow Transplantation Working Party for Acute and Chronic Leukemia studied the effect of DLI on acute and chronic leukemia in relapse after SCT. One hundred thirty-five patients were treated, including 22 patients with ALL (nine patients in CR1, five patients in CR2, and eight patients beyond CR2). The median age of the ALL patients was 21.5 yr. In contrast to 73% of CML patients achieving CR with DLI, no patients with ALL responded (67). Collins et al. reviewed data on 140 patients receiving DLI at a number of transplant centers. Fifteen patients with ALL were included; three patients in CR and 12 patients with progressive disease. There was an 18% response rate to DLI seen in the ALL group in contrast to 60% seen in the CML group (68).

Direct and indirect evidence suggests that donor T cells and natural killer (NK) cells are primary mediators of GVL after DLI, but the target antigens on the tumor cells are currently poorly defined. The disease specificity exhibited by DLI suggests that the target antigens of GVL may be tumor-specific. There may be differences in the ability of ALL cells to present

Table 5
Risk of Relapse Following Non-T Cell-Depleted Allogeneic Transplantation in Adult ALL

Study	No. of patients	Risk of relapse	(%)
Doney et al. *(24)*	192, Seattle		
	Transplanted in CR2	No GVHD	80
		Grade II–IV GVHD	40
Sullivan et al. *(64)*	200, Seattle		
	Transplanted in remission	No GVHD	56
		Acute GVHD	27
		Acute and chronic GVHD	22
	Transplanted in relapse	No GVHD	81
		Acute GVHD	39
		Acute and chronic GVHD	43
Horowitz et al. *(65)*	349, Intl Bone Marrow Transplant Registry		
	Transplanted in CR1	No GVHD	44
		Acute GVHD	17
		Chronic GVHD	20
		Acute and chronic GVHD	15

as antigen targets, differences in the frequency of T cell precursors that are reactive with minor antigens presented by ALL cells, or differences in the susceptibility of ALL targets to lysis. In addition to donor leukocyte preparations, G-CSF-mobilized PBSCs have also been investigated as an infusion source. The numbers of T cells and NK cells found in PBSC are comparable to those present in a DLI. Eleven patients (4 with CML, 5 with AML, 1 with ALL) received PBSC postrelapse; all patients with acute leukemia received cytoreductive therapy prior to PBSC. All 6 patients with acute leukemia achieved a CR, with the median remission duration of 24 wk. In contrast to the prolonged cytopenias observed post-DLI, patients did not sustain prolonged cytopenias, and some were treated successfully with repeat PBSC infusion. There are currently too few studies using this modality to draw any conclusions, but PBSC appears to be effective in inducing DLI, even in ALL patients. Perhaps the success noted in this study resulted, in part, from the cytoreduction prior to DLI, which may play an important role in determination of DLI efficacy for the acute leukemias. The combination of DLI and interleukin (IL)-2 appears to be another way of improving the efficacy of DLI in ALL patients. Slavin et al. demonstrated that patients with relapsed leukemia after allogeneic SCT had a response with DLI combined with IL-2 administration *(69)*. None of the 4 patients with ALL responded to DLI; whereas, all 4 responded to DLI with IL-2. Obviously, no conclusions can be drawn from a series of 4 patients, which included infants and adults. However, the additive or modulating effect of IL-2 with DLI on the GVL effect is intriguing. In conclusion, more clinical data are required to determine the best setting for administration of DLI (e.g., following cytoreduction, with other immunomodulators) and whether this modality will be a viable salvage option for ALL relapses following allogeneic transplants.

8. LONG-TERM COMPLICATIONS OF ALLOGENEIC SCT

Socie et al. *(70)* analyzed the characteristics of 6691 patients listed in the IBMTR who underwent allogeneic SCT for AML, ALL, CML, or aplastic anemia between January 1980 and December 1993. The median duration of follow-up was 80 months. Mortality rates in this cohort were compared with those of an age-, sex-, and nationality-matched general population. All patients were free of disease 2 yr posttransplant, with 89% survival at 5 yr. Mortality rates remained significantly higher than the general population throughout the study among patients who underwent transplantation for ALL or CML, and through the ninth year for patients who had AML. Specifically, for patients with ALL, the relative mortality rate was 20.1 2 yr after transplantation, 25.9 5 yr after transplantation, and 15.4 10 yr after transplantation. Not surprisingly, recurrent leukemia was the chief cause of death for patients who underwent SCT for leukemia, and GVHD the chief cause of death for patients who underwent SCT for aplastic anemia. Older age was associated with an increased risk of relapse in the ALL group, with 48% relapse observed in ALL compared with 11% relapses in the overall group. Chronic GVHD was the second leading cause of death overall, with 23% observed in the ALL cohort. A low incidence of secondary cancer was reported overall (6%), with a slightly higher rate observed in the ALL group (10%). Increased rates of secondary cancer may be noted with longer follow-up *(70)*.

With improvements in DFS following allogeneic SCT, psychosocial functioning after transplant becomes a more prominent issue. Broers et al. evaluated the psychological functioning and quality of life in a prospective study of 125 consecutive patients who underwent BMT at the Leiden University Medical Center in the Netherlands between 1987 and 1992 *(71)*. Patients were evaluated with questionnaires measuring quality of life, functional limitations, psychological distress, anxiety, depression, and self-esteem. Questionnaires were answered prior to the BMT, 1 mo after BMT following discharge, at 6 mo, 1 yr, and 3 yr after BMT. Nearly 90% of patients reported a good to excellent quality of life at 3 yr. Changes in quality of life and psychological distress could be explained entirely by changes in functional limitations and somatic symptoms. The minority of patients who reported a worse quality of life reported experiencing continued serious functional limitations. Thus, emphasis should be placed on interventions that help patients cope with their physical limitations.

9. NOVEL TRANSPLANT APPROACHES

9.1. CAMPATH-1H: Novel Method of T Cell Depletion

Studies have shown consistently that a major therapeutic effect of SCT is derived from the GVL effect. The difficulty lies in separating GVHD from the GVL effect. This objective is the basis of much laboratory and clinical work. One approach, to capitalize on this effect while sparing initial complications of acute GVHD, is to perform T cell depletion of donor stem cells and to follow up, at later time points, with infusions of donor lymphocytes to achieve an anti-leukemic effect. Recent studies are evaluating CAMPATH-1H, which is an antibody to CD52, as a novel method of T cell depletion. In ALL, Campath-1H treatment may have the added benefit of anti-leukemia activity since malignant lymphoblasts express CD52 *(72)*. Novitzky et al. evaluated 13 patients with ALL (8 patients in CR1) and 37 patients with AML (33 patients in CR1), who had undergone HLA-identical sibling transplants. The conditioning regimen consisted of TBI/cyclophosphamide. Bone marrow or PBSC were exposed to CAMPATH-1H ex vivo. Patients received no posttransplant immunosuppression. All but one patient engrafted, and only 22% of all patients developed grade I or II GVHD; there was no severe GVHD. Unfortunately, 54% (7 of 13) of the ALL patients relapsed *(73)*. Of note, these data are not significantly worse than many non-T cell-depleted allogeneic SCT series. Naparstek et al. *(74)* analyzed the factors associated with engraftment in 216 recipients of T cell-depleted allogeneic SCT using CAMPATH-1H. The patient population consisted of 168 patients with hematologic malignancies, 26 patients with aplastic anemia and 22 patients with hemoglobinopathies. Overall, 24 patients, including 17 with leukemia, had graft failure. Variables favorably associated with engraftment were older age and colony-forming unit granulocyte macrophage (CFU-GM) number. A higher concentration of CAMPATH-1H antibody in vitro and in vivo adversely affected engraftment *(74)*. Both of these studies indicate that satisfactory engraftment can be achieved in patients transplanted with CAMPATH-1H-treated allografts; however, relapse still poses a significant problem, and more selective T cell depletion may be necessary. Larger, randomized studies will be required to determine whether CAMPATH-1H represents a therapeutic advance for patients undergoing transplantation for ALL.

9.2. Nonmyeloablative SCT

Recent studies have demonstrated successful donor stem cell engraftment without the use of a myeloablative preparative regimen for patients undergoing SCT for hematologic and solid organ malignancies. These regimens use a combination of moderate doses of chemotherapy with immune suppression to facilitate donor engraftment and establish a donor derived anti-host tumor effect. Consistent chimerism should theoretically lead to durable long-term remission. Since there appears to be a GVL effect in ALL, non-myeloablative SCT may have a role in this disease. In addition, the relative decrease in upfront morbidity, secondary to decreased organ toxicity and a lower rate of neutropenic infection, makes it a theoretically attractive option in this disease where the median age is greater than 50 yr. This option would be particularly attractive for patients with Ph+ ALL, where the majority of these poor prognosis patients are older than 50 yr. Slavin et al. *(75)* investigated the feasibility of non-myeloablative SCT in combination with DLI in 26 patients with standard indications for allogeneic SCT, including two patients with ALL (1 patient in CR1 and 1 patient in CR2). The nonmyeloablative conditioning regiment consisted of fludarabine, ATG, and BU at 8 mg/kg. Cyclosporine A was used for GVHD prophylaxis; DLI was used for relapse. The preparative regimen was well tolerated, with neutrophil recovery on d 15 (median), and platelet recovery on d 12. Severe GVHD was the major toxicity and the cause of four deaths. DLI reversed relapse in 2 of 3 of cases. Eighty-five percent of patients are alive, with 81% disease free, during a very short follow-up observation period, with a median of 8 mo follow-up. Interestingly, the ALL patient in CR2 relapsed 4 mo after SCT and was treated successfully with DLI. The ALL patient in CR1 did not relapse after SCT *(75)*. This is a small, but encouraging, study demonstrating the feasibility of this approach. Unfortunately, complications of GVHD remain a significant problem with nonmyeloablative transplantation. A number of larger phase II studies are ongoing that are designed to demonstrate efficacy of this approach to transplantation and may provide more data about specific efficacy in patients with ALL.

In conclusion, allogeneic SCT has been demonstrated to have tremendous therapeutic benefit for selected patients with high-risk ALL. Since ALL is a relatively rare disease in adults, it will be very important to perform large prospective studies through cooperative groups or other large consortium to answer many of the outstanding questions regarding the promise of allogeneic transplantation as a therapeutic modality that will lead to improvements in survival for patients with this challenging disease.

REFERENCES

1. Rivera GK, Pinkel D, Simone JV, Hancock MI, Crist WM. Treatment of acute lymphoblastic leukemia. *N Engl J Med* 1993;329:1289–1295.
2. Charrin C. Cytogenetic abnormalities in adult acute lymphoblastic leukemia: correlations with hematologic findings and outcome. A collaborative study of the Groupe Francais de Cytogenetique Hematologique. *Blood* 1996;87:3135–3142.
3. Faderl S, Kantarjian HM, Talpaz M, Estrov Z. Clinical significance of cytogenetic abnormalities in adult acute lymphoblastic leukemia. *Blood* 1998;91(11):3995–4019.
4. Hoelzer D, Theil E, Loffler T, et al. Prognostic factors in a multicentric study for treatment of acute lymphoblastic leukemia in adults. *Blood* 1988;71:123–131.
5. Wetzler M, Dodge RK, MrUzek K, et al: Prospective karyotype analysis in adult acute lymphoblastic leukemia: the Cancer and Leukemia Group B experience. *Blood* 1999;93:3983–3993.

6. Wetzler, M. Cytogenetics in adult acute lymphocytic leukemia. *Hematol/Oncol Clin N Am* 2000;14(6):1237–1249.

7. Hoelzer D, Ludwig WD, Thiel E, et al. Improved outcome in adult B-cell acute lymphoblastic leukemia. *Leukemia* 1996;6(suppl 4):495–508.

8. Patte C, Michon J, Frappaz D, et al. Therapy of Burkitt and other B-cell acute lymphoblastic leukemia and lymphoma: Experience with LMB protocols of the SFOP (French Pediatric Oncology Society) in children and adults. *Bailliere's Clin Haematol* 1994;7:339–348.

9. Daliani D, Robertson L, O'brien S, et al. Adult B-cell acute lymphocytic leukemia (B-ALL): Results with short, dose-intensive therapy. Proc ASCO 1995;14:339.

10. Larson RA, Dodge RK, Bloomfield CD, et al. Treatment of biologically determined subsets of acute lympho-blastic leukemia in adults: cancer and leukemia group B studies. In: *Acute Leukemias VI: pPrognostic Factors and Treatment Strategies.* Springer-Verlag, Berlin, 1997.

11. Laport GF, Larson RA. Treatment of adult acute lymphoblstic leukemia. *Semin Oncol* 1997;24:70–82.

12. Cave H, van der Werff ten bosch J, Suciu S, et al. Clinical significance of minimal residual disease in childhood acute lymphoblastic leukemia. *N Engl J Med* 1998;339:591–598.

13. van Dongen JM, Seriu T, Panzer-Grumayer ER, et al. Prognostic value of minimal residual disease in acute lymphoblastic leukemia in childhood. *Lancet* 1998;352:1731–1738.

14. Brisco MJ, Hughes E, Neoh SH, et al. Relationship between minimal residual disease and outcome in adult acute lymphoblastic leukemia. *Blood* 1996;87:5251–5256.

15. Stock W, Estrov Z. Studies of minimal residual disease in acute lymphocytic leukemia. *Hematol/Oncol Clin N Am* 2000;14(6):1289–1305.

16. Horowitz MM, Messerer D, Hoelzer D, et al. Chemotherapy compared with bone marrow transplantation for adults with acute lymphoblastic leukemia in first complete remission. *Ann Intern Med* 1991;115:13–18.

17. Rowe JM, Richards S, Wienik PH, et al. Allogeneic bone marrow transplantation (BMT) for adults with acute lymphoblastic leukemia (ALL) in first complete remission (CR): early results from the International ALL Trial (MRC UKALL/ECOG 2993). *Blood* 1999;94(suppl. 1):168a.

18. Sebban C, Lepage E, Vernant J, et al. Allogeneic bone marrow transplantation in adult acute lymphoblastic leukemia in first complete remission: a comparative study. *J Clin Oncol* 1994;12:2580–2587.

19. Thiebaut A, Vernant JP, Degos L. Adult acute lyphocytic leukemia study testing chemotherapy and autologous and allogeneic transplantation. A follow-up report of the French protocol LALA 87. *Hematol/Oncol Clin N Am* 2000;14(6):1353–1365.

20. Oh H, Gale R, Zhang M, et al. Chemotherapy vs HLA-identical sibling bone marrow transplant for adults with acute lymphoblastic leukemia in first remission. *Bone Marrow Transplant* 1998; 22:253–257.

21. Wingard JR, Piantadosi S, Santos GW, et al. Allogeneic bone marrow transplantation for patients with high-risk acute lymphoblastic leukemia. *J Clin Oncol* 1990;8:820–830.

22. Blaise D, Gaspard MH, Stoppa AM, et al. Allogeneic or autologous bone marrow transplantation for acute lymphoblastic leukemia in first complete remission. *Bone Marrow Transplant* 1990;5:7–12.

23. Chao NJ, Schmidt GM, Forman SJ, et al. Allogeneic bone marrow tranplantation for high-risk acute lympho-blastic leukemia during first complete remission. *Blood* 1991;78:1923–1927.

24. Doney K, Fisher LD, Appelbaum FR, et al. Treatment of adult acute lymphoblastic leukemia with allogeneic bone marrow transplantation. Multivariate analysis of factors affecting acute graft-versus-host disease, relapse, and relapse-free survival. *Bone Marrow Transplant* 1991;7:453–459.

25. Sutton L, Kuentz M, Cordonnier C, et al. Allogeneic bone marrow transplantation for adult lymphoblastic leukemia in first complete remission. Factors predictive of transplant-related mortality and influence of total body irradiation modalities. *Bone Marrow Transplant* 1993;12:583–589.

26. Vey N, Blaise D, Stoppa AM, et al. Bone marrow transplantation in 63 adult patients with acute lymphoblastic leukemia in first complete remission. *Bone Marrow Transplant* 1994;14:383–388.

27. DeWitte T, Awwad B, Boezeman J, et al. Role of allogeneic bone marrow transplantation in adolescent or adult patients with acute lymphoblastic leukemia or lymphoblastic lymphoma in first remission. *Bone Marrow Transplant* 1994;14:767–774.

28. Advisory committee of the IBMTR. *Bone Marrow Transplant* 1989;4:221.

29. Barrett AJ, Horowitz MM, Gale RP, et al. Marrow transplantation for acute lymphoblastic leukemia: factors affecting relapse and survival. *Blood* 1989;74:862–871.

30. Greinix HT, Reiter E, Keil F, et al. Leukemia-free survival and mortality in patients with refractory or relapsed acute leukemia given marrow transplants from sibling and unrelated donors. *Bone Marrow Transplant* 1998;21(7):673–678.

31. Michallet M, Tanguy ML, Socie G. Second allogeneic hematopoietic stem cell transplantation in relapsed acute and chronic leukemias for patients who underwent a first allogeneic bone marrow transplantation: a survey of the Societe Francaise de Greffe de moelle (SFGM). *Br J Haematol* 2000;108(2):400–407.

32. Biggs JC, Horowitz MM, Gale RP, et al. Bone marrow transplants may cure patients with acute leukemia never achieving remission with chemotherapy. *Blood* 1992;80:1090–1093.

33. Forman SJ, Schmidt GM, Nademanee AP, et al. Allogeneic bone marrow transplantation as therapy for primary induction failure for patients with acute leukemia. *J Clin Oncol* 1991;9:1570–1574.
34. Grigg AP, Szer J, Beresford J, et al. Factors affecting the outcome of allogeneic bone marrow transplantation for adult patients with refractory or relapsed acute leukemia. *Br J Haematol* 1999;107:409-418.
35. Goldstone AH, Richards S, Wiernik PH, et al. Philadelphia chromosme +ve patients with adult acute lymphoblastic leukaemia (ALL). Early results from the International ALL Trial (MRC UKALL-XII/ECOG 2993), 1999;(suppl. 1):694a.
36. Snyder DS, Nademanee AP, O'Donnell MR. Long-term follow-up of 23 patients with Philadelphia chromosome-positive acute lymphoblastic leukemia treated with allogeneic bone marrow transplant in first complete remission. *Leukemia* 1999;13:2053–2058.
37. Dunlop LC, Powles R, Singhal S. Bone marrow transplantation for Philadelphia chromosome-positive acute lymphoblastic leukemia. *Bone Marrow Transplant* 1996;17(3):365–369.
38. Stockschlader M, Hegewisch-Becker S, Kruger W, et al. Bone marrow transplantation for Philadelphia chromosome-positive acute lymphoblastic leukemia. *Bone Marrow Transplant* 1995;16(5):663–667.
39. Deane M, Koh M, Foroni L. FLAG-idarubicin and allogeneic stem cell transplantation for Ph-positive ALL beyond first remission. *Bone Marrow Transplant* 1998;22:1137–1143.
40. Sierra J, Radich J, Hansen JA. Marrow transplants from unrelated donors for treatment of Philadelphia chromosome-positive acute lymphoblastic leukemia. *Blood* 1997;90:1410–1414.
41. Keil F, Kalhs P, Haas OA, et al. Relapse of Philadelphia chromosome positive acute lymphoblastic leukemia after marrow transplantation: sustained molecular remission after early and dose-escalating infusion of donor leukocytes. *Br J Haematol* 1997;97:161–164.
42. Yazaki M, Andoh M, Ito T. Successful prevention of hematological relapse for a patient with Philadelphia chrmosome-positive acute lymphoblastic leukemia after allogeneic bone marrow transplantation by donor leukocyte infusion. *Bone Marrow Transplant* 1997;19:393–394.
43. Glass B, Majolino I, Dreger P, et al. Allogeneic peripheral blood progenitor cells for treatment of relapse after bone marrow transplantation. *Bone Marrow Transplant* 1997;20:533–541.
44. Druker BJ, Sawyers CL, Kantarjian H, et al. Activity of a specific inhibitor of the BCR-ABL tyrosine kinase in the blast crisis of chronic myeloid leukemia and acute lymphoblastic leukemia with the Philadelphia chromosome. *N Engl J Med* 2001;344(14):1038–1042.
45. Gehly GB, Bryant AM, Lee AM, et al. Chimeric BCR-ABL messenger RNA as a marker for minimal residual disease in patients transplanted for Philadelphia chromosome-positive acute lymphoblastic leukemia. *Blood* 1991;78:458–465.
46. Miyamura K, Tanimoto M, Morishima Y, et al. Detection of Philadelphia chromosome-positive acute lymphoblastic leukemia by polymerase chain reaction: possible eradication of minimal residual disease by marrow transplantation. *Blood* 1992;79:1366–1370.
47. Preudhomme C, Henic N, Cazin B, et al. Good correlation between RT-PCR analysis and relapse in Philadelphia (Ph1)-positive acute lymphoblastic leukemia (ALL). *Leukemia* 1997;11:294–298.
48. Radich JP, Gehy G, Lee A, et al. Polymerase chain reaction detection of BCR-ABL fusion transcript after allogeneic marrow transplantation for CML: results and implications in 346 patients. *Blood* 1995;85:2632–2638.
49. Mitterbauer G, Nemeth P, Wacha S. Quantification of minimal residual disease in patients with BCR-ABL positive acute lymphoblastic leukaemia using quantitative competitive polymerase chain reaction. *Br J Haematol* 1999;106:634–643.
50. Stock W, Sher D, Dodge R, et al. Quantitative molecular monitoring of BCR/ABL transcripts in adult acute lymphoblastic leukemia (ALL) using real-time PCR assay: pilot study from the Cancer and Leukemia Group B (CALGB 8762). *Blood* 1999;94(suppl 1):287a.
51. Woods WG, Ramsay NK, Weisdorf DJ, et al. Bone marrow transplantation for acute lymphocytic leukemia utilizing total body irradiation followed by high doses of cytosine arabinoside: lack of superiority over cyclophosphamide-containing conditioning regimens. *Bone Marrow Transplant* 1990;6:9–16.
52. Blume KG, Forman SJ, O'Donnell MR, et al. Total body irradiation and high-dose etoposide: a new preparatory regimen for bone marrow transplantation in patients with advanced hematologic malignancies. *Blood* 1987;69:1015–1020.
53. Matthews DC, Appelbaum FR, Eary JF, et al. Phase I study of 131I-anti-CD45 antibody plus cyclophosphamide and total body irradiation for advanced acute leukemia and myelodysplastic syndrome. *Blood* 1999;94(4):1237–1247.
54. Blume KG, Kopecky KJ, Henslee-Downey JP, et al. A prospective randomized trial of total body irradiation-etoposide versus busulfan-cyclophosphamide as preparatory regimens for bone marrow transplantation in patients with recurrent leukemia: a SWOG study. *Blood* 1993;81:2187–2193.
55. Copelan EA, Deeg Hj. Conditioning for allogeneic marrow transplantation in patients with lymphohematopoietic malignancies without the use of total body irradiation. *Blood* 1992;80:1648–1658.

56. Bensinger WI, Martin PJ, Storer B, et al. Transplantation of bone marrow as compared with peripheral blood cells from HLA-identical relatives in patients with hematologic malignancies. *N Engl J Med* 2001;344(3):175–181.

57. Szydlo R, Goldman J, Klein J, et al. Results of allogeneic bone marrow transplants for leukemia using donors other than HLA-identical siblings. *J Clin Oncol* 1997;15:176,177.

58. Petersdorf EW, Gooley TA, Anasetti C, et al. Optimizing outcome after unrelated marrow transplantation by comprehensive matching of HLA class I and II alleles in the donor and recipient. *Blood* 1998;92:3515–3520.

59. Godder KT, Hazlett LJ, Abhyankar KY, et al. Partially mismatched related-donor bone marrow transplantation for pediatric patients with acute leukemia: younger donors and absence of peripheral blasts improve outcome. *J Clin Oncol* 2000;18(9):1856–1866.

60. Weisdorf DJ, Billet AL, Hannan P, et al. Autologous versus unrelated donor allogeneic marrow transplantation for acute lymphoblastic leukemia. *Blood* 1997;90:2962–2968.

61. Ringden O, Labopin M, Gluckman E, et al. Donor search or autografting in patients with acute leukemia who lack an HLA-identical sibling? A matched-pair analysis. Acute Leukemia Working Party of the European Cooperative Group for Blood and Marrow Transplantation (EBMT) and the International Marrow Unrelated Search and Transplant (IMUST) study. *Bone Marrow Transplant* 1997;19:963–968.

62. Aversa F, Terenzi A, Carotti A, et al. Improved outcome with T-cell-depleted bone marrow transplantation for acute leukemia. *J Clin Oncol* 1999;17(5):1545–1550.

63. Schattenberg A, Schaap N, Preijers F, et al. Outcome of T-cell depleted transplantation after conditioning with an intensified regimen in patients aged 50 years or more is comparable with that in younger patients. *Bone Marrow Transplant* 2000;26:17–22.

64. Sullivan KM, Weiden PL, Storb R, et al. Influence of acute and chronic graft-versus-host disease on relapse and survival after bone marrow transplantation from HLA-identical siblings as treatment of acute and chronic leukemia. *Blood* 1989;73:1720–1728.

65. Horowitz MM, Gale RP, Sondel PM, et al. Graft-versus-leukemia reactions after bone marrow transplantation. *Blood* 1990;75:555–562.

66. Appelbaum FR. Graft versus leukemia (GVL) in the therapy of acute lymphoblastic leukemia (ALL). *Leukemia* 1997;11:S15–17.

67. Hans-Jochem K, Schattenberg A, Goldman JM, et al. Graft-versus-leukemia effect of donor lymphocyte transfusions in marrow grafted patients. *Blood* 1995;86(5):2041–2050.

68. Collins RH, Shpilberg O, Drobyski WR, et al. Donor leukocyte infusions in 140 patients with relapsed malignancy after allogeneic bone marrow transplantation. *J Clin Oncol* 15(2);1997:433–444.

69. Slavin S, Naparstek E, Nagler A, et al. Allogeneic cell therapy with donor peripheral blood cells and recombinant human interleukin-2 to treat leukemia relapse after allogeneic bone marrow transplantation. *Blood* 1996;87(6):2195–2204.

70. Socie G, Stone J, Wingard J, et al. Long-term survival and late deaths after allogeneic bone marrow transplantation. *N Engl J Med* 1999;341(1):14–21.

71. Broers S, Kaptein A, Cessie S, et al. Psychological functioning and quality of life following bone marrow transplantation: a 3 year follow-up study. *J Psychosom Res* 2000;48:11–21.

72 Hale G, Xia MQ, Tighe HP, et al. The CAMPATH-1 antigen (CDw52). *Tissue Antigens* 1990:35:118–127.

73. Novitzky N, Thomas V, Hale G, Waldmann H. Ex vivo depletion of T cells from bone marrow grafts with CAMPATH-1 in acute leukemia: graft-versus-host disease and graft-versus-leukemia effect. *Transplantation* 1999;67(4):620–626.

74. Naparstek E, Delukina M, Or R. Engraftment of marrow allografts treated with Campath-1 monoclonal antibodies. *Exp Hematol* 1999;27(7):1210–1218.

75. Slavin S, Nagler A, Naparstek A. Nonmyeloablative stem cell transplantation and cell therapy as an alternative to conventional bone marrow transplantation with lethal cytoreduction for the treatment of malignant and nonmalignant hematologic diseases. *Blood* 1998;91(3):756–763.

76. Thomas ED, Buchner CD, Banaji M, et al. One hundred patients with acute leukemia treated by chemotherapy, total body irradiation, and allogeneic marrow transplantation. *Blood* 1977;49:511–533.

4 Chronic Myelogenous Leukemia

Edward Copelan

CONTENTS

1. INTRODUCTION

Chronic myelogenous leukemia (CML) is a malignant hematopoietic stem cell disorder characterized by the Philadelphia chromosome (Ph1), a balanced translocation of the long arms of chromosomes 9 and 22 *(1,2)*. This translocation results in the juxtaposition of the Bcr and Abl sequences and the creation of a Bcr-Abl fusion protein, a constitutively active cytoplasmic tyrosine kinase. The Bcr-Abl protein phosphorylates several substrates, which activate multiple signal transduction cascades, thus altering cell growth, differentiation, and apoptosis. These activities result in independence from normal growth constraints *(3,4)*.

The median age at presentation with CML is approx 53 *(4,5)*. Patients commonly present with fatigue, anorexia, and weight loss. Many patients are diagnosed solely on the basis of abnormal blood counts. Splenomegaly is usually found on physical examination. Leukocytosis, thrombocytosis, and anemia are typical. Most patients progress over a period of 2–6 yr, from chronic phase, often through an accelerated phase, into a rapidly fatal blastic phase.

2. NONTRANSPLANT TREATMENT

2.1. Standard Treatment

Control of blood counts can be achieved in nearly all patients with presently available agents, including hydroxyurea and interferon α. A small minority will achieve cytogenetic and even molecular remission using interferon *(6–9)*; less than 10% will remain in cytogenetic remission for a prolonged period. The addition of cytarabine to interferon results in higher rates of complete hematologic and cytogenetic remission and improved survival *(10,11)*.

From: *Current Clinical Oncology: Allogeneic Stem Cell Transplantation*
Edited by: Mary S. Laughlin and Hillard M. Lazarus © Humana Press Inc., Totowa, NJ

2.2. Investigational Treatment

The introduction of STI 571, a novel tyrosine kinase inhibitor, which "selectively" inactivates Bcr-Abl, has generated justified enthusiasm among physicians and patients. The drug's oral route of administration, minimal early toxicity, and dramatic and rapid responses in some patients with advanced disease have led to large numbers of patients seeking treatment with this agent *(12–14)*. A recently published Phase 1 dose-escalating trial of STI 571, in patients with chronic phase disease who had failed treatment with interferon α revealed that 29 of 54 patients (54%) treated with at least 300 mg daily had cytogenetic responses, including 7 with complete cytogenetic remission *(15)*. Cytogenetic responses occurred rapidly compared to those occurring with interferon α treatment. It appears that STI 571 will shortly be recognized as the best agent for treatment of CML. At present, there is no evidence that STI 571 alone is curative or will result in improved long-term survival. It is critical that appropriate studies with extended follow-up be performed and analyzed. Attempts to define its ultimate role must await the results of these studies.

3. HEMATOPOIETIC STEM CELL TRANSPLANTATION IN CML

3.1. Syngeneic Bone Marrow Transplantation

Between 1976 and 1981 the Seattle group performed 14 bone marrow transplantations (BMTs) in patients with CML using identical twin donors following a preparative regimen of dimethylbusulfan, cyclophosphamide (Cy), and total body irradiation (TBI). Eight remained in complete remission a median of approx 17 yr after transplantation *(16)*. A subsequent study by the International Bone Marrow Transplantation Registry revealed that while only 1 of 34 identical twins undergoing syngeneic transplantation for CML died from treatment-related causes, 17 of 34 relapsed *(17)*. These patients did not receive dimethylbusulfan in addition to Cy/TBI, as had the patients transplanted in Seattle.

3.2. Allogeneic BMT in Patients with Advanced Disease

These data using identical twin donors led to investigation of allogeneic transplantation using marrow from human leukocyte antigen (HLA)-identical sibling donors. In an initial study in blastic phase patients, 8 of 10 died due to transplant-related complications within 3 mo. There were no long-term survivors *(18)*. McGlave and colleagues reported some success in accelerated phase patients *(19)*, but significant incidences of transplant-related mortality and early relapses were reported by others *(18–21)*.

3.3. Allogeneic Transplantation from Sibling Donors in Patients with CML in Chronic Phase

The early results in patients with advanced disease compared unfavorably with results in chronic phase using syngeneic donors and in first remission acute myelogenous leukemia (AML) with HLA-identical sibling donors. These comparisons led to trials of BMT in chronic phase patients using HLA-identical sibling donors *(22–24)*. These studies demonstrated the profound influence of disease stage on outcome. Sustained disease-free survival was achieved in over 50% of chronic phase patients, but in only about 10% of blastic phase patients *(25)*. Transplant-related mortality rates however exceeded 30% in large groups of patients undergoing allogeneic transplantation for CML in all disease stages, which tempered the enthusiasm for this therapy.

3.3.1. INTERVAL FROM DIAGNOSIS TO TRANSPLANT

Based on the median survival of newly diagnosed patients (more than 3 yr) and the risk of early mortality with transplantation, many physicians chose not to recommend this procedure or recommended it only after a delay (usually approx 2 yr) following diagnosis. Subsequent data from multiple sources, however, demonstrate inferior outcome in patients who undergo transplantation after delay *(26–30)*. Prior treatment with busulfan (BU) *(26,27)*, and in some settings with interferon *(31,32)*, appear to particularly compromise results. It has been reported that if interferon is stopped at least 90 d before transplantation, it does not adversely influence outcome *(33)*. However, regardless of specific therapy, delay compromises outcome.

The inferior outcome in patients transplanted at longer intervals from diagnosis results predominantly from a higher incidence of transplant-related mortality *(26–30)*. In patients prepared for transplantation with BU, a significantly higher incidence of hepatic venoocclusive disease (VOD) occurs in those undergoing transplantation at longer intervals from diagnosis *(30)*. These data suggest clinically undetected injury to vital organs from prolonged administration of chemotherapy. Data from Seattle support this hypothesis: the higher incidence of VOD with BU compared to TBI in patients with CML occurs only in heavily pretreated patients *(34)*.

Most studies have compared the results of transplantation following delays of longer than 1 yr to those with lesser delays. As a result most clinicians recognize that transplantation less than 1 yr following diagnosis is associated with improved outcome. There is little appreciation for the further improvement in results achieved with less delay. The Seattle group has shown that patients transplanted less than 6 mo following diagnosis fare better than those transplanted later in the course of disease *(16)*. Results from Ohio State indicate that more than 90% of patients who undergo transplantation less than 3 mo from diagnosis achieve sustained disease-free survival and that transplantation within 3 mo of diagnosis is an independent, significant favorable prognostic factor *(30)*. Furthermore, the favorable results in patients transplanted earlier in the course of disease occur primarily because of lower rates of transplant-related mortality. Transplant-related mortality rates of approx 10% have been achieved in patients transplanted early in the course of disease in single- *(16,30)* and multi-institutional *(35)* trials.

Low mortality rates are exceptionally important, because early mortality (and not the possibility of relapse) is the dominant factor preventing or delaying transplantation in most patients. This is particularly true considering recent data demonstrating that donor lymphocyte infusion (DLI) is an effective treatment for patients who relapse following allogeneic transplantation, often resulting in sustained disease-free survival *(36–38)*.

The considerable heterogeneity in results, particularly transplant-related mortality, from different institutions and study groups have complicated decision making. For example, single institutional *(39)* and registry data *(40)*, inclusive of patients transplanted through 1990, demonstrated transplant-related mortality rates in excess of 40% for chronic phase patients with HLA-identical sibling donors. This is approximately quadruple the previously described rates from some single institutions and study groups. While mortality rates and leukemia-free survival (LFS) are clearly improving with time, results are better at some centers than at others.

3.3.2. PREPARATIVE REGIMENS

Present data indicate that BuCy2 is at least equivalent and may be preferable to Cy/TBI as preparation for allogeneic transplantation from HLA identical sibling donors in patients with CML. Although a significant survival advantage has not been detected in randomized trials *(34,41)*, BU is associated with less acute toxicity, including a shorter neutropenic interval *(34)*. Fewer relapses occurred following BU in one randomized study *(41)*. Further, BU appears to be associated with fewer delayed effects including second malignancies and sterility *(42)*.

The established favorable results with BU continue to be improved upon. There has been considerable heterogeneity in the administration of the BuCy2 regimen. The body size parameter utilized to establish dose and the timing of the drug administration, including the interval between Bu and Cy, have varied. These differences influence outcome: plasma BU levels affect the incidence of graft rejection *(43)*, hepatic VOD *(43–45)*, early transplant-related mortality *(46)*, and relapse *(45)*. Dose adjustment of BU based on first dose pharmacokinetics achieve desired levels within 10% of the target in 90% of patients *(45)*. Furthermore, the ability to prevent low steady-state levels, which have been associated with graft rejection, may make this regimen more applicable to unrelated transplants. Preliminary results from Seattle, using dose adjustment based on plasma levels, show that nearly 90% of patients with chronic phase CML receiving transplants from HLA identical siblings are surviving free of disease *(47)*.

Studies using intravenous BU suggest less interpatient variability *(48)*, more consistent achievement of desirable plasma levels, and less VOD *(49)*. It has been suggested that the low incidence of VOD might be due to the absence of a first pass effect. It seems more likely that the relatively low plasma levels of BU achieved with the standard 0.8 mg/kg dose (for iv BU) may be responsible for the low toxicity. Dose adjustment of oral BU appears to improve results. Whether intravenous BU offers additional advantages requires further study.

3.3.3. OLDER AGE

Many texts and reviews urge "caution" in considering patients who are older than 40 yr of age for allotransplantation. "Caution" translates to a delay or failure to perform transplantation in a substantial proportion of patients, since most patients with CML are older than 50. Ironically the fear of early mortality leads to delay, which in turn subjects patients to a higher risk of early mortality than does their age.

The view that older age subjects patients to a substantially higher risk of mortality is not supported by critical analysis of recent data. The association of older age with more severe graft-vs-host disease (GVHD), transplant-related mortality, and significantly poorer survival is largely based on comparisons of pediatric to adult patients *(50–52)*. Differences in outcome between younger and older adults are far less compelling, particularly in CML *(27,30,39, 40,52,53)*. Many studies have detected no difference in outcome between patients 50–65 and younger adults *(30,52)*. The Seattle group reported survival rates at 4 yr in excess of 75% among 47 patients with CML aged 50–60 *(16)*. At Ohio State, patients older than 40, and those aged 50–66, had virtually identical outcomes to younger adults *(30)*. Older patients who undergo transplantation within 1 yr of diagnosis, and particularly within 3 mo of diagnosis fare well. Any potentially adverse affect of older age on outcome is more than balanced by the beneficial influence of transplantation shortly after diagnosis.

In summary, patients younger than 18 yr of age fare extremely well with allogeneic transplant and fare better than adults. However, there appears to be little difference in survival between adults with CML less than 40 and those 40–65 undergoing allogeneic transplantation from sibling donors. Otherwise healthy individuals 65 yr or younger with sibling donors should be considered for early transplantation. Whether individuals older than 65 might tolerate allotransplantation has not been adequately studied.

3.3.4. NONMYELOABLATIVE PREPARATIVE REGIMENS

The use of sublethal doses of chemotherapy alone or in combination with a low dose of TBI as preparation for allogeneic transplantation has achieved growing popularity following the demonstration of engraftment and extended remissions in some patients *(54,55)*. Generally, these "minitransplants" have been performed in patients considered ineligible for transplantation with myeloablative preparative regimens because of older age (often >40 yr) or other factors. Cautious interpretation of results is warranted. At some centers, many of these individuals would undergo allogeneic transplant using standard preparative regimens. As previously stated, results in older patients are favorable using standard preparative regimens. Similarly, modest impairment of cardiac ejection fraction or minimally elevated liver function tests—criteria that have been utilized to select patients for minitransplantation—do not dramatically influence outcome with standard regimens. While it seems likely that this therapy will ultimately prove advantageous in some patients who cannot tolerate standard preparative regimens, its sustained effectiveness is unproven, and its appropriate role in CML awaits definition.

3.4. Patients Without Sibling Donors

Similar controversy surrounds the transplantation of patients who do not have sibling donors. Historically, results using unrelated donors have been much less favorable than those using sibling donors. For several years following the introduction of unrelated donors, high transplant-related mortality rates occurred even in healthy young patients (56–59). High incidences of regimen-related mortality and severe acute GVHD alarmed physicians and patients alike. Based on these results or on cumulative results that include these early studies, many clinicians recommend that transplantation not be considered in such patients until they fail chemotherapy.

3.4.1. SUPPORTIVE CARE

However, improvements in prevention of complications, including GVHD with the combination of cyclosporine and methotrexate, cytomegalovirus (CMV) infection with ganciclovir, and fungal infection with fluconazole, have led to better results.

3.4.2. HLA-TYPING

The development of DNA-based typing techniques for class I and II molecules and the application of these techniques to additional histocompatibility antigens is of even greater importance (60,61). Initial studies of unrelated transplantation used serologic methods to identify compatibility between donor and recipient at the A, B, and DR loci. Many patients identified as "matched" or "HLA identical" were not. Graft rejection (62) and overwhelming GVHD (63) occurred on the basis of unrecognized mismatches at specific antigens. The use of molecular techniques has defined a multiplicity of alleles for previously defined "single" antigens. Furthermore, the impact of additional foci, including HLA-C and DQB1, on outcome is now well documented (60,61).

Appropriate interpretation and application of HLA typing is critical. For donor–recipient pairs identical at all 10 antigens, results closely approach those using sibling donors (60,61). Graft failure occurs more frequently in instances of disparities of more than one class I (but not class II) molecule. GVHD occurs more frequently in the presence of class II mismatch. Severe GVHD occurs more frequently in association with combined class I and class II disparities. In a study of patients with a variety of diseases, patients matched at HLA-A, -B, -C, DRB1, and DQB1 had a 5-yr survival rate of 61%. Those with mismatches of single locus class I or class II mismatches had survivals of 56 and 57%, respectively. Those with mismatches of more than one class I or both class I and class II molecules had significantly poorer survival rates (33 and 28%, respectively) (60).

Data from Seattle demonstrate that matched unrelated donor transplants performed in patients with chronic phase CML, less than 1 yr from diagnosis, yield 5-yr survival rates of 74% (33). Appropriate use of currently available HLA -typing techniques can help choose better donors in patients with multiple potential donors and will substantially improve results. These techniques also identify patients whose outcome is likely to be poor and who should not undergo transplantation or in whom the procedure should be undertaken with appropriate skepticism.

3.4.3. PREPARATIVE REGIMENS

Generally, patients undergoing unrelated transplantation receive preparation with TBI and not with BU. However, results have been similar in unrelated transplants, regardless of whether

TBI or BU are utilized *(64–66)*. Dose adjustment to avoid low BU levels (associated with graft rejection) and intravenous BU (less heterogeneity in levels) may be of particular importance in the unrelated setting.

In summary, patients less than 50, with well-matched unrelated donors, should undergo transplantation in a timely manner following diagnosis. As with sibling donors, transplantation at shorter intervals following diagnosis has resulted in better outcomes *(30,32)*. Appropriate prevention and treatment of CMV and fungal infections are critical in the care of these patients. Appropriate application of modern typing techniques yields results in patients with well matched unrelated donors that closely resemble those obtained with sibling donors.

4. COMPARISON OF TRANSPLANTATION TO STANDARD CHEMOTHERAPY

Comparisons of results achieved with allogeneic transplantation to those attained with palliative chemotherapy are complex. The early risk of mortality with transplant must be balanced with its sustained survival advantage.

Transplant results are often portrayed by LFS, which is the main goal of this treatment. Relapse occurs in 10–30% of patients undergoing transplantation for CML in chronic phase with unmanipulated marrow from sibling donors. Patients with CML who relapse following allogeneic transplantation may have sustained LFS following treatment, using infusions of donor lymphocytes harvested from the original stem cell donor *(36–38)*. Responses are often complete and prolonged, yet patients who benefit from this salvage therapy are not reflected by LFS, but are defined as survival with relapse following transplantation. Patients who achieve sustained remission following DLI are classified as treatment failures. This "inaccuracy" has led to the recommendation for a new measurement of current LFS (CLFS) defined as survival without evidence of leukemia *(38)*. This measurement recognizes patients in original remission as well as those in subsequent remission following treatment for relapse after transplantation. Using this measure, long-term disease-free survival is improved by salvage therapy by roughly 10%.

Notably, patients transplanted in first chronic phase at short intervals following diagnosis are particularly likely to achieve long-term complete remission (CR) as a result of DLI. Measurement of LFS following allotransplant, as reported in most studies, underestimates the proportion of patients likely to achieve sustained remission and cure. Further, these measures understate the impact of early transplantation.

In patients lacking (9 of 10 antigen) matched unrelated donors, decision making is more complex. In most instances, high rates of early mortality should be expected, and significant reservation by physician and patient is appropriate. Still, if a decision to proceed is made, best results will be achieved with early transplantation. Delay in transplantation only further compromises these results and increases the risk of transplant-related complications and early mortality.

At present, the approach to patients with CML varies widely among clinicians and institutions. Several algorithms addressing treatment options in CML have been published in the last few years. Most attempt to provide a balanced approach. However, in many instances these algorithms are based on, but fail to specifically define, young vs old, early vs late, degree of HLA match, and other factors that profoundly influence transplant outcome. No algorithm can adequately define the best treatment for every patient. Individual risk factors and the wishes of the individual will determine appropriate treatment. However, allogeneic stem cell transplant is too often not recommended in patients with substantial chance for cure or performed late in the course of disease, thus compromising results.

The introduction of STI 571 has already had substantial impact on the treatment of CML. Initial trials suggest that it offers substantial advantages over other palliative therapies. Its use

Initial Treatment in Newly Diagnosed Patient with CML

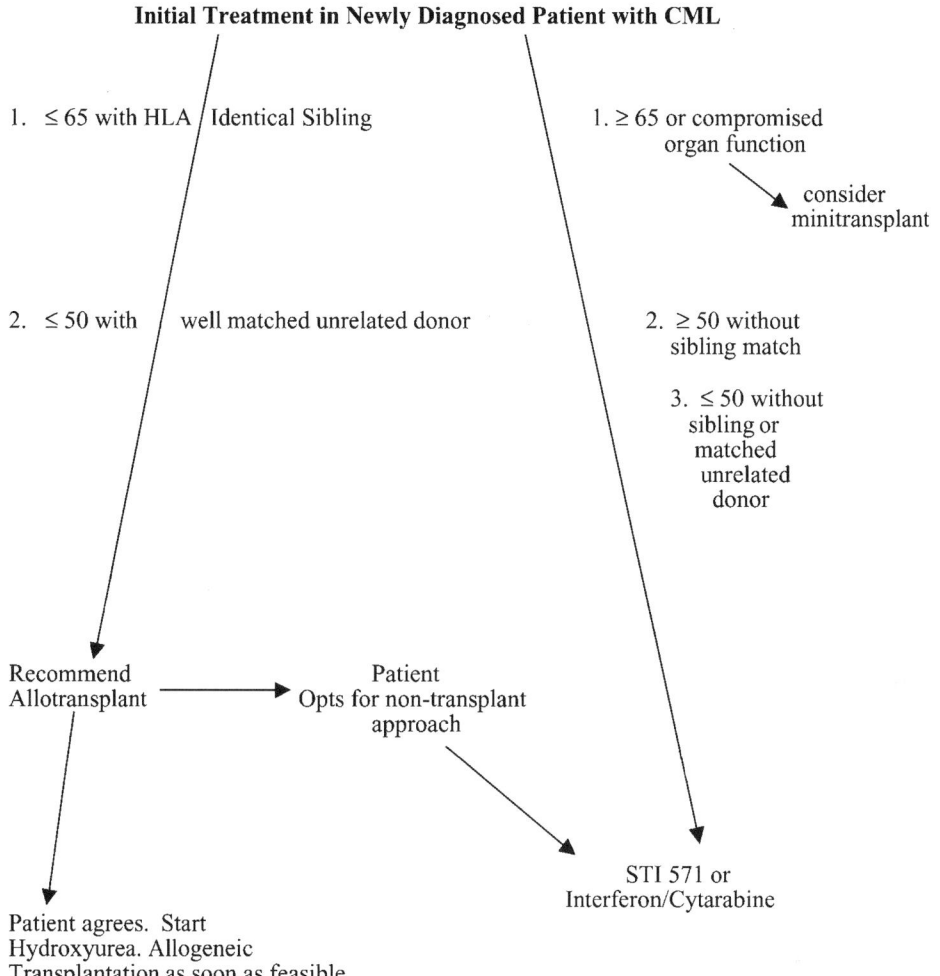

1. ≤ 65 with HLA / Identical Sibling

1. ≥ 65 or compromised organ function

consider minitransplant

2. ≤ 50 with / well matched unrelated donor

2. ≥ 50 without sibling match

3. ≤ 50 without sibling or matched unrelated donor

Recommend Allotransplant → Patient Opts for non-transplant approach

STI 571 or Interferon/Cytarabine

Patient agrees. Start Hydroxyurea. Allogeneic Transplantation as soon as feasible

Figure 1.

appears to have already resulted in a decreased number of patients referred for allotransplantation. Its Food and Drug Administration (FDA) approval will expand its use. Yet, there is no evidence that STI 571 prolongs life more than other available agents. It seems unlikely that, as a single agent, it will cure a substantial proportion of patients. Furthermore, similar to interferon α, initial treatment with STI 571 will significantly delay the interval from diagnosis to transplantation, subjecting those who undergo transplantation to a higher risk of early mortality. Present data does not justify this delay.

Patients with CML should be considered for allogeneic transplantation shortly after diagnosis. HLA typing of patients (≤65) and siblings should be performed in a timely manner. In the absence of a matched sibling, searches for unrelated donors should be initiated (for patients ≤50). Patients with HLA identical sibling donors and those whose initial searches indicate a high likelihood of finding a suitable unrelated donor, and who make informed decisions to proceed towards transplantation, should be placed on hydroxyurea. Some patients can be brought to transplantation without the institution of chemotherapy. At the author's institution, patients who are asymptomatic and with white blood counts below 60,000/μL are brought to transplantation quickly and without institution of chemotherapy.

There is substantial variability in results achieved with transplantation at different institutions. Multiple factors account for these differences, including patient selection, preparative therapy, supportive care, and skill of the transplant team. Rather than denying or delaying curative treatment for patients because of poor results at specific institutions, patients should be referred to institutions where verifiably favorable results in large number of patients have been achieved.

Figure 1 describes a reasonable treatment approach in individuals with newly diagnosed CML. It is intended to serve as a guide. The patient's clinical situation and unique perspective will determine treatment.

REFERENCES

1. Nowell P, Hungerford D. A minute chromosome in human chronic granulocytic leukemia. *Science* 1960;132:1497.
2. Rowley J. A new consistent chromosomal abnormality in chronic myelogenous leukemia identified by quinacrine fluorescence and Giemsa staining. *Nature* 1973;243:290–293.
3. Kabarowski J, Witte O. Consequences of bcr-abl expression within the hematopoietic stem cell in chronic myeloid leukemia. *Stem Cells* 2000;18:399–408.
4. Sawyers C. Chronic myeloid leukemia. *N Engl J Med* 1999;340:1330–1340.
5. Faderl S, Talpaz M, Estrov Z, et al. Chronic myelogenous leukemia: biology and therapy. *Ann of Internal Med* 1999;131:3:207–219.
6. Kantarjian HM, Smith TL, O'Brien S, et al. Prolonged survival in chronic myelogenous leukemia after cytogenetic response to interferon-a therapy. *Ann Internal Med* 1995;122:254–261.
7. Allan NC, Richards SM, Shepherd P, et al. UK Medical Research Council Randomised, multicentre trial of interferon-a for chronic myeloid leukemia: improved survival irrespective of cytogenetic response. *Lancet* 1995;345:1392–1397.
8. Kurzrock R, Estov Z, Kantarjian H, et al. Conversion of interferon-induced, long-term cytogenetic remissions in chronic myelogenous leukemia to polymerase chain reaction negativity. *J Clinical Oncol* 1998;16:1526–1531.
9. Lee S, Anasetti C, Horowitz M, et al. Initial therapy for chronic myelogenous leukemia: playing the odds. *J Clin Oncol* 1998;16:9:2897–2903.
10. Kantarjian H, O'Brien S, Smith T, et al. Treatment of Philadelphia chromosome- positive early chronic phase myelogenous leukemia with daily doses of interferon alpha and low-dose cytosine arabinoside. *J Clin Oncol* 1999;17:284–292.
11. Guilhot F, Chastang C, Michallet M, et al. Interferon alfa-2b combined with cytarabine versus interferon alone in chronic myelogenous leukemia. *N Engl J Med* 1997;337:223–229.
12. Talpaz M, Silver RT, Druker B, et al. The phase II study of STI 571 in adult patients with Philadelphia chromosome positive chronic myeloid leukemia in accelerated phase [abstract]. *Blood* 2000;96:469a.
13. Kantarjian H, Sawyers C, Hochhaus A, et al. Phase II study of STI571, a tyrosine kinase inhibitor, in patients with resistant or refractory Philadelphia chromosome positive chronic myeloid leukemia (Ph+CML) [abstract]. *Blood* 2000;96:470a
14. Hochhaus A, Feldman E, Goldman JM, et al. A phase II study to determine the safety and anti-leukemic effects of STI571 in patients with Philadelphia chromosome positive chronic myeloid leukemia in myeloid blast crisis [abstract]. *Blood* 2000;96:503a.
15. Druker J, Talpaz M, Resta D, et al. Efficacy and safety of a specific inhibitor of the BCR-ABL tyrosine kinase in chronic myeloid leukemia. *N Engl J Med* 2001;344:14:1031–1037
16. Appelbaum F, Clift R, Radich J, et al. Bone marrow transplantation for chronic myelogenous leukemia. *Semin Oncol* 1995;22:4:405–411.
17. Gale RP, Horowitz M, Ash R, et al. Identical-twin bone marrow transplants for leukemia. *Ann Intern Med* 1994;120:8:646–652.
18. Doney K, Buckner CD, Sale GE, et al. Treatment of chronic granulocytic leukemia by chemotherapy, total body irradiation and allogeneic bone marrow transplantation. *Exp Hematol* 1978:6:738–747.
19. McGlave PB, Arthur DC, Kim TH, et al. Successful allogeneic bone-marrow transplantation for patients in the accelerated phase of chronic granulocytic leukemia. *Lancet* 1982a;2:625–627.
20. Champlin R, Mitsuyasu R, Elashoff R, et al. Allogeneic bone marrow transplantation for chronic myelogenous leukemia in chronic or accelerated phase. *Blood* 1982;60:1038–1041.
21. Goldman J, Baughan A. Application of bone marrow transplantation in chronic granulocytic leukemia. *Clin Hematol* 1983;12:3:739–753.

22. Curtis JE, Messner HA. Bone marrow transplantation for leukemia and aplastic anemia: management of ABO incompatibility. *Can Med Assoc J* 1982;126:649–655.
23. Clift RA, Buckner CD, Thomas ED, et al. Treatment of chronic granulocytic leukemia in chronic phase by allogeneic marrow transplantation. *Lancet* 1982;2:621–623.
24. Goldman JM, Baughan AS, McCarthy DM, et al. Marrow transplantation for patients in the chronic phase of chronic granulocytic leukemia. *Lancet* 1982a;2:623–625.
25. Champlin R, Mitsuyasu R, Elashoff R, et al. The role of bone marrow transplantation in the treatment of chronic myelogenous leukemia. In: Gale RP, ed. *Recent Advances in Bone Marrow Transplantation.* Alan R Liss, New York, 1983.
26. Thomas ED, Clift RA, Fefer A, et al. Marrow transplantation for the treatment of chronic myelogenous leukemia. *Ann Internal Med* 1986;104:155–163.
27. Biggs JC, Szer J, Crilley P, et al. Treatment of chronic myeloid leukemia with allogeneic bone marrow transplantation after preparation with BuCy2. *Blood* 1992;80:5:1352–1357.
28. Horowitz MM, Rowlings PA, Passweg JR. Allogeneic bone marrow transplantation for CML: a report from the International Bone Marrow Transplant Registry. *Bone Marrow Transplant* 1996;17:Suppl 3:s5–s6.
29. Goldman JM, Szydlo R, Horowitz MM, et al. Choice of pre-transplant treatment and timing of transplants for chronic myelogenous leukemia in chronic phase. *Blood* 1993;82:2235–2238.
30. Copelan EA, Penza SL, Theil KS, et al. The influence of early transplantation, age, GVHD prevention regimen, and other factors on outcome of allogeneic transplantation for CML following BuCy. *Bone Marrow Transplant* 2000;26:1037–1043.
31. Beelen DW, Graeven U, Elmaagacli AH, et al. Prolonged administration of interferon-alpha in patients with chronic-phase Philadelphia chromosome-positive chronic myelogenous leukemia prior to allogeneic bone marrow transplantation may adversely affect transplant outcome. *Blood* 1994;84:6:2026–2043.
32. Hansen J, Gooley T, Martin P, et al. Bone marrow transplants from unrelated donors for patients with chronic myeloid leukemia. *N Engl J Med* 1998;338:962–968.
33. Hehlmann R, Hochhaus A, Kolb HJ, et al. Interferon-a before allogeneic bone marrow transplantation in chronic myelogenous leukemia does not affect outcome adversely, provided it is discontinued at least 90 days before the procedure. *Blood* 1999;94:11:3668–3677.
34. Clift RA, Buckner ED, Thomas WI, et al. Marrow transplantation for chronic myelogenous leukemia: a randomized study comparing cyclophosphamide and total body irradiation with busulfan and cyclophosphamide. *Blood* 1994;84:2036–2043.
35. Ringden O, Ruutu T, Remberger M, et al. A randomized trial comparing busulfan with total body irradiation as conditioning in allogeneic marrow transplant recipients with leukemia: a report from the Nordic bone marrow transplantation group. *Blood* 1994;83:2723–2730.
36. Dazzi F, Szydlo RM, Craddock C, et al. Comparison of single-dose and escalating-dose regimens of donor lymphocyte infusion for relapse after allografting for chronic myeloid leukemia. *Blood* 2000;95:1:67–71.
37. Guglielmi C, Arcese W, Hermans J, et al. Risk assessment in patients with Ph+ chronic myelogenous leukemia in first relapse after allogeneic stem cell transplant: an EBMT retrospective analysis. *Blood* 2000;95:11:3328–3334.
38. Craddock C, Szydlo R, Klein J, et al. Estimating leukemia-free survival after allografting for chronic myeloid leukemia: a new method that takes into account patients who relapse and are restored to complete remission. *Blood* 2000;96:1:86–90.
39. Bacigalupo A, Gualandi F, Van Lint MT, et al. Multivariate analysis of risk factors for survival and relapse in chronic granulocytic leukemia following allogeneic marrow transplantation: impact of disease related variables (Sokal score). *Bone Marrow Transplant* 1993;12: 443–448.
40. Gratwohl A, Hermans J, Niederwieser D, et al. Bone marrow transplantation for chronic myeloid leukemia: long term results. *Bone Marrow Transplant* 1993;12:509–516.
41. Devergie A, Blaise D, Attal M, et al. The French Society of Bone Marrow Graft (SFGM). Allogeneic bone marrow transplantation for chronic myeloid leukemia in first chronic phase: a randomized trial of busulfan-cytoxan versus cytoxan-total body irradiation as preparative regimen: a report from The French Society of Bone Marrow Graft (SFGM). *Blood* 1995;85:2263–2268.
42. Copelan E, Deeg HJ. Conditioning for allogeneic marrow transplantation in patients with lympho-hematopoietic malignancies without the use of total body irradiation. *Blood* 1992;80:7:1648–1658.
43. Slattery JT, Sanders JE, Buckner CD, et al. Graft-rejection and toxicity following bone marrow transplantation in relation to busulfan pharmacokinetics. *Bone Marrow Transplant* 1995;16:31–42.
44. Grochow LB. The role of therapeutic monitoring in bone marrow transplantation induction regimens. *Semin Oncol* 1993;20:18–25.
45. Slattery JT, Clift RA, Buckner CD, et al. Marrow transplantation for chronic myeloid leukemia: the influence of plasma busulfan levels on the outcome of transplantation. *Blood* 1997;89:3055–3060.
46. Copelan EA, Bechtal TP, Avalos BR, et al. Busulfan levels are influenced by prior treatment and are associated with hepatic veno-occlusive disease and early mortality but not with delayed complications following marrow transplantation. *Bone Marrow Transplantation* 2001;11:1121–1124.

47. Applebaum FR. The future of CML treatment. The American Society of Hematology Conference. San Francisco, CA, December 1, 2000.
48. Andersson B, Fernandez H, Cagnoni P, et al. IV busulfan, cyclophosphamide (BuCy) and hematopoietic stem cells for non-Hodgkin's lymphomas (NHL). Proceedings of the American Society for Blood and Marrow Transplantation and the International Bone Marrow Transplant Registry/Autologous Blood and Marrow Transplant Registry Tandem BMT Meetings, Keystone Resort, CO, February 28-March 6 [abstract]. 1999;2:3.
49. Vaughan W, Cagnoni P, Fernandez H, et al. Pharmacokinetics of intravenous busulfan in hematopoietic stem cell transplantation (HSCT). Proceedings of the American Society for Blood and Marrow Transplantation and the International Bone Marrow Transplant Registry/Autologous Blood and Marrow Transplant Registry Tandem BMT Meetings, Keystone Resort, CO, February 28-March 6 [abstract]. 1999;2:22.
50. Dinsmore R, Kirkpatrick D, Flomenberg N, et al. Allogeneic bone marrow transplantation for patients with acute nonlymphocytic leukemia. *Blood* 1984;63:649–656.
51. Geller RB, Saral R, Piantadosi S, et al. Allogeneic bone marrow transplantation after high-dose busulfan and cyclophosphamide in patients with acute nonlymphocytic leukemia. *Blood* 1989;73:2209–2218.
52. Bolwell B. Is bone marrow transplantation appropriate in older patients?In: Bolwell B, ed. *Current Controversies in Bone Marrow Transplantation.* Humana Press, Totowa, New Jersey, 2000.
53. McGlave P, Arthur D, Hakke R, et al. Therapy of chronic myelogenous leukemia with allogeneic bone marrow transplantation. *J Clin Oncol* 1987;5:1033–1040.
54. Giralt S, Gajewski J, Khouri I, et al. Induction of graft-vs-leukemia as primary treatment of chronic myelogenous leukemia. *Blood* 1997;1990(suppl):1857a.
55. Champlin R, Khouri I, Komblau S, et al. Reinventing bone marrow transplantation: nonmyeloablative preparative regimens and induction of graft-vs-malignancy effect. *Oncology* 1999;13:621–628.
56. Beatty PG, Ash R, Hows JM, et al. The use of unrelated bone marrow donors in the treatment of patients with chronic myelogenous leukemia: experience of four marrow transplant centers. *Bone Marrow Transplant* 1989;18:421–425.
57. McGlave PB, Beatty P, Ash R, et al. Therapy for chronic myelogenous leukemia with unrelated donor bone marrow transplantation: results in 102 cases. *Blood* 1990;75:1728–1732.
58. Mackinnon S, Hows JM, Goldman JM, et al. Bone marrow transplantation for chronic myeloid leukemia: the use of histocompatible unrelated volunteer donors. *Exp Hematol* 1990;18:421–425.
59. McGlave P, Bartsch G, Anasetti C, et al. Unrelated donor marrow transplantation therapy for chronic myelogenous leukemia: initial experience of the National Marrow Donor Program. *Blood* 1993;81:843–850.
60. Sasazuki T, Juji T, Morishima Y, et al. Effect of matching of class I HLA alleles on clinical outcome after transplantation of hematopoietic stem cells from an unrelated donor. *N Engl J Med* 1998;339:17:1177–1185.
61. Petersdorf EW, Gooley TA, Anasetti C, et al. Optimizing outcome after unrelated marrow transplantation by comprehensive matching of HLA class I and II alleles in the donor and recipient. *Blood* 1998;92:10:3515–3520.
62. Fleischauer K, Kernan NA, O'Reilly RJ, et al. Bone marrow-allograft rejection by T lymphocytes recognizing a single amino acid difference in HLA-B44. *N Engl J Med* 1990;323: 1818–1822.
63. Keever CA, Leong N, Cunnigham I, et al. HLA-B44-directed cytotoxic T cells associated with acute graft-versus-host disease following unrelated bone marrow transplantation. *Bone Marrow Transplant* 1994;14:137–145.
64. Klein JL, Avalos BR, Belt P, et al. Bone marrow engraftment following unrelated donor transplantation utilizing busulfan and cyclophosphamide preparatory chemotherapy. *Bone Marrow Transplant* 1996;17:479–483.
65. Bertz H, Potthoff K, Mertelsmann R, et al. Busulfan/cyclophosphamide in volunteers unrelated donor (VUD) BMT: excellent feasibility and low incidence of treatment-related toxicity. *Bone Marrow Transplant* 1997;19:1169–1173.
66. Kroger N, Zabelina T, Kruger W, et al. Comparison of total body irradiation vs busulfan in combination with cyclophosphamide as conditioning for unrelated stem cell transplantation in CML patients. *Bone Marrow Transplant* 2001;27:349–354.

5

Allogeneic Stem Cell Transplantation for Breast Cancer

Abby B. Siegel, MD *and Linda T. Vahdat,* MD

Contents

INTRODUCTION
RATIONALE FOR HIGH DOSE CHEMOTHERAPY IN BREAST CANCER
RATIONALE FOR ALLOGENEIC STEM CELL TRANSPLANT
ALLOGENEIC TRANSPLANT FOR BREAST CANCER: RATIONALE
LIMITATIONS OF ALLOGENEIC TRANSPLANTATION
FUTURE DIRECTIONS
CONCLUSIONS
REFERENCES

1. INTRODUCTION

Breast cancer will affect about 192,200 women in the United States in 2001, and about 40,200 will die from their disease. While mortality has been decreasing steadily by 0.8% per year since 1989, breast cancer remains the leading cause of cancer deaths in women in the 20–59-yr-old age group *(1)*. Although trends are towards diagnosis at an earlier stage of disease, 35% of Caucasian and 43% of African-American women still present with nonlocalized breast cancer. Furthermore, the mortality for those with 10 or more involved lymph nodes or inflammatory breast cancer still hovers in the 75% range at 10 yr with standard chemotherapy. For those with advanced disease, the median survival remains in the range of 2–2.5 yr *(2)*. As a consequence of the poor prognosis of this group, new strategies have been employed in an attempt to improve survival. The research trend over the past 13 yr has been to utilize higher doses of chemotherapy, and preliminary phase III data on this approach has been slowly emerging over the past 2 yr.

Allogeneic bone marrow transplantation has improved survival for many diseases, including aplastic anemia, myelodysplastic disorders, and leukemias, most notably chronic myelogenous leukemia (CML) *(3–5)*. For the hematological malignancies, the beneficial effect is considered twofold. First, there is replacement of the malignant clone without reintroducing contaminated cells as may happen in an autologous transplant. Second, after allogeneic transplantation, donor T cells can exert a graft-vs-tumor (GVT) effect by recognizing the host's tumor antigens. Allogeneic stem cell transplants might provide the same advantages in the treatment of solid tumors by harnessing this GVT effect while preventing the re-infusion of a stem cell product that may contain viable tumor cells. Similar to the hematological malignan-

From: *Current Clinical Oncology: Allogeneic Stem Cell Transplantation*
Edited by: Mary S. Laughlin and Hillard M. Lazarus © Humana Press Inc., Totowa, NJ

cies, the major constraint with this approach is that donor T cells can also lead to graft-vs-host disease (GVHD) by recognizing histocompatibility antigens that differ between host and donor. This inability to separate the toxic GVHD from the desirable GVT effect has been one of the main challenges associated with allogeneic stem cell transplantation. The ultimate goal is to preferentially activate the GVT reaction. Alternatively, it may be possible to modulate the damaging GVH effects with immunosuppressive drugs or donor lymphocyte infusions. This chapter will focus on the rationale and data for allogeneic transplant for breast cancer in the context of data generated in autologous stem cell transplantation.

2. RATIONALE FOR HIGH DOSE CHEMOTHERAPY IN BREAST CANCER

There is both pre-clinical and clinical evidence for a dose response relationship for many of the chemotherapeutic agents active in the treatment of breast cancer (6–8).

2.1. Dose Escalation with/without Hematopoietic Growth Factors

2.1.1. ADJUVANT TREATMENT FOR PRIMARY BREAST CANCER

Recent studies in the adjuvant setting assessing the impact of dose escalation within the standard dose range have produced mixed results (9–11). Certainly with anthracyclines and cyclophosphamide there appears to be a threshold dose for efficacy, and escalation above that level does not appear improve disease-free survival (DFS) or overall survival (OS) to date.

2.1.2. TREATMENT IN ADVANCED BREAST CANCER

Randomized clinical trials in advanced breast cancer, in which dose intensity is the sole or most important variable are difficult to interpret because the increased doses planned varied from 10% to fourfold greater than the low-dose arms. Because serum levels for a given drug commonly vary at least fivefold, serum levels of drug may overlap. Still, about one-half of these trials have shown a statistically significant increase in response rate for regimens with greater dose intensity, with several of the trials showing a modest survival advantage (12).

2.2. Dose Escalation with Stem Cell Support

2.2.1. SUMMARY OF PHASE I–III STUDIES OF HIGH DOSE CHEMOTHERAPY WITH STEM CELL SUPPORT

2.2.1.1. Advanced Breast Cancer.
During the late 1980s and 1990s, there were many studies in advanced breast cancer in which myeloablative chemotherapy was administered with either autologous bone marrow and/or peripheral blood stem cells to circumvent the hematological toxicity of the conditioning regimens. The complete response rates ranged from 45 to 80%. However, the majority of patients relapsed, with only 15–20% remaining disease-free at 5 yr (12). As the field progressed, increased use of peripheral blood stem cells (instead of bone marrow) and hematopoietic growth factors facilitated rapid engraftment and contributed to decreased mortality rates to 2% nationwide.

From this research, several consistent themes emerged. First, those who have complete responses (CR) to therapy have improved DFS over those with partially responding (PR) or nonresponding disease (13). In addition, other factors may play a role in the maintenance of response, including extent of disease and length of induction therapy (14). When patterns of relapse were assessed, it appeared that patients tended to relapse at sites of prior bulk disease. Three possible explanations for this phenomenon have been proposed: relapse may either be due to resistant disease to the inability of immune effector cells to eradicate minimal residual disease, or autologous stem cell graft contamination by tumor cells that contribute to relapse. To date, this last hypothesis has not been substantiated with stem cell purging gene-marking

Table 1
Randomized High Dose Breast Cancer Studies

| | % Toxic deaths | | | |
	Randomized	BMT	Control	Comments (ref.)
Adjuvant:				
CALGB 9082	785	7.4	0	too early (22)
Dutch adjuvant	885	1.0	0	too early,positive trend (23)
NCI Milan	382	0.5	0	no difference (25)
Pegase I	314	0.6	0	improved DFS at 3 yr (24)
Metastatic :				
NCIC (Ma 16)	224	0	6	equivalent (19)
Philadelphia	199	1	0	equivalent (18)
Pegase 04	61	0	0	positive trend (17)
Duke CR study	98	NA	NA	positive DFS (21)
Duke bone only	69	NA	NA	positive PFS (20)

trials (15,16). Hence, it is rational to suggest that these limitations might be overcome with an allogeneic stem cell transplant capitalizing on a tumor-free graft and a GVT effect.

As shown in Table 1, five randomized trials assess the role of increased dose with stem cell support as a component of the overall treatment in women with responding metastatic breast cancer. Three of these trials demonstrate the equivalence of a single high-dose cycle of chemotherapy with stem cell support to maintenance chemotherapy (17–19). Survival was doubled in the small French trial (Pegase 04), a difference that was not statistically significant (17). The two Duke University trials compare a single high dose cycle of chemotherapy after four cycles of conventional therapy to observation alone, with the high-dose therapy producing superior DFS (20,21). There are at least two trials assessing high-dose chemotherapy with stem cell support in this setting which will be reported in the next 1–3 yr (German and IBDIS Trials).

2.2.2. HIGH-RISK PRIMARY BREAST CANCER: SUMMARY OF PHASE III TRIALS

There are seven randomized trials assessing the worth of high dose chemotherapy with stem cell support compared to conventional-dose chemotherapy for patients with four or more lymph nodes involved with breast cancer. Although all are touted as "adjuvant" trials, only six are really adjuvant, as the Scandinavian Trial included those with abnormal bone scans and/or positive bone marrows. In addition, only 4 of the 6 have sufficient numbers of patients enrolled to answer the question they pose (which is a different question in most of these studies).

2.2.3. CALGB 9082 INTERGROUP TRIAL

This study compares high- vs intermediate-dose cyclophosphamide, BCNU, and cisplatin (CBP) after a cyclophosphamide, adriamycin, and 5-flurouracil (CAF) induction in women with 10 or more positive lymph nodes. Seven hundred and eighty-five women with primary breast cancer initially received four cycles of CAF. They were then randomized to receive either high-dose CBP with marrow and peripheral stem cell support, or the same chemotherapy at a lower dose requiring only hematopoietic growth factors. Fewer relapses were seen in the high-dose arm (28 vs 39%). With a median follow-up of 5.1 yr, there was a trend for improved progression-free survival, but no statistically significant difference in DFS or OS (22). There was also a 7.4% treatment-related death rate in the high-dose arm vs none in the intermediate-dose arm. If in fact a difference exists between these two treatment arms, the difference will need to be large to compensate for the high toxic death rate in the high-dose arm.

2.2.4. Dutch Adjuvant Trial

This study is a comparison between standard dose chemotherapy and the same with high-dose chemotherapy followed by stem cell support. Eight hundred and eighty-five women with four or more lymph nodes involved with breast cancer were randomized to FEC (5-flourouracil, epirubicin, and cyclophosphamide) × 5 vs FEC × 4 followed by high dose chemotherapy with stem cell support consisting of cyclophosphamide, thiotepa, and carboplatin (CTCb). An interim analysis was mandated by the Dutch Insurance Council to evaluate the first 284 patients entered on the study. With a median follow-up of 52 mo there was a 15% DFS (62 vs 77%, $p = 0.009$) and a 10% OS (79 vs 89%, $p = 0.05$) advantage favoring the high-dose arm. When looking at the entire group with a median follow-up of 30 mo, these differences are not statistically significant. Day 100 mortality was 1% *(23)*.

2.2.5. French Adjuvant Trial

Pegase 01 was designed to assess the worth of a single high dose cycle of chemotherapy with stem cell support following epirubicin-based chemotherapy in women with seven or more lymph nodes involved with breast cancer. The primary endpoint was disease-free survival at 3 yr. Three hundred and fourteen patients were randomized to FEC × 4 vs the same followed by high dose chemotherapy with stem cell support (cyclophosphamide, mitoxantrone, melphalan). At a median follow-up of 39 mo there was a 15 % disease-free survival advantage observed in patients receiving the high dose chemotherapy vs. standard dose therapy (55 vs 70.8%, $p < 0.003$). Survival was similar for both groups at 86 vs 84% ($p = 0.33$), respectively and the toxic death rate was <1% *(24)*. Longer follow-up will be needed to assess if a survival difference is observed.

2.2.6. NCI Milan

This trial looked at high dose sequential chemotherapy versus standard dose chemotherapy in women with four or more involved lymph nodes. Three hundred and eighty-two patients were randomized to either epirubicin × 3 followed by CMF × 6 versus high dose sequential (HDS) chemotherapy. HDS chemotherapy consisted of cyclophosphamide (7 g/m^2) followed by methotrexate (8 g/m^2) plus leucovorin, followed by epirubicin (at 120 mg/m^2) × 2, followed by thiotepa (600 mg/m^2) + melphalan (160 or 180 mg/m^2) with stem cell support. At a median follow-up of 52 mo both treatments produced similar disease-free and overall survival results. The DFS for the Epi/CMF vs HDS was 62 vs 65% and overall survival was 77 vs 76%, respectively *(25)*.

There are at least six trials of sufficient size, which will be analyzed over the next 3–5 yr, which address the role of increased dose in this population.

2.3. Trials of Immunomodulation

In an effort to mimic the GVT effect observed in allogeneic stem cell transplants for the hematological malignancies, several investigators have initiated clinical trials of immuno-modulatory agents in the post-high-dose chemotherapy and autologous stem cell transplant setting. In summary, there appears to be no clinical benefit derived when compared to historical data sets.

2.3.1. Trials to Induce GVHD

Preliminary studies in humans have shown that an autologous GVHD may be introduced in patients with hematological malignancies following the infusion of autologous marrow *(26–28)*. Kennedy and colleagues at Johns Hopkins demonstrated that GVHD may be induced with cyclosporine A in a dose-dependent fashion in up to 92% of breast cancer patients undergoing autologous transplanatation. They also reported that the combination of cyclosporine and γ interferon (which increases the expression of human leukocyte antigen (HLA)-DR on target tissues) produced a biopsy-proven grade II GVHD of the skin in 43% of patients, and 79% of patients showed evidence of autolytic activity directed against pretransplant lymphoblasts. In addition, the in vitro lytic activity correlated with the histologic grade of GVHD *(29,30)*.

2.3.2. TRIALS TO INCREASE EFFECTOR CELL NUMBER AND FUNCTION

Interleukin (IL)-2 amplifies the number of effector T cells, and has also been used to create GVHD in autologous transplant settings. Georgetown investigators incubated peripheral blood progenitors with IL-2 for 24 h, and then gave subcutaneous IL-2 injections to breast cancer patients after autologous transplantation for 5 of 7 d for 4 wk. Clinical cutaneous GVHD was seen in 23% of patients. DFS with immunomodulation seems comparable to that reported in the literature without immunomodulation *(31)*.

Kennedy et al. added IL-2 to cyclosporine in order to augment the effects of GVHD after high-dose chemotherapy in women with advanced breast cancer. Twenty-nine patients with stage IIIB or IV breast cancer were treated with cyclosporine A and interferon γ after stem cell infusions. Patients then received one of three different dose levels of IL-2 (10,000, 100,000, or 500,000 $\mu/M^2/d$). Lytic activity against autologous lymphoblasts was decreased at all dose levels for unclear reasons *(32)*.

3. RATIONALE FOR ALLOGENEIC STEM CELL TRANSPLANT

There is ample clinical evidence for a graft-vs-leukemia effect in allogeneic stem cell transplant for the hematologic malignancies *(33)*. The incidence of leukemic relapse is lower after allogeneic bone marrow transplantation (BMT) than after syngeneic transplant. The incidence of relapse is also lower in allogeneic marrow recipients who develop GVHD than those who do not. Further, identical twin transplants for acute myelogenous leukemia (AML) and CML are associated with increased relapse risk compared with HLA-identical sibling transplants *(34,35)*. In patients in the chronic phase of CML, the incidence of relapse was 10% in recipients of non-T cell-depleted (TCD) marrow that had moderate to severe acute GVHD, and 50% in recipients of T cell-depleted marrow that had no or mild GVHD *(36)*. These studies suggest that an antileukemic effect is associated with donor T cells and that the same mechanism which effects host destruction seems to work to destroy tumor cells. In addition, although GVHD effects are important predictors of a lower relapse rate, clinical GVHD is not required for the graft-vs-leukemia effect.

4. ALLOGENEIC TRANSPLANT FOR BREAST CANCER: RATIONALE

Many human cancers are intensely infiltrated with T cells. Flow cytometric analysis of cellular infiltrates in solid primary breast cancers has shown that CD8+ T lymphocytes are the predominant cell infiltrating these tumors. Cytotoxic T lymphocytes recognize short peptide antigens presented on the cell-surface by Class I major histocompatibility complex (MHC) alleles. Linehan et al. *(33)* have shown that highly tumor-specific CD8+ tumor-associated lymphocytes can be isolated and expanded from metastatic effusions of patients with breast cancer. Furthermore, these cells can selectively lyse autologous and allogeneic tumor cells in a tumor-specific HLA-A2-restricted fashion. In addition, tumor-specific lymphocytes derived from breast cancer patients can selectively lyse HLA-A2+ pancreatic and ovarian tumor cell targets, suggesting a common HLA-A2-restricted tumor-associated antigen between these distinct epithelial tumors *(37)*.

In vitro studies have shown that exposure of tumor infiltrating lymphocytes to IL-2 will generate activated T lymphocytes with MHC-restricted and non-MHC-restricted cytotoxicity towards a panel of tumor target cells. Tumor infiltrating lymphocytes from primary tumors of breast carcinoma and effusion-associated mononuclear cells from metastatic disease increased in number by more than 300-fold when cultured with recombinant IL-2 and exhibited mostly potent autologous tumor cell-specific cytotoxicity *(38)*. This preclinical evidence suggests the possibility of harnessing an immune response against breast cancer cell targets.

4.1. Clinical Data: Breast Cancer

In a case report by Eibl et al. *(35)*, the development of circulating minor histocompatability, antigen-specific cytotoxic T lymphocytes recognizing breast carcinoma targets appeared to coincide with the clinical disappearance of liver metastases, suggesting a GVT effect in breast cancer in a human subject *(39)*. In this study, a 32-yr-old patient with metastatic breast cancer was transplanted with bone marrow from her HLA identical sister. Peripheral blood mononuclear cells were obtained from the donor and from the patient before transplantation, and again during acute GVHD. A cytotoxic T cell line was established using posttransplant recipient PBMC harvested during GVHD which was stimulated with irradiated pretransplant recipient PBMC and cultured. The cells were then stimulated with IL-2. Successful engraftment was achieved on d 13. On d 27, the patient developed biopsy-proven GVHD of the skin. On the same day, the patient's CT scan documented complete resolution of the liver metastases. At the time of GVHD, cytotoxic T lymphocytes were identified which recognized host pretransplant cells but not the donor cells (which were HLA identical). These cells were thus defined as minor histocompatability antigen specific. They were also MHC class I-antigen restricted. The presence of these circulating, minor histocompatability antigen-specific CTL, recognizing breast carcinoma target cells at the time of metastasis regression support the idea that a GVT effect may have at least contributed to the disappearance of the hepatic metastases.

Slavin's group in Jerusalem conducted a clinical pilot study of allogeneic transplantation in six patients with metastatic breast cancer. The patients were cytoreduced with high-dose chemotherapy and autologous stem cell transplantation. They were then given HLA-matched donor peripheral blood lymphocytes activated in vivo with human recombinant IL-2. Five of the six patients then received additional activated donor lymphocytes when they showed signs of progression. Four patients displayed transient improvement of disease parameters, with a progression-free interval between allo-SCT and disease progression of 7–12 mo. One patient with metastatic disease in the liver responded markedly to the activated lymphocytes and was given a second dose, but still died with an overall survival of 18+ mo. One patient was alive with evidence of disease at 32 mo, while one patient is alive with no evidence of disease at 34 mo. Toxicity seen in all patients was mild, including fever, anorexia, and a pruritic maculopapular rash. No patient was hospitalized for toxicity. The group suggests that perhaps the transient response in five of the six patients was due to the inability to induce durable chimerism in any of the patients *(40)*.

Dr. Ueno and colleagues at MD Anderson Cancer Center conducted a trial in which ten breast cancer patients underwent HLA identical sibling-matched allogeneic peripheral blood stem cell transplantation *(41)*. The patients had bone and/or liver metastases, and the conditioning regimen consisted of cyclophosphamide, carmustine and thiotepa. GVHD prophylaxis consisted of cyclosporine and methylprednisolone in the first two patients. The other eight patients received tacrolimus and micromethotrexate (minidose at 5 mg/m^2). Patients who developed grade II or greater GVHD were treated with methylprednisolone 2 mg/kg/d in divided doses and tapered as tolerated. Patients who entered the trial with residual or recurrent breast cancer had immunosuppressive therapy rapidly tapered. If GVHD was not present, additional donor lymphocytes were infused.

Response to therapy was evaluated at 3, 6, and 12 mo and as clinically indicated. The disease endpoints included response, time to treatment failure and survival. Six patients had recurrent disease and four initially presented with advanced disease. Four patients had bone marrow involvement, five patients had liver involvement, and one patient had both. All patients received standard-dose induction chemotherapy with 5-flourouracil, cyclophosphamide, and doxorubicin (FAC) and/or a paclitaxel-containing regimen. The overall response rate was 50%, and the median remission duration was 238 d. All ten patients achieved complete hematopoetic engraftment by d 24. Eight assessable patients were confirmed to have complete chimerism by RFLP. The 100-d mortality was 10%. Three patients have died- one of fungal infection, another from GVHD and sepsis, and a third of progressive disease. The median progression-free survival from the initial treatment of metastatic breast cancer was 495 d. The median survival had not been reached at the time of publication, with seven patients alive at a median of 602 d. Four patients with progressive disease had immunosuppressive therapy reduced, and one received a donor lymphocyte infusion in an attempt to enhance the graft-vs-tumor effect. Regression of tumor was observed in two of the four patients who had immunosuppression tapered with concomitant development of GVHD. The patient who received the DLI did not develop GVHD and died of progressive disease at d 64.

As compared to high dose chemotherapy with autologous stem cell support, the response rates in this study appear similar and the toxicity appears greater. However, when the field of high dose chemotherapy and autologous stem cell transplant began, toxic death rates where much higher than the 10% noted in this group.

The International Bone Marrow Transplant Registry is collecting full data on 33 patients who have undergone high dose chemotherapy with allogeneic stem cell transplant as treatment for advanced breast cancer. Table 2 lists some of the trials which have begun to evaluate high dose chemotherapy with allogeneic stem cell transplantation for breast cancer.

5. LIMITATIONS OF ALLOGENEIC TRANSPLANTATION

This approach is currently limited by the toxicity of the high-dose chemotherapy preparative regimens and the complications surrounding the profound immunosuppression that is involved. For these reasons, many older patients with co-morbid illnesses are ineligible for this approach. Immunosuppressive agents are used after hematopoetic cell transplantation in order to reduce the cytokine cascade, which is thought to be responsible for much of the damage incurred with GVHD. Various combinations of corticosteroids, methotrexate, cyclosporine, and tacrolimus (FK506) have been used to prevent and treat GVHD, as have antibodies such as intravenous immunoglobulin and antithymocyte globulin *(42–45)*. Newer immunosuppressive agents being studied are compounds such as thalidomide and the anticytokines *(46,47)*. Perhaps reducing the chemotherapy dose, as is done in nonmyeloablative stem cell transplants (mini-allotransplants) or further optimizing the immunosuppressive regimens will overcome the limitations of this approach.

6. FUTURE DIRECTIONS

There is much ongoing research geared towards minimizing the dose of chemotherapy and optimizing the degree of immunosuppression. There is also emphasis on teasing out the GVH problems from the desirable GVT effect. While these are crucial to improving the success of allogeneic transplantation for breast cancer, there are other potential approaches that may incorporate these concepts as part of an overall treatment strategy for women with advanced breast cancer.

6.1. Advances in the Treatment of GVHD

Preparative regimens damage end organs and trigger inflammatory cytokines, such as TNF-α *(28,46)*. For this reason, reducing TNF-α is being studied in the context of allogeneic trans-

Table 2
Ongoing Trials of Allotransplantation for Solid Tumors
Including Breast

Tumor type	Center	Phase
Solid tumors	Northwestern	I
Breast stage 4 mini-allo	Ireland Ca Ctr	II
Solid tumors with CAMPTH 1-H	Duke University	II
Solid tumors mini-allo	NIH	II

plantation as a way to lower the toxicity associated with GVHD. IL-11 may also help to decrease inflammation associated with GVHD. Hill et al. *(43)* have shown that IL-11 can reduce small bowel damage, reduce cytokine levels, and improve survival in a mouse model of GVHD *(48)*. The same group then found that IL-11 selectively inhibited CD4-mediated GVHD while retaining CD4 and CD8 mediated graft-vs-leukemia effects, suggesting that IL-11 may be able to separate graft-vs-leukemia from GVH effects *(49)*. The use of the minitransplant (nonmyeloablative allotransplant) is also being evaluated as a way to decrease toxicity while capitalizing on the GVT effects of the transplanted T cells *(50,51)*.

6.2. Gene Therapy

Human marrow progenitors may be transduced with the human multidrug resistance gene, which may then be positively selected for after treatment with chemotherapy. The ability to maintain expression of the transduced cell may be utilized to correct cancers with a genetic basis, the myeloablative allotransplant might serve as a vehicle to "switch" stem cells *(52)*.

Other gene therapy experiments have focused on transferring a suicide gene into donor lymphocytes so that they may be eradicated in the face of GVHD. Bonini et al. transduced donor lymphocytes with a herpes simplex virus thymidine kinase suicide gene *(48)*. Eight patients who experienced complications after T cell-depleted allogeneic BMT for hematologic malignancy or immunodeficiency were treated with these donor lymphocytes. The lymphocytes survived for up to 12 mo, and resulted in antitumor activity in five patients. Three patients developed GVH disease, which was effectively controlled by gancyclovir-induced elimination of the transduced cells. This offers another possible way to separate the effects of GVH from the GVT effect *(53)*.

6.3. Adoptive Immunotherapy

Adoptive immunotherapy involves transferring lymphoid cells with antitumor activity to a tumor-bearing host. Suppressor, helper and cytotoxic T lymphocytes, natural killer (NK) cells, and B cells all may be activated by IL-2. Adoptive immunotherapy with IL-2 and in vitro lymphokine-activated killer cells, as well as tumor-infiltrating lymphocytes are being studied as potential antitumor agents (54–56).

In one study, 25 patients with advanced cancer were treated with recombinant human IL-2 by continuous infusion with adoptive transfer of autologous lymphocytes activated in vitro with IL-2 *(55)*. Nine patients had objective tumor regressions for a median duration of 16 wk. deMagalhaes–Silverman et al. *(49)* evaluated fifteen patients with metastatic breast cancer who received autologous stem cell transplants, and divided them into three groups to receive (i) recombinant IL-2, (ii) recombinant IL-2 and activated NK cells, or (iii) neither. The overall toxicities did not differ between the three groups and the IL-2 and NK cells did not adversely affect engraftment. The response rate (six out of 15) is similar to that observed in trials of high dose chemotherapy with stem cell support without immunomodulation *(54)*.

Donor lymphocyte infusions have also been shown to be effective in treating relapsed CML via a graft-vs-leukemia effect, and are just beginning to be studied in solid tumors *(41,57)*.

6.4. Tumor Vaccines

Cancer vaccine trials are now focusing on presenting tumor antigens to specific antigen-presenting cells so that the cellular (rather than humoral system) is activated to kill tumor cells. This first involves finding antigens that are specific to different tumor types. Mucin-related antigens have been studied in breast cancer, and vaccines to these peptides are being developed *(58–60)*. The MAGE genes code for other distinct antigens that are recognized by many cancer cell types, including breast cancer cells. They are not expressed in any normal tissue except testes and placenta, which may facilitate the development of targeted tumor vaccines *(61)*.

In addition to identifying and incorporation tumor antigens, research has also focused on combining cytokines such as granulocyte-macrophage colony-stimulating factor (GM-CSF) with cancer cells, which are then used to immunize a patient. The use of GM-CSF may help to activate the patient's cellular immune response in the environment of the tumor cells *(62,63)*.

6.5. Dendritic Cells

Dendritic cells (DCs) play an important role as antigen-presenting cells (APCs) in immune responses. Human dendritic cells can differentiate from myeloid or lymphoid precursors with the use of differentiating agents, but the myeloid precursors have been the focus of applications to stimulate immunity against cancer *(64)*. In the first published human DC trial, patients with malignant B cell lymphoma who failed conventional chemotherapy, were treated with DCs isolated from their peripheral blood and pulsed with tumor-specific Id antigen. Two of ten patients with relapsed, measurable, indolent lymphoma treated with DC infusions had CRs. A third had a molecular response with BCL-2+ bone marrow converting to negative *(65)*. DCs are now being studied in a wide variety of tumors, including breast cancer. In a Phase I study, Morse et al. gave dendritic cells loaded with carcinoembryonic antigen (CEA) peptide (CAP-1) to 21 patients with CEA-expressing malignancies including breast cancer. One patient had a minor response, and another patient had stable disease *(66)*.

7. CONCLUSIONS

Allogeneic stem cell transplant is a worthwhile research strategy for advanced breast cancer for several reasons. Despite advances in the field with the incorporation of new drugs and immunotherapies, the majority of patients with advanced disease relapse and ultimately die from their disease. If their disease could be maximally cytoreduced by chemotherapy, then perhaps the residual disease could be treated utilizing the GVT effect from donor effector cells. This could be accomplished by allotransplant, mini-transplant, or possibly donor lymphocyte infusion. Moreover, as we learn more about immunomodulation, we will hopefully be able to limit the toxicities of GVHD. We are still learning which patients benefit most from allotransplantation for solid tumors, and from GVT effects. It is crucial to direct patients to centers with ongoing research studies in order to learn more about this potentially valuable therapy for breast cancer.

REFERENCES

1. Greenlee RT, Hill-Harmon MB, Murray T, Thun M. Cancer statistics. *CA Cancer J Clin* 2001;51:15–36.
2. Clark G, Sledge GW, Osborne CK, McGuire WL. Survival from first recurrence: relative importance of prognostic factors in 1,015 breast cancer patients. *J Clin Oncol* 1987;5:55–61.

3. Anderson JE. Bone marrow transplantation for myelodysplasia. *Blood Rev* 2000;14(2):63–77.

4. Ball SE. The modern management of severe aplastic anemia. *Br J Haematol* 2000;110:41–53.

5. Savage DG, Goldman JM. Chronic myelogenous leukemia. In: Armitage JO, Antman KH, eds. *High-Dose Cancer Therapy Pharmacology, Hematopoetins, Stem Cells.* 3rd ed. Lippincott, Philadelphia, PA, 2000, pp. 705–732.

6. Frei III E, Canellos GP. Dose, a critical factor in cancer chemotherapy. *Am J Med* 1980;69:585–594.

7. Teicher BA, III EF. Development of alkylating agent-resistant human tumor cell lines. *Cancer Chemother Pharmacol* 1988;21:292–298.

8. Hryniuk WM, Bush H. The importance of dose intensity in chemotherapy of metastatic breast cancer. *J Clin Oncol* 1984;2:1281–1287.

9. Fisher B, Anderson S, DeCillis A, et al. Further evaluation of intensified and increased total dose of cyclophosphamide for the treatment of primary breast cancer: findings from national surgical adjuvant breast and bowel project B-25. *J Clin Oncol* 1999;17(11):3374–3388.

10. Fisher B, Anderson S, Wickerham DL, et al. Increased intensification and total dose of cyclophosphamide in a doxorubicin-cyclophosphamide regimen for the treatment of primary breast cancer: findings from National Surgical Adjuvant Breast and Bowel Project B-22. *J Clin Oncol* 1997;15(5):1858–1869.

11. Henderson I, Berry D, Demetri G, et al. Improved disease free and overall survival from the addition of sequential paclitaxel but not from the escalation of doxorubicin dose level in the adjuvant chemotherapy of patients with node positive primary breast cancer. *Proc Am Soc Clin Oncol* 1998;17:101a (abstract 390A).

12. Vahdat L, Antman K. Dose-intensive chemotherapy in breast cancer. In: Armitage J, Antman K, eds. *High-Dose Cancer Therapy Pharmacology, Hematopoetins, Stem Cells.* 3rd ed. Lippincott, Philadelphia, PA, 2000, pp. 821–840.

13. Antman K, Rowlings P, Vaughn W, et al. High dose chemotherapy with autologous hematopoietic stem cell support for breast cancer in North America. *J Clin Oncol* 1997;15(5):1870–1879.

14. Nieto Y, Cagnoni PJ, Shpall EJ, et al. Phase II trial of high-dose chemotherapy with autologous stem cell transplant for stage IV breast cancer with minimal metastatic disease. *Clin Cancer Res* 1999;5:1731–1737.

15. Rill D, Santana V, Roberts W, et al. Direct demonstration that autologous bone marrow transplantation for solid tumors can return a multiplicity of tumorigenic cells. *Blood* 1994;84(2):380–383.

16. Shpall E, Franklin W, Jones R, et al. Transplantation of CD34+ selected progenitor cells into breast cancer patients following high dose chemotherapy. *Am Soc Blood Marrow Transplant* 1995;1 (abstract).

17. Lotz JP, Cure H, Janvier M, et al. High-dose chemotherapy with hematopoietic stem cells transplantation for metastatic breast cancer: results of the French protocol Pegase 04. *Proc Am Soc Clin Oncol* 1999;18:43a (abstract 161).

18. Stadtmauer EA, O'Neill A, Goldstein LJ, et al. Conventional-dose chemotherapy compared with high-dose chemotherapy plus autologous hematopoietic stem-cell transplantation for metastatic breast cancer. Philadelphia Bone Marrow Transplant Group. *N Engl J Med* 2000;342(15):1069–1076.

19. Crump M, Gluck S, Stewart D, et al. A randomized trial of high dose chemotherapy wih autologous peripheral blood stem cell support compared to standard therapy in women with metastatic breast cancer : a National Cancer Institute of Canada (NCIC) Clinical Trials Group Study. *Proc Am Soc Clin Oncol* 2001;20:21a (abstract 82).

20. Madan B, Broadwater G, Rubin P, et al. Improved survival with consolidation high-dose cyclophosphamide, cisplatin and carmustine (HD-CPB) compared with observation in women with metastatic breast cancer (MBC) and only bone metastases treated with induction adriamycin, 5-flourouracil, and methotrexate (AFM): a phase three prospective randomized comparative trial. *Proc Am Soc Clin Oncol* 2000;19:48a (abstract 184).

21. Peters W, Jones R, Vredenburgh J, et al. A large prospective randomized trial of high-dose combination alkylating agents (CPB) with autologous cellular support as consolidation for patients with metastatic breast cancer achieving complete remission after intensive doxorubicin-based induction therapy (AFM). *Proc Am Soc Clin Oncol* 1996;15:121 (abstract 149).

22. Peters W, Rosner G, Vredenburgh J, et al. Updated results of a prospective, randomized comparison of two doses of combination alkylating agents as consolidation after CAF in high-risk primary breast cancer involving ten or more axillary lymph nodes: CALGB 9082/SWOG 9114/NCIC Ma13. *Proc Am Soc Clin Oncol* 2001;20:21a(abstract 81).

23. Rodenhuis S, Bontenbal M, Beex L, et al. Randomized phase III study of high-dose chemotherapy with cyclophosphamide, thiotepa and carboplatin in operable breast cancer patients with 4 or more axillary lymph nodes. *Proc Am Soc Clin Oncol* 2000;19:74a (abstract 286).

24. Roche H, Pouillart P, Meyer N, et al. Adjuvant high dose chemotherapy improves early outcome for high risk (N>7) breast cancer patients: The Pegase 01 trial. *Proc Am Soc Clin Oncol* 2001;20:26a(abstract 102).

25. Gianni A, Bonadonna G. Five-year results of the randomized clinical trial comparing standard versus highdose myeloablative chemotherapy in the adjuvant treatment of breast cancer with >3 positive nodes. *Proc Am Soc Clin Oncol* 2001;20:21a(abstract 80).

26. Marin G, Porto A, Prates V, et al. Graft versus host disease in autologous stem cell transplantation. *J Exp Clin Cancer Res* 1999;18(2):201–208.

27. Miura Y, Ueda M, Zeng W, et al. Induction of autologous graft-versus-host disease with cyclosporin A after peripheral blood stem cell transplantation: analysis of factors affecting induction. *J Allergy Clin Immunol* 2000;106:51–57.
28. Vogelsang G. Advances in the treatment of graft-versus-host disease. *Leukemia* 2000;14:509,510.
29. Kennedy M, Vogelsang G, Beveridge R, et al. Phase I trial of intravenous cyclosporine to induce graft-versus-host disease in women undergoing autologous bone marrow transplantation for breast cancer. *J Clin Oncol* 1993;11:478–484.
30. Kennedy M, Hess A, Passos Coelho J, et al. Cyclosporine A induces autologous graft vs. host disease following high dose chemotherapy supported with peripheral blood progenitor cell infusions alone. *Proc Am Soc Clin Oncol* 1996;15:335 (abstract 964).
31. Meehan K, Verma U, Cahill R, et al. Interleukin-2-activated hematopoietic stem cell transplantation for breast cancer: investigation of dose level with clinical correlates. *Bone Marrow Transplant* 1997;20:643–651.
32. Kennedy M, Davidson N, Fetting J, et al. Phase I and immunologic study of interleukin-2 to augment cyclosporine A- induced autologous graft-versus-host disease after high dose chemotherapy in women with advanced breast cancer. *Proc Am Soc Clin Oncol* 1997;16:106a (abstract 372).
33. Fefer A. Graft-versus-tumor responses. In: Thomas ED, Blume KG, Forman SJ, eds. *Hematopoetic Cell Transplantation*. 2nd ed. Blackwell Science, Malden, 1999, 316–326.
34. Weiden PL, Flournoy N, Tomas ED, et al. Antileukemic effect of graft-versus-host diseases in human recipients of allogeneic marrow grafts. *N Engl J Med* 1979;330:1068–1073.
35. Gale R, Horowitz M, Ash R, et al. Identical-twin bone marrow transplants for leukemia. *Ann Intern Med* 1994;120(8):646–652.
36. Goldman JM, Gale RP, Horowitz MM, et al. Bone marrow tansplantation for chronic myelogenous leukemia in chronic phase: increased risk of relapse associated with T-cell depletion. *Ann Intern Med* 1988;108:806–814.
37. Linehan DC, Goedgebuure PS, Peoples GE, Rogers SO, Eberlein TJ. Tumor-specific and HLA-A2-restricted cytolysis by tumor-associated lymphocytes in human metastatic breast cancer. *J Immunol* 1995;155:4486–4491.
38. Baxevanis CN, Dedoussis GVZ, Papodopoulos NG, et al. Tumor-specific cytolysis by tumor infiltrating lymphocytes in breast cancer. *Cancer* 1994;74(4):1275–1282.
39. Eibl B, Schwaighofer H, Nachbaur D, et al. Evidence for a graft-versus-tumor effect in a patient treated with marrow ablative chemotherapy and allogeneic bone marrow transplantation for breast cancer. *Blood* 1996;88(4):1501–1508.
40. Or R, Ackerstein A, Nagler A, et al. Allogeneic cell-mediated immunotherapy for breast cancer after autologous stem cell transplantation: a clinical pilot study. *Cytokines Cell Molec Ther* 1997;4(1):1–6.
41. Ueno N, Randon G, Mirza N, et al. Allogeneic peripheral blood progenitor cell transplantation for poor risk patients with metastatic breast cancer. *J Clin Oncol* 1998;16(3):986–993.
42. Feinstein L, Seidel K, Jocum J, et al. Reduced dose of intravenous immunoglobulin does not decrease transplant-related complications in adults given related donor marrow allografts. *Biol Blood Marrow Transplant* 1999;5(6):369–378.
43. Dugan M, DeFor T, Steinbuch M, Filipovich A, Weisdorf D. ATG plus corticosteroid therapy for acute graft-versus-host disease: predictors of response and survival. *Ann Hematol* 1997;75(1–2):41–46.
44. Nash R, Antin J, Karanes C, et al. Phase 3 study comparing methotrexate and tacrolimus with methotrexate and cyclosporine for prophylaxis of acute graft-versus-host disease after marrow transplantation from unrelated donors. *Blood* 2000;96(6):2062–2068.
45. Zikos P, Van Lint M, Frassoni F, et al. Low transplant mortality in allogeneic bone marrow transplantation for acute myeloid leukemia: a randomized study of low-dose cyclosporin versus low-dose cyclosporin and low-dose methotrexate. *Blood* 1998;91(9):3503–3508.
46. Cooke K, Hill G, Crawford J, et al. Tumor necrosis factor-alpha production to lipopolysaccharide stimulation by donor cells predicts the severity of acute graft-versus-host disease. *J Clin Invest* 1998;102(10):1882–1891.
47. Vogelsang G, Farmer E, Hess A, et al. Thalidomide for the treatment of chronic graft-versus-host disease. *N Engl J Med* 1992;326(16):1055–1058.
48. Hill G, Cooke K, Teshima T, Crawford J, Keith J, Brinson Y. Interleukin 11 promotes T cell polarization and prevents acute graft-versus-host disase after allogeneic bone marrow transplantation. *J Clin Invest* 1998;102(1):115–123.
49. Teshima T, Hill G, Brinson Y, van den Brink M, Cooke K, Ferrara J. IL-11 separates graft-versus-leukemia effects from graft-versus-host disease after bone marrow transplantation. *J Clin Invest* 1999;104(3):317–325.
50. Bishop M. Non-myeloablative allogenic hematopoetic stem cell transplantation as adoptive cellular therapy. *Updates: Princ Prac Biol Ther Cancer* 2001;2(1):1–9.
51. Slavin S, Nagler A, Naparstek E, et al. Nonmyeloablative stem cell transplantation and cell therapy as an alternative to conventional bone marrow transplantation with lethal cytoreduction for the treatment of malignant and nonmalignant hematologic diseases. *Blood* 1998;91(3):756–763.

52. Hesdorffer C, Ayello J, Ward M, et al. A phase I trial of retroviral-mediated transfer of the human MDR-1 gene as marrow chemoprotection in patients undergoing high dose chemotherapy and autologous stem cell transplantation. *J Clin Oncol* 1998;16:165–172.

53. Bonini C, Ferrari G, Verzeletti S, et al. HSV-TK gene transfer into donor lymphocytes for control of allogeneic graft-vs-leukemia. *Science* 1997;276(5319):1719–1724.

54. deMagalhaes-Silverman M, Donnenberg A, Lembersky B, et al. Posttransplant adoptive immunotherapy with activated natural killer cells in patients with metastatic breast cancer. *J Immunother* 2000;23(1):154–160.

55. Paciucci PA, Holland JF, Glidewell O, Odchimar R. Recombinant interleukin-2 by continuous infusion and adoptive transfer of recombinant interleukin-2-activated cells in patients with advanced cancer. *J Clin Oncol* 1989;7(7):869–878.

56. Topalian SL, Solomon D, Avis FP, et al. Immunotherapy of patients with advanced cancer using tumor-infiltrating lymphocytes and recombinant Interleukin-2: a pilot study. *J Clin Oncol* 1988;6(5):839–853.

57. Kolb H-J, Holler E. Adoptive immunotherapy with donor lymphocyte transfusions. *Curr Opin Oncol* 1997;9:139–145.

58. Holmberg L, Oparin D, Gooley T, et al. Clinical outcomes of breast and ovarian cancer patients treated with high-dose chemotherapy, autologous stem cell rescue and THERATOPE STn-KLH cancer vaccine. *Bone Marrow Transplant* 2000;25(12):1233–1241.

59. Gilewski T, Adluri S, Ragupathi G, et al. Vaccination of high-risk breast cancer patients with mucin-1 (MUC-1) keyhole limpet hemocyanin conjugate plus QS-21. *Clin Cancer Res* 2000;6:1693–1701.

60. Brossart P, Heinrich K, Stuhler G, et al. Identification of HLA-A2-restricted T-cell epitopes derived from the MUC1 tumor antigen for broadly applicable vaccine therapies. *Blood* 1999;12:4309–4317.

61. Fujie T, Mori M, Sugimachi K, Akiyoshi T. Expression of MAGE and BAGE genes in Japanese breast cancers. *Ann Oncol* 1997;8(4):369–372.

62. Bank A. Gene therapy. In: Armitage J, Antman K, eds. *High-Dose Cancer Therapy Pharmacology, Hematopoetins, Stem Cells.* 3rd ed. Lippincott, Philadelphia, PA, 2000, pp. 167–184.

63. Borrello I, Sotomayor EM, Rattis F-M, Cooke SK, Gu L, Levitsky HI. Sustaining the graft-versus-tumor effect through posttransplant immunization with granulocyte-macrophage colony-stimulating factor (GM-CSF) producing tumor vaccines. *Blood* 2000;95(10):3011–3019.

64. Weber J, Schultz W. Clinical trials of dendritic cells for cancer. *Updates: Princ Prac Biol Ther Cancer* 2000;1(1):1–11.

65. Hsu FJ, Benicke C, Fagnoni F, et al. Vaccination of patients with B-cell lymphoma using autologous antigen-pulsed dendritic cells. *Nat Med* 1996;2(1):52–58.

66. Morse M, Deng Y, Coleman D, et al. A phase I study of active immunotherapy with carcinoembryonic antigen peptide (CAP-1)-pulsed, autologous human cultured dendritic cells in patients with metastatic malignancies expressing carcinoembryonic antigen. *Clin Cancer Res* 1999;5:1331–1338.

6

Allogeneic Transplantation for the Treatment of Multiple Myeloma

Stefano Tarantolo, MD and Philip J. Bierman, MD

CONTENTS

1. INTRODUCTION

Multiple myeloma is a disorder characterized by the neoplastic proliferation of a single clone of plasma cells. The annual incidence of multiple myeloma in the United States is approx 4 per 100,000 *(1)*. Approximately 14,400 new cases will be diagnosed in the year 2001 in the United States with 11,200 deaths attributable to multiple myeloma. Multiple myeloma represents slightly over 1% of all malignancies and 13% of all hematologic malignancies. It is predominantly a disease of older people with a median age at diagnosis of 66 yr However, approx 80% of patients are under the age of 70 and 18% are less than 50 yr of age *(2)*.

The treatment of myeloma remains a challenge. Conventional-dose chemotherapy regimens are not curative. The use of combination chemotherapy regimens is associated with improved response rates, but long-term outcomes are comparable to treatment with melphalan and prednisone *(3,4)*. High-dose therapy with autologous hematopoietic stem cell rescue is associated with an improved event-free survival and overall survival in selected patients when compared to conventional chemotherapy, although patients are not cured with this approach *(5–8)*.

In contrast, allogeneic stem cell transplantation has been shown to be curative in 15–20% of patients with multiple myeloma *(9,10)*. However, limited donor availability, the advanced age of most patients, and high treatment-related mortality limit the widespread use of allogeneic transplantation for patients with multiple myeloma.

The curative potential of allogeneic transplantation lies primarily in the development of a graft-vs-myeloma (GVM) effect to eradicate minimal residual disease after transplantation

From: *Current Clinical Oncology: Allogeneic Stem Cell Transplantation*
Edited by: Mary S. Laughlin and Hillard M. Lazarus © Humana Press Inc., Totowa, NJ

(11,12). Patients are generally treated prior to transplant to achieve a state of minimal residual disease. A preparative regimen is used that immunosuppresses the host sufficiently to allow engraftment of a tumor-free donor graft. The concept of a GVM effect is based on indirect evidence demonstrating lower relapse rates after allogeneic transplantation when compared to autologous transplantation *(13,14)*. Donor lymphocyte infusions (DLI) may reestablish complete remissions in patients who have relapsed after an allogeneic transplant, further substantiating the concept of a GVM effect *(15–22)*.

2. BACKGROUND OF THERAPY

Malignant plasma cells are sensitive to chemotherapy. Since the early 1960s, akylating agents in combination with corticosteroids have been the benchmark to which all other therapies have been compared. Standard-dose chemotherapy yields a 40–60% response rate but without a curative potential *(3)*. A meta-analysis of 6633 myeloma patients treated in 27 randomized trials showed the median survival to be 29 mo. No survival advantages were noted when treatment with melphalan and prednisone was compared with combination chemotherapy regimens *(4)*.

Escalating doses of chemotherapy induce higher remission rates, and high-dose therapy with autologous hematopoietic stem cell rescue yields additional improvements in complete remission rates. Attal and colleagues *(5)* conducted a randomized trial on 200 patients with stage II and III myeloma comparing high-dose therapy vs standard chemotherapy. Overall response rates (81 vs 57%), disease-free survival (28 vs 10%), and overall survival (52 vs 10%) were significantly higher in patients receiving high-dose therapy. Fermand et al. *(6)* conducted a randomized trial comparing conventional chemotherapy to high-dose therapy for myeloma. An improvement in event-free survival and quality of life were seen, but no significant overall survival advantages were demonstrated. It should be cautioned that the major benefit of high-dose therapy was noted in patients who responded to standard therapy prior to transplant *(6)*.

Several institutions have investigated the use of tandem autologous transplants for multiple myeloma. Investigators from the University of Arkansas reported on 1000 consecutive patients treated in a nonrandomized trial with tandem transplantation. Their results suggest that tandem transplants are superior to standard treatment *(7)*. Patients in a French study (IFM 94) were randomized between one or two autologous transplants. Preliminary data on 405 previously untreated patients did not demonstrate a significant difference in complete remission rate, overall survival, or event-free survival between arms. However, subset analysis suggested that patients with low β-2 microglobulin levels might have a survival advantage *(8)*.

Despite improved response rates, recurrent disease is the main reason for failure following autologous transplantation for myeloma. In selected patients, attention has been focused on utilizing allogeneic transplantation in an attempt to improve outcomes and potentially cure patients with myeloma.

3. EVIDENCE SUPPORTING A GVM EFFECT

There is both direct and indirect evidence supporting the existence of a GVM effect. Relapse after allogeneic transplantation is lower than after autologous transplantation. In some cases, remission has been reestablished after withdrawal of immunosuppression or with the development of graft-vs-host disease (GVHD) *(23)*. In addition, patients with persistent disease after allogeneic transplantation will show evidence of continued response as donor hematopoiesis is established. Finally, vaccinating donors with idiotypic protein can facilitate development of donor immunity against myeloma and transfer to recipient *(24)*.

A number of investigators have demonstrated clinical evidence of GVM following DLI to myeloma patients who relapse after allogeneic transplantation *(15–22)*. A review of published data demonstrated that 50–70% of myeloma patients treated with DLI achieved a response. GVM may occur without GVHD, but the association of a response with the occurrence of GVHD is very strong. One report reviewing the use of DLI for relapsed myeloma clearly demonstrated the GVM effect. Eighteen of 22 patients who developed GVHD had a response to DLI, compared to two of seven patients who did not develop GVHD ($p = 0.02$) *(12)*.

4. ALLOGENEIC TRANSPLANTATION

4.1. Criteria for Response

One major limitation in interpreting the results of allogeneic transplantation for multiple myeloma is the lack of consistent staging and response criteria. The variability in staging and response criteria prompted the International Bone Marrow Transplant Registry (IBMTR), the European Group for Blood and Marrow Transplantation (EBMT), and the Autologous Blood and Marrow Transplant Registry (ABMTR) to recommend the following criteria for determining response:

1. Complete remission (CR) is the disappearance of the monoclonal protein for a minimum of 6 wk, less than 5% plasma cells in the bone marrow, and no increase in the size or number of lytic lesions.
2. A partial response (PR) requires a 50% reduction in monoclonal protein for at least 6 wk and greater than 90% reduction in Bence-Jones protein for a minimum of 6 wk.
3. Progressive disease is defined as a 25% increase in the level of serum monoclonal protein *(9,25)*.

4.2. Syngeneic Transplants

Two studies have reported results of syngeneic transplantation for multiple myeloma. Bensinger et al. reported on 11 patients treated with syngeneic transplants *(26)*. The preparative regimen consisted of cyclophosphamide and total body irradiation (TBI) followed by bone marrow ($n = 10$) or peripheral blood stem cell rescue ($n = 1$). Two early deaths occurred due to treatment-related mortality. Five of the nine evaluable patients achieved a CR after transplantation, three patients achieved PR, and one patient was a nonresponder. Of the five patients who achieved a CR, three relapsed and a fourth died of myelodysplasia (MDS). One patient remained in remission with a small monoclonal spike at 15 yr after transplant *(26)*.

A review of EBMT data identified 25 patients with myeloma who were transplanted with a syngeneic graft *(27)*. The results obtained with this group of patients were compared in a case-matched analysis with 125 autologous and 125 allogeneic transplant patients. This analysis showed that survival after syngeneic transplantation was superior to autologous transplants and significantly better than allogeneic transplants. At 4 yr, the actuarial overall survival after syngeneic transplantation was 77%, as compared with 46% after autologous transplantation and 31% following allogeneic transplantation. Low treatment-related mortality for the syngeneic group was largely responsible for the improved outcome when compared to allogeneic transplants *(27)*.

These limited data suggest that syngeneic donor stem cells are the preferred stem cell source in the rare cases when these donors are available.

4.3. Allogeneic Bone Marrow Transplantation

The majority of available data on the treatment of myeloma with allogeneic transplantation is derived from transplant registry data and single-institution trials. Interpretation of results is hindered by the lack of uniform staging, the absence of strict stratification criteria, the use of

Table 1
Comparison of Published Reports Using Allogeneic Transplantation for Multiple Myeloma

Reference	No. of patients	CR	TRM	Survival
EBMT (9)	1368	45–50%	25%	RFS at 6 yr 34% OS 32% (4 yr), 18% (9 yr)
Seattle (10)	136	34%	48%	RFS at 5 yr 14%, OS 22%
Dana-Faber (31)	61	23%	10%	Median OS 22 mo
Mehta (13)	42	41%	43% (at 1yr)	PFS at 3 yr 31% Median OS 20 mo
Kulkurni (33)	33	37%	54% (at 1 yr)	DFS 39% (3 yr) OS 35.7% (3yr)
Couban (35)	22	62%	27%	OS at 3 yr 32%, EFS 22%
Russell (34)	13	76%	15%	DFS at 3 yr 65%
Cavo (32)	19	42%	37%	OS at 4 yr 26%, EFS 21%
Reece (36)	19	58%	16%	PFS 40% at median 14 mo
Majolino (38)	10	71%	20%	Median 18.5 mo

CR, complete remission; TRM, treatment related mortality; EFS, event-free survival; RFS, relapse-free survival; OS, overall survival; DFS, disease-free survival; PFS, progression-free survival.

heterogeneous transplant regimens, variable GVHD prophylaxis regimens, and differences in supportive care.

Table 1 summarizes the results of the largest reports of allogeneic transplantation for multiple myeloma. The overall CR rate for patients treated with allogeneic transplantation ranges from 23 to 76%. Transplant-related mortality ranges from 10 to 54%. The incidence of GVHD following allogeneic transplantation for myeloma appears to be higher than rates following allogeneic transplantation for other hematologic malignancies. The reasons for this occurrence are unclear even when adjusted for factors such as age.

In 1991, Gahrton et al. reported on the EBMT data and showed a poor median survival of 1.5 yr and long-term actuarial survival of 30% with a high relapse rate of 70%, including late relapses occurring many years after transplant (28). In these reports, a variety of preparative regimens were used, howeve, the majority of patients received high-dose cyclophosphamide with TBI or melphalan with TBI. A uniform approach for GVHD prophylaxis was not followed, although acceptable prophylaxis programs were dictated per institution. The treatment-related mortality rate was 25%, primarily due to GVHD, infection, or interstitial pneumonia. The incidence of both acute and chronic GVHD was higher than expected. The overall CR rate was 44%, and the actuarial survival at 4 and 9 yr was 32 and 18%, respectively. In patients who achieved a CR, the 6-yr relapse-free survival was estimated to be 34%. Factors associated with a favorable prognosis included female gender, low β-2 microglobulin level, stage I disease at the time of initial diagnosis, minimal therapy prior to transplantation, and CR after transplantation (29).

These EBMT data were updated in 2001 to include 1368 patients with myeloma who underwent allogeneic transplantation. CR rates reported ranged between 45–50%. It should be noted, however, that less strict response criteria were used in this report (9). Withing this report, a comparison analysis between 225 allogeneic bone marrow transplants performed from 1994 to 1990 with 339 patients, transplanted from 1983 to 1993, was undertaken. This analysis demonstrated a reduction in transplant-related deaths, a reduction of total mortality from 50 to 30%, and a reduction in early mortality from 30 to 20% over that time frame. The actuarial survival was improved to 50% at 4 yr compared to 30% in the group transplanted prior to 1994. A decrease in infections and interstitial pneumonitis, as well as transplanting patients earlier in the course of disease, appear to account for this improvement.

In 1996, using EBMT registry data, Bjorkstrand et al. reported a retrospective analysis that compared 189 allogeneic transplant patients with 189 case-matched autologous transplants as controls. This analysis showed significantly improved survival after autologous transplantation compared to allogeneic transplantation with a median survival of 34 mo compared to 18 mo, respectively. Seventy percent of the autologous patients relapsed compared to 50% of the allogeneic patients. Transplant-related mortality was 41% in the allogeneic group compared to 13% in the autologous group. This study did not identify a specific group of patients that would benefit from allogeneic transplantation *(14)*.

Investigators from Seattle reported the largest single-institution results of allogeneic transplantation for 136 myeloma patients transplanted between 1987 and 1999 *(10)*. One hundred fourteen patients received bone marrow from an HLA-matched sibling, and 22 patients received marrow from mismatched or unrelated donors. Most patients had refractory disease at the time of transplant. Several preparative regimens were used, but the majority received busulfan and cyclophosphamide with or without TBI incorporating shielding of liver and lung. GVHD prophylaxis consisted of cyclosporine and methotrexate. Within the first 100 d, the treatment-related mortality was 48%. The major causes of death included venoocclusive disease of the liver, infection, and GVHD. During the first year, an additional 15% of patients died from complications related to chronic GVHD and infections. The CR was 34%, and the 5-yr probability of survival and progression-free survival were estimated to be 22 and 14%, respectively *(10,30)*.

The Dana-Farber Cancer Center reported 61 patients who underwent allogeneic transplant. All patients had chemotherapy-sensitive disease prior to transplant. The preparative regimens included cyclophosphamide and TBI (80%) or busulfan and cyclophosphamide (20%). Bone marrow was collected from HLA-matched siblings. The marrow was T cell-depleted with anti-CD6 monoclonal antibody and complement for primary GVHD prophylaxis. Only 17% of patients developed grade III–IV acute GVHD (7% developed grade III–V acute GVHD) with this approach. No deaths were attributable to GVHD. The incidence of chronic GVHD was 20%. In addition, treatment-related mortality was only 10%. The overall response rate was 82%, with 23% achieving CR and 60% achieving a PR. The median progression-free survival was 12 mo, and the median overall survival was 22 mo. Although toxicity was low, relapse was problematic *(31)*.

Mehta et al. *(12)* compared allogeneic transplantation with repeat autologous transplants for patients who had failed their first autologous transplant. Although the response rate was higher in the allogeneic group, mortality was significantly higher at 43 vs 10% in the autologous group. Unfortunately, among patients who had allogeneic transplants, a plateau was not yet seen at 5-yr posttransplant *(13)*.

Kulkarni et al. *(32)* reported 33 patients who received HLA-identical allogeneic bone marrow transplants for myeloma. Nineteen patients had received prior chemotherapy and 14 patients had progressed after an autologous transplant. Twenty-eight patients were conditioned with a TBI-containing regimen, and five patients received chemotherapy alone. The source of allogeneic cells was bone marrow in 26 patients, and two patients received peripheral blood stem cells. Seventy-eight percent developed acute GVHD, and treatment-related mortality at 1 yr was 54%. Twelve of the 28 patients (42.8%) with matched sibling donors remained alive. The 2-yr event-free survival was significantly lower in patients who had received an autologous transplant prior to their allogeneic transplant, as compared with patients who had only received an allogeneic transplant (16.7 vs 47.9%; $p = 0.019$) *(32)*.

Couban et al. *(33)* reported on 22 patients who received allogeneic bone marrow transplants from HLA-matched donors. The majority of patients (73%) had chemosensitive disease. Conditioning consisted of TBI and cyclophosphamide ($n = 13$), melphalan and TBI ($n = 1$), or busulfan and cyclophosphamide ($n = 8$). The majority of patients (88%) received cyclosporine and methotrexate for GVHD prophylaxis, while the remainder received cyclosporine, methotrexate, or prednisone alone or in combination. Twenty patients received bone marrow, and two pateints received granulocyte clony-stimulating factor (G-CSF)-mobilized peripheral blood stem cells. The 90-d mortality rate was 27%. The CR rate was 62% and the 3-yr overall survival and event-free survival rates were 32 and 22%, respectively. A high incidence of acute GVHD was observed (86%) with four patients developing grade III–IV acute GVHD *(33)*.

Russell et al. performed allogeneic transplants on 13 patients using TBI (12 gy in six fractions) and melphalan (110 mg/m^2) ($n = 12$) or cyclophosphamide and TBI ($n = 1$) as conditioning regimens. Patients also received radiotherapy to major sites of bone disease the week before admission for transplant. Twelve patients were transplanted from HLA-identical siblings, and one patient was transplanted from an HLA-B-mismatched sister. The stem cell rescue product was from bone marrow in 12 patients ,and blood stem cells were in one. Prophylaxis of GVHD consisted of cyclosporine and methotrexate. Of the 13 patients, 11 were evaluable for response. Ten patients achieved a CR and 9 were disease-free between 7 and 70 mo after transplant. Treatment-related mortality was 15% *(34)*.

Cavo and colleagues reported on 19 patients who received allogeneic transplants for multiple myeloma following high-dose therapy with busulfan and cyclophosphamide *(35)*. Sixty-three percent of patients had refractory disease at the time of transplant. The CR rate was 42%, and the overall survival and event-free survival at 4 yr were estimated at 26 and 21%, respectively. Treatment-related mortality was 37% *(35)*.

The Vancouver group reported on 26 patients who received allogeneic bone marrow transplants. Nineteen patients received HLA-matched sibling donor, and seven patients with a mismatched or unrelated donor. The majority of the patients had chemosensitive disease at the time of transplant. Several different conditioning regimens were administered, and the majority of the patients received cyclosporine and methotrexate for GVHD prophylaxis. The overall treatment-related mortality for related sibling transplants was 16%. The overall response rate was 73%, with 58% of the patients achieving a CR and 23% a PR. At a medium follow-up of 14 mo, the progression-free survival was 40% *(36)*.

4.4. Allogeneic Peripheral Blood Stem Cell Transplantation

Peripheral blood stem cells have largely replaced bone marrow as a source of hematopoietic stem cells for allogeneic transplantation. Several advantages exist for the donor and recipient. The major advantage to the donor is convenience. Advantages to the recipient include more rapid engraftment with shorter hospital stays. Despite the infusion of large number of T cells, the incidence of acute GVHD is not increased following allogeneic peripheral blood stem cell transplantation, although the incidence of chronic GVHD appears to be greater *(37)*.

There is less experience with allogeneic peripheral blood stem cell transplantation for multiple myeloma as compared with bone marrow. One small trial evaluated 10 patients with a median age of 45 yr. Four patients had progressed after an autologous transplant. Donors were HLA-identical and mobilized with filgrastim. Nine patients were conditioned with busulfan and melphalan, and one patient was conditioned with busulfan and cyclophosphamide. Four patients developed grade II or greater acute GVHD, and two patients died from GVHD. The CR rate was 71% with eight patients alive and six in CR at a median of 18.5 mo (range: 7–28 mo) from the transplant. Two patients died and one patient is alive with progressive disease. Polymerase chain reaction (PCR) analysis of immunoglobulin heavy-chain (IgH) rearrangements showed that residual disease was not detectable in four of seven patients *(38)*.

A retrospective study reported by EBMT compared 133 allogeneic blood stem cell transplants to 333 bone marrow transplants matched for prognostic factors and transplanted during the same time period. This study failed to show a difference in overall survival, progression-free survival, transplant-related mortality, or relapse rates *(9)*. This observation differs from the results reported on the prospective randomized trial for other hematologic malignancies that demonstrated reduced relapses and lower transplanted-related mortality in patients that received peripheral blood stem cells *(39,40)*.

4.5. Nonmyeloablative Allogeneic Stem Cell Transplantation

Due to the high treatment-related toxicity seen in allogeneic transplantation and the advanced age of most patients, investigators have begun evaluating the use of nonmyeloablative regimens *(41)*. The rationale for this approach is to minimize the toxicity related to a myeloablative regimen, while instituting a sufficiently immunosuppressive regimen to allow donor cell engraftment. As donor chimerism is achieved, GVM would ensue, which is considered to be the curative mechanism of allogeneic transplantation.

While many trials are ongoing at various institutions, only one published report exists to date. Badros et al. *(42)* reported their results in 16 poor-risk patients with multiple myeloma. The preparative regimen was melphalan 100 mg/m^2. The donors were HLA-matched siblings in 14 patients and mismatched siblings in two patients. DLI were given posttransplant to patients who did not demonstrate clinical GVHD or to attain full donor chimerism ($n = 14$) *(42)*. No treatment-related deaths were observed in the first 100 d. Fifteen patients achieved myeloid engraftment, and 12 patients had full donor chimerism by d 21. Ten patients developed acute GVHD, with one patient dying from grade IV acute GVHD. Seven of these patients went on to develop chronic GVHD. Follow-up was relatively short (median follow-up of 1 yr). Five patients achieved and sustained a CR, three had a "near" CR and four had a PR. Four patients progressed after transplant but three of these patients achieved remission after further chemotherapy with DLI. Two patients died of progressive disease and three patients died of complications related to GVHD.

These results are encouraging particularly in light of the responses seen in this group of poor-risk patients, all of whom had failed one or two prior autologous transplants. Nonetheless, GVHD continues to be a problem although the absence of any treatment-related deaths in the first 100 d is a definite improvement over traditional allogeneic transplant regimens.

The preliminary results with nonmyeloablative allogeneic transplants have enabled clinicians to sequence autologous transplants with nonmyeloablative allogeneic transplants *(43)*.

4.6. Alternative Donors (Unrelated or Mismatched Related Donors)

It is estimated that fewer than 25–35% of patients with multiple myeloma have an HLA-identical sibling who is a suitable donor for allogeneic transplantation. Therefore most patients who are candidates for allogeneic transplantation will require alternative donors. There are relatively little data on allogeneic transplantation using alternative donor transplants for myeloma. The EBMT reported on six alternative donor transplants. Three were from HLA-mismatched related donors, and three were from HLA-matched unrelated donors. Early mortality was high, with five of six patients dying before d 33.

Investigators from Seattle reported on 26 patients transplanted with alternative donors. Twelve patients received either one-antigen-mismatched ($n = 8$) or two-antigen-mismatched ($n = 4$) grafts from related donors. The remaining patients received HLA-matched bone marrow from unrelated donors. Five of the eight one-antigen-mismatched patients died of transplant-related complications. A single patient had progressive disease. Two of eight patients are alive and disease-free at 7 yr after transplantation. Overall, nine of 12 patients who received HLA-matched unrelated donor transplants died of transplant-related complications including GVHD in three patients, regimen-related toxicity in three patients, and infection in three patients. One patient had progressive disease. Two patients were alive and disease-free at 18 mo and 7 yr after transplant *(10)*.

The Vancouver group reported on seven patients who received transplants from unrelated donors or mismatched related donors. Grade II–IV acute GVHD occurred in all seven patients and was the primary cause of death in two. Two patients died of chronic GVHD, and one patient died of progressive disease *(36)*.

Kulkarni et al.reported results from one haploidentical and four matched unrelated bone marrow transplants for myeloma. One patient was alive more than 12 mo following transplantation *(32)*.

These reports represent a limited select group of heavily pretreated patients and further studies are obviously required to determine the efficacy of this approach.

5. DLI FOR RELAPSED MULTIPLE MYELOMA AFTER ALLOGENEIC TRANSPLANTATION

DLI are an important strategy to restore remissions in patients with hematologic malignancies who relapse after an allogeneic transplant. Several studies have demonstrated that patients with myeloma relapsing after an allogeneic transplant can achieve a clinical remission by DLI. As mentioned earlier, this provides support for the existence of a GVM effect *(11,12)*. These observations have prompted several investigators to utilize DLI to treat or prevent relapses in myeloma (Table 2).

Lokhorst et al. *(17)* treated 13 myeloma patients who had relapsed after an allogeneic transplant with DLI. The T-cell dose ranged between 1×10^6/kg and 33×10^7/kg. Eight of 13 patients responded, with four patients achieving a CR and four patients achieving a partial remission *(17)*. Expanding on this initial observation, 27 more patients were treated with 52 courses of DLI at a median of 30 mo after the initial allogeneic transplant. Thirteen patients required reinduction therapy. Fourteen patients (52%) responded to DLI and six patients (22%) achieved a CR. Five patients remained in remission more than 30 mo following DLI. In addition, two patients achieved a molecular remission. Major toxicity associated with DLI included acute GVHD (55%), chronic GVHD (26%), aplasia (19%), and treatment-related mortality (11%). Factors that were predictive of a response to DLI included a T cell dose greater than 1.1×10^8 cells/kg and chemotherapy-sensitive disease before DLI. There was no clinical evidence of GVHD among the 14 patients who responded to DLI *(19)*.

Interestingly, a number of investigators have reported on extramedullary relapses with plasmacytomas in patients treated with DLI who had normal marrow findings and low paraprotein levels at the time of infusion. These observations suggest that extramedullary sites may be a sanctuary for myeloma cells *(44)*.

Alyea and colleagues reported on a prospective trial for 24 patients with myeloma who underwent allogeneic transplantations. Patients received bone marrow transplant with a CD-6 T cell-depleted graft from HLA-identical sibling donors *(20)*. The goals of this trial was for eligible patients to receive prophylactic CD4+ DLI 6–9 mo after bone marrow transplantation in an attempt to reduce treatment-related mortality and induce GVM. The preparative regimen included cyclophosphamide and TBI. T cell depletion was the only GVHD prophylaxis. Acute GVHD developed in five patients (17% grade II and 4% grade III). Fourteen patients received DLI, three patients with CR and 11 patients with persistent disease. GVM was documented in 10 patients with persistent disease, with six patients achieving a CR and patients achieving a partial response. Following DLI, half of the patients developed acute or chronic GVHD. The estimated 2-yr overall survival and progression-free survival for all 24 patients is 55 and 42%, respectively. Of the 14 patients who received DLI, the estimated 2-yr progression-free survival was 65% *(18,20)*.

Current strategies being explored to reduce the significant toxicity of DLI include selective depletion of other T cell subsets or transduction of donor T cells with suicide genes or infusion of antigen-specific T cells *(45,46)*. The optimal timing and dose of DLI to maximize efficacy and minimize toxicity after bone marrow transplantation remains to be defined.

Table 2
DLI for Relapsed Myeloma

Reference	No. of patients	Cell dose range	Chemotherapy	GVHD	Response	Survival
Lokhorst (19)	27	1×10^6/kg–33×10^7/kg	13 patients	14 patients	RR 52% PR 30% CR 22%	Median OS 18 mo
Salama (22)	25	$> 1 \times 10^8$	3 patients	13 patients 13 acute 11 chronic	RR 20% CR 8% PR 13%	OS 48% median 56 wk
Alyea (18)	6	CD4+ 0.3–1.5×10^8	No	3 patients	RR 83% CR 50% PR 33%	Median F/u 26 wk
Alyea (20)	14	CD4+ 0.3–1.5×10^8	No	7 patients	RR 71% CR 2% PR 28%	2-yr PFS 65%

OS, overall survival; RR, response rate; CR, complete remission; PR, partial response; PFS, progression free survival; GVHD, graft-vs-host disease.

Table 3
Prognostic Factors for Allogeneic Transplantation

Favorable Prognostic Factors

EBMTR (9)	Female gender
	Female donor
	IgA myeloma
	Low β-2 microglobulin
	Durie stage I
	Minimal prior chemotherapy
	Complete remission prior to transplant

Unfavorable Prognostic Factors

Bensinger (10)	Albumin <3 g/dL
	Male donors
	Greater than 6 cycles of prior chemotherapy
	Advanced stage Durie III
	Resistant disease
	β-2 microglobulin >2.5 mg/dL
Mehta (13)	Previous Autologous transplant

6. PROGNOSTIC FACTORS FOR ALLOGENEIC TRANSPLANTATION

Several prognostic factors that are associated with the outcome following allogeneic transplantation for multiple myeloma have been identified (Table 3). Recognition of these factors may improve treatment strategies for this disease. After autologous transplantation, a number of poor prognostic indicators have been identified, including elevated β-2 microglobulin and abnormalities in chromosomes 11q and 13 (47,48). These patients should be considered for early allogeneic transplantation if eligible.

The EBMT has defined prognostic factors for response and survival. Favorable prognostic factors include female gender, use of only one treatment regimen prior to transplant, IgA myeloma, low β-2 microglobulin, stage I disease at diagnosis, and CR status prior to transplant *(29)*. In a recent EBMT analysis, donor gender was a significant factor with a female donor and a female recipient having the best outcome and female donor with a male recipient the worst outcome *(9)*. Not all studies support this observation.

The Seattle group identified adverse prognostic factors as transplantation more than 1 yr after diagnosis, β-2 microglobulin >2.5 mg/dL, female gender, transplant from male donors, use of more than eight cycles of chemotherapy, Durie-Salmon stage III disease at the time of transplant and a serum albumin less than 3 g/dL. In addition, several groups have shown that a previous autologous transplant is associated with a poor prognosis. Severe acute GVHD after transplantation is also associated with a poor survival. Achieving a CR predicts for long-term disease-free survival *(10,30)*.

7. TREATMENT-RELATED MORTALITY

Treatment-related mortality is extremely high after allogeneic transplantation, resulting in relatively poor overall and event-free survival. An EBMT analysis compared autologous and allogeneic transplants performed before 1995. This comparison showed that autologous transplant results were superior, due, in part, to higher treatment-related mortality in allogeneic transplant recipients. The causes of treatment-related mortality were acute GVHD (10%), bacterial and fungal infections (18%), and interstitial pneumonia (17%) *(9,28)*. Allogeneic transplants performed between 1983 and 1993 were then compared to transplants done between 1994 and 1998. Transplants in the latter period were associated with a higher CR rate as well as improvement in both overall and event-free survival. Between 1983 and 1993, early treatment-related mortality and total mortality rates were 30 and 50%, respectively. Between 1994 and 1998, these rates had declined to 20 and 30%, respectively. Reductions in the rate of interstitial pneumonitis from lung shielding and use of prophylactic antibiotics to reduce the rates of bacterial and fungal infections were thought to explain the improved outcomes over time *(9)*.

8. MOLECULAR REMISSIONS

Allogeneic transplantation offers the only known curative therapy for myeloma and molecular remissions are frequently obtained. The rearranged IgH is a sensitive tumor marker for detecting minimal residual disease. PCR-based methods can detect patient-specific clonal rearrangements. Two groups have evaluated minimal residual disease by PCR techniques in a small number of patients after allogeneic and autologous transplantation *(49,50)*.

Corradini et al. performed molecular monitoring following allogeneic transplantation (*n* = 14) and autologous transplantation (*n* = 15) *(49)*. Seven allogeneic recipients and one autologous transplant recipient achieved a molecular CR. Martinelli et al. performed molecular monitoring in 44 patients who had achieved a clinical CR after either autologous or allogeneic stem cell transplantation for myeloma *(50)*. Molecular CR was defined as having more than one consecutive negative PCR test. Twelve of 44 patients achieved a molecular CR. Fourteen of 26 patients in clinical CR after allogeneic transplantation were evaluated. Seven (50%) achieved a molecular CR and remained in remission. Thirty of 47 patients in clinical CR after autologous transplantation were evaluated. Only five (16%) of 30 achieved a molecular CR. Molecular CR was observed in a higher percentage of allogeneic transplant recipients and translated into a durable remission. These data support the curative potential of allogeneic transplantation for myeloma.

Cavo evaluated 13 patients who had undergone allogeneic stem cell transplantation for myeloma *(51)*. Patient-specific PCR primers were generated from complementary-determining regions two and three of the rearranged IgH gene. Nine of 12 patients who achieved a CR remained persistently PCR negative for a median of 36 mo and four patients remained PCR negative at 48, 72, and 120 mo after allogeneic transplantation. None of the PCR negative subgroup experienced a relapse, and only one of four PCR positive patients have relapsed. These results demonstrate that allogeneic stem cell transplantation has the potential to induce sustained serological and molecular CR in selected patients with multiple myeloma.

9. FUTURE DIRECTIONS

Current efforts are being directed at improving the outcome for patients undergoing allogeneic transplantation for myeloma. The role of nonmyeloablative allogeneic transplants, either as a single modality or in tandem following an autologous transplant in patients with high-risk features, is being explored. Incorporation of allogeneic transplants for high-risk patients (chromosome 13 abnormalities or failure to achieve a remission with standard dose therapy) at an earlier point in the treatment algorithm is also being evaluated.

Although the results with donor lymphocytes are encouraging, toxicity associated with GVHD remains limiting. Early reports utilizing nonmyeloablative regimens for a variety of hematologic malignancies are encouraging. Graft engineering, donor vaccination with patient-specific vaccines, and suicide gene insertion are all potential methods to reduce transplant-related toxicity and improving outcome.

REFERENCES

1. Landis SH, Murray T, Bolden S, Wingo PA. Cancer statistics. *CA Cancer J Clin* 1999;49:8–31.
2. Kyle RA. Newer approaches to the management of multiple myeloma. *Cancer* 1993;72:3489–3494.
3. Gregory WM, Richards MA, Malpas JS. Combination chemotherapy versus melphalan and prednisone in the treatment of multiple myeloma: an overview of published trials. *J Clin Oncol* 1992;10:334–342.
4. Myeloma Trialists' Collaborative Group. Combination chemotherapy versus melphalan plus prednisone as treatment for multiple myeloma: an overview of 6,633 patients from 27 randomized trials. *J Clin Oncol* 1998;16:3832–3842.
5. Attal M, Harousseau JL, Stoppa AM, et al. Autologous bone marrow transplantation versus conventional chemotherapy in multiple myeloma: a prospective, randomized trial. *N Engl J Med* 1996;335:91–97.
6. Fermand J-P, Ravaud P, Chevret S, et al. High-dose therapy and autologous peripheral blood stem cell transplantation in multiple myeloma: up-front or rescue treatment? Results of a multicenter sequential randomized clinical trial. *Blood* 1998;92:3131–3136.
7. Barlogie B, Jagannath S, Desikan KR, et al. Total therapy with tandem transplants for newly diagnosed multiple myeloma. *Blood* 1999;93:55–65.
8. Attal M, Harousseau JL. Randomized trial experience of the Intergroupe Francophone du Myelome. *Semin Hematol* 2001;38:226–230.
9. Bjorkstrand B. European Group for Blood and Marrow Transplantation Registry studies in multiple myeloma. *Semin Hematol* 2001;38:219–225.
10. Bensinger WI, Maloney D, Storb R. Allogeneic hematopoietic cell transplantation for multiple myeloma. *Semin Hematol* 2001;38:243–249.
11. Tricot G, Vesole DH, Jagannath S, Hilton J, Munshi N, Barlogie. Graft-versus-myeloma effect: proof of principle. *Blood* 1996;87:1196–1198.
12. Mehta J, Singhal S. Graft-versus-myeloma. *Bone Marrow Transplant* 1998;22:835–843.
13. Mehta J, Tricot G, Jagannath S, et al. Salvage autologous or allogeneic transplantation for multiple myeloma refractory to or relapsing after a first-line autograft? *Bone Marrow Transplant* 1998;21:887–892.
14. Bjorkstrand B, Ljungman P, Svensson H, et al. Allogeneic bone marrow transplantation versus autologous stem cell transplantation in multiple myeloma—a retrospective case-matched study from the European Group for Blood and Marrow Transplantation. *Blood* 1996;88:4711–4718.
15. Kolb HJ, Schattenberg A, Goldman JM, et al. Graft-versus-leukemia effect of donor lymphocyte transfusions in marrow grafted patients. *Blood* 1995;86:2041–2050.
16. Collins R, Shpilberg O, Drobyski W, et al. Donor leukocyte infusions in 140 patients with relapsed malignancy after allogeneic bone marrow transplantation. *J Clin Oncol* 1997;13:433–444.

17. Lokhorst HM, Schattenberg JJ, Cornelissen JJ, Thomas LLM, Verdonck LF. Donor lymphocyte infusions are effective in relapsed multiple myeloma after allogeneic transplantation. *Blood* 1997;90:4206–4211.
18. Alyea E, Soiffer RJ, Canning C, et al. Toxicity and efficacy of defined doses of CD 4 (+). donor lymphocytes for treatment of relapse after allogeneic bone marrow transplant. *Blood* 1998; 91:3671–3680.
19. Lokhorst HM, Schattenberg A, Cornelissen JJ, et al. Donor lymphocyte infusions for relapsed multiple myeloma after allogeneic stem-cell transplantation: predictive factors for response and long-term outcome. *J Clin Oncol* 2000;18:3031–3037.
20. Alyea E, Weller E, Schlossman R, et al. T-cell-depleted allogeneic bone marrow transplantation followed by donor lymphocyte infusion in patients with multiple myeloma: induction of graft-versus-myeloma effect. *Blood* 2001;98:934–939.
21. Orsini E, Alyea EP, Schlossman R, et al. Changes in T cell receptor repertoire associated with graft-versus-tumor effect and graft-versus-host disease in patients with relapsed multiple myeloma after donor lymphocyte infusion. *Bone Marrow Transplant* 2000;25:623–632.
22. Salama M, Nevill T, Marcellus D, et al. Donor leukocyte for multiple myeloma. *Bone Marrow Transplant* 2000;26:1179–1184.
23. Libura J, Hoffmann T, Passweg JR, et al. Graft-versus-myeloma after withdrawal of immunosuppression following allogeneic peripheral stem cell transplantation. *Bone Marrow Transplant* 1999;24:925–927.
24. Kwak LW, Taub DD, Duffy PL, et al. Transfer of myeloma idiotype-specific immunity from an actively immunized marrow donor. *Lancet* 1995;345:1016–1020.
25. Durie BGM, Dixon Do, Carter S, et al. Improved survival duration with combination chemotherapy induction for multiple myeloma: a Southwest Oncology Group Study. *J Clin Oncol* 1986;4:1227–1237.
26. Bensinger WI, Demirer T, Buckner CD, et al. Syngeneic marrow transplantation in patients with multiple myeloma. *Bone Marrow Transplant* 1996;18:527–531.
27. Gahrton G, Svensson H, Bjorkstrand B, et al. Syngeneic transplantation in multiple myeloma—a case-matched comparison with autologous and allogeneic transplantation. *Bone Marrow Transplant* 1999;24:741–745.
28. Gahrton G, Tura S, Ljungman P, et al. Allogeneic bone marrow transplantation in multiple myeloma. *N Engl J Med* 1991;325:1267–1273.
29. Gahrton G, Tura S, Ljungman P, et al. Prognostic factors in allogeneic bone marrow transplantation for multiple myeloma. *J Clin Oncol* 1995;13:1312–1322.
30. Bensinger WI, Buckner CD, Anasetti C, et al. Allogeneic Marrow Transplantation for Multiple Myeloma: an Analysis of Risk Factors on Outcome. *Blood* 1996;88:2787–2793.
31. Schlossman SF, Alyea E, Orsini E, et al. Immune based strategies to improve hematopoietic stem cell transplantation in multiple myeloma. In: Dicke KA, Keating A, eds. *Autologous Marrow and Blood Transplantation*. Carden, Jennings, Charlottesville, VA, 1999, pp. 207–221.
32. Kulkarni S, Powles RL, Treleaven JG, et al. Impact of previous high-dose therapy on outcome after allografting for multiple myeloma. *Bone Marrow Transplant* 1999;23:675–680.
33. Couban S, Stewart AK, Loach D, Panzarella T, and Meharchand J. Autologous and allogeneic transplantation for multiple myeloma at a single center. *Bone Marrow Transplant* 1997;19:783–789.
34. Russell NH, Miflin G, Stainer C, et al. Allogeneic bone marrow transplant for multiple myeloma. *Blood* 1997;89:2610–2611.
35. Cavo M, Bandini G, Benni M, et al. High dose busulfan and cyclophosphamide are an effective conditioning regimen for allogeneic bone marrow transplantation in chemosensitive multiple myeloma. *Bone Marrow Transplant* 1998;22:27–32.
36. Reece DE, Shepard JD, Klingemann HG, et al. Treatment of myeloma using intensive therapy and allogeneic bone marrow transplantation. *Bone Marrow Transplant* 1995;15:117–123.
37. Schmitz N, Bacigalupo A, Hasenclever D, et al. Allogeneic bone marrow transplantation vs filgrastim-mobilized peripheral blood progenitor cell transplantation in patients with early leukemia: first results of a randomized multicentre trial of the European Group of Blood and Marrow Transplantation. *Bone Marrow Transplant* 1998;21:995–1003.
38. Majolino I, Corradini P, Scime R, et al. Allogeneic transplantation of unmanipulated peripheral blood stem cells in patients with multiple myeloma. *Bone Marrow Transplant* 1998;22:449–455.
39. Bensinger WI, Clift R, Martin P, et al. Allogeneic peripheral blood stem cell transplantation in patients with advanced hematologic malignancies: a retrospective comparison with marrow transplantation. *Blood* 1996;88:2794–2000.
40. Bensinger WI, Martin PJ, Storer B, et al. Transplantation of bone marrow as compared with peripheral-blood cells from HLA-identical relatives in patients with hematologic cancers. *N Engl J Med* 2001;344:175–181.
41. Slavin S, Nagler A, Naparstek E, et al. Nonmyeloablative stem cell transplantation and cell therapy as an alternative to conventional bone marrow transplantation with lethal cytoreduction for the treatment of malignant and nonmalignant hematologic diseases. *Blood* 1998;91:756–763.

42. Bardros A, Barlogie B, Morris C, et al. High response rate in refractory and poor-risk multiple myeloma after allotransplantation using a nonmyeloablative regimen and donor lymphocte infusions. *Blood* 2001;97:2574–2579.
43. Molina A, Sahebi F, Maloney DG, et al. Non-myeloablative peripheral blood stem cell (PBSC) alloggrafts following cytoreductive autotransplants for treatment of multiple myeloma (MM). *Blood* 2000;96(suppl 1):480a.
44. Zomas A, Stefanoudak K,Fisfis, M et al. Graft-versus-myeloma after donor leukocyte infusion: maintenance of marrow remission but extramedullary relapse with plasmacytomas. *Bone Marrow Transplant* 1998;21:1163–1165.
45. Soiffer RJ, Murray C, Mauch P, et al. Prevention of graft-versus-host disease by selective depletion of CD6-positive T lymphocytes from donor bone marrow. *J Clin Oncol* 1992;10:1191–1200.
46. Bonini C, Ferrari G, Verzeletti S, et al. HSV-TK gene transfer into donor lymphocytes for control of allogeneic graft-versus-leukemia. *Science* 1997;276:1719–1724.
47. Zojer N, Konigsberg R, Ackermann J, Fritz E, et al. Deletion of 13q14 remains an independent adverse prognostic variable in multiple myeloma despite its frequent detection by interphase flurescence in situ hybridization. *Blood* 2000;95:1925–1930.
48. Facon T, Avet-loiseau H, Guillerm G, et al. Chromosome 13 abnormalities identified by FISH analysis and serum B-2 microglobulin produce a powerful myeloma staging system for patients receiving high-dose therapy. *Blood* 2001;97:1566–1571.
49. Corradini P, Voena C, Tarella C, et al. Molecular and clinical remission in multiple myeloma: role of autologous and allogeneic transplantation of hematopoietic cells. *J Clin Oncol* 1999;17:208–215.
50. Martinelli G, Terragna C, Zamagni E, et al. Molecular remission after allogeneic or autologous transplantation of hematopoietic stem cells for multiple myeloma. *J Clin Oncol* 2000;18:2273–2281.
51. Cavo M, Terragna C, Martinelli G, et al. Molecular monitoring of minimal residual disease in patients in long-term complete remission after allogeneic stem cell transplantation for multiple myeloma. *Blood* 2000;96:355–357.

7

Non-Hodgkin's Lymphoma

Igor Espinoza-Delgado, MD and Dan L. Longo, MD

1. INTRODUCTION

It is estimated that 56,200 new cases of non-Hodgkin's lymphoma (NHL) were diagnosed in the United States in 2001, and approx 26,300 people died from NHL, which makes it the fifth leading cause of cancer death in men and the sixth leading cause of cancer death among women *(1)*. NHLs represent around 5% of all newly diagnosed cancers and, in contrast with other malignancies that are decreasing in incidence, the overall incidence of NHL has been increasing at 3–5%/yr since 1950 and increased by 81% between 1973 and 1997. The reasons for this overall increase in the incidence are not clear. However, the combined influences of several factors such as a rise in the number of patients with immunocompromised states and an increase in the aging population may contribute to this trend *(2,3)*. The increased incidence of NHL combined with a stable Hodgkin's disease incidence and noticeably improved survival has dramatically changed the composition of total lymphoma mortality. Indeed, Hodgkin's disease accounted for nearly 40% of lymphoma deaths in 1950, but now represents less than 7%. The 5-yr survival of patients with NHL is 51%. These significant changes warrant that major efforts be undertaken both at the clinical and the basic research level to define steps that may help us to control and improve the outcome of patients with NHL.

NHL are a heterogeneous group of malignancies with complex biological features resulting in a variety of clinical manifestations. The new World Health Organization classification of lymphoid malignancies identifies at least 33 named entities, including lymphoid leukemias and myeloma *(4)*. Nevertheless, about 70% of patients with NHL in the United States have either follicular lymphoma (indolent, natural history measured in years) or diffuse large B cell lymphoma (aggressive, natural history measured in months). Most patients with NHL have advanced-stage disease at the time of diagnosis, and despite a relatively high rate of response to treatment, a significant percentage of patients will relapse and eventually die as a consequence of the NHL. There is great interest in the development of innovative therapeutic approaches for NHL, because only about half of patients will be cured with standard treatments, and the overall survival in some subtypes has remained stable for many years *(5)*.

From: *Current Clinical Oncology: Allogeneic Stem Cell Transplantation*
Edited by: Mary S. Laughlin and Hillard M. Lazarus © Humana Press Inc., Totowa, NJ

High dose chemotherapy (HDCT) followed by the transplantation of hematopoietic stem cells is increasingly being used in the treatment of aggressive hematological malignancies, such as acute leukemia and aggressive NHL. Both bone marrow and peripheral blood stem cells are effective in treating these diseases, as are both autologous and allogeneic sources for the grafts. The role of HDCT followed by autologous transplantation in NHL has been explored in several clinical trials and should be considered in patients who do not achieve complete remission with initial therapy or in those who develop early relapses. The Parma trial, in which autologous bone marrow transplantation (BMT) was compared with conventional-dose salvage chemotherapy in patients with chemotherapy-sensitive relapses of NHL, demonstrated that 46% of the patients in the transplant arm were alive and disease-free 5 yr after therapy compared to only 12% in the salvage chemotherapy arm (6). Comparable results were also obtained in a phase II clinical trial conducted by the Southwest Oncology Group Trial in a similar group of patients (7). Therefore, this approach has become the gold standard in patients with chemotherapy-sensitive relapsed aggressive histology NHL. Requirements for demonstrated disease chemosensitivity, restrictions on the age of eligibility, a high relapse rate after transplant, and late complications such as second malignancies and myelodysplasia, limit the number of patients who may benefit from this approach.

The role of HDCT with autologous stem cells in the primary treatment of patients with NHL is more controversial, with some studies concluding that this approach has no role in primary management and others concluding that patients with high or high-intermediate risk factors may benefit (8).

There is renewed interest in the role of allogeneic stem cell transplantation (alloSCT) for patients with NHL. A major advantage of alloSCT is the potential to exploit a graft-vs-lymphoma (GVL) effect. Although allogeneic transplantation was initially designed to treat aggressive recurrent acute leukemia, it also has been demonstrated to be effective in the treatment of less aggressive hematological malignancies, such as chronic myeloid leukemia (CML) and multiple myeloma. The success of this approach has prompted researchers to investigate the role of transplantation in other malignancies with indolent behavior, and promising results have been reported in follicular lymphoma and CLL (5,9,10). Although HDCT followed by alloSCT represents an attractive approach for the treatment of NHL, its full therapeutic potential has not been reached for several reasons, including the occurrence of graft-vs-host disease (GVHD), toxicity of the preparative regimen, the lack of full immune reconstitution, infections, and most important, the inability to completely eliminate tumor cells. In this chapter, we shall discuss potential clinical interventions designed to circumvent some of the above-mentioned obstacles and, therefore, improve the outcome of patients with NHL undergoing allogeneic SCT.

2. ALLOGENEIC BMT FOR NHL?

The optimal management of patients with low-grade lymphoma remains controversial, because of the absence of evidence that treatment influences the natural history of the disease and because of the patients' prolonged survival even without treatment, and in the presence of advanced-stage disease. However, most patients with advanced-stage disease will go on to relapse and die of their lymphoma, often after a change in pattern of growth (to diffuse) and an acceleration in natural history. The treatment of advanced-stage patients (III and IV) has generally followed two divergent approaches (11,12): (i) an aggressive approach that has included radiation therapy, combination chemotherapy, or combined modality therapy; and (ii) a conservative approach that involves no initial treatment followed by single-agent chemotherapy or involved-field radiotherapy if required (12,13). This dichotomy is due to the fact that most forms of systemic therapy have produced high complete response rates, but have failed to produce long-term disease-free survival or prolong overall survival. In an attempt to improve the outcome of these patients, HDCT with either autologous or allogeneic stem cells is being evaluated.

Patients with advanced-stage follicular NHL are very likely to have involvement of the bone marrow and peripheral blood by tumor cells. Therefore, one of the major obstacles to the use of autologous stem cell transplantation (autoSCT) is the potential for reinfusing tumor cells to the recipient, which is associated with an increased risk of relapse (14–16). Indeed, patients with lymphoid malignancies that are treated with HDCT and autoSCT suffer more relapses than those undergoing allogeneic SCT (17,18), though it is not clear whether the difference reflects reinfusing tumor cells with the stem cells. Furthermore, long-term follow-up of patients with NHL who have undergone autoSCT substantiates a high incidence of myelodysplastic syndromes (MDS), especially in those patients who received total body irradiation as part of their conditioning regimen (19–21). The limitations of autoSCT for NHL have become evident, and a revitalized interest in allogeneic SCT is evolving. There is significant evidence that in NHL, allogeneic SCT has predominantly yielded excellent relapse-free survival superior to that of autoSCT (10,18,22–25); however, the adverse effects associated with allografting, particularly GVHD, lack of immune reconstitution, and toxicity of the preparative regimen, have masked the advantage so that the overall survival is comparable to autoSCT (17). Allografting is also becoming increasingly used as a salvage treatment for patients relapsing after autologous BMT. In this particular setting, the results have been mixed, with some groups reporting a dismally low disease-free survival and advising against this approach (26). On the other hand, Bierman et al. (27) reported 16 patients who had failed autologous transplantation and received either an allogeneic bone marrow or peripheral blood progenitor cell transplant. Forty-four percent of patients died within 100 d of the transplant, and the overall treatment-related mortality was more than 60%. There were no deaths for any reason other than treatment-related complications. Remarkably, no patient died of recurrent lymphoma (27). Recently, the International Bone Marrow Transplant Registry group reported the results of an observational study conducted in 50 centers in patients with advanced-stage low-grade lymphoma (28). Eighty-one percent of the patients had stage IV disease, most commonly due to bone marrow involvement, 38% had refractory disease, and 30% had poor performance status. More than one-third of the patients were felt to have chemotherapy-resistant disease (i.e., they had achieved less than a partial remission to the last chemotherapy regimen administered before transplant). The 3-yr probabilities of recurrence, survival, and disease-free survival were 16, 49, and 49%, respectively. Most of the mortality was treatment-related, and recurrence was uncommon (only one recurrence among 33 patients followed for more than 2 yr). This rate of recurrence is lower than that reported for autologous transplantation and is consistent with other reports (29,30). It is possible that the low recurrence rate is due to multiple factors, including a GVL effect that has been reported by others (22,24,31,32), and/or lack of tumor contamination in the allogeneic graft. The characteristics of the patients in this study and their outcome are similar to those reported in single institution series (33–35), suggesting that the observed consistent benefits are genuine and warrant further investigation of this approach.

3. PROBLEMS ASSOCIATED WITH ALLOGENEIC SCT

Although allogeneic transplantation is a very appealing therapeutic approach for patients with advanced-stage NHL, its results are far from being optimal, and several drawbacks need to be addressed if allogeneic SCT is to become a widely used therapeutic tool for NHL. The most difficult therapeutic goals are: (i) ameliorating the toxicities of and improving the efficacy of the preparative regimens; (ii) preventing and treating GVHD without compromising bone marrow engraftment or immune reconstitution; and (iii) promoting both general and tumor-specific immune reconstitution of the recipient.

3.1. Alloresponse and the Case for Nonmyeloablative SCT

Allogeneic SCT classically has used high doses of chemotherapy and/or radiation therapy for both eradication of the underlying malignancy and suppression of the patient's immune system to allow engraftment of the donor hematopoietic stem cells. These preparative regimens are associated with severe hematologic and nonhematologic toxicities, which result in significant morbidity and mortality *(36)*. Until recently, SCT was considered a supportive-care modality for restoring hematopoiesis. However, a significant part of the curative potential of allogeneic SCT is due to another effect of the donor stem cell population, the development of an immune-mediated graft-vs-tumor (GVT) effect *(37,38)*. The efficacy of the antitumor activity of the donor immune system (allograft) is supported by evidence of an increased rate of relapse in recipients of T cell-depleted allografts, a higher relapse risk after syngeneic marrow transplantation, and an inverse correlation between relapse rate and severity of GVHD *(39–44)*. The most compelling evidence of a GVT effect is the finding that donor lymphocyte infusions (DLI), can reinduce remission in patients with leukemia who have relapsed after allogeneic SCT *(45–47)*. The GVT effect has been observed in other malignancies including multiple myeloma *(48–51)*, renal cell cancer *(52)*, CLL *(53)*, and NHL *(31,32,54,55)*.

The data suggested that GVT effects contribute to therapeutic efficacy of allogeneic SCT. In addition, independent evidence suggested that higher doses of drugs and radiation therapy in the preparative regimen exacerbated the severity of GVHD through increased tissue damage and associated inflammation with systemic cytokine production *(56–58)*. Furthermore, some authors felt that GVHD and GVT were separable effects. These lines of thought led to the hypothesis that a reduction in the doses of the preparative regimen might reduce the collateral damage to normal tissue, reduce GVHD, and rely more heavily on the adoptively transferred lymphocytes to eliminate the tumor. Nonmyeloablative preparative regimens were designed to suppress the immune system of the patient to allow the engraftment of the donor stem cells and development of a GVT effect. This relatively low dose preparative regimen should produce less toxicity and be effective in settings in which GVT effects are operative, such as NHL. The approach is called nonmyeloablative SCT (NMS). If this approach were effective and reduced the treatment-related complications, it would open the possibility of allogeneic SCT for the elderly and for patients with comorbid conditions, which are contraindications to high dose allogeneic SCT that preclude the participation of a significant percentage of patients with NHL.

The development of purine analogs, fludarabine and 2-chlorodeoxyadenosine, with impressive toxicity directed at lymphocytes has helped to advance the field of NMS. The toxic effects of nucleosides are more prominent in T cells than in B cells or CD34+ precursors *(59,60)*. Fludarabine has the additional advantages of having a significant antilymphoma activity and low toxicity to other tissues *(61,62)*; hence, it has been incorporated into the majority of the nonmyeloablative regimens described thus far. Investigators from the M.D. Anderson Cancer Center reported results observed in 15 patients with lymphoid malignancies treated with a fludarabine-based low dose conditioning regimen *(54,55)*. At the time of transplant, 12 patients had active disease with either primary refractory disease or recurrent disease after primary chemotherapy and they were treated with fludarabine and cyclophosphamide or fludarabine, cyclophosphamide and cisplatin. These regimens were given at nonmyeloablative doses, so mixed hematopoietic chimerism (i.e., blood cells derived from both the donor and the host) was anticipated. Eleven patients achieved engraftment of donor cells with the percentage of donor

Table 1
Characteristics of Patients and Clinical Outcome of Minitransplant Approaches

No. of patients	Median age	Engraftment	Responses	> Grade II toxicity	References
15	55	11 (73%)	CR 8 (53%) PR 3 (20%)	0	54
11	51	11 (100%)	CR 11 (100%)	0	63

CR, complete remission; PR, partial response.

cells, in the marrow ranging from 50 to 100% at 4 wk after transplant. One patient had 75% donor cells in the marrow at 6 wk posttransplant and converted to 100% donor cells after DLI. The four patients who had failed to engraft were those who received the lower dose level of chemotherapy, and they experienced prompt recovery of autologous hematopoiesis without serious adverse effects. The regimen was well-tolerated, with no patient developing > grade II nonhematologic toxicity. All 11 patients with donor engraftment have experienced antitumor responses, with eight patients achieving complete remission. Responses were slow in developing and took up to 1 yr to be achieved in some patients. Interestingly, responses were observed even in patients with mixed chimerism.

Based on these promising results, Khouri et al. conducted a phase II clinical trial using NMS in patients with recurrent NHL (63). Eleven patients with a median age of 51 yr were enrolled in the study, nine patients had chemotherapy-sensitive disease, and two had chemotherapy-refractory disease (Table 1). The median duration of severe neutropenia was 6 d, and infection was limited to three episodes of fever of unknown origin. Eight patients never required platelet transfusion, and engraftment was achieved in all patients. The median percentage of donor cells in patients' bone marrow was 80% (range 5–100%). No patient had a nonhematologic toxicity > grade II. Two patients developed acute GVHD limited to the skin, and one of the patients with grade III GVHD responded to antithymocyte globulin (ATG). All patients achieved complete remission, and no relapses have been observed with a median follow up of 16 mo.

Given the protracted natural history of low-grade lymphoma, it is too early to make a definitive statement regarding the role of NMS in indolent lymphoma. However, the preliminary results are very encouraging and warrant further investigation of NMS for the treatment of NHL. One interesting observation derived from this study is that durable responses were obtained in patients who had a minimal number of donor cells, suggesting that in low-grade lymphoma, full chimerism may not be required to achieve optimal results. This finding may have important implications, because there is evidence that mixed donor chimerism is associated with a lower incidence of acute GVHD (64).

Despite the optimism raised by the initial experiences with NMS, there are some concerns that need to be addressed. For instance, it remains unclear how much of a tumor burden can be treated with NMS. Patients with active bulky disease or those with primary refractory disease may have difficulty in achieving significant responses to NMS. These patients may need to be cytoreduced first (by either conventional chemotherapy or HDCT and autologous transplantation) and then undergo NMS. Carella et al. reported this layered approach in 15 patients, 10 patients had Hodgkin's disease, and five patients had NHL (65). All five patients with NHL had stage IV bulky disease and were a median of 25 mo from diagnosis. Two had primary refractory disease, and one each was in first, third, and fourth relapse. All five patients achieved a partial response after autologous transplantation and underwent NMS at a median of 61 d after the autoSCT. Four patients attained complete remission, and one had progressive disease. These preliminary results are very encouraging and further studies are required to ascertain whether similar results can be accomplished with conventional-dose salvage chemotherapy instead of HDCT followed by autoSCT.

3.2. Immune Reconstitution and Minimal Residual Disease

Tumor relapse is one of the major barriers for successful transplantation in lymphomas. The relapses following HDCT with either autoSCT or allogeneic SCT are associated with persistent chemoresistant minimal residual disease (MRD), suggesting that these patients will not benefit from further chemotherapy-based approaches. Therefore, novel strategies for posttransplantation therapy are required. One approach to reduce relapse rates is to amplify immune-mediated mechanisms against lymphomas. This could potentially be accomplished by immunization with lymphoma-specific vaccine, by administration of cytokines, which may facilitate immunological recognition or activate antilymphoma effector mechanisms, or perhaps by using targeted immunotherapy with monoclonal antibodies (mAbs).

3.2.1. Lymphoma Vaccination

Immunoglobulin molecules (Ig) contain highly specific unique peptide sequences in their variable regions at their antigen-combining sites in the complementarity determining regions (CDRs). The variable region of heavy and light chains combine to form the unique antigen recognition site of the Ig protein. These variable regions contain determinants that can themselves be recognized as antigens or idiotypes. NHLs are usually (85%) clonal proliferations of B cells synthesizing a single type of antibody molecule with unique variable regions, which can serve as a tumor-specific antigen (66). These unique idiotypic determinants can be targeted for cancer vaccination. Follicular lymphomas are also associated with a characteristic chromosomal translocation that brings the bcl-2 gene in chromosome 18 under the transcriptional influence of the Ig heavy chain gene located in chromosome 14. This translocation t(14;18) involving the major breakpoint region has been used as a molecular marker for MRD (67,68). Most patients with follicular lymphoma in complete remission after conventional dose chemotherapy still have cells bearing the t(14;18) detectable by polymerase chain reaction (PCR) (68) and they seem to be at increased risk of relapse.

A pilot clinical trial has been reported using a new idiotype protein vaccine that eradicates residual t(14;18)+ lymphoma cells from the peripheral blood in a significant number of patients in complete remission after a ProMACE-based chemotherapy regimen called PACE (prednisone, doxorubicin, cyclophosphamide, etoposide) (69). Twenty previously untreated patients with stage III/IV follicular lymphoma underwent lymph node collection and were then uniformly treated with combination chemotherapy to complete remission plus two additional cycles. After at least 6 mo of immune recovery, each patient received 4-monthly vaccinations with the lymphoma-associated Ig idiotype with keyhole limpet hemocyanin (KLH) plus granulocyte-macrophage colony stimulating factor (GM-CSF) as adjuvant. Eleven out of 20 patients were found to have detectable translocation in their primary tumor. All 11 patients had evidence of the malignant clone detectable in their blood by PCR both at diagnosis and after chemotherapy, despite being in complete clinical remission. Eight of the 11 patients achieved and sustained molecular remission after the vaccinations. Tumor-specific CD8+ cells were uniformly found in 19 of 20 patients. Furthermore, CD4+ tumor-specific cells, which may be required for the generation and maintenance of the CD8+ cells, were also induced by vaccination. Although the long-term clinical relevance of molecular remission in follicular lymphoma patients remains to be ascertained (68,70), it is clear that vaccination either reduces the tumor burden beyond that already achieved by chemotherapy or led to the redistribution of residual tumor cells to sites other than peripheral blood. This trial provides definitive evidence for an antitumor effect of lymphoma-specific vaccination and will require a randomized trial comparing chemotherapy alone with chemotherapy plus vaccination to determine the long-term clinical benefit of this approach. The study also suggests that a similar approach may be taken in the context of MRD after NMS in patients with NHL. It is possible that elicitation of lymphoma-specific T cells, both CD8+ and CD4+, may result in long-term antitumor immunity and possibly prolonged remission.

A second approach to vaccination in lymphoma is based on animal and human studies that have established the principle that immunity to certain antigens can be transferred from the marrow donor to the recipient *(71–74)*. This strategy entails the immunization of the immunologically normal allogeneic donor with the idiotype vaccine derived from the recipient's tumor before harvesting the stem cells to be used in the transplant. This strategy may generate in the donor highly specific antilymphoma T cells that are capable of transferring antitumor idiotype-specific immunity from bone marrow transplant donor to recipient. This approach has been already successfully used in a patient with multiple myeloma, and it was clearly demonstrated that a *de novo* anti-idiotype response was transferred to the recipient *(75)*. This approach is applicable when the host's immune system is suppressed by HDCT. It is tempting to speculate that the use of nonmyeloablative regimens and the use of booster immunizations of the recipient may allow the reconstituted immune system to mount a more vigorous and efficacious antitumor response. Another potential benefit of transferring highly specific anti-idiotype effector cells is the possibility of decreasing the severity of GVHD. This approach could be optimized by ex vivo expansion of the anti-idiotype-specific T cells. Ex vivo-expanded antigen-specific T cells have been successfully used in patients with advanced metastatic melanoma *(76,77)*. Such cells have also been used for the treatment of cytomegalovirus and Epstein-Barr virus infections after alloSCT *(78,79)* and in refractory CML *(80)*.

Alternatively, immunization against lymphomas could be accomplished by using monocyte-derived dendritic cells (DCs) as carriers of idiotype. A DC-based vaccine has been already successfully applied in NHL *(81)*. DCs are potent professional antigen-presenting cells (APCs) and have the potential for priming naive T cells and eliciting an antigen-specific T-cell response. This unique feature of DCs could be further exploited in the context of a lymphoma whole-cell vaccine. This strategy may target potential lymphoma antigens other than idiotype that are not yet defined and thus widening the T cell repertoire against the lymphoma. Finally, genetically modified lymphoma cells could be used as their own APC *(82)*. Further research is required to ascertain the benefits of the above-mentioned approaches, particularly in a peritransplant setting.

3.2.2. CYTOKINE THERAPY

Multiple immune alterations, including decreased T cell responses to mitogen, antigens, or allogeneic stimulation and impairment of interleukin (IL)-2 production has been reported in patients following BMT or intensive chemotherapy *(83–88)*. The ineffective immune reconstitution post-SCT related in part to the inability of the involuted thymus to generate new antigen-naive T cells may account for the inability of the patient to eliminate MRD and reduce the clinical response rate and duration of response. It is now clear that T cells are mainly responsible for the GVT effect observed in the allogeneic SCT and after DLI. Therefore, it seems reasonable to design and to investigate strategies to improve the immune-mediated mechanisms that are already in place in the allogeneic setting.

IL-2, is a potent activator of T cells, natural killer (NK) cells, B cells, and monocytes *(89–91)* that may play an important role in recognizing and mounting an effective immune response against MRD. The rationale for IL-2-based immunotherapy after SCT for hematological malignancies is based on preclinical and clinical data. IL-2 has been shown to induce effector cells against lymphoma cells in vitro *(92,93)* and preliminary pilot clinical trials demonstrated antitumor effects in Hodgkin's disease and NHL *(94–97)*. Investigators have also used IL-2 alone or in conjunction with either cellular therapy or interferon (IFN)-α in the context of autoSCT *(98–100)*, with encouraging but inconclusive results. A major advantage of IL-2 immunotherapy is a lack of cross-resistance to chemotherapy or radiotherapy *(101)*.

Biotherapy with IL-2 should be more efficacious in a setting of low tumor burden, i.e., MRD or no evidence of disease (NED) after conventional dose chemotherapy or HDCT plus SCT. The posttransplant setting may be more suitable than the post-conventional dose chemotherapy setting, because in the former, there may be fewer residual malignant cells. In a leukemia murine model, Slavin et al. has demonstrated that the efficacy of GVL effects can be substantially enhanced by the in vivo administration of IL-2 *(102–105)*. Although these animal studies are very encouraging, we need to be careful in translating these findings into clinical trials in humans, because of the possibility that IL-2 could exacerbate GVHD. The use of IL-2 after allogeneic SCT is based on the assumption that a GVL effect can be augmented without concurrently increasing GVHD.

IL-2 therapy after T cell-depleted SCT has been reported to decrease the relapse rate without increasing GVHD, as compared to historical controls who received T cell-depleted SCT without IL-2 therapy *(106)*. However, IL-2 given after non-T cell-depleted SCT could potentially induce a greater GVL and a greater GVHD. Fefer et al. conducted a phase I trial of IL-2 after non-T cell-depleted allogeneic SCT in children with leukemia beyond first complete remission *(107)*. The aim was to identify a dose of IL-2 that could be used in the allogeneic SCT setting. Because IL-2 could conceivably exacerbate GVHD, and because the immunosuppressive agents used to prevent GVHD in adults could interfere with any immunologic antitumor effect of IL-2 therapy, IL-2 was administered only to children who had no GVHD when immunosuppressive drugs were discontinued. The study identified a dose of IL-2 that could be administered safely early after unmodified human leukocyte antigen (HLA)-identical SCT to children without GVHD. Clearly, there is a need to perform similar studies in adults with NHL that eventually will lead to prospective randomized studies addressing the question whether IL-2 post-allogeneic SCT can reduce the incidence of relapse without increasing the incidence of GVHD. Until then, IL-2 in a peritransplant setting should be used only within the context of well-designed clinical trials.

One other major obstacle with IL-2-based therapy is the substantial acute toxicity observed in patients receiving high dose IL-2. One approach to decrease IL-2-induced toxicity, and simultaneously increase its antitumor activity in patients with NHL and MRD after SCT, is to combine low dose IL-2 with a biological with intrinsic antitumor activity and the potential of synergizing with IL-2. Bryostatin-1 exhibits a unique pattern of biological activities, including antitumor activity and immunomodulatory activity. In preclinical models, we have demonstrated that Bryostatin-1 by itself has significant antilymphoma activity *(108)*. Furthermore, our group reported that Bryostatin-1 synergizes with low dose IL-2 in activating human monocytes *(109)*. In a murine model, it was demonstrated that Bryostatin-1 plus low dose IL-2 exerted significant antitumor activity without the toxicity associated with high dose IL-2 *(110)*. We are currently conducting a phase I trial to establish the safety profile of the combination of Bryostatin and low dose IL-2 in adults. These results are very promising and warrant further investigation of this combination in a posttransplant setting.

In summary, a significant body of evidence demonstrates the presence of many alterations in the immune system of patients undergoing SCT. Future studies in this area should focus on strategies aimed to harness the allograft to enhance GVT without worsening GVHD. At the present time, a role for IL-2 in a peritransplant setting is not clearly established. It is possible that the ultimate role of IL-2 in the treatment of hematological malignancies may be in the generation and clonal expansion of T cells with lymphoma-specific reactivity.

3.2.3. Monoclonal Antibodies

Despite the potential benefits that patients with NHL may derive from allogeneic transplantation a significant percentage of patients undergoing this procedure will relapse. Treating patients with a non-cross-resistant immunotherapy, e.g., directed monoclonal antibody therapy, may offer the opportunity of eradicating MRD after transplantation and therefore it has the potential for increasing both the number and the duration of complete responses that may lead to an improve survival in NHL. Unlabeled and labeled mAbs targeted to CD20, CD52, CD19 and CD25 have been investigated for several years for the treatment of patients with NHL. The anti-lymphoma activity observed in early clinical trials using murine mAbs was more limited than initially anticipated. The lack of efficacy was probably related to: 1) the immunogenicity of the murine mAb that led to a short half-live and prevented repeated administration, 2) defects in murine antibodies directing antibody-mediated cytotoxicity, and 3) inadequate fixation of human complement. Most recently, major advances in molecular biology and chelation chemistry have led to the development of chimeric and humanized mAbs with a better therapeutic profile. Rituximab, alemtuzumab, and tositumomab are probably the most commonly used mAbs in the setting of NHL. Early trials with rituximab, a chimeric antiCD-20 mAb, have reported encouraging results when used either alone *(111)* or in combination with chemotherapy *(112–114)*. The experience with rituximab as an adjuvant in the alloSCT setting is much more limited *(115)* and delayed immune reconstitution is a major concern when using this approach. B-cell reconstitution may take more than six months *(116)* and the long-term consequences of this depletion need to be studied in detail. Additionally, the efficacy of rituximab may be decreased in the postransplant setting if antibody-dependent cellular cytotoxicity is an important mechanism of action for this antibody.

Alemtuzumab, a humanized mAb, recognizes the CD52 antigen that is highly expressed on virtually all B- and T-cells lymphomas and leukemias and also on normal leukocytes. The use of alemtuzumab in recurrent CLL and NHL has resulted in response rates of 40% and 14% respectively *(117,118)*. In both studies, the responses were commonly observed in the peripheral blood and in the bone marrow. However, this antibody did not significantly affect malignant cells located in the lymph nodes. Alemtuzumab has also been investigated in allogeneic SCT to prevent GVHD and graft rejection. In this setting, T-cell depletion with alemtuzumab has clearly resulted in a significant reduction in the risk of acute and chronic GVHD *(119,120)*. It is noteworthy that whereas deaths from GVHD are greatly reduced, it appears that there is an important risk of developing clinically relevant infectious complications *(120,121)*. A high rate of infections has been reported in a phase II multicenter study evaluating alemtuzumab in previously treated patients with nonbulky NHL (118). The trial was terminated early due to the excessive number of infectious complications observed. More recently it has been reported that 50% of the patients receiving alemtuzumab (30 mg dose) developed CMV reactivation (121). It is clear from these early clinical trials that immune reconstitution and infectious complications need to be formally addressed before directed mAb therapy becomes of commonly used in the setting of alloSCT. At the present time the clinical benefit of unlabeled- or labeled- mAbs in the context of MRD after alloSCT remains to be determined.

3.3. GVHD: The Challenge Continues

Twenty-six yr ago, Thomas et al. catalogued GVHD as one of the major obstacles to successful transplantation *(122)*. Today GVHD continues to be responsible for a significant percentage of the morbidity and mortality associated with alloSCT. The basic model of GVHD, in which T cells, APC, and NK cells become activated and produce cytokines in response to both allogeneic recognition and the tissue damage done by the conditioning regimen, has evolved over the last several years. Although the core of the model has not fundamentally changed, the details have been further elucidated. GVHD is now defined as a complex multistep process *(123)*, in which T cells have a major role in the induction or initiation of GVHD. In this induction stage, the T cells from the donor are exposed to dissimilar alloantigens from the recipient and then become activated and clonally expanded. The expanded T cells release multiple cytokines and chemokines creating a cytokine storm *(56,58,124)*, which is then responsible for the recruitment of other regulatory and effector cells (macrophages, NK cells, DC, etc.). Finally, the activated effector cells are responsible for targeting the host tissue, producing a well-defined clinical picture that we recognize as GVHD. These well-defined phases of GVHD (induction, expansion, recruitment, and effector phases) have allowed a better comprehension of GVHD and, more importantly, have generated specific models of therapeutic intervention *(123)*. We will mention just few of them that may be relevant to the area of NHL. An exhaustive discussion will be found in Chapter 24 of this book.

3.3.1. GVT without GVHD—Is that Possible?

The principal purpose of allogeneic SCT is to create a state of tolerance between donor and recipient, which concurrently allows the development of an efficient GVT effect with a minimum of GVHD. The targets for GVT effect seem to be minor histocompatibility antigens shared by the tumor cells and the tissues involved in GVHD *(125,126)*. However, some patients may have GVT effect without GVHD, suggesting either an immune response against tumor target antigens or the presence of differential sensitivity of tumor cells and normal tissues to a common immunologic mechanism. Given the intricate relationship between GVT and GVHD, the task of separating these two phenomena has proven difficult. If we are going to be successful in this formidable mission, significant efforts should be directed toward understanding the basic biology of these closely related phenomena.

3.3.2. Induction of Anergy

One potential approach to achieve the above-mentioned goal is to simultaneously generate two different subpopulations of cells in the graft. One subset will contain highly specific anti-idiotype (or tumor antigen-specific) T cells, and a second subset will be composed of cells that have been anergized against the recipient alloantigens. The first group of cells will be mainly responsible for the antitumor effects, and the anergized cells will be responsible for supporting marrow repopulation and immune reconstitution.

The use of the anti-idiotype vaccination approach that we have previously discussed may allow us to generate the specific antilymphoma effector cells that may preferentially target tumor cells and spare normal tissue. The induction of anergy in the second subset of donor cells could be accomplished by using molecules capable of blocking co-stimulatory signals. Cytotoxic T lymphocyte-associated antigen (CTLA)-4, a counterreceptor for B7, is a potent regulatory molecule that is expressed on the surface of activated helper T cells *(127)* and blocks the interaction between B7 proteins and CD28 *(128–130)*. Administration of CTLA-4Ig, a soluble fusion protein consisting of the extracellular domain of CTLA-4 and the constant region of IgG1, allows animals to accept foreign grafts without using immunosuppressive drugs *(130,131)*. Soluble CTLA-4Ig induces anergy in T cells from human marrow when the cells are co-cultured with allogeneic cells; the marrow T cells afterward fail to react against the allogeneic cells with which they were initially cultured, but they react normally when presented with different allogeneic cells *(130)*. Recently, Guinan et al. confirmed this finding in a clinical setting in which they successfully induced ex vivo anergy before the transplantation of histoincompatible bone marrow *(132)*. The authors found that the CTLA-4Ig-treated marrow supported the hematologic reconstitution of the recipient. Strikingly, the occurrence of GVHD was very low, only two patients with mild gastrointestinal GVHD, despite the fact that all patients had multiple risk factors for GVHD. This study demonstrated that suppressing a segment of the alloreactive T cell repertoire is possible. However, we need to be cautious in interpreting these data because of the small number of patients and the lack of information regarding the success of immune reconstitution.

As can be seen from the two above-mentioned studies *(69,132)*, it may be possible to generate two well-defined subsets of graft cells that could be used in NHL patients in an allogeneic setting. The timing and sequence of administration of these two subsets need to be established in well-designed preclinical studies before this approach is taken to a clinical setting.

Other approaches to inhibit or decrease GVHD involve the blockade of the CD40-CD40 ligand (CD40L) interactions. Ex vivo incubation of donor T-cells with antibodies to CD40L in the presence of host alloantigens has been shown in preclinical models to induce tolerance while allowing the T cells to remain responsive to nominal antigens *(133)*, suggesting that GVT effects could be separated from GVHD. More recently, Ito et al. demonstrated that interfering with CD40-CD40L pathway reliably overcomes the CD4 T cell-mediated resistance to fully major histocompatibility complex (MHC)-mismatched allogeneic bone marrow engraftment *(134)*. These interesting observations in mice need to be tested in large animals as a next step to developing human clinical trials.

The success of DLI in posttransplant settings has prompted investigators to identify which cells are responsible for the observed GVT effect. NK cells have been implicated as one of the mediators of GVL effects *(135–137)*. Indeed, it has been demonstrated that activated NK cells may have a dual role in a peritransplant strategy by inhibiting GVHD, through a transforming growth factor (TGF)-β-mediated mechanism, and promoting immune reconstitution and GVT effects *(138)*. These results confirm previous observations suggesting that GVHD and GVT effects are dissociable phenomena. However, more research needs to be done to unequivocally identify the NK cell subsets responsible for each effect before clinical trials are initiated.

4. CONCLUSION

The use of allogeneic SCT in the treatment of NHL and other tumors is becoming feasible for a broader spectrum of cancer patients because of advances in the transplantation procedure. Preparative regimens can be made safer by using lower doses of less toxic drugs aimed at immune suppression rather than myeloablation. Humanized monoclonal antibodies can be incorporated into treatment regimens before and after transplantation in light of their specific antitumor effects and mild toxicities. Strategies to improve immune reconstitution in the recipient include vaccinating the donor and the host to tumor-specific antigens, adding immune stimulatory cytokines, and adoptively transferring effector lymphocytes, among others. Donors may be tolerized to host minor histocompatibility antigens; a number of such strategies are in development. Adoptive transfer of activated NK cells may facilitate tolerance induction and immune reconstitution. Experimental efforts to promote the regeneration of the thymus are also worth considering for human application to facilitate the generation of a broad spectrum of T cell responses to infectious organisms as well as the tumor.

Given the abundance of ideas emerging from the laboratories, the next decade promises unprecedented growth in the development of safe and effective protocols for using allogeneic SCT in cancer treatment.

REFERENCES

1. Greenlee RT, Murray T, Bolden S, Wingo PA. Cancer statistics, 2000. *CA Cancer J Clin* 2000;50(1):7–33.
2. Weisenburger, D.D. Epidemiology of non-Hodgkin's lymphoma: recent findings regarding an emerging epidemic. *Ann Oncol* 1994;5:S19–S24.
3. Lyons SF, Liebowitz DN. The roles of human viruses in the pathogenesis of lymphoma. *Semin Oncol* 1998;25(4):461–475.

 4. Harris NL, Jaffe, ES, Diebold J, Flandrin G, Muller-Hermelink HK, et al. World Health Organization classification of neoplastic diseases of the hematopoietic and lymphoid tissues: report of the clinical advisory committee meeting–Airlie House, Virginia, November, 1997. *J Clin Oncol* 1999;17:3835–3849.

 5. Horning SJ. Natural history of and therapy for the indolent non-Hodgkin's lymphomas. *Semin Oncol* 1993;20(5 Suppl 5):75–88.

 6. Philip T, Guglielmi C, Hagenbeek A, Somers R, Van Der LH, Bron D, et al. Autologous bone marrow transplantation as compared with salvage chemotherapy in relapses of chemotherapy-sensitive non-Hodgkin's lymphoma. *N Engl J Med* 1995;333(23):1540–1545.

 7. Stiff PJ, Dahlberg S, Forman SJ, McCall AR, Horning SJ, Nademanee AP, et al. Autologous bone marrow transplantation for patients with relapsed or refractory diffuse aggressive non-Hodgkin's lymphoma: value of augmented preparative regimens—a Southwest Oncology Group trial. *J Clin Oncol* 1998;16(1):48–55.

 8. Shipp MA, Abeloff MD, Antman KH, Carroll G, Hagenbeek A, Loeffler M, et al. International Consensus Conference on high-dose therapy with hematopoietic stem-cell transplantation in aggressive non-Hodgkin's lymphomas: report of the jury. *Ann Oncol* 1999;10:13–19.

 9. Khouri IF, Keating MJ, Vriesendorp HM, Reading CL, Przepiorka D, Huh YO, et al. Autologous and allogeneic bone marrow transplantation for chronic lymphocytic leukemia: preliminary results. *J Clin Oncol* 1994;12(4):748–758.

10. van Besien KW, Mehra RC, Giralt SA, Kantarjian HM, Pugh WC, Khouri IF, et al. Allogeneic bone marrow transplantation for poor-prognosis lymphoma: response, toxicity and survival depend on disease histology. *Am J Med* 1996;100(3):299–307.

11. Longo DL, Young RC, DeVita V. What is so good about the "good prognosis" lymphomas? In: Williams CJ, Whitehouse J, eds. *Recent Advances in Clinical Oncology*. Churchill-Livingstone, Edinburgh, 1982, pp. 223–231.

12. Portlock CS. "Good risk" non-Hodgkin lymphomas: approaches to management. *Semin Hematol* 1983;20(1):25–34.

13. Horning SJ, Rosenberg SA. The natural history of initially untreated low-grade non-Hodgkin's lymphomas. *N Engl J Med* 1984;311(23):1471–1475.

14. Gribben JG, Freedman AS, Neuberg D, Roy DC, Blake KW, Woo SD, et al. Immunologic purging of marrow assessed by PCR before autologous bone marrow transplantation for B-cell lymphoma. *N Engl J Med* 1991;325(22):1525–1533.

15. Brenner MK, Rill DR, Holladay MS, Heslop HE, Moen RC, Buschle M, et al. Gene marking to determine whether autologous marrow infusion restores long-term haemopoiesis in cancer patients. *Lancet* 1993;342(8880):1134–1137.

16. Sharp JG, Kessinger A, Mann S, Crouse DA, Armitage JO, Bierman P, et al. Outcome of high-dose therapy and autologous transplantation in non-Hodgkin's lymphoma based on the presence of tumor in the marrow or infused hematopoietic harvest. *J Clin Oncol* 1996;14(1):214–219.

17. Karanes C, Du W, Abella E, Klein JP, Dansey R, Cassels L, et al. Single institution cohort analysis of allogeneic and autologous stem cell transplantation for non-Hodgkin's lymphoma. *Blood* 1998;92(Suppl 1):266a.

18. Verdonck LF, Dekker AW, Lokhorst HM, Petersen EJ, Nieuwenhuis HK. Allogeneic versus autologous bone marrow transplantation for refractory and recurrent low-grade non-Hodgkin's lymphoma. *Blood* 1997;90(10):4201–4205.

19. Friedberg JW, Neuberg D, Stone RM, Alyea E, Jallow H, LaCasce A, et al. Outcome in patients with myelodysplastic syndrome after autologous bone marrow transplantation for non-Hodgkin's lymphoma. *J Clin Oncol* 1999;17(10):3128–3135.

20. Milligan DW, Ruiz De Elvira MC, Kolb HJ, Goldstone AH, Meloni G, Rohatiner AZ, et al. Secondary leukaemia and myelodysplasia after autografting for lymphoma: results from the EBMT. EBMT Lymphoma and Late Effects Working Parties. European Group for Blood and Marrow Transplantation. *Br J Haematol* 1999;106(4):1020–1026.

21. Krishnan A, Bhatia S, Bhatia R, Slovak ML, Arber D, Niland J, et al. Risk factors for development of therapy-related leukemia (t-MDS/t-AML) following autologous transplantation for lymphoma. *Blood* 1998;92(10):1588–1593.

22. Jones RJ, Ambinder RF, Piantadosi S, Santos GW. Evidence of a graft-versus-lymphoma effect associated with allogeneic bone marrow transplantation. *Blood* 1991;77(3):649–653.

23. Chopra R, Goldstone AH, Pearce R, Philip T, Petersen F, Appelbaum F, et al. Autologous versus allogeneic bone marrow transplantation for non- Hodgkin's lymphoma: a case-controlled analysis of the European Bone Marrow Transplant Group Registry data. *J Clin Oncol* 1992;10(11):1690–1695.

24. Ratanatharathorn V, Uberti J, Karanes C, Abella E, Lum LG, Momin F, et al. Prospective comparative trial of autologous versus allogeneic bone marrow transplantation in patients with non-Hodgkin's lymphoma. *Blood* 1994;84(4):1050–1055.

25. Appelbaum F. Treatment of aggressive non-Hodgkin's lymphoma with marrow transplantation. *Marrow Transplant Rev* 1993;3:1–16.

26. Radich JP, Gooley T, Sanders JE, Anasetti C, Chauncey T, Appelbaum F. Second allogeneic transplants after failure of autologous first transplant. *Blood* 1998;92(10):494a.

27. Bierman P, Kottaridis P, Kollath J, Vose J, Linch D, Mackinnon S, et al. Allogeneic transplantation following failure of autologous transplantation for lymphoma. *Blood* 1998;92(10):321a.

28. van Besien K, Sobocinski KA, Rowlings PA, Murphy SC, Armitage JO, Bishop MR, et al. Allogeneic bone marrow transplantation for low-grade lymphoma. *Blood* 1998;92(5):1832–1836.

29. Attal M, Socie G, Molina L, Jouet J, Pico J, Kuentz M, et al. Allogeneic bone marrow transplantation for refractory and recurrent follicular lymphoma: a case-matched analysis with autologous transplantation from the French bone marrow transplant group registry data. *Blood* 1997;20(suppl 1):1120a.

30. Pleniket A, Ruiz de Elvira M, Taghipour G, de Witte T, Tazelaar P, Carella AM, et al. Allogeneic transplantation for lymphoma produces a lower relapse rate than autologous transplantation but survival has no risen because of higher treatment-related mortality. A report of 764 cases from the EBMT lymphoma registry. *Blood* 1997;20(Suppl 1):1121a.

31. van Besien KW, de Lima M, Giralt SA, Moore DF, Jr., Khouri IF, Rondon G, et al. Management of lymphoma recurrence after allogeneic transplantation: the relevance of graft-versus-lymphoma effect. *Bone Marrow Transplant* 1997;19(10):977–982.

32. Mandigers CM, Meijerink JP, Raemaekers JM, Schattenberg AV, Mensink EJ. Graft-versus-lymphoma effect of donor leucocyte infusion shown by real-time quantitative PCR analysis of t(14;18). *Lancet* 1998;352(9139):1522,1523.

33. van Besien KW, Khouri IF, Giralt SA, McCarthy P, Mehra R, Andersson BS, et al. Allogeneic bone marrow transplantation for refractory and recurrent low-grade lymphoma: the case for aggressive management. *J Clin Oncol* 1995;13(5):1096–1102.

34. Mandigers C, Raemaekers J, Schattenperg A, Bogman J, Mensik E, de Witte T. Allogeneic bone marrow transplantation in patients with relapse low-grade follicular non-Hodgkin's lymphoma. *Blood* 1995;86:208a.

35. Molina I, Nicolini F, Viret F, Pegourie-Bandelier B, Leger J, Sotto JJ. Allogeneic bone marrow transplantation for refractory and recurrent low grade non-Hodgkin's lymphoma. *Blood* 1995;86:209a.

36. Bearman SI, Appelbaum FR, Back A, Petersen FB, Buckner CD, Sullivan KM, et al. Regimen-related toxicity and early posttransplant survival in patients undergoing marrow transplantation for lymphoma. *J Clin Oncol* 1989;7(9):1288–1294.

37. Buckner CD, Clift RA, Fefer A, Lerner KG, Neiman PE, Storb R, et al. Marrow transplantation for the treatment of acute leukemia using HLA-identical siblings. *Transplant Proc* 1974;6(4):365,366.

38. Maraninchi D, Gluckman E, Blaise D, Guyotat D, Rio B, Pico JL, et al. Impact of T-cell depletion on outcome of allogeneic bone-marrow transplantation for standard-risk leukaemias. *Lancet* 1987;2(8552):175–178.

39. Weiden PL, Sullivan KM, Flournoy N, Storb R, Thomas ED. Antileukemic effect of chronic graft-versus-host disease: contribution to improved survival after allogeneic marrow transplantation. *N Engl J Med* 1981;304(25):1529–1533.

40. Horowitz MM, Gale RP, Sondel PM, Goldman JM, Kersey J, Kolb HJ, et al. Graft-versus-leukemia reactions after bone marrow transplantation. *Blood* 1990;75(3):555–562.

41. Sullivan KM, Storb R, Buckner CD, Fefer A, Fisher L, Weiden PL, et al. Graft-versus-host disease as adoptive immunotherapy in patients with advanced hematologic neoplasms. *N Engl J Med* 1989;320(13):828–834.

42. Gale RP, Champlin RE. How does bone-marrow transplantation cure leukaemia? *Lancet* 1984;2(8393):28–30.

43. Fefer A, Cheever MA, Greenberg PD. Identical-twin (syngeneic) marrow transplantation for hematologic cancers. *J Natl Cancer Inst* 1986;76(6):1269–1273.

44. Gale RP, Horowitz MM, Ash RC, Champlin RE, Goldman JM, Rimm AA, et al. Identical-twin bone marrow transplants for leukemia. *Ann Intern Med* 1994;120(8):646–652.

45. Kolb HJ, Schattenberg A, Goldman JM, Hertenstein B, Jacobsen N, Arcese W, et al. Graft-versus-leukemia effect of donor lymphocyte transfusions in marrow grafted patients. European Group for Blood and Marrow Transplantation Working Party Chronic Leukemia. *Blood* 1995;86(5):2041–2050.

46. Antin JH. Graft-versus-leukemia: no longer an epiphenomenon. *Blood* 1993;82(8):2273–2277.

47. Drobyski WR, Keever CA, Roth MS, Koethe S, Hanson G, McFadden P, et al. Salvage immunotherapy using donor leukocyte infusions as treatment for relapsed chronic myelogenous leukemia after allogeneic bone marrow transplantation: efficacy and toxicity of a defined T-cell dose. *Blood* 1993;82(8):2310–2318.

48. Lokhorst HM, Schattenberg A, Cornelissen JJ, Thomas LL, Verdonck LF. Donor leukocyte infusions are effective in relapsed multiple myeloma after allogeneic bone marrow transplantation. *Blood* 1997;90(10):4206–4211.

49. Tricot G, Vesole DH, Jagannath S, Hilton J, Munshi N, Barlogie B. Graft-versus-myeloma effect: proof of principle. *Blood* 1996;87(3):1196–1198.

50. Verdonck LF, Lokhorst HM, Dekker AW, Nieuwenhuis HK, Petersen EJ. Graft-versus-myeloma effect in two cases. *Lancet* 1996;347(9004):800,801.

51. Collins RH, Jr., Shpilberg O, Drobyski WR, Porter DL, Giralt S, Champlin R, et al. Donor leukocyte infusions in 140 patients with relapsed malignancy after allogeneic bone marrow transplantation. *J Clin Oncol* 1997;15(2):433–444.

52. Childs R, Chernoff A, Contentin N, Bahceci E, Schrump D, Leitman S, et al. Regression of metastatic renal-cell carcinoma after nonmyeloablative allogeneic peripheral-blood stem-cell transplantation. *N Engl J Med* 2000;343(11):750–758.

53. Rondon G, Giralt S, Huh Y, Khouri I, Andersson B, Andreeff M, et al. Graft-versus-leukemia effect after allogeneic bone marrow transplantation for chronic lymphocytic leukemia. *Bone Marrow Transplant* 1996;18(3):669–672.

54. Khouri IF, Keating M, Korbling M, Przepiorka D, Anderlini P, O'Brien S, et al. Transplant-lite: induction of graft-versus-malignancy using fludarabine- based nonablative chemotherapy and allogeneic blood progenitor-cell transplantation as treatment for lymphoid malignancies. *J Clin Oncol* 1998;16(8):2817–2824.

55. Champlin R, Khouri I, Komblau S, Molidrem J, Giralt S. Reinventing bone marrow transplantation. Nonmyeloablative preparative regimens and induction of graft-vs-malignancy effect. *Oncology* (Huntingt) 1999;13(5):621–628.

56. Antin JH, Ferrara JL. Cytokine dysregulation and acute graft-versus-host disease. *Blood* 1992;80(12):2964–2968.

57. Hill GR, Krenger W, Ferrara JL. The role of cytokines in acute graft-versus-host disease. *Cytokines Cell Mol Ther* 1997;3(4):257–266.

58. Krenger W, Hill GR, Ferrara JL. Cytokine cascades in acute graft-versus-host disease. *Transplantation* 1997;64(4):553–558.

59. Carrera CJ, Saven A, Piro LD. Purine metabolism of lymphocytes. Targets for chemotherapy drug development. *Hematol Oncol Clin N Am* 1994;8(2):357–381.

60. Goodman ER, Fiedor PS, Fein S, Sung RS, Athan E, Hardy MA. Fludarabine phosphate and 2-chlorodeoxyadenosine: immunosuppressive DNA synthesis inhibitors with potential application in islet allo- and xenotransplantation. *Transplant Proc* 1995;27(6):3293–3294.

61. Keating MJ, Kantarjian H, Talpaz M, Redman J, Koller C, Barlogie B, et al. Fludarabine: a new agent with major activity against chronic lymphocytic leukemia. *Blood* 1989;74(1):19–25.

62. Estey E, Plunkett W, Gandhi V, Rios MB, Kantarjian H, Keating MJ. Fludarabine and arabinosylcytosine therapy of refractory and relapsed acute myelogenous leukemia. *Leuk Lymphoma* 1993;9(4-5):343–350.

63. Khouri I, Lee M-S, Palmer L, Giralt SA, McLaughlin P, Korbling M, et al. Transplant-lite using fludarabine-cyclophosphamide and allogeneic stem cell transplant for low-grade lymphoma. *Blood* 1999;94(Suppl 1):348a.

64. Hill RS, Petersen FB, Storb R, Appelbaum FR, Doney K, Dahlberg S, et al. Mixed hematologic chimerism after allogeneic marrow transplantation for severe aplastic anemia is associated with a higher risk of graft rejection and a lessened incidence of acute graft-versus-host disease. *Blood* 1986;67(3):811–816.

65. Carella AM, Cavaliere M, Lerma E, Ferrara R, Tedeschi L, Romanelli A, et al. Autografting followed by nonmyeloablative immunosuppressive chemotherapy and allogeneic peripheral-blood hematopoietic stem-cell transplantation as treatment of resistant Hodgkin's disease and non- Hodgkin's lymphoma. *J Clin Oncol* 2000;18(23):3918–3924.

66. Stevenson GT, Stevenson FK. Antibody to a molecularly-defined antigen confined to a tumour cell surface. *Nature* 1975;254(5502):714–716.

67. Lee MS, Chang KS, Cabanillas F, Freireich EJ, Trujillo JM, Stass SA. Detection of minimal residual cells carrying the t(14;18) by DNA sequence amplification. *Science* 1987;237(4811):175–178.

68. Gribben JG, Freedman A, Woo SD, Blake K, Shu RS, Freeman G, et al. All advanced stage non-Hodgkin's lymphomas with a polymerase chain reaction amplifiable breakpoint of bcl-2 have residual cells containing the bcl-2 rearrangement at evaluation and after treatment. *Blood* 1991;78(12):3275–3280.

69. Bendandi M, Gocke CD, Kobrin CB, Benko FA, Sternas LA, Pennington R, et al. Complete molecular remissions induced by patient-specific vaccination plus granulocyte-monocyte colony-stimulating factor against lymphoma. *Nat Med* 1999;5(10):1171–1177.

70. Lopez-Guillermo A, Cabanillas F, McLaughlin P, Smith T, Hagemeister F, Rodriguez MA, et al. The clinical significance of molecular response in indolent follicular lymphomas. *Blood* 1998;91(8):2955–2960.

71. Grosse-Wilde H, Krumbacher K, Schuning F, Doxiadis I, Mahmoud HK, Emde C, et al. Immune transfer studies in canine allogeneic marrow graft donor- recipient pairs. *Transplantation* 1986;42(1):64–67.

72. Starling KA, Falletta JM, Fernbach DJ. Immunologic chimerism as evidence of bone marrow graft acceptance in an identical twin with acute lymphocytic leukemia. *Exp Hematol* 1975;3(4):244–248.

73. Lum LG, Munn NA, Schanfield MS, Storb R. The detection of specific antibody formation to recall antigens after human bone marrow transplantation. *Blood* 1986;67(3):582–587.

74. Lum LG, Seigneuret MC, Storb R. The transfer of antigen-specific humoral immunity from marrow donors to marrow recipients. *J Clin Immunol* 1986;6(5):389–396.

75. Kwak LW, Taub DD, Duffey PL, Bensinger WI, Bryant EM, Reynolds CW, et al. Transfer of myeloma idiotype-specific immunity from an actively immunised marrow donor. *Lancet* 1995;345(8956):1016–1020.

76. Rosenberg SA, Packard BS, Aebersold PM, Solomon D, Topalian SL, Toy ST, et al. Use of tumor-infiltrating lymphocytes and interleukin-2 in the immunotherapy of patients with metastatic melanoma. A preliminary report. *N Engl J Med* 1988;319(25):1676–1680.

77. Rosenberg SA, Yannelli JR, Yang JC, Topalian SL, Schwartzentruber DJ, Weber JS, et al. Treatment of patients with metastatic melanoma with autologous tumor- infiltrating lymphocytes and interleukin 2. *J Natl Cancer Inst* 1994;86(15):1159–1166.

78. Rooney CM, Smith CA, Ng CY, Loftin S, Li C, Krance RA, et al. Use of gene-modified virus-specific T lymphocytes to control Epstein- Barr-virus-related lymphoproliferation. *Lancet* 1995;345(8941):9–13.

79. Walter EA, Greenberg PD, Gilbert MJ, Finch RJ, Watanabe KS, Thomas ED, et al. Reconstitution of cellular immunity against cytomegalovirus in recipients of allogeneic bone marrow by transfer of T-cell clones from the donor. *N Engl J Med* 1995;333(16):1038–1044.

80. Smit WM, Rijnbeek M, van Bergen CA, Willemze R, Falkenburg JH. Generation of leukemia-reactive cytotoxic T lymphocytes from HLA- identical donors of patients with chronic myeloid leukemia using modifications of a limiting dilution assay. *Bone Marrow Transplant* 1998;21(6):553–560.

81. Hsu FJ, Benike C, Fagnoni F, Liles TM, Czerwinski D, Taidi B, et al. Vaccination of patients with B-cell lymphoma using autologous antigen- pulsed dendritic cells. *Nat Med* 1996;2(1):52–58.

82. Levitsky HI, Montgomery J, Ahmadzadeh M, Staveley-O'Carroll K, Guarnieri F, Longo DL, et al. Immunization with granulocyte-macrophage colony-stimulating factor- transduced, but not B7-1-transduced, lymphoma cells primes idiotype- specific T cells and generates potent systemic antitumor immunity. *J Immunol* 1996;156(10):3858–3865.

83. Lum LG. Immune recovery after bone marrow transplantation. *Hematol Oncol Clin N Am* 1990;4(3):659–675.

84. Atkinson K. Reconstruction of the haemopoietic and immune systems after marrow transplantation. *Bone Marrow Transplant* 1990;5(4):209–226.

85. Witherspoon RP, Kopecky K, Storb RF, Flournoy N, Sullivan KM, Sosa R, et al. Immunological recovery in 48 patients following syngeneic marrow transplantation or hematological malignancy. *Transplantation* 1982;33(2):143–149.

86. Ault KA, Antin JH, Ginsburg D, Orkin SH, Rappeport JM, Keohan ML, et al. Phenotype of recovering lymphoid cell populations after marrow transplantation. *J Exp Med* 1985;161(6):1483–1502.

87. Velardi A, Terenzi A, Cucciaioni S, Millo R, Grossi CE, Grignani F, et al. Imbalances within the peripheral blood T-helper (CD4+) and T-suppressor (CD8+) cell populations in the reconstitution phase after human bone marrow transplantation. *Blood* 1988;71(5):1196–1200.

88. Mackall CL, Fleisher TA, Brown MR, Andrich MP, Chen CC, Feuerstein IM, et al. Distinctions between CD8+ and CD4+ T-cell regenerative pathways result in prolonged T-cell subset imbalance after intensive chemotherapy. *Blood* 1997;89(10):3700–3707.

89. Muraguchi A, Kehrl JH, Longo DL, Volkman DJ, Smith KA, Fauci AS. Interleukin 2 receptors on human B cells. Implications for the role of interleukin 2 in human B cell function. *J Exp Med* 1985;161(1):181–197.

90. Caligiuri MA, Zmuidzinas A, Manley TJ, Levine H, Smith KA, Ritz J. Functional consequences of interleukin 2 receptor expression on resting human lymphocytes. Identification of a novel natural killer cell subset with high affinity receptors. *J Exp Med* 1990;171(5):1509–1526.

91. Espinoza-Delgado I, Ortaldo JR, Winkler-Pickett R, Sugamura K, Varesio L, Longo DL. Expression and role of p75 interleukin 2 receptor on human monocytes. *J Exp Med* 1990;171(5):1821–1826.

92. Morecki S, Revel-Vilk S, Nabet C, Pick M, Ackerstein A, Nagler A, et al. Immunological evaluation of patients with hematological malignancies receiving ambulatory cytokine-mediated immunotherapy with recombinant human interferon-alpha 2a and interleukin-2. *Cancer Immunol Immunother* 1992;35(6):401–411.

93. Morecki S, Nagler A, Puyesky Y, Nabet C, Condiotti R, Pick M, et al. Effect of various cytokine combinations on induction of non-MHC- restricted cytotoxicity. *Lymphokine Cytokine Res* 1993;12(3):159–165.

94. Dutcher JP, Wiernik PH. The role of recombinant interleukin-2 in therapy for hematologic malignancies. *Semin Oncol* 1993;20(6 Suppl 9):33–40.

95. Duggan DB, Santarelli MT, Zamkoff K, Lichtman S, Ellerton J, Cooper R, et al. A phase II study of recombinant interleukin-2 with or without recombinant interferon-beta in non-Hodgkin's lymphoma. A study of the Cancer and Leukemia Group B. *J Immunother* 1992;12(2):115–122.

96. Bernstein ZP, Vaickus L, Friedman N, Goldrosen MH, Watanabe H, Rahman R, et al. Interleukin-2 lymphokine-activated killer cell therapy of non-Hodgkin's lymphoma and Hodgkin's disease. *J Immunother* 1991;10(2):141–146.

97. Gisselbrecht C, Maraninchi D, Pico JL, Milpied N, Coiffier B, Divine M, et al. Interleukin-2 treatment in lymphoma: a phase II multicenter study. *Blood* 1994;83(8):2081–2085.

98. Fefer A, Benyunes M, Higuchi C, York A, Massumoto C, Lindgren C, et al. Interleukin-2 +/- lymphocytes as consolidative immunotherapy after autologous bone marrow transplantation for hematologic malignancies. *Acta Haematol* 1993;89(Suppl 1):2–7.

99. Fefer A, Benyunes MC, Massumoto C, Higuchi C, York A, Buckner CD, et al. Interleukin-2 therapy after autologous bone marrow transplantation for hematologic malignancies. *Semin Oncol* 1993;20(6 Suppl 9):41–45.

100. Mazumder A. Experimental evidence of interleukin-2 activity in bone marrow transplantation. *Cancer J Sci Am* 1997;3(Suppl 1):S37–S42.

101. Allavena P, Damia G, Colombo T, Maggioni D, D'Incalci M, Mantovani A. Lymphokine-activated killer (LAK) and monocyte-mediated cytotoxicity on tumor cell lines resistant to antitumor agents. *Cell Immunol* 1989;120(1):250–258.

102. Weiss L, Reich S, Slavin S. Use of recombinant human interleukin-2 in conjunction with bone marrow transplantation as a model for control of minimal residual disease in malignant hematological disorders: I. Treatment of murine leukemia in conjunction with allogeneic bone marrow transplantation and IL-2- activated cell-mediated immunotherapy. *Cancer Invest* 1992;10(1):19–26.

103. Weiss L, Lubin I, Factorowich I, Lapidot Z, Reich S, Reisner Y, et al. Effective graft-versus-leukemia effects independent of graft-versus- host disease after T cell-depleted allogeneic bone marrow transplantation in a murine model of B cell leukemia/lymphoma. Role of cell therapy and recombinant IL-2. *J Immunol* 1994;153(6):2562–2567.

104. Slavin S, Ackerstein A, Kedar E, Reich S, Gomez S, Naparstek E, et al. Induction of cell-mediated IL-2-activated antitumor responses in conjunction with autologous and allogeneic bone marrow transplantation. *Transplant Proc* 1991;23(1 Pt 1):802,803.

105. Leshem B, Vourka-Karussis U, Slavin S. Correlation between enhancement of graft-versus-leukemia effects following allogeneic bone marrow transplantation by rIL-2 and increased frequency of cytotoxic T-lymphocyte precursors in murine myeloid leukemia. *Cytokines Cell Mol Ther* 2000;6(3):141–147.

106. Soiffer RJ, Murray C, Gonin R, Ritz J. Effect of low-dose interleukin-2 on disease relapse after T-cell-depleted allogeneic bone marrow transplantation. *Blood* 1994;84(3):964–971.

107. Fefer A, Robinson N, Benyunes MC, Bensinger WI, Press O, Thompson JA, et al. Interleukin-2 therapy after bone marrow or stem cell transplantation for hematologic malignancies. *Cancer J Sci Am* 1997;3(Suppl 1):S48–S53.

108. Hornung RL, Pearson JW, Beckwith M, Longo DL. Preclinical evaluation of bryostatin as an anticancer agent against several murine tumor cell lines: in vitro versus in vivo activity. *Cancer Res* 1992;52(1):101–107.

109. Bosco MC, Rottschafer S, Taylor LS, Ortaldo JR, Longo DL, Espinoza-Delgado I. The antineoplastic agent bryostatin-1 induces proinflammatory cytokine production in human monocytes: synergy with interleukin-2 and modulation of interleukin-2Rgamma chain expression. *Blood* 1997;89(9):3402–3411.

110. Espinoza-Delgado I, Rottschafer S, Garcia CS, Curiel R, Bravo JC, Skrepkin N, et al. Bryostatin-1 and low-dose IL-2 is as efficientas high-dose IL-2 without the acute toxicity. *J Clin Oncol* 1999;18:452a.

111. McLaughlin P, Grillo-Lopez AJ, Link BK, Levy R, Czuczman MS, Williams ME, et al. Rituximab chimeric anti-CD20 monoclonal antibody therapy for relapsed indolent lymphoma: half of patients respond to a four-dose treatment program. *J Clin Oncol* 1998;16: 2825–2833.

112. Czuczman MS, Grillo-Lopez AJ, White CA, Saleh M, Gordon L, LoBuglio AF, et al. Treatment of patients with low-grade B-cell lymphoma with the combination of chimeric anti-CD20 monoclonal antibody and CHOP chemotherapy. *J Clin Oncol* 1999;17: 268–276.

113. Wilson WH, Frankel SR, Drbohlav N, Hedge U, Gutierrez M, Janik J, et al. Phase II study of dose-adjusted EPOCH-Rituximab in untreated patients with high-risk large B-cell lymphomas. *J Clin Oncol* 2001;20:290a.

114. Coiffier B, Lepage E, Briere J, Herbrecht, Tilly H, Boubdallah R, et al. CHOP chemotherapy plus rituximab compared with CHOP alone in elderly patients with diffuse-large-B-cell lymphoma. *N Engl J Med* 2002;346:235–242.

115. Seropian S, MsGuirk JP, and Cooper DL. Rituximab antibody therapy for non-Hodgkin's lymphoma following allogeneic stem cell transplantation. *Blood* 1999;94(Supple 1):387b.

116. Flinn IW, O'Donnell, Goodrich A, Vogelsang G, Abrams R, Noga S. Immunotherapy with rituximab during peripheral blood stem cell transplantation for Non-Hodgkin's lymphoma. *Biol Blood Marrow Transplant* 2000;6:628–632.

117. Osterborg A, Dyer MJ, Bunies D, Pangalis GA, Bastion Y, Catovsky D. Phase II multicenter study of uman CD52 antibody in previously treated Chronic lymphocytic leukemia. *J Clin Oncol* 1997;15:1567–1574

118. Khorama A, Bunn P, McLaughlin P, Vose J, Stewart C, Czuczman MS. Leul A phase II multicenter study of campath-1h antibody in previously treated patients with non-bulky non-hodgkin's lymphoma. *Leuk Lymphoma* 2001;41(1-2):77–87

119. Hale G, Jacobs P, Wood L, Fibbe WE, Barge R, Novitzky N. CD52 antibodies for prevention of graft-versus-host disease and graft rejection following transplantatio of allogeneic peripheral blood stem cells. *Bone Marrow Transplant* 2000;26:69–76.

120. Davison GM, Novitsky N, Kline A, Thomas V, Abrahams L, Hale G, et al. Immune reconstitution after allogeneic bone marrow transplantation depleted of T-cells. *Transplantation* 2000;69:1341–1347.

121. O'Brien SM, Thomas DA, Cortes J, Gilles FJ, Kornblau M, Willians H, et al. Campath-1H for minimal residual disease in CLL. *J Clin Oncol* 2001;20:1132.

122. Thomas E, Storb R, Clift RA, Fefer A, Johnson FL, Neiman PE, et al. Bone-marrow transplantation (first of two parts). *N Engl J Med* 1975;292(16):832–843.

123. Murphy WJ, Blazar BR. New strategies for preventing graft-versus-host disease. *Curr Opin Immunol* 1999;11(5):509–515.

124. Serody JS, Cook DN, Kirby SL, Reap E, Shea TC, Frelinger JA. Murine T lymphocytes incapable of producing macrophage inhibitory protein-1 are impaired in causing graft-versus-host disease across a class I but not class II major histocompatibility complex barrier. *Blood* 1999;93(1):43–50.

125. Goulmy E, Schipper R, Pool J, Blokland E, Falkenburg JH, Vossen J, et al. Mismatches of minor histocompatibility antigens between HLA-identical donors and recipients and the development of graft-versus-host disease after bone marrow transplantation. *N Engl J Med* 1996;334(5):281–285.

126. Behar E, Chao NJ, Hiraki DD, Krishnaswamy S, Brown BW, Zehnder JL, et al. Polymorphism of adhesion molecule CD31 and its role in acute graft- versus-host disease. *N Engl J Med* 1996;334(5):286–291.

127. Scheipers P, Reiser H. Role of the CTLA-4 receptor in T cell activation and immunity. Physiologic function of the CTLA-4 receptor. *Immunol Res* 1998;18(2):103–115.

128. Walunas TL, Lenschow DJ, Bakker CY, Linsley PS, Freeman GJ, Green JM, et al. CTLA-4 can function as a negative regulator of T cell activation. *Immunity* 1994;1(5):405–413.

129. Schwartz RH. Costimulation of T lymphocytes: the role of CD28, CTLA-4, and B7/BB1 in interleukin-2 production and immunotherapy. *Cell* 1992;71(7):1065–1068.

130. Gribben JG, Guinan EC, Boussiotis VA, Ke XY, Linsley L, Sieff C, et al. Complete blockade of B7 family-mediated costimulation is necessary to induce human alloantigen-specific anergy: a method to ameliorate graft-versus-host disease and extend the donor pool. *Blood* 1996;87(11):4887–4893.

131. Lin H, Bolling SF, Linsley PS, Wei RQ, Gordon D, Thompson CB, et al. Long-term acceptance of major histocompatibility complex mismatched cardiac allografts induced by CTLA4Ig plus donor-specific transfusion. *J Exp Med* 1993;178(5):1801–1806.

132. Guinan EC, Boussiotis VA, Neuberg D, Brennan LL, Hirano N, Nadler LM, et al. Transplantation of anergic histoincompatible bone marrow allografts. *N Engl J Med* 1999;340(22):1704–1714.

133. Blazar BR, Taylor PA, Noelle RJ, Vallera DA. CD4(+) T cells tolerized ex vivo to host alloantigen by anti-CD40 ligand (CD40L:CD154) antibody lose their graft-versus-host disease lethality capacity but retain nominal antigen responses. *J Clin Invest* 1998;102(3):473–482.

134. Ito H, Kurtz J, Shaffer J, Sykes M. CD4 T cell-mediated alloresistance to fully MHC-mismatched allogeneic bone marrow engraftment is dependent on CD40-CD40 ligand interactions, and lasting T cell tolerance is induced by bone marrow transplantation with initial blockade of this pathway. *J Immunol* 2001;166(5):2970–2981.

135. Hauch M, Gazzola MV, Small T, Bordignon C, Barnett L, Cunningham I, et al. Anti-leukemia potential of interleukin-2 activated natural killer cells after bone marrow transplantation for chronic myelogenous leukemia. *Blood* 1990;75(11):2250–2262.

136. Zeis M, Uharek L, Glass B, Gaska T, Steinmann J, Gassmann W, et al. Allogeneic NK cells as potent antileukemic effector cells after allogeneic bone marrow transplantation in mice. *Transplantation* 1995;59(12):1734–1736.

137. Murphy WJ, Reynolds CW, Tiberghien P, Longo DL. Natural killer cells and bone marrow transplantation. *J Natl Cancer Inst* 1993;85(18):1475–1482.

138. Asai O, Longo DL, Tian ZG, Hornung RL, Taub DD, Ruscetti FW, et al. Suppression of graft-versus-host disease and amplification of graft-versus-tumor effects by activated natural killer cells after allogeneic bone marrow transplantation. *J Clin Invest* 1998;101(9):1835–1842.

III ALLOGENEIC GRAFT SELECTION

8

Blood vs Marrow Allogeneic Stem Cell Transplantation

Daniel Anderson, MD and Daniel Weisdorf, MD

CONTENTS

INTRODUCTION
BIOLOGY OF PERIPHERAL BLOOD PROGENITOR AND STEM CELLS
CLINICAL ASPECTS OF PBSC TRANSPLANTATION
DONOR CONSIDERATIONS
COST
CONCLUSION
REFERENCES

1. INTRODUCTION

Peripheral blood stem cells (PBSCs) are increasingly being used in allogeneic transplantation. While the first report describing the use of peripheral blood for allogeneic transplantation appeared in 1989 *(1)*, case series demonstrating its feasibility in the allogeneic setting did not appear until the mid-1990s *(2–4)*.

As more data emerged suggesting advantages over traditional marrow stem cell transplantation, peripheral blood transplantation rapidly became widely used *(5)*. In 1999, the International Bone Marrow Transplant Registry (IBMTR) reports that of 6093 allogeneic transplants performed, 34% used PBSCs *(6)*. Preliminary IBMTR results for 2000 estimate that this percentage increased to 43%. Most allogeneic transplants reported to date have involved matched sibling donors, although experience with unrelated donor transplants is accumulating *(7)*.

Despite the rapid acceptance of PBSCs for transplantation, only recently have data from randomized trials *(8–12)* and large registry-based data *(13)* become available. This chapter will focus on the known biological and clinical characteristics of PBSC transplantation, with an emphasis on information obtained from randomized trials and large registry analyses.

2. BIOLOGY OF PERIPHERAL BLOOD PROGENITOR AND STEM CELLS

Without cytokine priming, very low numbers of hematopoietic progenitor cells circulate in peripheral blood, with CD34+ cells representing 0.06% of all nucleated cells *(14)* Administration of cytokines, however, increases not only the total peripheral leukocyte count, it preferentially increases the concentration of peripheral blood progenitor and stem cells *(14,15)*. Direct comparison of granulocyte colony-stimulating factor (G-CSF) to granulocyte-macrophage colony-stimulating factor (GM-CSF) found G-CSF to be superior in mobilizing stem

From: *Current Clinical Oncology: Allogeneic Stem Cell Transplantation*
Edited by: Mary S. Laughlin and Hillard M. Lazarus © Humana Press Inc., Totowa, NJ

cells for harvest, although GM-CSF may effectively mobilize more primitive progenitor cells *(16)*. Other cytokines, such as flt-3 ligand, used alone and in combination with G-CSF to mobilize PBSCs, are currently the subject of investigation *(17,18)*. G-CSF at concentrations up to 10 μg/kg/d has been shown to produce dose-dependent increases in CD34+ cells and is generally is administered in doses of 10–16 μg/kg/d when used clinically to ensure adequate donor harvests.

After administration of G-CSF to normal individuals, peripheral leukocyte counts begin increasing within 4 h and remain elevated throughout the duration of treatment *(19)*. Progenitor cell mobilization is delayed, however, with peripheral blood CD34+ cells beginning to increase in concentration after 3 d of administration and peaking after 5 or 6 d of treatment *(20)*. This increase in cytokine-mediated PBSC concentration is transient, falling to one-third of peak levels after 10 d.

The increase in circulating hematopoietic progenitor cells after cytokine priming has been demonstrated both phenotypically and via stem cell culture *(14,15)*. Administration of G-CSF to normal donors has been shown to increase the peripheral concentration of CD34+ cells by 16-fold at d 4 and more primitive CD34+Thy-1dim cells and CD34+Thy-1dimCD38- cells increased by 24- and 23-fold, respectively *(14)*. Examination of PBSCs from normal donors in culture demonstrated that the number of long-term culture initiating cells (LTC-IC) measured in 5-wk cultures was 60-fold greater after G-CSF priming than at steady state *(15)*. Longer term, more primitive LTC-IC decreased by 85%, suggesting that while G-CSF is able to mobilize primitive progenitor cells, it is most potent at mobilizing progenitor cells of intermediate maturity. Subsequent analysis from the same investigators suggests that despite these limitations, the absolute yield of LTC-IC obtained after mobilization from peripheral blood is similar to that obtained from steady-state bone marrow *(21)*. The mechanism of action by which G-CSF mobilizes stem cells to circulate in peripheral blood is not entirely clear, but may be related in part to downregulation of $\alpha4\beta1$ integrin on CD34+ cells, which reduces the adhesive interaction between progenitors and the marrow stroma *(22)*.

Although peripheral blood progenitor cell concentrations increase dramatically after cytokine priming, the concentration achieved varies greatly among individuals *(23)*. Reasons for the wide variation are unclear. Some data suggest that older donors do not mobilize PBSCs as well as younger donors *(24,25)*, but in these series, poor mobilization occurred within all age groups, suggesting that other factors contribute as well. In mice, genetic factors have been demonstrated to play a role in numbers of stem cells mobilized *(26)*, though in humans, no similar genetic factors have been identified. Generally, yields of CD34+ cells have been significantly higher in peripheral blood grafts than in marrow grafts *(10–12)* (Table 1).

Up to one log more lymphocytes are contained within grafts obtained from peripheral blood compared to marrow. As a consequence, there has been both concern that incidence of graft-vs-host disease (GVHD) may be increased in blood recipients, along with hope that more prominent graft-vs-leukemia effects will enhance outcomes *(13)*. Results of clinical trials and large registry analyses have supported both of these concepts *(10,13,27)*.

Some data regarding immune reconstitution after peripheral blood and marrow grafting has been reported. One group has published data demonstrating that patients receiving PBSC grafts have higher memory T cell counts and T cell proliferative responses to phytohemagglutinin, pokeweed, Tetanus, and Candida than patients receiving marrow grafts *(28)*. In these patients, both the higher T-cell counts and increased T-cell proliferative activity persisted in PBSC recipients for at least 11 mo.

Another group has shown that while absolute T cell counts are higher in PBSC recipients, T cell proliferation in response to phytohemaglutinin and herpes virus antigens, is higher at d 30 posttransplant in PBSC recipients, but becomes similar for PBSC and marrow recipients

Table 1
Biologic Differences between Blood and Marrow as Stem Cell Sources

Characteristic	Peripheral blood allografts	Bone marrow allografts	Fold increase
Nucleated cells ($\times 10^8$/kg)	13.3	2.9	4.6
CD34+ cells ($\times 10^6$/kg)	11.7	3.2	3.7
CD3+ cells ($\times 10^6$/kg)	393.2	24.4	16.1
(Adapted with permission from ref. 14.)			

Characteristic	Peripheral blood allografts	Bone marrow allografts	Fold increase
Nucleated cells ($\times 10^8$/kg)	11.6 (1.5–24.6)	2.3 (0.02–14.6)	5.0
CD34+ cells ($\times 10^6$/kg)	7.3 (1.0–29.8)	2.4 (0.8–10.4)	3.0
CD3+ cells ($\times 10^6$/kg)	279 (143–788)	23.8 (1.2–30.5)	11.7
(Adapted with permission from ref. 12.)			

throughout the remainder of the first year following transplantation (29). In these patients, median serum IgG levels were shown to be similar between groups, suggesting that clinical differences in infection rates (discussed in Subheading 3.4.) are due primarily to enhanced cell-mediated immune function.

3. CLINICAL ASPECTS OF PBSC TRANSPLANTATION

Knowledge of the clinical aspects of PBSC transplantation has increased dramatically in recent years with the proliferation of studies comparing it to traditional marrow transplantation. While early results have become clear, late outcomes continue to require further investigation and longer patient follow-up.

3.1. Graft Characteristics

The evidence that greater CD34+ cell numbers are obtained using peripheral blood harvesting is strong. Four of five randomized trials published to date have harvested greater numbers of CD34+ cells from peripheral blood donors than from marrow donors (8,10–12). Three of these studies demonstrated a statistically significant difference in blood progenitors, with twice the number collected by apheresis as were collected from marrow (10–12). Graft composition data was not uniformly available in a recent comparison of peripheral blood vs marrow stem cell transplantation reported from the IBMTR (13), but several smaller series comparing PBSC recipients with historical or nonrandomized controls have shown higher CD34+ cell concentrations in peripheral blood (7,14,24).

The minimum number of cells needed for successful engraftment remains unclear. It has been estimated that approx 2.5–5 $\times$ 10^6 CD34+ cells/kg are required for consistently rapid engraftment (3), but no experimental evidence confirms this hypothesis. With regard to speed of engraftment, a higher CD34+ cell dose has been reported to facilitate more rapid platelet engraftment in allogeneic transplants (30), as was also shown in autologous transplants (31). Data from clinical trials of PBSC suggest that higher CD34+ counts promote more rapid neutrophil and platelet engraftment in the allogeneic setting as well.

3.2. Engraftment

Both neutrophil and platelet engraftment consistently occur more rapidly when using peripheral blood grafts as opposed to marrow grafts. All five published randomized trials found a shorter time to both neutrophil and platelet engraftment (Table 2), as do virtually all smaller series with nonrandomized controls.

Table 2
Summary of Randomized Clinical Trials Investigating PBSC vs BMT

Trial (ref.)	Year	N	Diseases included	GVHD prophylaxis	Neutrophil engraftment PBSC	Neutrophil engraftment BMT	Platelet recovery PBSC	Platelet recovery BMT	2-yr survival PBSC	2-yr survival BMT	Acute GVHD (grade II–IV) PBSC	Acute GVHD (grade II–IV) BMT	Chronic GVHD PBSC	Chronic GVHD BMT	Median follow-up PBSC	Median follow-up BMT
EBMT (8)	1998	33 PBSC 33 BMT	AML, ALL in 1st or 2nd remission, CML in 1st chronic phase	CSA/MTX[b] CSA/ prednisone	14 d	15 d	15 d	19 d	Not available		54%	48%	Not available		400 d	
Brazil (9)	1998	18 PBSC 19 BMT	CML, AML, ALL, MDS, NHL, MM Early and advanced disease	CSA/MTX	16 d	18 d	12 d	17 d[a]	51%	47%	27%	19%	71%	53%	355 d	631 d
France (10)	2000	48 PBSC 52 BMT	ALL, AML in 1st or 2nd CR CML in 1st CP	CSA/MTX[b]	15 d	21 d[a]	15 d	26 d[a]	67%	65%	44%	42%	50%	28%[a]	20 mo	
U.K. (11)	2000	20 PBSC 19 BMT	ALL, AML, CML, NHL, MDS, MM Low risk: PBSC 9, BMT 12 High risk: PBSC 11, BMT 7	CSA/MTX	17 d	23 d[a]	11 d	18 d[a]	70%	63%	50%	47%	44%	40%	33 mo	
U.S. (12)	2001	81 PBSC 91 BMT	AML, ALL, NHL, HD, CML, MM, MDS, CLL, Waldenström's Macroglobulinemia, Mycosis Fungoides	CSA/MTX	16 d	21 d[a]	13 d	19 d[a]	66% (p = 0.06)	54%	64%	57%	46%	35%	26 mo	

[a]Indicates p < 0.05 for given result.
[b]Methotrexate given on d 1, 3, and 6, but not d 11.
Abbreviations: ALL, acute lymphoblastic leukemia; CSA, cyclosporine; NHL, non-Hodgkin's lymphoma; MM, multiple myeloma; CR, complete remission; HD, Hodgkin's disease.

In the five published randomized trials, neutrophil engraftment occurred 1–6 d earlier in PBSC transplants than in marrow transplants. Differences were statistically significant in three of the five trials. In the larger IBMTR analysis, neutrophil engraftment occurred 5 d earlier in PBSC transplants than in marrow transplants *(13)*.

Platelet engraftment also occurs more rapidly using peripheral blood allografts. All randomized trials found more rapid platelet recovery, with the median differences ranging from 4 to 7 d. The IBMTR analysis found that platelet engraftment occurred a median of 7 d earlier in the PBSC transplants than in traditional marrow transplants. As with neutrophil engraftment, numerous smaller series have shown similar results.

Four of the five randomized trials included information about transfusions administered during the observational period. In the largest trial, the median number of platelet transfusions required in peripheral blood recipients was less than that in marrow recipients (30 vs 46), but the number of red blood cell (RBC) transfusions was the same (six in both groups) *(12)*. The largest European trial published found similar results, with fewer platelet transfusions occurring during the first 180 d after transplantation (PBSC median 3 vs bone marrow transplantation [BMT] 6) *(10)*. A smaller trial found that fewer platelet transfusions were required in peripheral blood recipients (PBSC 12.5, BMT 17.5), but similar RBC transfusions in the two groups (PBSC 5, BMT 6) *(9)*. One European trial found that PBSC recipients required more platelet transfusions than marrow recipients (PBSC 12, BMT 10) *(8)*.

3.3. GVHD

Since the earliest reports of peripheral blood allografting, there has been considerable concern that because such high numbers of lymphocytes are transplanted in peripheral blood grafts, GVHD would occur at high rates *(1–4)*. In clinical studies to date, however, consistent data has emerged suggesting little, if any, difference in overall rates of acute GVHD *(9,10-12)*. Chronic GVHD, in contrast, has been shown to occur more commonly in patients receiving peripheral blood allografts *(13,32)*. Because of the length of follow-up involved in ascertaining the incidence of chronic GVHD, data are not complete in all studies.

3.3.1. ACUTE GVHD

Overall rates of acute GVHD are generally similar in patients receiving peripheral blood or marrow transplants. Four of five randomized trials have found a 44–64% rate of grade II–IV acute GVHD in patients receiving peripheral blood transplants compared with a 42–57% rate in patients receiving marrow transplants *(8,10-12)*. In one randomized trial *(9)*, rates of acute GVHD were lower in both peripheral blood and marrow recipients when compared to other trials (PBSC 27%, BMT 19%). IBMTR analyses (Fig. 1) found that grades II–IV acute GVHD occurred in 40% of patients receiving peripheral blood transplants and 35% of patients receiving marrow transplants *(13)*. No study reported the difference in acute GVHD between peripheral blood and marrow to be statistically significant. In all cases, however, the reported rate was slightly higher in peripheral blood recipients.

One randomized trial published only in abstract form to date, found similar rates of grade II–IV acute GVHD in peripheral blood and marrow transplant recipients (PBSC 54% BMT 48%), but found that PBSC patients were more likely to have steroid-dependent or refractory disease. (PBSC 50%, BMT 14%, $p = 0.003$) *(27)*. In this trial, grade III–IV acute GVHD was also higher in patients receiving peripheral blood transplants (PBSC 46%, BMT 17%, $p = 0.02$). Rates of grade III–IV acute GVHD were not found to be different in patients included in the largest randomized trial *(12)* or in the IBMTR analysis *(13)*.

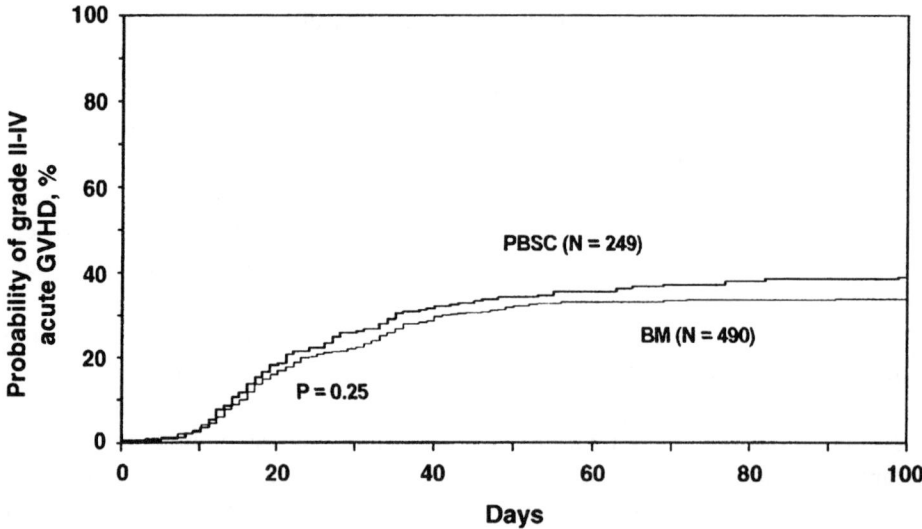

Fig. 1. Probabilities of grades II–IV acute GVHD after human leukocyte antigen (HLA) identical sibling PBSC transplantation compared with BMT for acute leukemia and CML. Probabilities were derived from multivariate Cox proportional hazards models and adjusted for effects of other significant covariates. Adapted with permission from ref. *13*.

3.3.2. Chronic GVHD

A growing body of evidence suggests that the occurrence of chronic GVHD is greater in patients receiving peripheral blood allografts than in those receiving marrow transplants. Results from several randomized trials show an increased risk of chronic GVHD *(9,10,12)*, but follow-up periods in these trials are generally short and may not represent the true burden of disease in study participants. One trial, designed to determine differences in GVHD based on stem cell source, closed enrollment early because the incidence of extensive chronic GVHD was significantly greater in patients receiving peripheral blood (77 vs 27%) *(27)*. The IBMTR analysis (Fig. 2) also found a statistically significant difference in the rate of chronic GVHD based on graft source (65 vs 53%, $p = 0.05$) *(13)*. As seen in Fig. 2, in this analysis the difference between groups did not become evident until 10–12 mo after transplant. Moreover, rates of chronic GVHD did not plateau until 12–15 mo after treatment, suggesting that shorter follow-up times are inadequate for determining true incidence of chronic GVHD. Experience with another smaller cohort was similar, with no difference in chronic GVHD found between peripheral blood and marrow grafts at a median follow-up of less than 1 yr *(33)*, but more chronic GVHD was noted in peripheral blood recipients when follow-up was extended to 2 yr *(34)*.

Risk factors for developing chronic GVHD in the IBMTR analysis include gender, no GVHD prophylaxis, and age equal to 40. Also of note is that a significant center effect was found for incidence of chronic GVHD but not for acute GVHD. In two trials that reported an increased risk of chronic GVHD, prophylactic regimens consisted of a shorter course of methotrexate than in other trials *(9,10)*, suggesting that prophylaxis with four doses of methotrexate plays an important role in preventing chronic GVHD in peripheral blood transplants.

In the IBMTR analysis, sites of chronic GVHD involvement did not differ substantially between treatment groups. Gastrointestinal involvement occurred at higher rates in patients receiving marrow transplants (35 vs 25%), and skin involvement was more frequent in patients receiving peripheral blood transplants (74 vs 66%). Other organ involvement occurred at essentially the same rates in the two treatment groups. Overall, available data suggests no

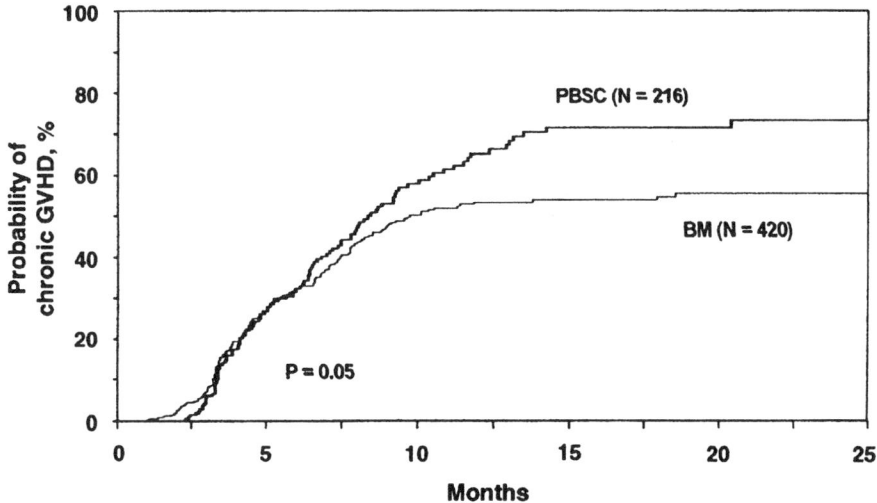

Fig. 2. Probabilities of chronic GVHD (limited or extensive disease) after HLA identical sibling PBSC transplantation compared with BMT for acute leukemia and CML. Probabilities were derived from multivariate Cox proportional hazards models and adjusted for effects of other significant covariates. Adapted with permission from ref. *13*.

major differences in the clinical presentation of chronic GVHD after allografts using marrow or peripheral blood.

3.4. Infections

Emerging data suggests that PBSC recipients have fewer infectious complications than marrow recipients. Data from the Seattle trial show that the overall rate of culture-proven infections was 1.7× higher in marrow recipients compared to PBSC recipients between d 30 and 365 of transplant ($p = 0.001$) *(29)*. Additionally, the rate of infections requiring inpatient treatment was 2.4× higher in marrow recipients ($p = 0.002$). The difference in rates of infection between groups was greatest for fungal infections (rate ratio [RR] 5.5, $p = 0.03$), but was also apparent for bacterial infections (RR 1.8, $p = 0.03$) and viral infections (RR 1.44, $p = 0.10$). Deaths associated with a definite infection between d 30 and 365 occurred in nine BMT recipients and three PBSC recipients ($p = 0.17$). If only deaths from bacterial and fungal pathogens were considered, nine deaths occurred among BMT recipients compared to none in PBSC recipients ($p = 0.008$).

3.5. Survival

Currently data do not demonstrate a clear benefit in overall survival with peripheral blood transplantation. The largest randomized trial published to date found a 2-yr survival rate of 66% in patients receiving peripheral blood and 54% in patients receiving standard marrow ($p=0.06$) (Fig. 3) *(12)*. Another trial with more patients available for 2-yr follow-up, however, found no difference in 2-yr survival between treatment groups (PBSC 67%, BMT 65%) *(10)*. Other published trials are limited in their ability to predict survival because of small patient numbers and short observational periods *(8,9,11)*.

Patients with advanced cancers, on the other hand, do seem to have better overall survival with peripheral blood allografts. IBMTR analyses show lower rates of treatment-related mortality at 1 yr for patients with acute leukemia in second remission and chronic myeloid leukemia (CML) in acute phase when transplanted with peripheral blood *(13)*. In the Seattle

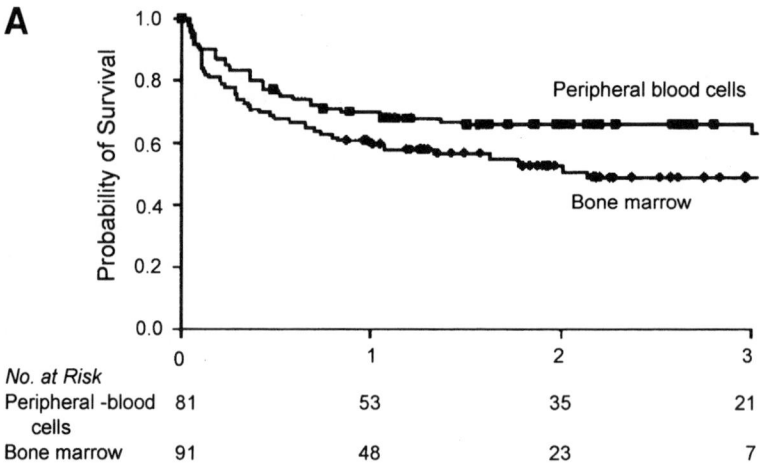

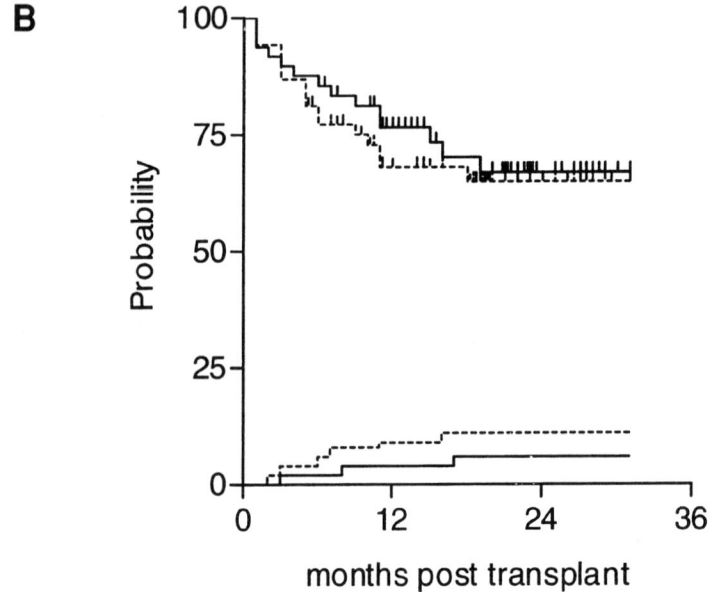

Fig. 3. Probability of overall survival in the largest randomized trials of peripheral blood vs marrow transplantation. (**A**) Overall survival in a major US trial. (**B**) Overall survival and relapse in a European trial (solid line, peripheral blood cells; dashed line, bone marrow). Adapted with permission from refs. *10* and *12*.

series, patients with advanced malignancies receiving peripheral blood transplants had a 57% 2-yr survival rate compared to a 33% 2-yr survival rate in marrow patients (*12*). It is not known why peripheral blood grafts improve survival for these patients, although some have hypothesized that more rapid neutrophil engraftment is of more benefit in more heavily pretreated or seriously ill patients (*13*). It is hypothesized that a more vigorous allogeneic response may reduce relapse rates after peripheral blood allotransplantation without more severe or more frequent GVHD.

Limited information is available comparing cause of death in patients receiving peripheral blood and marrow transplants. In the largest U.S. and European trials published to date (*10,12*), there were more deaths from disease relapse in marrow recipients, but otherwise cause of death was similar between groups. In the IBMTR analysis, there were no significant differences in cause of death between peripheral blood and marrow recipients *(13)*.

3.6. Disease-Free Survival

Evidence has emerged that peripheral blood recipients have improved disease-free survival over marrow recipients. In the Seattle report, rates of disease-free survival at 2 yr were 65% in peripheral blood recipients and 45% in marrow recipients *(12)*. A smaller European trial also found lower rates of relapse in peripheral blood recipients, despite small overall numbers *(11)*.

In the IBMTR analyses, patients with advanced disease who received peripheral blood allografts had fewer relapses by a substantial margin, but relapse was similar in patients with early disease *(13)*. A small nonrandomized series, in contrast, found that patients with CML in first chronic phase had improved survival after peripheral blood transplants *(35)*. Another series comparing acute myeloid leukemia (AML) and myelodysplasia (MDS) patients, who received peripheral blood transplants with historical marrow controls, also found improved survival in low risk patients due to lower rates of relapse *(32)*. Further research is needed to systematically investigate these observations.

3.7. Quality of Life

A few studies have analyzed quality of life in survivors of peripheral blood transplants. Generally, data comes from series comparing recent peripheral blood transplant recipients with historical controls who received marrow, limiting the validity of measures that may vary depending on length of follow-up.

In a comparison of peripheral blood recipients with historical controls who received marrow allografts, 48% of surviving peripheral blood recipients were found to have Karnofsky scores of 80 or less, while only 5% of those surviving marrow transplants had scores less than 80 *(32)*. Another uncontrolled series found that 64% of blood allograft progression-free survivors had Karnofsky scores between 70 and 80, compared to 29% between 90 and 100 *(36)*. In both series, chronic GVHD was responsible for most of the excess morbidity accompanying blood allotransplants. No data on quality of life was included in any of the trials published to date.

3.8. Unrelated Peripheral Blood Transplants

All randomized trials performed to date have included only related donors, but a series comparing 45 unrelated peripheral blood recipients with historical marrow controls has been published *(7)*. In this series, although neutrophil and platelet engraftment were more rapid in PBSC recipients, there was little difference in survival at 1 yr (PBSC 54%, BMT 53%) and in relapse-free survival at 2 yr (PBSC 46%, BMT 41%). Grade II–IV acute GVHD occurred at a rate of 30% in the PBSC group and 20% in the marrow group (p = ns), and chronic GVHD occurred at 59% in the PBSC group and 85% in the marrow group.

Research continues, examining this series of transplant recipients, with 107 PBSC recipients now included (O. Ringden, personal communication). Results in this expanded series are similar to those published earlier, with no substantial differences in grade II–IV acute GVHD, chronic GVHD, and disease-free survival. Overall survival remains comparable with 46% of PBSC recipients alive at 3 yr compared to 51% of BMT patients (p = ns).

3.9. Cytokine-Primed Marrow Transplantation

A few nonrandomized studies have investigated using G-CSF-primed marrow as an alternative source of stem cells for transplant. The rationale for marrow priming is based on murine

(37) and human *(38,39)* studies, demonstrating improved repopulating ability of G-CSF-primed bone marrow. A series comparing 26 primed bone marrow transplantation (pBMT) recipients with a historical cohort of 20 peripheral blood transplant recipients found that neutrophil recovery between groups was similar, but platelet recovery was more rapid in the peripheral blood recipients (PBSC 13 d, pBMT 16 d) *(40)*. Chronic GVHD occurred at a lower rate in patients receiving marrow (PBSC 68%, pBMT 37% $p = 0.049$), but survival was similar at 2 yr (PBSC 60%, pBMT 54%, $p = 0.9$).

Another small study compared transplantation of G-CSF-primed marrow in 29 patients with historical unprimed marrow controls *(41)*. It found more rapid granulocyte and platelet recovery in primed marrow recipients, but no difference in secondary endpoints, such as platelet and red cell transfusions, days on antibiotics, and length of hospital stay between groups. In contrast, a study of 17 patients receiving primed marrow compared with historical marrow controls found more rapid neutrophil recovery and shortened hospital stay in primed marrow recipients *(42)*.

With chronic GVHD and its negative impact on quality of life becoming a greater concern in patients receiving PBSC transplants, attention may shift to cytokine-primed marrow as an alternative. While early results show potential, controlled trials are needed to demonstrate any substantive benefit in clinical outcomes.

4. DONOR CONSIDERATIONS

Concerns regarding the safety for PBSC donors have not been completely addressed. Although short-term effects of G-CSF in normal donors are mild *(43)*, little is known about long-term effects of G-CSF in normal donors. Doses of G-CSF used in PBSC harvests range from 2–24 µg/kg/d (44). In clinical trials, doses of 10–16 µg/kg/d have been used for allogeneic stem cell harvesting *(8–12)*. A dose of 10 µg/kg/d was recently recommended for use in harvesting by some investigators, but evaluation of higher doses was recommended in the context of clinical trials *(44)*. In the one randomized trial that used a dose of 16 µg/kg/d *(12)*, a higher median yield of CD34+ cell counts was obtained, but no improvement in neutrophil recovery was demonstrated when compared with other trials.

A comparison of 30 blood and 38 marrow donor experiences from the Seattle randomized trial was recently published *(45)*. In this study, donors completed questionnaires describing their experiences prior to, during, and after donation, with weekly questionnaires completed until donors felt they had returned to their baseline state of health. For both donor groups, emotional status was essentially unchanged throughout donation and follow-up. Physical status, however, deteriorated after donation in both groups, primarily as a result of pain associated with the procedure. PBSC donors reported a considerable amount of pain during the days G-CSF was administered, with a generally rapid return to baseline after completion of the harvest procedure. Marrow donors reported average and maximal levels of pain similar to PBSC donors as a result of the procedure. All PBSC donors, but only 80% of marrow donors reported good physical status by 14 d after donation. It should be noted that donors in this series were given 16 µg/kg/d of G-CSF, which is higher than the 10 µg/kg/d used in most other series.

The most common short-term adverse effects of G-CSF administration include bone pain, headache, fatigue, and nausea. Less commonly, noncardiac chest pain, insomnia, night sweats, fluid retention, and dizziness have been reported *(44)*. Severe side effects requiring discontinuation of G-CSF are uncommon, occurring in 1–3% of donors *(20)*. Laboratory abnormalities, including transient elevations of alkaline phosphatase and lactate dehydrogenase and less commonly, electrolyte disturbances, have also been noted. Both thrombocytopenia and granulocytopenia have been reported after donation, but these findings result from the leukapheresis procedure itself, not from administration of G-CSF *(44)*. In general, adverse effects appear to be dose-related. A case of episcleritis *(46)* and a case of iritis *(47)* exacerbation following the administration of G-CSF have been reported, leading to concern that donors with inflammatory diseases of all types could experience worsening of their condition. Additionally, the G-CSF package insert states that animal studies have shown that cerebral ischemia may occur related to G-CSF induced 15- to 28-fold increases in leukocyte count. In the randomized trials published to date, one donor had a moderate anemia requiring transfusion, but otherwise no serious complications were noted in the 200 PBSC donors observed.

In 1997, an ad hoc committee was organized and convened by the University of Texas M.D. Anderson Cancer Center to discuss issues related to donor safety in allogeneic PBSC transplantation. The committee included representatives from more than 40 transplant teams, as well as from the IBMTR, the National Marrow Donor Program (NMDP), and the European Group for Blood and Marrow Transplantation (EBMT). It concluded that possible contraindications to donation include the presence of inflammatory, autoimmune, or rheumatologic disorders, as well as atherosclerotic or cerebrovascular disease *(44)*. This committee also recommended the formation of an international PBSC donor registry to facilitate monitoring of the long-term effects of donation. Routine laboratory testing for follow-up of donors was not recommended.

5. COST

One randomized trial included an economic analysis of peripheral blood transplants compared with marrow transplants *(10)*. It found that overall costs of peripheral blood transplants during the first 180 d were 16% less than costs of marrow transplants. The difference was primarily a result of lower room costs in the peripheral blood group, although cost was also reduced because of fewer platelet transfusions, fewer laboratory costs, and lower overall drug costs. Graft collection costs were higher in peripheral blood donors.

6. CONCLUSION

Our understanding of PBSC allogeneic transplantation has increased markedly during the past several years. Benefits of peripheral blood transplantation include more rapid engraftment and improved early survival in patients with advanced leukemia. Early data also suggests that infections occur less frequently in peripheral blood recipients. Unfortunately, chronic GVHD may occur more commonly in peripheral blood recipients, potentially compromising their long-term quality of life or their survival.

As research continues, more will be learned about long-term survival, late effects, and the use of peripheral blood grafts from both related and unrelated donors. While marrow currently remains the standard source of allografts, the safety and utility of peripheral blood will validate its expanded use in the future.

REFERENCES

1. Kessinger A, Smith DM, Strandjord SE, Landmark JD, Dooley DC, Law P, et al. Allogeneic transplantation of blood-derived, T cell-depleted hemopoietic stem cells after myeloablative treatment in a patient with acute lymphoblastic leukemia. *Bone Marrow Transplant* 1989;4:643–646.
2. Korbling M, Przepiorka D, Huh YO, Engel H, van Besien K, Giralt S, et al. Allogeneic blood stem cell transplantation for refractory leukemia and lymphoma: potential advantage of blood over marrow allografts. *Blood* 1995;85:1659–1665.
3. Bensinger WI, Weaver CH, Appelbaum FR, Rowley S, Demirer T, Sanders J, et al. Transplantation of allogeneic peripheral blood stem cells mobilized by recombinant human granulocyte colony-stimulating factor. *Blood* 1995;85:1655–1658.
4. Schmitz N, Dreger P, Suttorp M, Rohwedder EB, Haferlach T, Loffler H, et al. Primary transplantation of allogeneic peripheral blood progenitor cells mobilized by filgrastim (granulocyte colony-stimulating factor). *Blood* 1995;85:1666–1672.

5. Gratwohl A, Passweg J, Baldomero H, Hermans J. Blood and marrow transplantation activity in Europe 1996. European Group for Blood and Marrow Transplantation (EBMT). *Bone Marrow Transplant* 1998;22:227–240.
6. IBMTR Statistical Center. February 2001. Personal communication.
7. Ringden O, Remberger M, Runde V, Bornhauser M, Blau IW, Basara N, et al. Peripheral blood stem cell transplantation from unrelated donors: a comparison with marrow transplantation. *Blood* 1999;94:455–464.
8. Schmitz N, Bacigalupo A, Hasenclever D, Nagler A, Gluckman E, Clark P, et al. Allogeneic bone marrow transplantation vs filgrastim-mobilised peripheral blood progenitor cell transplantation in patients with early leukaemia: first results of a randomised multicentre trial of the European Group for Blood and Marrow Transplantation. *Bone Marrow Transplant* 1998;21:995–1003.
9. Vigorito AC, Azevedo WM, Marques JF, Azevedo AM, Eid KA, Aranha FJ, et al. A randomised, prospective comparison of allogeneic bone marrow and peripheral blood progenitor cell transplantation in the treatment of haematological malignancies. *Bone Marrow Transplant* 1998;22:1145–1151.
10. Blaise D, Kuentz M, Fortanier C, Bourhis JH, Milpied N, Sutton L, et al. Randomized trial of bone marrow versus lenograstim-primed blood cell allogeneic transplantation in patients with early-stage leukemia: a report from the Societe Francaise de Greffe de Moelle. *J Clin Oncol* 2000;18:537–546.
11. Powles R, Mehta J, Kulkarni S, Treleaven J, Millar B, Marsden J, et al. Allogeneic blood and bone-marrow stem-cell transplantation in haematological malignant diseases: a randomised trial. *Lancet* 2000;355:1231–1237.
12. Bensinger WI, Martin PJ, Storer B, Clift R, Forman SJ, Negrin R, et al. Transplantation of bone marrow as compared with peripheral-blood cells from HLA-Identical relatives in patients with hematologic cancers. *N Engl J Med* 2001;344:175–181.
13. Champlin RE, Schmitz N, Horowitz MM, Chapuis B, Chopra R, Cornelissen JJ, et al. Blood stem cells compared with bone marrow as a source of hematopoietic cells for allogeneic transplantation. IBMTR Histocompatibility and Stem Cell Sources Working Committee and the European Group for Blood and Marrow Transplantation (EBMT). *Blood* 2000;95:3702–3709.
14. Korbling M, Huh YO, Durett A, Mirza N, Miller P, Engel H, et al. Allogeneic blood stem cell transplantation: peripheralization and yield of donor-derived primitive hematopoietic progenitor cells (CD34+ Thy- 1dim) and lymphoid subsets, and possible predictors of engraftment and graft-versus-host disease. *Blood* 1995;86:2842–2948.
15. Prosper F, Stroncek D, Verfaillie CM. Phenotypic and functional characterization of long-term culture- initiating cells present in peripheral blood progenitor collections of normal donors treated with granulocyte colony-stimulating factor. *Blood* 1996;88:2033–2042.
16. Lane TA, Law P, Maruyama M, Young D, Burgess J, Mullen M, et al. Harvesting and enrichment of hematopoietic progenitor cells mobilized into the peripheral blood of normal donors by granulocyte-macrophage colony-stimulating factor (GM-CSF) or G-CSF: potential role in allogeneic marrow transplantation. *Blood* 1995;85:275–282.
17. Brasel K, McKenna HJ, Charrier K, Morrissey PJ, Williams DE, Lyman SD. Flt3 ligand synergizes with granulocyte-macrophage colony-stimulating factor or granulocyte colony-stimulating factor to mobilize hematopoietic progenitor cells into the peripheral blood of mice. *Blood* 1997;90:3781–3788.
18. Molineux G, McCrea C, Yan XQ, Kerzic P, McNiece I. Flt-3 ligand synergizes with granulocyte colony-stimulating factor to increase neutrophil numbers and to mobilize peripheral blood stem cells with long-term repopulating potential. *Blood* 1997;89:3998–4004.
19. Stroncek DF, Confer DL, Leitman SF. Peripheral blood progenitor cells for HPC transplants involving unrelated donors. *Transfusion* 2000;40:731–741.
20. Stroncek DF, Clay ME, Petzoldt ML, Smith J, Jaszcz W, Oldham FB, et al. Treatment of normal individuals with granulocyte-colony-stimulating factor: donor experiences and the effects on peripheral blood CD34+ cell counts and on the collection of peripheral blood stem cells. *Transfusion* 1996;36:601–610.
21. Prosper F, Vanoverbeke K, Stroncek D, Verfaillie CM. Primitive long-term culture initiating cells (LTC-ICs) in granulocyte colony-stimulating factor mobilized peripheral blood progenitor cells have similar potential for ex vivo expansion as primitive LTC-ICs in steady state bone marrow. *Blood* 1997;89:3991–3997.
22. Prosper F, Stroncek D, McCarthy JB, Verfaillie CM. Mobilization and homing of peripheral blood progenitors is related to reversible downregulation of alpha4 beta1 integrin expression and function. *J Clin Invest* 1998;101:2456–2467.
23. Russell NH, Gratwohl A, Schmitz N. Developments in allogeneic peripheral blood progenitor cell transplantation. *Br J Haematol* 1998;103:594–600.
24. Dreger P, Haferlach T, Eckstein V, Jacobs S, Suttorp M, Loffler H, et al. G-CSF-mobilized peripheral blood progenitor cells for allogeneic transplantation: safety, kinetics of mobilization, and composition of the graft. *Br J Haematol* 1994;87:609–613.
25. Anderlini P, Przepiorka D, Seong C, Smith TL, Huh YO, Lauppe J, et al. Factors affecting mobilization of CD34+ cells in normal donors treated with filgrastim. *Transfusion* 1997;37:507–512.
26. Roberts AW, Foote S, Alexander WS, Scott C, Robb L, Metcalf D. Genetic influences determining progenitor cell mobilization and leukocytosis induced by granulocyte colony-stimulating factor. *Blood* 1997;89:2736–2744.

27. Durrant S, Morton AJ. A randomized trial of filgrastim (G-CSF) stimulated donor marrow (BM) versus peripheral blood (PBPC) for allogenic transplantation: increased extensive chronic graft versus host disease following PBPC transplantation. *Blood* 1999;10:608a.

28. Ottinger HD, Beelen DW, Scheulen B, Schaefer UW, Grosse-Wilde H. Improved immune reconstitution after allotransplantation of peripheral blood stem cells instead of bone marrow. *Blood* 1996;88:2775–2779.

29. Storek J, Dawson MA, Storer B, Stevens-Ayers T, Maloney DG, Marr KA, et al. Immune reconstitution after allogeneic marrow transplantation compared with blood stem cell transplantation. *Blood* 2001;97:3380–3389.

30. Lickliter JD, McGlave PB, DeFor TE, Miller JS, Ramsay NK, Verfaillie CM, et al. Matched-pair analysis of peripheral blood stem cells compared to marrow for allogeneic transplantation. *Bone Marrow Transplant* 2000;26:723–728.

31. Bensinger WI, Longin K, Appelbaum F, Rowley S, Weaver C, Lilleby K, et al. Peripheral blood stem cells (PBSCs) collected after recombinant granulocyte colony stimulating factor (rhG-CSF): an analysis of factors correlating with the tempo of engraftment after transplantation. *Br J Haematol* 1994;87:825–831.

32. Russell JA, Larratt L, Brown C, Turner AR, Chaudhry A, Booth K, et al. Allogeneic blood stem cell and bone marrow transplantation for acute myelogenous leukemia and myelodysplasia: influence of stem cell source on outcome. *Bone Marrow Transplant* 1999;24:1177–1183.

33. Bensinger WI, Clift R, Martin P, Appelbaum FR, Demirer T, Gooley T, et al. Allogeneic peripheral blood stem cell transplantation in patients with advanced hematologic malignancies: a retrospective comparison with marrow transplantation. *Blood* 1996;88:2794–2800.

34. Storek J, Gooley T, Siadak M, Bensinger WI, Maloney DG, Chauncey TR, et al. Allogeneic peripheral blood stem cell transplantation may be associated with a high risk of chronic graft-versus-host disease. *Blood* 1997;90:4705–4709.

35. Elmaagacli AH, Beelen DW, Opalka B, Seeber S, Schaefer UW. The risk of residual molecular and cytogenetic disease in patients with Philadelphia-chromosome positive first chronic phase chronic myelogenous leukemia is reduced after transplantation of allogeneic peripheral blood stem cells compared with bone marrow. *Blood* 1999;94:384–389.

36. Brown RA, Adkins D, Khoury H, Vij R, Goodnough LT, Shenoy S, et al. Long-term follow-up of high-risk allogeneic peripheral-blood stem-cell transplant recipients: graft-versus-host disease and transplant-related mortality. *J Clin Oncol* 1999;17:806–812.

37. Bodine DM, Seidel NE, Orlic D. Bone marrow collected 14 days after in vivo administration of granulocyte colony-stimulating factor and stem cell factor to mice has 10-fold more repopulating ability than untreated bone marrow. *Blood* 1996;88:89–97.

38. Johnsen HE, Hansen PB, Plesner T, Jensen L, Gaarsdal E, Andersen H, et al. Increased yield of myeloid progenitor cells in bone marrow harvested for autologous transplantation by pretreatment with recombinant human granulocyte-colony stimulating factor. *Bone Marrow Transplant* 1992;10:229–234.

39. Martinez C, Urbano-Ispizua A, Rozman M, Rovira M, Marin P, Montfort N, et al. Effects of short-term administration of G-CSF (filgrastim) on bone marrow progenitor cells: analysis of serial marrow samples from normal donors. *Bone Marrow Transplant* 1999;23:15–19.

40. Serody JS, Sparks SD, Lin Y, Capel EJ, Bigelow SH, Kirby SL, et al. Comparison of granulocyte colony-stimulating factor (G-CSF)—mobilized peripheral blood progenitor cells and G-CSF—stimulated bone marrow as a source of stem cells in HLA-matched sibling transplantation. *Biol Blood Marrow Transplant* 2000;6:434–440.

41. Couban S, Messner HA, Andreou P, Egan B, Price S, Tinker L, et al. Bone marrow mobilized with granulocyte colony-stimulating factor in related allogeneic transplant recipients: a study of 29 patients. *Biol Blood Marrow Transplant* 2000;6:422–427.

42. Isola L, Scigliano E, Fruchtman S. Long-term follow-up after allogeneic granulocyte colony-stimulating factor—primed bone marrow transplantation. *Biol Blood Marrow Transplant* 2000;6:428–433.

43. Anderlini P, Przepiorka D, Champlin R, Korbling M. Biologic and clinical effects of granulocyte colony-stimulating factor in normal individuals. *Blood* 1996;88:2819–2825.

44. Anderlini P, Korbling M, Dale D, Gratwohl A, Schmitz N, Stroncek D, et al. Allogeneic blood stem cell transplantation: considerations for donors. *Blood* 1997;90:903–908.

45. Rowley SD, Donaldson G, Lilleby K, Bensinger WI, Appelbaum FR. Experiences of donors enrolled in a randomized study of allogeneic bone marrow or peripheral blood stem cell transplantation. *Blood* 2001;97:2541–2548.

46. Huhn RD, Yurkow EJ, Tushinski R, Clarke L, Sturgill MG, Hoffman R, et al. Recombinant human interleukin-3 (rhIL-3) enhances the mobilization of peripheral blood progenitor cells by recombinant human granulocyte colony-stimulating factor (rhG-CSF) in normal volunteers. *Exp Hematol* 1996;24:839–847.

47. Parkkali T, Volin L, Siren MK, Ruutu T. Acute iritis induced by granulocyte colony-stimulating factor used for mobilization in a volunteer unrelated peripheral blood progenitor cell donor. *Bone Marrow Transplant* 1996;17:433,434.

9

Haploidentical Stem Cell Transplantation

Hillard M. Lazarus, MD
and Jacob M. Rowe, MD

CONTENTS

1. INTRODUCTION

Allogeneic stem cell transplantation has been performed clinically for more than 30 yr as therapy for a number of different hematologic malignancies, genetic disorders, and immunologic deficiency syndromes *(1,2)*. In most instances, the donor stem cells were obtained from sibling-matched donors. Patient outcome after transplant has been influenced by many factors, such as patient age, disease type, duration and stage at transplant, and cytomegalovirus (CMV) serologic status of the patient and donor. The best results with allogeneic transplant have been obtained in patients who have disease responsive to chemotherapy and who received hematopoietic stem cells obtained from human leukocyte antigen (HLA)-matched sibling donors. Even in this setting, this proceedure has been associated with substantial morbidity and mortality, predominantly due to the occurrence of acute and chronic graft-vs-host disease (GVHD), opportunistic infection, visceral organ dysfunction, or a combination of these. Until recently, the vast majority of patients received bone marrow as the source of hematopoietic stem cell graft. Recent data support the use of donor hematopoietic stem cells obtained from peripheral blood rather than bone marrow, especially in more advanced disease states *(3)*. Despite the drawbacks noted above, allogeneic stem cell transplantation remains a treatment modality that has provided curative therapy for many patients.

Unfortunately, only about one-quarter of patients have a histocompatible sibling donor. Over the past decade, the need for alternative donors has pushed the scientific frontiers. As a result, sensitive molecular methods of tissue typing have been developed, including DNA

From: *Current Clinical Oncology: Allogeneic Stem Cell Transplantation*
Edited by: Mary S. Laughlin and Hillard M. Lazarus © Humana Press Inc., Totowa, NJ

oligonucleotide sequencing, which provide an opportunity to use matched, but unrelated, donors. Improvements in the precision of HLA-typing methologies allow identification of more closely matched donors, which will result in a lower incidence and severity of GVHD and improved survival *(4–6)*. Additionally, various centralized registries have been developed that can identify potential donors and procure hematopoietic stem cells from these matched unrelated individuals. Such registries can furnish bone marrow, peripheral blood, and umbilical cord blood units, thus enabling appropriate candidates to undergo alternative donor allogeneic transplant procedures.

The morbidity and mortality associated with the use of alternative donor transplants, however, is significantly greater than that observed with sibling-matched donors. Also, the time necessary to locate and procure unrelated donor stem cells often is long, which may limit availability for the majority of patients who urgently require allograft therapy.

2. HAPLOIDENTICAL TRANSPLANTS

A genetically haploidentical family member represents another potential alternative donor. These individuals are readily available for nearly 90% of patients. Due to the ease of donor accessibility in most instances, haploidentical transplants have been attempted over the past two decades. The initial efforts, however, were largely unsuccessful due to an excessively high treatment-related mortality. Table 1 depicts the main problems. Due to the marked disparity between donor and recipient, refractory GVHD has been a significant problem *(7,8)*. T cell depletion of the donor graft is often performed to prevent this problem; engraftment failure may occur due to the fact that standard conditioning regimens are not sufficiently immunosuppressive to eradicate host cytotoxic T lymphocytes *(9–12)*. An additional drawback of haploidentical transplants includes the slow immune reconstitution, which puts the patient at risk for life-threatening infectious complications. This effect persists for a significantly longer period of time when compared to an HLA-matched sibling donor transplant, despite adequate engraftment and absent or adequate control of GVHD *(13–15)*.

In the past decade, significant strides in allogeneic transplantation have markedly increased the feasibility of using these donor grafts for transplantation. Recent data suggest that procedures utilizing haploidentical grafts may have a role in patients who do not have markedly advanced disease, which has confounded interpretation of the data (Table 2) *(16–21)*. Most reports describe enrollment and treatment of poor-risk patients resulting in high transplant-related morbidity and mortality and high rates of relapse. Over the past decade, several investigators have aggressively approached haploidentical transplants in earlier stage, or responsive-disease, acute leukemia patients, focusing on the safety and improved long-term efficacy of the procedure. This communication reviews these data.

3. GVHD

GVHD has been one of the major problems which has plagued the success of haploidentical transplantation *(7,8)*. The risk of acute GVHD was increased significantly in patients who received marrow grafts obtained from donors incompatible at one, two, or three HLA loci. The degree of HLA incompatibility correlated directly with the risk for the development of acute GVHD *(5)*. Patients who received marrow grafts from donors incompatible at one or more HLA loci had a relative-risk of 3.23 for the development of GVHD compared to controls. More than 80% of patients incompatible for three HLA loci developed severe acute GVHD.

A variety of approaches have been attempted to reduce the high rate of GVHD, including removal or suppression donor T cells in the graft *(22–25)*. Infusions of grafts, which contain less than $1–5 \times 10^4$ CD3 cells/kg recipient weight usually are not associated with the develop-

Table 1
Barriers to Successful Haploidentical Stem Cell Transplantation

Barriers	Current or potential solutions (ref.)
Graft failure	Megadoses of CD34 donor cells (47,49).
	Immunosuppresive conditioning regimen (44).
	Selective myeloablative conditioning (35,36).
Refractory GVHD	Maximal donor-cell immune suppression (44).
	T cell depletion of the donor graft (22–25).
	Co-stimulatory blockade of the donor graft (21), i.e., CTLA-4.
Delayed immune reconstitution	Cytokine manipulation (56).
	Adoptive cellular immunotherapy (59).
	Use of nonalloreactive CTL (27).
Decreased graft-vs-tumor effect	NK cell alloreactivity (KIR epitope-mismatching) (73,74).

GVHD, graft-vs-host disease; KIR, donor NK cell killer inhibitory receptors.

Table 2
Logistic Advantages of Haploidentical Family Member Allografts

Immediate donor availability.
No racial or ethnic restrictions.
Multiple donors: select for gender, age, and CMV status.
Continued donor access: additional cells for later immunologic initiatives.
Decreased costs: no banking or registration fees and less HLA typing.

ment of GVHD; in fact, this degree of T cell depletion may obviate the need for the use of posttransplant immunosuppression as GVHD prophylaxis (26,27). Other factors, however, may play a role in likelihood of developing GVHD, including the previous patient cytotoxic agent exposure and the intensity of the immunosuppression afforded by the conditioning regimen. Thus, the positve and negative effects of T cell depletion cannot be considered in isolation (28).

Recent advances in prevention of GVHD utilize inactivation of a select segment of the alloreactive T cell repertoire. This strategy is executed via blockade of B7-mediated T cell co-stimulation, which appears to result in a significant reduction in the risk of GVHD without increasing the risk for graft failure. Donor bone marrow cells can be treated ex vivo in co-culture with irradiated recipient cells in the presence of CTLA-4-Ig, which is an agent that inhibits B7:CD28-mediated co-stimulation and induces anergy to recipient alloantigens. Although only relatively few transplants have been conducted in this fashion, GVHD rates have been quite low, thus encouraging further investigation of this approach (21,29).

Selection depletion of effector cells such as CD8+ T lymphocytes have been utilized by ex vivo treatment of donor bone marrow with anti-Leu-2 monoclonal antibody and complement (30). Although this maneuver may abrogate the severity of GVHD, there are as yet no data in haploidentical transplantation, demonstrating that such a manipulation will reduce the risk of graft failure after T cell depletion (31).

4. GRAFT FAILURE

Despite implementation of strategies designed to reduce the likelihood for developing GVHD, haploidentical transplants remain a high risk procedure. Donor T cells facilitate engraftment and assist in immunological reconstitution of the host. These actions prevent opportunistic infections, as well as contribute to the direct antitumor effect of the graft. Thus, T cell depletion of a graft could prevent GVHD, but such benefit was offset by infection and recurrence of malignancy. Some investigators believed that barriers to engraftment in haploidentical transplantation could be overcome by increasing the intensity of the conditioning regimen, especially with the use of higher doses of total body irradiation (TBI) alone or in combination with other myeloablative and immunosuppressive regimens (19,32–34). Such intensive preparative regimens lead to significant visceral organ toxicity, especially in subjects who previously have received large doses of cytotoxic therapy for advanced disease states.

Graft failure also may be mediated by competition between host hematopoietic progenitor cells, which survive the conditioning and donor stem cells (35,36). Potent stem cell toxic agents such as melphalan, busulphan (36), and thiotepa (37), provide relatively selective myeloablative therapy and can facilitate successful engraftment in the absence of TBI (20,38). In an attempt to facilitate engraftment without excessive toxicity and GVHD, a variety of immunosuppressive agents have been incorporated into conditioning regimens, including fludarabine (20), high dose methylprednisolone (39), total nodal irradiation (10), anti-T cell antibodies (40,41), and antithymocyte globulin (ATG) (20,39,42,43).

One of the most difficult issues in performing a haploidentical transplantation has been balancing the necessary degree of myeloablation and immunosuppression against the resulting regimen-related toxicity. One approach has been to utilize a sequential administration of myeloablative drugs and immunosuppressive therapy, recognizing that the toxic effects of the procedure may be reduced if these essential components are not given simultaneously. The group at the University of South Carolina reported a favorable experience in 210 patients in whom the addition of ATG to a TBI based conditioning regimen resulted in a 16-d median time to engraftment (44).

The University of Perugia has contributed significantly to advancing the field in haploidentical transplantation (20). This group developed a relatively nontoxic conditioning regimen by incorporating thiotepa, single-fraction TBI dose (800 cGy), fludarabine, and ATG. This regimen is associated with an approx 10% treatment-related mortality at 30 d after stem cell infusion. This approach relies upon the concept that escalation of stem cell dose directly contributes to the likelihood of establishing donor-type chimerism. Cells within the CD34 subset possess potent "veto activity," which enable these cells to neutralize cytotoxic T lymphocyte-precursors (CTL-p) directed against veto-cell antigens. The greater the number of CD34 stem cells infused, the greater the induction of tolerance in the host (45,46).

The concept of stem cell dose escalation in humans could be tested only after technologies for the mobilization and collection of peripheral blood progenitor cells became available as a result of cytokine therapy (47,48). Megadoses of CD34 cells, in the range 10^7 CD34 cells/kg recipient weight or greater, could be collected and T cell-depleted in vitro. After infusion, these cells engraft successfully and are not associated high GVHD rates (49). This method has been replicated at other institutions and offers great promise for current and future studies of haploidentical transplantation (50).

T cell-depleted allografts, however, appear to have only a limited capacity to reconstitute bone marrow mesenchymal stem cells (51). This cell type not only contributes to fabricating the bone marrow microenvironment, but also may possess immunosuppressive properties that can attenuate GVHD (52). Future transplant strategies may incorporate infusions of ex vivo culture-expanded mesenchymal stem cells as a supplement to T cell-depleted hematopoietic stem cell allografts in order to improve bone marrow stromal reconstitution (52).

5. DELAYED IMMUNE RECONSTITUTION

As the problems of engraftment and prevention of excessive GVHD have become more manageable, investigators performing haploidentical transplants have focused on the marked delay in immune reconstitution, which persists for months and even years after transplant. Recovery of CD4 cells may take 6–18 mo or longer to recover. Immune recovery after intensive T cell depletion has been associated with a very high risk for viral, fungal, and other opportunistic infections *(13,53,54)*. This delay represents the most important cause of mortality in adults undergoing haploidentical bone marrow transplantation and may approach a rate of 40% in the posttransplant setting *(20)*.

Delayed immunity results from the low number of infused donor T cells and diminished thymic function in the adult and defective antigen-presenting cell function (including monocytes and dendritic cells) are significant factors *(55)*. The use of granulocyte colony-stimulating factor (G-CSF) to speed engraftment has been demonstrated recently to block interleukin (IL)-12 production by the antigen-presenting cells; IL-12 is a key participant in the initiation of protective Th1 immunity against opportunistic infections and viruses *(53)*. Preliminary clinical data indicate that avoidance of G-CSF after transplant results in an enhanced rate of immune reconstitution, including the recovery of CD4 cells without adversely affecting rate of engraftment *(45,56)*.

Adoptive transfer of specific T cell clones is a tool that has been used to a limited extent to restore specific immunity against *Candida* sp., *Aspergillus* sp., and *Toxoplasma* after transplantation *(27,57)*. Investigators at the Fred Hutchinson Cancer Research Center in Seattle have developed a reliable method for the adoptive transfer of haploidentical donor CMV-specific T cell clones targeted against infected host T cells *(58,59)*. The process is extremely time-consuming, labor-intensive, and technically complex; however, infusion of these donor T cells, which are specifically reactive for CMV antigens, has resulted in very specific targeted immunity. At present the use of such adoptive therapy is not a routine laboratory procedure, but this technique represents another promising clinical avenue to reduce infection-related morbidity and mortality after transplant.

6. INDUCING TOLERANCE

Another approach to improving haploidentical transplantation might involve the induction of tolerance. GVHD is initiated by adoptive transfer of donor T cells that recognize host alloantigens and produce a characteristic reaction, but use of T cell depletion strategies in the donor graft may lead to engraftment failure and a prolongation of the immunodeficiency after transplant. The more common method of preventing GVHD, via the application of nonspecific immunosuppressive medications given as prophylaxis after transplantation, can lead to the development of opportunistic infection, tumor recurrence, and onset of secondary malignancy *(60–63)*.

Several investigators have addressed such problems by attempting specifically to suppress alloreactive T cells, without inhibiting the entire T cell repetoire, by blocking the initial steps of immune recognition that induce GVHD. Immune activation of T cells requires two signals from antigen-presenting cells, i.e., one specific antigen signal and a nonspecific costimulatory signal *(64,65)*. These two signals include delivery of an immunogenic peptide presented within the major histocompatibility locus to the T cell receptor and the interaction of cell surface proteins present on antigen presenting cells and T cells. If the latter signal is not present or is blocked, the T cells become incapable of responding to the antigen presented to them, i.e., the state of anergy.

An example of one critical co-stimulatory signal occurs between the B7 protein on antigen-presenting cells and the CD28 molecule on the T cell surface. If this interaction is blocked, i.e., B7 blockade, anergy ensues *(66)*. In preclinical systems interfering with B7:C28, interaction permits successful transplantation of histoincompatible allografts without the need for pharmacologic immunosuppression *(67)*. Another method to produce anergy is to interfere with donor T cell recognition of host antigens as targets potentially leading to GVHD, the agent CTL-associated antigen (CTLA)-4 Ig can be used to create a situation of anergy in the patient. One group has successfully reported that donor bone marrow mismatched at one HLA haplotype could be treated ex vivo with CTLA-4 Ig to induce anergy and a low risk of GVHD in the recipient without impairing hematopoiesis *(21,66,68)*. These methods for co-stimulatory blockade provide a theoretical means to induce tolerance and are likely to be more extensively studied over the next few years. Some authors, however, have urged caution, since efforts to induce tolerance might result in the development of severe GVHD if any of the CTL-p escape deletion or anergy induction and committed CTLs are generated. Once primed, the alloreactivity of these antihost CTLs is extremely difficult to suppress in vivo *(27)*.

Another approach currently being evaluated is based on earlier studies that showed that CD8[+] CTL clones possess extremely high veto activity *(69)*. Preliminary data from the Weizmman Institute in Israel has focused on depleting such veto cells of alloreactive activity by generating nonalloreactive anti-third-party CTL clones. These cells, evaluated by their capacity to facilitate engraftment of purified Sca-1[+]Lin[-] hematopoietic progenitors in sublethally irradiated mismatched recipients, can be used to induce tolerance *(27,50,70–72)*. If this strategy can be successfully implemented, many complications of haploidentical transplantation can be avoided making this type of transplant approach more commonplace.

7. IMPAIRED ANTITUMOR RESPONSE

T cell depletion carries with it a high risk of leukemic relapse, in part due to abrogation of the graft-vs-leukemia effect. This phenomenon made it difficult to reconcile the finding of a relatively low relapse rate in advanced acute myeloid leukemia patients undergoing T cell-depleted allogeneic transplants *(20)*. Recent studies, however, suggest that donor natural killer (NK) cell alloreactivity may play a significant role in providing a graft-vs-leukemia effect *(73,74)*. This donor NK cell alloreactivity probably is unique to the mismatched transplant situation; donor NK cell killer inhibitory receptors (KIR) do not appear to recognize the major histocompatibility complex (MHC) allotypes of the recipient as "self." Thus, these donor cells lyse the recipients' hematopoietic cells. The NK cells, which generate in vivo after donor graft infusion and which arise from the donor stem cells, do not exhibit tolerance towards the new host, and a significant number of donor-type NK cells clones are alloreactive against the recipient *(74)*. This alloreactivity usually depends upon the recognition of a particular epitope shared by specific HLA allotypes.

In long-term follow-up of 75 high risk acute myeloid leukemia patients, this donor cell NK alloreactivity effect appears quite potent *(75)*. Only one of 28 patients transplanted from donors with the potential to transfer anti-recipient NK alloreactivity has relapsed. In contrast, 14 of 47 patients have relapsed when donor grafts were unable to provide anti-recipient NK cell alloreactivity in vivo *(75)* ($p < 0.05$). Thus, these clinical data strongly support the hypothesis that only mismatched transplants can provide a graft-vs-leukemia effect, independent of T cell-mediated GVHD reactions, when KIR epitope incompatibility is in the GVHD direction. These authors suggest that donor-vs-recipient NK cell alloreactivity may become a major criteria for donor selection in mismatched hematopoietic stem cell transplants.

8. CLINICAL PERSPECTIVE

Although the number of sibling-matched allogeneic stem cell transplants performed has steadily increased over the past four decades, this type of procedure can be offered only to a minority of patients, since most subjects do not have an HLA-matched sibling donor and many individuals are beyond the age where this approach can be performed within a reasonable

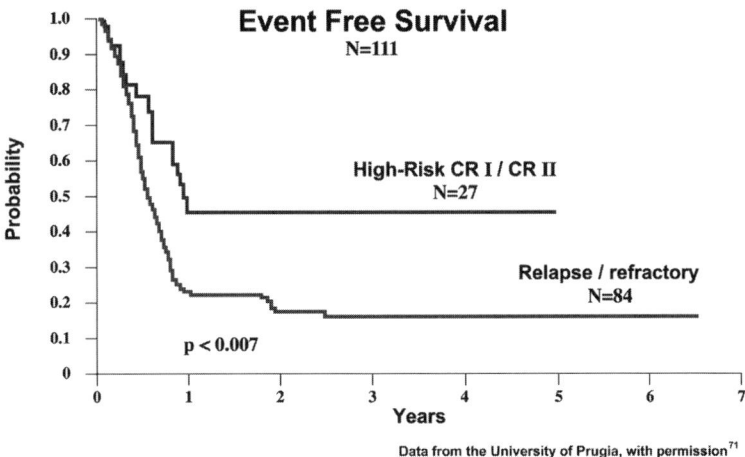

Fig. 1. Event-free survival for 111 patients with acute leukemia who underwent haploidentical transplantation April 1993 through June 2000 at the University of Perugia, Italy.

degree of safety. For those patients who lack an acceptable matched donor and are otherwise suitable candidates, a matched unrelated donor transplant usually is performed. Although success rates are increasing, this procedure is associated with a high transplant-related mortality (30–40%) and a high long-term morbidity *(76–79)*. In the setting of advanced leukemia, this approach rarely is successful, as many such patients do not survive the long waiting period (3–6 mo) until a suitable donor can be found.

One of the largest series reporting results of matched unrelated donor transplants has been updated demonstrating that long-term leukemia-free survival in 81 relapsed acute myelogenous leukemia patients was only 7% *(80)*. These less-than-desired results paradoxically reflect an inherent patient selection bias. Those individuals who could "survive" the long waiting period required to identify a suitable donor likely provided a better group to undergo the procedure. The logistics of donor identification have precluded undertaking an intent-to-treat analysis comparing matched unrelated donor transplants with other approaches for advanced acute myeloid leukemia patients.

Haploidentical hematopoietic stem cell transplantation presents a better logistic and practical alternative to matched unrelated donor transplants. About 90% of patients have a suitable, willing family member donor readily available (parent, sibling, offspring) and the procedure can be arranged and undertaken within a very short period of time. The most recent experience published from the University of Perugia, Italy, suggests that not only does the morbidity and mortality not exceed the values reported for matched unrelated donor transplants, but in acute myeloid leukemia there is no excessive risk of relapse *(20,50)*. The results in 111 acute leukemia patients transplanted April 1993 through June 2000 are shown in Figs. 1 and 2 *(81)*. The 5-yr event-free survival for refractory disease patients (N = 84) was disappointing at 15%. These data, however, do not reflect a lead-time bias since all refractory disease patients are reported, including those who would never have survived long enough to wait for an unrelated donor to be located and the stem cells collected. In contrast, Figs. 1 and 2 show a 45% 5-yr event-free survival and 12% relapse rate for very high-risk acute leukemia patients (N = 27) in first or second complete remission who received haploidentical transplants. The Perugia group results reflect the fact that they utilize the CliniMACS (Miltenyi Biotech, Bergisch Gladbach, Germany) stem cell selection instrument for providing a donor graft, enriched for CD34 and depleted of T cells, which is associated with reduced transplant-related

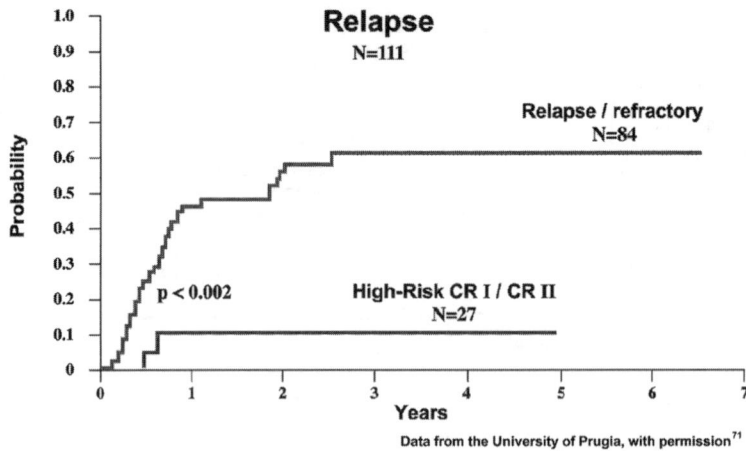

Data from the University of Prugia, with permission[71]

Fig. 2. Risk for relapse of leukemia in 111 patients who underwent haploidentical transplantation April 1993 through June 2000 at the University of Perugia, Italy.

mortality. Of great import, these investigators showed in sequential studies that the transplant-related mortality was reduced from 63%, using the Isolex 300 device (Baxter, Deerfield, IL), to 42%, with the Ceprate instrument (CellPro, Bothell, WA), to only 20% with the CliniMACS apparatus *(82)*. These data are not prospective comparisons, and the patient sample sizes are limited. These results, using the CliniMACS device, have been confirmed by another group, while use of other technologies has proven inferior in approaching haploidentical transplants *(83,84)*. As other groups continue to utilize differing approaches, such as the blockade of B7-mediated T cell co-stimulation, the improved results with haploidentical transplantation may lead to greater acceptance as a therapeutic alternative *(21,66,68)*.

9. SUMMARY

Haploidentical hematopoietic stem cell transplantation is a viable option for acute leukemia patients who do not have a suitable HLA-compatible sibling donor. Since most patients have a genetically haploidentical family member, identification and collection of donor cells and subsequent transplant may be performed without delay. In the past, this approach proved too toxic due uncontrolled GVHD, failure to engraft, delayed immune reconstitution, and late opportunistic infection, often resulting in an unacceptably high treatment-related morbidity and mortality. Recent modifications and new technologic developments have largely overcome the problems of excessive GVHD and high rates of nonengraftment. The most promising data utilize "megadoses" of CD34[+] and CD3-depleted donor cells obtained from peripheral blood. In some T cell-depleted haploidentical transplants, an NK-mediated graft-vs-leukemia effect may lead to a low rate of relapse. Encouraging clinical results have shifted the focus to resolve the delay in immune reconstitution and to prevent late infectious complications. Although highly specialized, new directions include applying adoptive cellular therapy to restore defective immunity and more efficient and selective instruments for CD34 enrichment of the graft. Additional advances may include use of anti-third-party nonalloreactive CTLs, which may improve immunologic reconstitution in dramatic fashion; these preclinical data await testing in humans.

Haploidentical transplantation is an option immediately available to the majority of patients with acute leukemia and may be an acceptable alternative to matched unrelated donor transplantation. Most HLA-mismatched donor hematopoietic stem cell transplants have been undertaken in acute leukemia patients. One group, however, has reported results in five bone marrow transplant procedures from haploidentical-related donors (sharing at least one HLA-A, -B, or -DR allele on the mismatched haplotype) in refractory non-Hodgkin's lymphoma patients using nonmyeloablative conditioning *(85)*. Mixed hematopoietic chimerism was established, with a predominance of donor lymphoid tissue and varying degrees of myeloid chimerism. Two patients were in GVHD-free states of complete and partial clinical remission at 460 and 103 d, respectively, after bone marrow transplantation. Prospective, multicenter, controlled clinical trials, and companion translational studies in acute leukemia and other disorders undoubtedly should further improve upon this modality.

REFERENCES

1. Armitage JO. Bone marrow transplantation. N *Engl J Med* 1994;330:827–838.
2. Thomas ED. Bone marrow transplantation:a review. *Semin Hematol* 1999;36(Suppl 7):95–103.
3. Bensinger WI, Martin PJ, Storer B, et al. Transplantation of bone marrow as compared with peripheral-blood cells from HLA-identical relatives in patients with hematologic cancers. *N Engl J Med* 2001;344:175–181.
4. Petersdof EW, Gooley T, Anasetti C, et al. Optimizing outcome after unrelated marrow transplantation by comprehensive matching of HLA class I and II alleles in the donor and recipient. *Blood* 1998;92:3515–3520.
5. Sasazuki T, Juji T, Morishima Y, et al. Effect of matching of class I HLA alleles on clinical outcome after transplantation of hematopoietic stem cells from an unrelated donor. *N Engl J Med* 1998;339:1177–1185
6. Lamparelli T, Van Lint MT, Gualandi F, et al. Bone marrow transplantation for chronic myeloid leukemia from unrelated and sibling donors:Single center experience. *Bone Marrow Transplant* 1997;20:1057–1062.
7. Beatty PG, Clift RA, Mickelson EM, et al. Marrow transplantation from related donors other than HLA-identical siblings. *N Engl J Med* 1985;313:765–771.
8. Anasetti C, Amos D, Beattyp PG, et al. Effect of HLA compatibility on engraftment of bone marrow transplants in patients with leukemia or lymphoma. *N Engl J Med* 1989;320:197–204.
9. Kernan NA, Flomenberg N, Dupont B, O'Reilly RJ. Graft rejection in recipients of T-cell-depleted HLA-nonidentical marrow transplants for leukemia. Identification of host-derived antidonor allocytotoxic lymphocytes. *Transplantation* 1987;43:842–847.
10. Soiffer RJ, Mauch P, Tarbell NJ, et al. Toal lymphoid irradiation to prevent graft rejection in recipients of HLA non-identical T cell-depleted allogeneic marrow. *Bone Marrow Transplant* 1991;7:23–33.
11. Reisner Y, Ben-Bassat I, Douer D, et al. Demonstration for clonable alloreactive host T cells in a primate model for bone marrow transplantation. *Proc Natl Acad Sci USA* 1986;83:4012–4015.
12. Butturini A, Seeger RC, Gale RP. Recipient immune competent T lymphocytes can survive intensive conditioning for bone marrow transplantation. *Blood* 1986;68:954–956.
13. Kook H, Goldman F, Padley D, et al. Reconstruction of the immune system after unrelated or partially matched T-cell-depleted bone marrow transplantation in children:immunophenotypic analysis and factors affecting the speed of recovery. *Blood* 1996;88:1089–1097.
14. Ochs L, Shu XO, Miller J, et al. Late infections after allogeneic bone marrow transplantation: comparison of incidence in related and unrelated donor transplant recipients. *Blood* 1995;10:3979–3986.
15. Sullivan KM, Mori M, Sanders J, et al. Late complications of allogeneic and autologous marrow transplantation. *Bone Marrow Transplant* 1992;10(Suppl 1):127–134.
16. Fleming DR, Henslee-Downey PJ, Romond EH, et al. Allogeneic bone marrow transplantation with T-cell-depleted partially matched related donors for advanced acute lymphoblastic leukemia in children and adults: a comparative matched cohort study. *Bone Marrow Transplant* 1996;17:917–922.
17. Powles RL, Morgenstern GR, Kay HE, et al. Mismatched family donors for bone marrow transplantation for treatment for acute leukemia. *Lancet* 1983;i:612–615.
18. Szydlo R, Goldman JM, Klein JP, et al. Results of allogeneic bone marrow transplants for leukemia using donors other than HLA-identical siblings. *J Clin Oncol* 1997;15:1767–1777.
19. Henslee-Downey PJ, Abhyankar SH, Parrish RS, et al. Use of partially mismatched related donors extends access to allogeneic marrow transplant. *Blood* 1997;89:3864–3872.
20. Aversa F, Tabilio A, Velardi A, et al. Treatment of high risk acute leukemia with T cell-depleted stem cells from related donors with one fully mismatched HLA haplotype. *N Engl J Med* 1998;339:1186–1193.
21. Guinan EC, Boussiotis VA, Neuberg D, et al. Transplantation of anergic histoincompatible bone marrow allograft. *N Engl J Med* 1999;340:1704–1714.
22. O'Reilly RJ, Collins NH, Kernan N, et al. Transplantation of marrow-depleted T cells by soybean lectin agglutination an E-rosette depletion:Major histocompatibility complex-related graft resistance in leukemic transplant recipients. *Transplant Proc* 1985;17:455,456.

23. Ferrara JL, Deeg HJ. Graft-versus-host disease. *N Engl J Med* 1991;324:667–674.
24. Korngold R, Sprent J. T-cell subsets and graft-versus-host disease. *Transplantation* 1987;44:335–339.
25. Reisner Y, Kapoor N, Kirkpatrick D, et al. Transplantation for severe combined immunodeficiency with HLA-A, B, D, DR incompatible parental marrow cells fractionated by soybean agglutinin and sheep red blood cells. *Blood* 1983;61:341–348.
26. Mackinnon S, Papadopoulos EB, Carabasi MH, et al. Adoptive immunotherapy evaluating escalating doses of donor leukocytes for relapsed of chronic myeloid leukemia after bone marrow transplantation:separation of graft-versus-leukemia responses from graft-versus-host disease. *Blood* 1995;86:1261–1268.
27. Reisner Y, Martelli MF. Transplantation tolerance induced by "mega dose" CD34$^+$ cell transplants. *Exp Hematol* 2000;28:119–127.
28. Drobyski WR, Ash RC, Casper JT, et al. Effect of T- cell depletion as a graft-versus-host disease prophylaxis on engraftment, relapse, and disease-free survival in unrelated marrow transplantation for chronic myelogenous leukemia. *Blood* 1994;83:1980–1987.
29. Guinan E. Costimulatory Blockade as a Mechanism of Inducing Tolerance in the allograft setting. *Educ Book Am Soc Hematol* 1999;383–88.
30. Champlin R, Ho W, Gajewski J, et al. Selective depletion of CD8+ T lymphocytes for prevention of graft-versus-host disease after allogeneic bone marrow transplantation. *Blood* 1990;76:418–423.
31. Lamb L, Gee A, Parrish R, et al. Acute rejection of marrow grafts in patients transplanted from a partially mismatched related donor:clinical and immunologic characteristics. *Bone Marrow Transplant* 1996;17:1021–1027.
32. Soderling CC, Cong CW, Blazer BR, Vallera DA. A correlation between conditioning and engraftment in recipients of MHC mismatched T cell-depleted murine bone marrow transplants. *Immunology* 1985;135:941–946.
33. Sondel TM, Bozdech MJ, Trigg ME, et al. Additional immunosuppression allows engraftment following HLA-mismatched T cell-depleted bone marrow transplantation for leukemia. *Transplant Proc* 1985;17:460–462.
34. Champlin RE, Ho WG, Mitsuyasu R, et al. Graft failure and leukemia relapse following T lymphocyte-depleted bone marrow transplants:effect of intensification of immunosuppressive conditioning. *Transplant Proc* 1987;19:2616–2619.
35. Lapidot T, Singer TS, Reisner Y. Transient engraftment of T cell depleted allogeneic bone marrow in mice improves survival rate following lethal irradiation. *Bone Marrow Transplant* 1988;3:157–164.
36. Lapidot T, Terenzi A, Singer TS, Salomon O, Reisner Y. Enhancement by dimethyl myleran of donor type chimerism in murine recipients of bone marrow allografts. *Blood* 1989;73:2025–2032.
37. Terenzi A, Lubin I, Lapidot T, et al. Enhancement of T-cell depleted bone marrow allografts in mice by thiotepa. *Transplantation* 1990;50:717–720.
38. Godder K, Pati AR, Abhyankar S, et al. Partially mismatched related donor transplants as salvage therapy for patients with refractory leukemia who relapse post-BMT. *Bone Marrow Transplant* 1996;17:49–53.
39. Kernan NA, Emanuel D, Castro-Malaspina H, et al. Posttransplant immunosuppression with antithymocyte globulin and methylprednisolone prevents immunologically mediated graft failure following a T-cell depleted marrow transplant. *Blood* 1989;74:123a.
40. Fischer A, Griscelli C, Blanche S, et al. Prevention of graft failure by an anti-HLFA-1 monoclonal antibody in HLA-mismatched bone marrow transplantation. *Lancet* 1986;ii:1058–1061.
41. Henslee-Downey PJ, Parrish RS, Macdonald JS, et al. Combined ex-vivo and in-vivo T-lymphocyte depletion for the control of graft-versus-host disease following haplo-identical marrow transplant. *Transplantation* 1996;61:738–745.
42. Malilay GP, Sevenich EA, Condie RM, Filipovich AH. Prevention of graft rejection in allogeneic bone marrow transplantation: I. Preclinical studies with antithymocyte globulins. *Bone Marrow Transplant* 1989;4:107–112.
43. Henslee-Downey PJ. Allogeneic related partially mismatched transplantation. In: Barrett J, Treleaven J (eds.), *The Clinical Practice of Stem-Cell Transplantation* Isis Medical Media, Oxford, 1998, pp. 391.
44. Henslee-Downey PJ, Godder K, Abhyankar S, Chiang KY, Lamb LS, Geier SS, Van Rhee F, Singhal S, Metha J. Sequential immuno- modulation to achieve engraftment and control graft-versus-host disease across mismatched mhc barriers. *Educ Book Am Soc Hematol* 1999;389–394.
45. Reisner Y, Martelli MF. Tolerance induction by "megadose" transplants of CD34$^+$ stem cells:a new option for leukemia patients without an HLA-matched donor. *Curr Opin Immunol* 2000;12:536–541.
46. Rachmim N, Gan J, Segall R, et al. Tolerance induction by "megadose" hematopoietic transplants: donor-type human CD34 stem cells induce potent specific reduction of host anti-donor cytotoxic T lymphocyte precursors in mixed lymphocytes culture. *Transplatation* 1998;65:1386–1393.
47. Aversa F, Tabilio A, Terenzi A, et al. Successful engraftment of T cell-depleted haploidentical "three-loci" incompatible transplants in leukemia patients by addition of recombinant human granulocyte colony-stimulating factor-mobilized peripheral blood progenitor cells to bone marrow inoculum. *Blood* 1994;84:3948–3955.
48. Reisner Y, Martelli MF. Bone marrow transplantation across HLA barriers by increasing the number of transplanted cells. *Immunol Today* 1995;16:437–440.

49. Bachar-Lustig E, Rachamim N, Li HW, Lan F, Reisner Y. Megadose of T cell-depleted bone marrow overcomes MHC barriers in sublethally irradiated mice. *Nature Med* 1995;1:1268–1273.

50. Reisner Y, Aversa F, Bachar-Lustig E, Velardi A, Gur H, Tabilio A, Reich-Zeliger S, Krauthgamer R, Martelli MF. The role of megadose CD34 haploidentical transplantation:Potential application to tolerance induction. Educ Book Am Soc Hematol 1999;376–382.

51. Cilloni D, Carlo-Stella C, Falzetti F, et al. Limited engraftment T capacity of bone marrow-derived mesenchymal cells following T-cell-depleted hematopoietic stem cell transplantation. *Blood* 2000;96:3637–3643.

52. Lazarus HM, Koc ON. Culture-expanded human marrow-derived MSCs in clinical hematopoietic stem cell transplantation. *Graft* 2001;3:329–333.

53. Lamb LS, Szafer F, Henslee-Downey, et al. Characterization of acute bone marrow graft rejection in T cell-depleted, partially mismatched related donor bone marrow transplantation. *Exp Hematol* 1995:23:1595–1600.

54. Lamb LS, Gee AP, Henslee-Downey PJ, et al. Phenotypic and functional reconstitution of peripheral blood lymphocytes following T cell-depleted bone marrow transplantation from partially mismatched related donors. *Bone Marrow Transplant* 1998;21:461–471.

55. Roux E, Dumont-Girard F, Starobinski M, et al. Recovery of immune reactivity after T-cell-depleted bone marrow transplantation depends on thymic activity. *Blood* 2000;96:2299–2303.

56. Volpi I, Perruccio K, Ruggeri L, et al. G-CSF blocks IL-12 production by antigen presenting cells:implications for improved immune reconsstitution after haploidentical hematopoietic transplantation. *Blood* 1999;10(Suppl 1):2841a.

57. Perruccio K, Tosti A, Posati S, et al. Transfer of functional immune responses to aspergillus and CMV after haploidentical hematopoietic transplantation. *Blood* 2000;96(11):2383a.

58. Walter EA, Greenberg PD, Gilbert MJ, et al. Reconstitution of cellular immunity against cytomegalovirus in recipients of allogeneic bone marrow by transfer of T-cell clones from the donor. *N Engl J Med* 1995;333:1038–1044.

59. Riddell SR, Greenberg PD. Adoptive immunotherapy with antigen-specific T cells. In: Thomas ED Blume KJ, Forman SJ, eds. *Hematopoietic Cell Transplantation*. Blackwell Science, Malden, 1999, pp. 327–341.

60. Bacigalupo A, Van Lint MT, Occhini D, et al. Increased risk of leukemia relapse with high-dose cyclosporine A after allogeneic marrow transplantation for acute leukemia. *Blood* 1991;77:1423–1428.

61. Weaver CH, Clift RA, Deeg HJ, et al. Effect of graft-versus-host disease prophylaxis on relapse in patients transplanted for acute myeloid leukemia. *Bone Marrow Transplant* 1994:14:885–893.

62. Craig F, Gulley ML, Banks PM. Posttransplantation lymphoproliferative disorders. *Am J Clin Pathol* 1993;99:265–276.

63. Sullivan KM, Witherspoon RP, Storb R, et al. Alternate-day cyclosporine and prednisone for treatment of high-risk chronic graft-v-host disease. *Blood* 1988;72:555–561.

64. Jenkins MK, Johnson JG. Molecules involved in T-cell costimulation. *Curr Opin Immunol* 1993;5:361–367.

65. Steinman RM, Young JW. Signals arising from antigen-presenting cells. *Curr Opin Immunol* 1991;3:361–372.

66. Boussiotis VA, Gribben JG, Freeman EJ, Nadler LM. Blockade of the CD 28 co-stimulatory pathway:a means to induce tolerance. *Curr Opin Immunol* 1994;6:797–807.

67. Blazar BR, Taylor PA, Noelle RJ, Vallera DA. CD4(+) T cells tolerized ex vivo to host alloantigen by anti-CD40 ligand (CD40L:CD154) antibody lose their graft-versus-host disease lethality capacity but retain nominal antigen responses. *J Clin Invest* 1998:102:473–482.

68. Gribben JG, Guinan EC, Boussiotis VA, et al. Complete blockade of B7 family-mediated costimulation is necessary to induce human alloantigen-specific anergy:a method to ameliorate graft-versus-host disease and extend the donor pool. *Blood* 1996;87:4887–4893.

69. Sambhara SR, Miller RG. Programmed cell death of T cells signaled by the T-cell receptor and the a3 domain of class I MHC. *Science* 1991;252:1424–1427.

70. Reisner Y, Bachar-Lustig E, Li HW, et al. Purified Sca-1+Lin-stem cells can tolerize fully allogeneic host T cells remaining after sublethal TBI. *Blood* 1997;90:563a.

71. Bachar-Lustig E, Li HW, Marcus H, Reisner Y. Tolerance induction of megadose stem cell transplants: synergism between Sca-1+Lin cells and non-alloreactive T-cells. *Transplant Proc* 1998;30:4007,4008.

72. Bachar-Lustig E, Li HW, Gur H, et al. Induction of donor-type chimerism and transplantation tolerance across major histocompatibility barriers in sublethally irradiated mice by Sca-1 (+) Lin (-) bone marrow progenitor cells:synergism with non-alloreactive (Host x donor)F (1) T cells. *Blood* 1999;94:3212–3221.

73. Lee LA, Sergio JJ, Sykes M. Natural killer cells weakly resist engrafment of allogeneic, long-term, multilineage-repopulating hematopoietic stem cells. *Transplantation* 1996;61:125–132.

74. Ruggeri L, Capanni M, Casucci M, et al. Role of natural killer cell alloreactivity in HLA-mismatched hematopoietic stem cell transplantation. *Blood* 1999;94:333–339.

75. Ruggeri L, Capanni M, Urbani E, et al. KIR epitope incompatibility in their GvH direction predicts control of leukemia relapse after mismatched hematopoietic transplantation. *Blood* 2000;96(11):2059a.

76. Davies SM, Kollman C, Anasetti C, et al. Engraftment and survival after unrelated-donor bone marrow transplantation: a report from the National Marrow Donor Program. *Blood* 2000;96:4096–4102.

77. McGlave PB, Shu XO, Wen W, et al. Unrelated donor marrow transplantation for chronic myelogenous leukemia: 9 year's experience of the national marrow donor program. *Blood* 2000;95:2219–2225.

78. Anasetti C. Transplantation of hematopoietic stem cells from alternate donors in acute myelogenous leukemia. *Leukemia* 2000;14:502–504.

79. Lazarus HM, Pérez WS, Weisdorf D, Keating A, Bate-Boyle B, Klein JP, Kollman C. Autologous versus unrelated donor (URD) transplantation for acute myeloid leukemia (AML) in first or second remission (CR1 or CR2) (abstract # 1781). *Blood* 2000;96:414a.

80. Sierra J, Storer B, Hansen JA, et al. Unrelated donor marrow transplantation for acute myeloid leukemia: an update of the Seattle experience. *Bone Marrow Transplant* 2000;26:397–404.

81. Aversa F, Velardi A, Tabillo A, Reisner Y, Martelli MF. Haploidentical stem cell transplantation in leukemia. *Blood Rev* 2001;15:111–119.

82. Aversa F, Tabilio A, Velardi A, et al. Advances in full-haplotype mismatched transplants in acute leukemia. *Blood* 1999;94(Suppl 1):2522a.

83. Bunjes D, Duncker C, Wiesneth M, et al. CD34 + selected cells in mismatched stem cell transplantation: a single centre experience of haploidentical peripheral blood stem cell transplantation. *Bone Marrow Transplant* 2000;25(Suppl 2):9–11.

84. Passweg JR, Kuhne T, Gregor M, et al. Increased stem cell dose, as obtained using currently available technology, may not be sufficient for engraftment of haploidentical stem cell transplants. *Bone Marrow Transplant* 2000;26:1033–1036.

85. Sykes M, Preffer F, McAfee S, et al. Mixed lymphohaemopoietic chimerism and graft-versus-lymphoma effects after non-myeloablative therapy and HLA-mismatched bone-marrow transplantation. *Lancet* 1999;353:1755–1759.

10

Umbilical Cord Blood Transplantation

Juliet Barker, MBBS *(Hons) and John E. Wagner,* MD

Contents

1. INTRODUCTION

Transplantation of allogeneic hematopoietic stem cells (HSC) derived either from sibling or unrelated donor bone marrow (BM) or mobilized peripheral blood (PB) have been successfully utilized in the treatment of high risk or recurrent hematological malignancies, BM failure syndromes, hemoglobinopathies, selected hereditary immunodeficiency states, and inborn errrors of metabolism *(1)*. However, a number of limitations exist that impede the successful use of such HSC transplant therapy. The first of these is the unavailability of suitable donors. With current trends in family size in the U.S. fewer than 35% of patients will have an human leukocyte antigen (HLA)-matched sibling *(2)*. While there are currently more than 5 million HLA-typed marrow donors registered in BM donor registries worldwide, substantial numbers of patients are still unable to find an available, suitably HLA-matched BM donor. For example, although an initial search may identify at least one potential HLA-matched donor for 85% of Caucasian patients, 40% of African-American or Asian-Pacific-Islanders will not have a matched donor *(3–5)*. Further, because of the heterogeneity of HLA haplotypes seen in some racial groups, such as African-Americans, HLA-matched BM may be unavailable regardless of registry size *(6)*. Also, the unrelated BM donor search process can be lengthy, taking 3.7 mo on average *(5)*.

A further problem of unrelated donor BM transplantation (BMT) is graft-vs-host disease (GVHD), particularly if HLA-mismatch is present *(5,7)*. This results in high transplant-related mortality that is substantial in children and potentially prohibitive in adults. While T cell

From: *Current Clinical Oncology: Allogeneic Stem Cell Transplantation*
Edited by: Mary S. Laughlin and Hillard M. Lazarus © Humana Press Inc., Totowa, NJ

Table 1
Diseases Treated by UCBT[a]

Malignant diseases
    Acute myelocytic leukemia
    Chronic myelogenous leukemia
    Myelodysplasia
    Acute lymphoblastic leukemia
    Non-Hodgkin's lymphoma
    Neuroblastoma
    Histiocytic disorders
Nonmalignant diseases
    Disorders of hematopoiesis
        Fanconi anemia
        Blackfan-Diamond syndrom
        Dyskeratosis congenita
        Sever aplastic anemia
        Amegakaryocytic thrombocytopenia
        Thalassemia
        Sickle cell anemia
    Congenital metabolism disorders
        Hurler syndrome
        Hunter syndrome
        Gunther syndrome
        Osteoporosis
        Globoid cell leucodystrophy
        Adrenoleucodystrophy
        Lesch-Nyhan syndrome
        Other (unspecified)
    Congenital immunodeficiencies
        Kostmann syndrome
        Severe combined immunodeficiency
        Leucocyte adhesion deficiency
        Chronic granulomatous disease
        X-linked lymphoproliferative disorder
        Wiskott-Aldrich syndrome
        Other (unspecified)

[a]Reported to the ICBTR and EuroCord.

depletion (TCD) of unrelated donor BM has reduced the incidence of GVHD, it has not resulted in an increased long-term survival due to the other complications of graft failure, delayed immune reconstitution, and relapse *(5,8)*.

Thus, a convincing rationale can be made to investigate alternative strategies in HSC transplantation. Umbilical cord blood transplantation (UCBT) represents an exciting new source of HSC that has the potential to address these limitations. Therefore, UCB banking programs were initiated in 1993 and now exist throughout North America, Europe, Japan, and Australia. In 1992–1993, the International Cord Blood Transplant Registry (ICBTR) (USA) and the EuroCord Transplant Registry were established as repositories of clinical data on the outcomes of UCBT in an attempt to determine the true attributes of this new HSC source. In 1997, the ICBTR was integrated with the International Bone Marrow Transplant Registry.

As of 2001, UCB from sibling and unrelated donors has been used to reconstitute hematopoiesis in an estimated 2000 patients with malignant and nonmalignant disorders. Diseases for which UCBT has been used are summarized in Table 1. UCB has the advantages of: (i) rapid availability; (ii) absence of donor risk; (iii) absence of donor attrition (except by use of the UCB unit); and (iv) very low risk of some transmissible infectious, diseases such as cytomegalovirus (CMV) and Epstein-Barr virus (EBV). In addition, clinical experience has shown HLA disparity is tolerated with lower than expected rates of GVHD *(9–13)*. Therefore, this novel source of HSC has a number of important attributes that may potentially make a major contribution to the field of HSC transplantation. This chapter will overview the current state of knowledge regarding UCBT with emphasis on new areas of interest, including the comparison of outcomes of UCBT and BMT, the application of UCBT to adults, and methods to overcome the problem of limited UCB cell dose.

2. HISTORICAL BACKGROUND

Use of human UCB as a source of transplantable HSC was first suggested in 1983 by Professor Edward A. Boyse in conversations with Dr. Hal Broxmeyer and Ms. Judith Bard. In 1984–1985, the hypothesis that UCB contained long-term reconstituting HSC was tested in a mouse model *(14)*. Broxmeyer et al. then established practical and efficient methods of collecting and storing UCB for clinical use *(15)*. The first UCB transplant took place in Paris in 1988, in which UCB was used as the sole source of HSC in a child with Fanconi anemia who was conditioned with cyclophosphamide and limited field radiation *(16)*. This resulted in complete and sustained chimerism in multiple lymphohematopoietic lineages, thus demonstrating that pluripotential HSC existed in human UCB. This child remains alive and well 12.5 yr after UCBT (Kurtzberg et al., personal communication).

3. BIOLOGICAL CHARACTERISTICS OF UCB

3.1. Primitive Progenitor Cells

Ontologically, hematopoiesis begins in the ventral aspect of the fetal aorta and primitive yolk sac early after conception. Subsequently, after an hepatic phase, hematopoietic cells migrate, via the blood, to the BM space at the end of the second gestational trimester, where hematopoiesis subsequently remains. The exact reason why cord blood is so enriched with hematopoietic cells is not known. This phenomenon has not been explained by the characterization of cell surface adhesion molecules thus far *(17)*. Broxmeyer et al. *(15)* have shown that these progenitors disappear from the circulation shortly after birth. The reasons for this are also unknown, but could be triggered by changes in hormonal levels or oxygen tension.

The fact that humans can be reliably reconstituted after myeloablative conditioning with a >1 log less UCB cells than are used in allogeneic BMT from an adult donor is the greatest testament to the unique nature of UCB HSC. Numerous laboratories have investigated the biological characteristics of UCB and demonstrated a higher proportion of primitive hematopoietic progenitors in UCB, with superior in vitro proliferative responses and in vivo engraftment capacity in comparison to adult BM *(18–22)*. These are summarized in Table 2. The functional differences in UCB primitive progenitors as compared to BM appear to relate to their relative positions in ontogeny, as fetal liver cells have even superior performance in some stem cell assays *(21)*. The mechanisms underlying functional differences between UCB and BM progenitors may include differing ability of UCB cells to exit the G0/G1 phase of the cell cycle, UCB autocrine production of stimulatory cytokines, and longer telomere length in UCB *(18,22)*.

3.2. Ex Vivo Expansion and Gene Transfer

As discussed elsewhere in this chapter, there are compelling clinical data relating engraftment and survival after UCBT to cell dose *(9,11,12)*. For this reason, numerous investigators

Table 2
Laboratory Characteristics of Primitive UCB Progenitors

Characteristic	Comments and comparison to BM
Phenotype	• CD34+ comprising approx 1% nucleated cells: similar to BM. • CD34+HLADR+ or -: differs from BM in which primitive cells are CD34+HLADR-. • CD34+CD38-: fourfold higher than BM. • Primitive CD34+CD38- cells also positive for flt3, thy1, AC133 with low levels of rhodamine 123 and c-kit.
Proliferation in vitro	• UCB cells demonstrate superior performance as compared to BM in terms of frequency and size of colonies in CFC and LTC-IC assays with greater self-renewal capacity.
Proliferation in vivo	• UCB cells engraft NON-SCID mice more efficiently than BM. • Frequency of SRC threefold higher than BM.
Telomere length	• Significantly longer than adult BM cells.
Cell cycling	• Primitive UCB cells are more likely in G0/G1 phase of cell cycle as compared with more rapid cell cycling of similar BM cells.

are exploring the possibility of ex vivo expansion of HSC in UCB. Thus far, no investigator has convincingly expanded true HSCs from UCB or other source. However, primitive progenitors may be expanded. Lewis et al., for example, have shown that primitive CD34+CD38- UCB progenitors may be expanded in a stromal-based noncontact culture supplemented with murine hematopoietic-supportive stroma, and early acting cytokines such as fetal liver tyrosine kinase-3-ligand (Flt3-L), interleukin (IL)-7, stem cell factor and thrombopoietin (Tpo) (23). Such cultures may expand both myeloid and lymphoid long-term culture-initiating cells (LTC-IC) for 5 wk and maintain severe combined immunodeficiency (SCID)-repopulating cells (SRC) for at least 2 wk that engraft in two sequential non-obese diabetic SCID (NOD-SCID) or fetal sheep recipients. The identification of the hematopoietic supportive factors secreted by the murine stromal feeders (24,25) has allowed the development of a stroma-free expansion system that supports a 19.8-fold expansion in colony folming cells (CFC), a 2.6-fold expansion in LTC-IC, and maintenance of SRC, which is now ready for clinical application (26).

Regardless of the exact culture system employed, it is not yet clear whether UCB hematopoietic progenitors expanded in culture are functionally equivalent to their unmanipulated counterparts. It is concerning that ex vivo culture systems have been shown to interfere with homing and engraftment of HSC in NOD-SCID mice, for example. The underlying mechanisms for this may relate to changes in the cell cycle status of the hematopoietic progenitor (27). This may explain why clinical trials of ex vivo-expanded UCB have not yet been shown to be efficacious in terms of rate of leucocyte recovery. For example, the largest series to date reported neutrophil engraftment to a count of $0.5 \times 10^9/L$ at a median of 26 d (range 15–45) in 31 of 33 patients (28). Of concern, this series was associated with higher than expected rates of severe acute grades III–IV (8 of 32 patients) and extensive chronic GVHD (9 of 15 patients), raising the possibility that this could be due to the ex vivo manipulation of the graft. Further clinical trials with ex vivo-expanded UCB HSC are currently underway.

Many possible methods to improve results with ex vivo expansion could be explored, as there are multiple variables in these culture systems including the media, sera, cytokines, glycosaminoglycans, culture bags, and culture time. Carow et al. have demonstrated the replating ability of UCB multipotential progenitors (colony-forming unit-granulocyte erythoid mancrophage [CFU-GEM]) was enhanced by UCB plasma as compared to fetal bovine serum

(29). Therefore, autologous neonatal serum collected from the cord blood unit could be used to substitute for other serum sources during culture, as tested by Kogler et al. *(30)*. Another possible approach could be cotransplantation of stromal cells with UCB, as has been suggested for in utero transplantation and demonstrated to be beneficial in the preimmune fetal sheep model *(31)*.

Gene transfer of UCB HSC would be highly useful for tracking the fate of expanded cells in ex vivo expansion protocols and in the correction of congenital disorders due to single gene defects. In families with a known genetically determined disease affecting hematopoiesis or the immune system, subsequent children should have their UCB collected at birth. If the child is normal, then these HSCs may be used for transplantation of the affected sibling, and if affected, the child may be able to undergo autologous transplant with genetically corrected cells. In this scenario, a further advantage of using HSC from UCB over other sources is that UCB has shown to be more readily transduced ex vivo *(32)*. An example of such an approach is the treatment of adenoside deaminase (ADA)-deficient neonates by Kohn et al. who used autologous genetically manipulated CD34+ UCB cells *(33)*.

Steady progress is being made in the field of gene therapy. For example, French physicians have recently treated two children with SCID due to defective IL-2 receptor common γ chain using a retroviral vector *(34)*. However, a number of challenges remain. For example, the application of gene marking using retroviral vectors to ex vivo expansion has proven to be problematic as the optimal expansion conditions are not necessarily the optimal conditions for transduction *(35)*. Also, because of concerns that the ex vivo culture required for retroviral marking may interfere with the homing and engraftment capacity of HSC *(27)*, alternative vector systems, such as lentiviral vectors, which can transduce nondividing cells, are currently being developed. Woods et al. have demonstrated efficient transduction of CD34+ UCB cells after overnight incubation with 16–28% of resultant colony-forming unit-granulocyte macrophage (CFU-GM) colonies being transduced *(36)*. Transduction of SRC were also seen with over 50% of CFU-GM colonies derived from primary and secondary NOD-SCID transplant recipients being transduced. However, no results from clinical studies utilizing such vectors are available as yet.

4. IMMUNE FUNCTION

The fact that 2 and 3 antigen HLA-mismatched unrelated donor UCB can be transplanted without inducing life-threatening GVHD suggests that significant differences exist between the neonatal and adult immune systems. However, the exact reasons why GVHD is lower than expected are not well understood. It may be partly accounted for by the reduced number of T cells in UCB grafts. UCB grafts contain a median of 8×10^6 CD3+ T cells/kg recipient body weight, as compared to an unmanipulated BM graft with $3–4 \times 10^7$ CD3+ T cells/kg. However, this is not sufficient to explain the relatively low GVHD rates, as most studies in BMT would suggest that a CD3 cell dose of $< 0.1 \times 10^6$ CD3+ cells/kg is required to eliminate the risk of severe acute GVHD, particularly in the setting of HLA disparity.

The alternative explanation is the "immunologic naiveté" of UCB immune cells. Numerous investigators have demonstrated complex differences between UCB and adult BM or blood. These include higher levels of CD4+CD 45RA+ cells, lower alloantigen and mitogen-specific T cell proliferation, lower inflammatory cytokine production and responses, a polyclonal T cell receptor repertoire, increased susceptibility to tolerance induction, and differences in natural killer (NK) cell and dendritic cell biology *(37–45)*. However, whether it is these properties that account for the reduced capacity of transplanted UCB cells to mediate GVHD remains to be determined. Furthermore, it is possible to hypothesize additional reasons for this phenomenon.

For example, circulating suppressor cell,s such as trophoblasts, could exert an immunomodulatory effect. Also of relevance, as suggested by results in haploidentical UCBT, is the role of partial tolerance to the HLA of noninherited maternal alleles (NIMA) *(46)*. This phenomenon has already been shown to impact the outcomes of mismatched BMT *(47)*.

There has been concern that a reduced number and/or function of UCB immune cells may raise the risk of opportunistic infection, relapse. and EBV-associated posttransplant lymphoproliferative disorder (PTLD), as has been observed in recipients of TCD BMT. The most compelling argument to counter this concern is that the human neonate does not die of opportunistic infection. Nonetheless, case series have suggested a high incidence of opportunistic infection in UCBT recipients. For example, a comparison of outcomes of HLA identical sibling donor UCB and BM by Rocha et al. demonstrated a higher incidence of death due to infection and bleeding in the UCB recipients compared to higher rates of GVHD, interstitial pneumonitis, and organ failure in the BM cohort *(48)*. While this may be due to a relative delay in neutrophil engraftment in UCBT, this may also reflect delayed immune reconstitution.

Thus far, clinical studies in this area are currently limited to small case series, predominantly in pediatric patients. Locatelli et al. *(81)* suggested that the kinetics of immune recovery of three recipients of related UCB was similar to that seen after BMT, except for a relative expansion of B cells in the peripheral blood. Normal or elevated B cell numbers were also noted by Giraud et al. *(49)*. Abu-Ghosh et al. showed recovery of B and NK cells within the first 90 d after transplant in seven pediatric unrelated donor UCBT recipients *(50)*. However, both CD4+ and CD8+ T cell subsets were significantly depressed during this period. Giraud et al. documented prolonged depression of CD3+CD8+ T cells until around 12 mo after transplant, with less impairment of CD3+CD4+ T cells (49). Thomson et al. *(51)* reviewed the experience of 27 children receiving unrelated donor UCBT. CD19 and NK cell recovery were seen at a median of 6 and 2 mo, respectively, whereas CD4 and CD8 T cell recovery were relatively delayed at a median of 12 and 9 mo, respectively *(51)*.

Immune reconstitution after unrelated donor transplantation is a relatively new area of analysis in HSC transplantation, and carefully controlled prospective studies will be required to determine if UCBT and BMT differ in this respect. Of interest, Talvvensaari et al. have compared the immune recovery of pediatric UCBT recipients (related and unrelated) with age-matched controls who received HLA identical non-TCD BMT for the treatment of hematologic malignancy *(52)*. They found similar disturbance of T cell repertoire and low levels of thymic emigrants as measured by T cell receptor excision circles (TREC) in the first year after transplant in both groups. Subsequently, however, reconstitution of the T cell compartments progressed with higher diversity of the T cell repertoire seen in the UCBT group. Weinberg et al. studied factors affecting thymic function after allogeneic HSC transplantation. Chronic GVHD was the most important factor that predicted low TREC levels, even years after transplant. In this regard it is, therefore, possible to hypothesize that UCB recipients may have an advantage due to the low incidence of chronic GVHD *(9–12)*. Notably, UCBT has also been associated with fully reconstituted T cell repertoires in adult recipients *(53)*. Overall, progress is being made in identifying factors that could improve T cell reconstitution after HSC transplantation, such as IL-7 *(54)* or keratinocyte growth factor *(55)*, and these could be applied to UCBT to assist in immune recovery.

One question that remains is whether differences in alloreactivity after UCBT may affect the incidence of malignant relapse. While it is too early to make a definitive statement about relapse risk in UCBT as compared to BMT, it is encouraging that the incidence of relapse has remained low after UCBT, suggesting that UCB can mediate a graft-vs-leukemia (GVL) effect. Furthermore, evidence of a UCB-mediated GVL can be obtained from case reports of the efficacy of sibling donor lymphocyte infusions (DLI) or induction of GVHD/GVL with cytokines *(56–59)*. Similarly, the incidence of EBV-associated posttransplant lymphoproliferative disorder (EBV-PTLD) is not increased relative to that seen with other allogeneic stem cell sources. Marshall et al. recently found impaired reconstitution of EBV-specific T lymphocytes in four UCB transplant recipients, although in none of these patients were EBV viral titers elevated *(60)*. Furthermore, a recent review of 272 unrelated donor UCBT done at the Universities of Minnesota and Duke revealed five cases of EBV-PTLD giving a cumulative incidence (CI) of 2% (95% CI: 0.3–3.7) at 2 yr *(61)*. This incidence compares favorably with that reported after TCD BMT.

5. RELATED DONOR UCBT

Although the greatest potential utility of UCB is as a source of unrelated donor HSC, clinical experience in UCBT was initially achieved in the setting of sibling donors. In this section, results of two sibling UCBT case series are summarized *(9,46)*, as well as a recent analysis by Rocha et al. in which the comparison between the outcomes of pediatric HLA-identical sibling BMT vs HLA identical sibling donor UCBT is described *(48)*.

5.1. Clinical Results: Case Series (Tables 3 and 4)

5.1.1. HEMATOPOIETIC RECOVERY

An analysis of ICBTR data revealed that the actuarial probability of neutrophil recovery by d 60 for 56 recipients of 0–1 HLA-mismatched sibling grafts was 0.91 (95% CI: 0.89–0.93) *(46)*. Platelet recovery to $\geq 50 \times 10^9$/L was 51 d (range 15–117). Of five patients that experienced graft failure, four patients were transplanted for a BM failure syndrome and one patient was transplanted for the treatment of Hunter syndrome. In the EuroCord analysis, the median time to achieve neutrophil recovery was 30 d (range 8–56) for 143 UCBT patients, with no differences between recipients of related and unrelated donor grafts *(9)*. The probability of neutrophil recovery by d 60 was 0.79, and for platelets was 0.62 for the related donor recipients, with 15 of 78 patients experiencing graft failure (malignancy 7 out of 46 vs nonmalignancy 8 out of 32). Neutrophil engraftment was influenced by age ($p = 0.02$) and weight ($p = 0.02$), and there was a trend toward the effect of cell dose ($p = 0.06$). In contrast, for platelet recovery, the most important factor was HLA identity between donor and recipient ($p < 0.001$).

The striking feature of these series was absence of a strong relationship between cell dose and hematopoietic recovery, which is in marked contrast to the unrelated donor UCBT experience. This difference may be explained by the homogeneity in recipient weights and/or ages. and the fact that the majority of pediatric sibling recipients had a UCB graft cell dose that exceeded the threshold required for engraftment. Although the data are limited, these data may suggest a higher risk of graft failure in recipients with nonmalignant diseases. Despite this, some promising results have been reported with sibling donor UCBT for hemoglobinopathy which are summarized in Table 5 *(62–66)*.

5.1.2. GVHD

The ICBTR analysis revealed very low rates of grade II–IV GVHD of 0.03 in the 56 recipients of 0–1 HLA-mismatched sibling donor grafts. Similarly, the rate of chronic GVHD was very low, with no patients having extensive disease. In the EuroCord analysis, the estimated probability of patients with an HLA-matched sibling donor experienced grade II–IV acute GVHD was 0.09. In this series, the only factor to impact on the incidence of GVHD was HLA disparity, with an acute GVHD incidence of 0.50 in recipients of HLA-mismatched UCB. Eight of 56 patients who survived more than 100 d experienced chronic GVHD. Overall, the incidence of GVHD in these series appears to be low, and this has been confirmed in a formal comparison of outcomes in UCBT and BMT recipients as detailed below.

Table 3
Summary of Patient and UCB Graft Characteristics of Two Case Series of Sibling Donor UCBT

Series	Total N	Age (yr) (range)	Cell dose[a] (range)	HLA-mismatch: N
ICBTR Wagner et al.	74	4.9 (0.5–16.3)	4.7 (1.0–33)	0–1: 56 2–3: 18
Eurocord Gluckman et al.	78 Malignancy: 46 Nonmalignancy: 32	5 (0.2–20)	3.7 (0.7–30)	0–1: 63 2–3: 14 4: 1

[a] $\times 10^7$ Nucleated cells/kg recipient body weight.

Table 4
Summary of Outcomes of Two Case Series of Sibling Donor UCBT

Outcomes	ICBTR[a] Wagner et al.	Eurocord[b] Gluckman et al.
N	56	78
Hematopoietic recovery		
Median days to ANC >0.5×10^9/L	22	30
Probability: ANC >0.5×10^9/L D + 60	0.91	0.79
Median d to plat. >20×10^9/L	NA	49
Median d to plat. >50×10^9/L	51	NA
GVHD		
Acute: grade III–IV	0.03	4 out of 78 patients (5%)
Chronic	None with extensive disease	8 out of 56 patients (14%)
Survival	0.61 at 2 yr	0.63 at 1 yr

[a]Data for 0–1 mismatch.
[b]Data for 0–4 HLA mismatch.

Table 5
Outcome of HLA Identical Sibling Donor UCBT for Patients with Hemoglobinopathies

1st Author	Disease	N	Engraftment	Outcome
Miniero	βthal	7	3 out of 7	7 out of 7 alive: 3 100% donor, 4 auto recovery.
	Sickle	3	2 out of 3	3 out of 3 alive: 2 100% donor, 1 100% donor after sibling BMT.
Issaragrisil	βthal	6	5 out of 5	5 out of 6 alive: 1 death d 25, 5 out of 6 engrafted (% donor N/A).
Li	Thal	1	0 out of 1	1 out of 1 alive: auto recovery.
Graphacos	βthal/HbLepore	1	1 out of 1	1 out of 1 alive: donor engrafted (% donor N/A).

βthal, βthalassemia; Sickle, sickle cell anemia; Auto, autologous.

5.1.3. SURVIVAL

At a median follow-up of 2 yr, the actuarial probability of survival for recipients of 0–1 HLA-mismatched grafts in the ICBTR analysis was 0.61 (95% CI: 0.81–0.49). In the EuroCord analysis, the 1-yr survival was 0.63 (95% CI: 0.57–0.69), with the only variables associated with longer survival being age <6 yr weight <20 kg, negative recipient CMV serology, and HLA identity. Notably, there was a high mortality in recipients of 2–3 HLA-mismatched-related donor grafts in both series.

Table 6
Comparison of Outcomes of Sibling Donor UCBT vs BMT *(48)*

Stem cell source	Neutrophil recovery d CI[a] at d 60	Platelet recovery d CI at d 180	Grade II–IV acute GVHD CI at d 100	Chronic GVHD CI at 3 yr	Survival CI at 3 yr
UCB	26 d	44 d	0.14	0.06	0.64
(N = 113)	0.89	0.86			
BM	18 d	24 d	0.24	0.15	0.66
(N = 2052)	0.98	0.96			

[a]Cumulative incidence.

5.2. Comparison of HLA Identical Sibling Donor UCBT vs BMT

Rocha et al. recently compared the outcomes of engraftment, GVHD, and survival in children transplanted with HLA-identical sibling BM vs HLA identical sibling donor UCB (Table 6) *(48)*. In this study, 113 recipients of UCBT between 1990 and 1997 were compared to 2052 BMT recipients transplanted over the same time period. The proportion of patients transplanted for malignancy were similar in the two groups (0.54 in UCB vs 0.62 in BM, $p = 0.11$). There were important differences in terms of age (UCB patients having a median age of 5 yr vs 8 yr in BM, $p < 0.001$) and time to transplant (25 mo in UCB recipients vs 10 mo in the BM group, $p < 0.001$), although these were adjusted for in the multivariate analysis. UCB and BM recipients received similar conditioning regimens, but UCB patients were less likely to receive methotrexate for GVHD prophylaxis, and more likely to receive prophylactic growth factors (0.40 in UCBT vs 0.21 in BMT, $p < 0.001$). UCB recipients received grafts with a median cell dose of 4.7×10^7 nucleated cells/kg recipient body weight.

The median number of days to reach an absolute neutrophil count of $\geq 0.5 \times 10^9/L$ was significantly longer in UCB recipients at 26 d, compared to 18 d for those receiving BM. In addition, the CI of neutrophil recovery by d 60 was lower in UCB recipients, being 0.89 (95% CI: 0.82–0.94) vs 0.98 (95% CI: 0.97–0.99) in BM recipients ($p < 0.001$). Similar findings were seen with platelet recovery at d 180, with a CI of 0.86 (95% CI: 0.78–0.92) vs 0.96 (95% CI: 0.94–0.97) ($p < 0.001$). In contrast, the CI of grades II–IV acute GVHD were significantly lower in UCBT vs BMT: 0.14 (95% CI: 0.08–0.22) vs 0.24 (95% CI: 0.22–0.26) ($p = 0.02$). Patients receiving UCB also had less severe acute GVHD. Also, lower incidences of chronic GVHD were seen in UCBT recipients at 3 yr: 0.06 (95% CI: 0.02–0.13) compared with 0.15 (95% CI: 0.13–0.17) in recipients of BM.

Adjusting for differences between the two cohorts, multivariate analysis confirmed the significant differences in outcomes between the two HSC sources in regard to engraftment and GVHD. However, 3-yr survival was 0.64 (95% CI: 0.53–0.74) vs 0.66 (95% CI: 0.64–0.68) in recipients of UCB and BM, respectively. Despite slower engraftment in recipients of UCB, no differences were detected in 100-d mortality. Although this study was not designed to analyze effects of graft type on leukemic relapse, it was encouraging that no difference in the relapse-related deaths was discerned in the two groups.

5.3. Summary

HLA-identical sibling donor UCB contains sufficient numbers of HSC to engraft most related donor recipients with survival comparable to pediatric sibling donor BMT. While UCBT and BMT survival rates were similar in the Rocha study *(48)*, the lower rates of chronic GVHD after UCBT may be beneficial in terms of quality of life. The role of HLA disparity in survival after related donor UCBT is yet to be fully determined. Although haploidentical transplants have been performed with a relatively low rate of severe GVHD, numbers are small, and few survivors have been reported. Therefore, related donor transplants using ≥ 3 HLA-mismatched grafts should be limited to those with high-risk disease when no other sources of HSC are available.

5.4. Practical Issues: When to Choose UCB Over BM from a Sibling Donor?

Despite the finding of equivalent survival in recipients of HLA identical sibling donor UCBT and BMT in the Rocha analysis *(48)*, the choice of whether to use UCB or BM as the source of HSC involves complex decision-making. In the situation where a mother of a patient with a hematological disorder requiring HSC transplantation is pregnant, or may become pregnant soon, and no other HLA identical siblings are available for BM donation, a decision whether to collect, store and subsequently use the UCB unit for sibling donor UCBT must be made. Key factors in this process are summarized in Fig. 1 and include the urgency of the transplant and whether the fetus is an ideal candidate for UCB donation (0–2 HLA-mismatched to the patient and, for genetically determined diseases, whether the fetus is affected). Although not directly compared, if timing is appropriate, it is reasonable to select an HLA-identical sibling donor UCB over an unrelated source of HSC. Also, although a strong association between cell dose and outcome in sibling donor UCBT has not been demonstrated, it may be appropriate to utilize UCB only if the cell dose is at least $\geq 1.5 \times 10^7$ nucleated cells/kg, based on unrelated donor UCBT experience. This is usually not a problem in younger recipients, but may arise if the patient is >20 kg. If the cell dose is limited, UCB may be supplemented with BM from the same donor. However, there is no published data concerning this approach.

A second possible scenario is that a three HLA-mismatched sibling UCB unit has or will be collected, but there is a possibility of obtaining an HLA-matched unrelated donor BM or a 0–2 HLA-mismatched unrelated donor UCB unit. In this situation, given the limited data concerning haploidentical sibling donor transplant, a closely matched unrelated donor may be preferable.

6. UNRELATED DONOR UCBT

In 1996, Kurtzberg et al. and Wagner et al. reported preliminary clinical results of unrelated donor UCBT in 25 and 18 patients, respectively *(67,68)*. Together, the clinical data suggested that banked unrelated donor UCB contained sufficient numbers of progenitors to achieve hematopoietic recovery and sustained engraftment, with lower than anticipated risk of acute GVHD, in children and young adults. In 1997, Gluckman et al reported the results of unrelated donor UCBT in 65 patients, as reported to the EuroCord Registry *(9)*. In this series, multiple regression analysis revealed that: (i) a higher graft nucleated cell dose and HLA identity predicted more rapid rate of neutrophil engraftment; (ii) recipient CMV seropositive status predicted higher risk of acute GVHD; and (iii) recipient CMV seronegative status and higher graft nucleated cell dose predicted better survival after unrelated donor UCBT.

The largest series to date, by Rubinstein et al. described the first large registry experience of unrelated donor UCBT in 562 patients *(11)*. UCBT recipients were predominantly small children with hematological malignancies (67%) or genetic diseases (24%) transplanted prior to 1998. UCB grafts were largely 1–2 HLA-mismatched (86%). The incidence of neutrophil engraftment was 0.81 by d 42 (median time to engraftment d 28) and 0.85 by d 180 for platelets (median time, d 90). The speed of neutrophil engraftment was primarily associated with the nucleated cell content of the graft. Grades III–IV acute GVHD occurred in 0.23 and 0.25 experienced chronic GVHD (predominantly limited). For patients with leukemia the rate of relapse was 0.26 at 1 yr. At 100 d, 218 of 562 patients (39%) had died, with infection contrib-

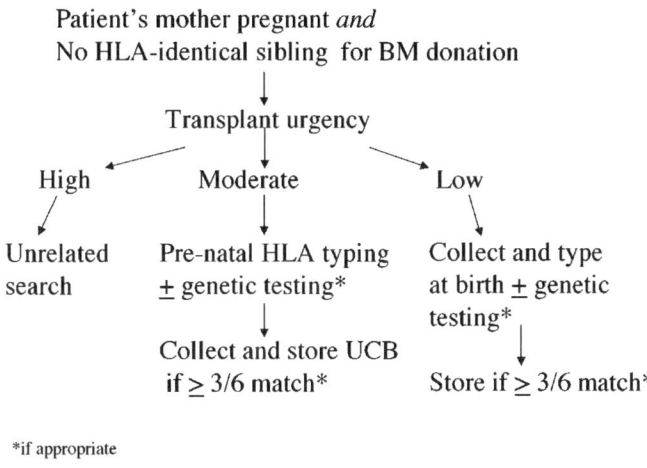

Fig. 1. UCB collection for sibling donor UCBT.

uting to death in 47% and GVHD in 11% of cases. Event-free survival in the first 100 d and the overall incidence of transplantation-related events (other than relapse) correlated with the recipient's age, diagnosis, the nucleated cell dose, the extent of the HLA disparity and the location of the transplant center in both univariate and multivariate analyses.

6.1. Clinical Results from the University of Minnesota

Between 1994 and 1999, 65 patients have been transplanted with unrelated donor UCB at the University of Minnesota. For the purpose of this analysis, patients with <42 d follow-up, history of prior allogeneic HSC transplantation ($n = 6$) or an immunodeficiency state not requiring myeloablative conditioning ($n = 1$) were excluded. The patients were treated for various malignant ($n = 36$) and nonmalignant ($n = 29$) disorders. The median age of recipients was 6.7 yr (0.2–52.9). The median weight of patients was 21.6 kg (range 5.0–102.8). UCB units, obtained from the Placental Blood Programs at the New York Blood Center, the St. Louis Cord Blood Bank, and through Netcord, had a median nucleated cell dose of 2.9×10^7/kg (range 0.7–57.9). The median CFU-GM dose in the UCB graft at the time of collection was 2.5×10^4/kg (range 0.1–89.1). The median CD34 and CD3 postthaw doses were 2.4×10^5/kg (range 0.4–21.6) and 7.0×10^6/kg (range 0.0–90.0), respectively. Confirmatory HLA typing was performed by serology for HLA-A and -B antigens and by high-resolution DNA techniques for HLA-DR antigens. In this series, the HLA disparity was 6 out of 6 in 10 patients, 5 out of 6 in 33 patients, 4 out of 6 in 20 patients, and 3 out of 6 in 2 patients.

All patients were conditioned with cyclophosphamide (CY) 120 mg/kg, fractionated total body irradiation (TBI) 1320–1375 cGy, except for a minority in whom TBI was contraindicated who received CY 200 mg/kg and busulphan 16 mg/kg ($N = 4$), and patients with Fanconi anemia who received a dose-reduced CY/TBI preparative regimen. All UCB recipients received antithymocyte globulin (ATG) 15 mg/kg d −3 to −1 every 12 h for six doses, and 66% received granulocyte-colony-stimulating factor (G-CSF) 5 µg/kg daily from d 0 until neutrophil engraftment. GVHD prophylaxis consisted of cyclosporine (CSA) for 6 mo, maintaining a trough blood level of >200 µg/L, and methylprednisone (MP) 1 mg/kg every 12 h d 5–19 after transplant and then taper.

6.1.1. HEMATOPOIETIC RECOVERY AND ENGRAFTMENT

The overall probability of neutrophil recovery by d 45 and platelet recovery by 6 mo were 0.91 (95% CI: 0.83–0.98) and 0.60 (95% CI 0.46–0.74), respectively. The median time required

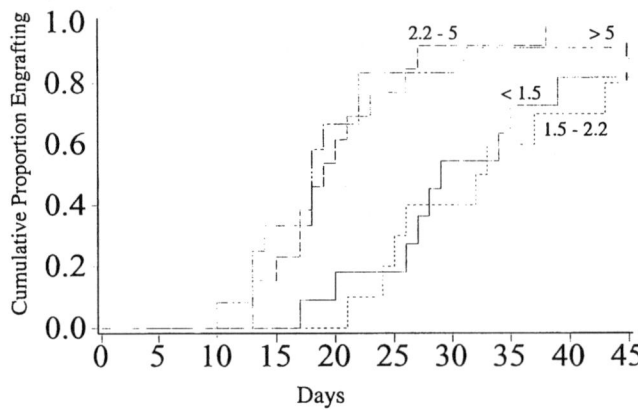

Fig. 2. Neutrophil engraftment in unrelated donor UCBT recipients by quartile of CD34+ cell dose (× 10^5/kg). University of Minnesota p <0.01.

to achieve an absolute neutrophil count (ANC) >0.5 × 10^9/L and platelet count >50 × 10^9/L was 26 d (range 10–54) and 2.7 mo (range 1–7), respectively. Of note, all patients engrafting after unrelated donor UCBT without relapse continue to have complete chimerism, and no secondary graft failures have been observed. For both neutrophil and platelet recovery, there was no difference in probability of recovery for patients with 0–1 vs 2–3 HLA disparate grafts. However, time to neutrophil recovery and overall neutrophil engraftment strongly correlated with the dose of thawed CD34 cells (p <0.01) (Fig. 2).

6.1.2. GVHD

The overall probabilities of grade II–IV and grade III–IV acute GVHD for the entire group of patients was 0.38 (95% CI: 0.26–0.50) and 0.09 (95% CI: 0.02–0.16) by d 100 after unrelated donor UCBT, respectively. In univariate analysis, degree of HLA disparity was not significantly associated with risk of acute GVHD. Notably, the probability of chronic GVHD was low at 0.05 (95% CI: 0.0–0.10).

6.1.3. SURVIVAL

With a median follow-up of 617 d (171–2087), the probabilities of survival at 1 and 4 yr was 0.58 (0.46–0.70) and 0.40 (0.22–0.58). While HLA disparity did not significantly impact on survival, harvested graft nucleated cell dose (p = 0.01) and thawed graft CD34 dose (p <0.01) were associated with improved survival (Fig. 3).

6.2. Comparison of Unrelated Donor UCBT and BMT

As many patients have access to both unrelated donor BM and UCB, and as experience in unrelated donor UCBT is increasing, the comparison of the relative merits of UCB and BM as HSC sources for unrelated donor transplantation is of great interest. A preliminary study performed at the University of Minnesota, using the matching criteria of age, diagnosis, and donor–recipient HLA disparity, demonstrated superior survival in UCBT recipients, suggesting HLA disparity is better tolerated in UCBT than BMT *(69)*. Therefore, a further study was performed comparing the outcomes of recipients of 0–3 HLA-mismatched UCB to recipients of HLA-A, -B, -DRB1-matched BM *(13)*. The matching criteria were age, diagnosis and disease stage. UCB patients, who received CSA and MP as GVHD prophylaxis, were matched with BM patients, who received either methotrexate (MTX) and CSA (26 pairs: UCB vs BM-MTX), or TCD and CSA/MP (31 pairs: UCB vs BM-TCD). Patients were predominantly

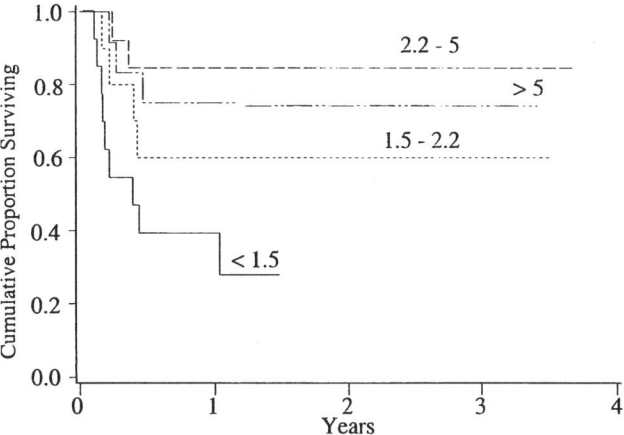

Fig. 3. Overall survival in recipients of unrelated donor UCBT by quartile of CD34+ cell dose (x 10^5/ kg). University of Minnesota p <0.01.

Table 7

Analysis of the Outcomes of Recipients of Unrelated Donor 0–3 HLA-Mismatched UCB vs HLA-Matched BM: Results of a Matched Pair Analysis

HSC source	N	Neutrophil recovery d 45	Platelet recovery d 180	Grades II–IV acute GVHD	Chronic GVHD	2-yr survival
UCB	2	0.88	0.72	0.42	0.05	0.53
	6	(0.75–1.00)	(0.50–0.94)	(0.23–0.61)	(0.0–0.13)	(0.31–0.75)
BM-MTX	2	0.96	0.76	0.35	0.20	0.41
	6	(0.89–1.00)	(0.54–0.98)	(0.17–50.3)	(0.05–0.35)	(0.22–0.60)
UCB	3	0.85	0.84	0.36	0.07	0.52
	1	(0.72–0.98)	(0.64–1.00)	(0.19–0.53)	(0.0–0.16)	(0.30–0.73)
BM-TCD	3	0.90	0.84	0.35	0.13	0.56
	1	(0.80–1.00)	(0.64–1.00)	(0.18–0.52)	(0.01–0.25)	(0.38–0.79)

( ), 95% confidence intervals. All outcomes were comparable (p >0.05).

children (median age 5 yr) transplanted for malignancy, storage diseases, BM failure, and immunodeficiency syndromes between 1991 and 1999.

Results are summarized in Table 7. Although neutrophil recovery was significantly slower after UCBT, the probability of donor-derived engraftment at d 45 was 0.88 in UCB vs 0.96 in BM-MTX recipients (p = 0.41) and 0.85 in UCB vs 0.90 in BM-TCD recipients (p = 0.32), respectively. Platelet recovery was similar in UCB vs BM pairs. Notably, incidences of acute and chronic GVHD were similar in UCB and BM recipients, with 0.53 of UCB vs 0.41 of BM-MTX recipients alive (p = 0.40) and 0.52 of UCB vs 0.56 of BM-TCD recipients alive at 2 yr (p >0.80), respectively (Fig. 4).

This study has the advantages of being from a single institution, where there is a standard-ized approach to HLA typing, including high resolution typing of HLA-DR, and homogeneity in both supportive care and toxicity and GVHD grading and long-term follow-up of patients. The data suggest that despite increased HLA disparity, probabilities of engraftment, GVHD, and survival after UCBT are comparable to those observed after HLA-matched BMT. A prospective randomized trial with larger patient numbers and longer follow-up will be required to firmly establish the relative merits of unrelated donor UCBT and BMT. However, these

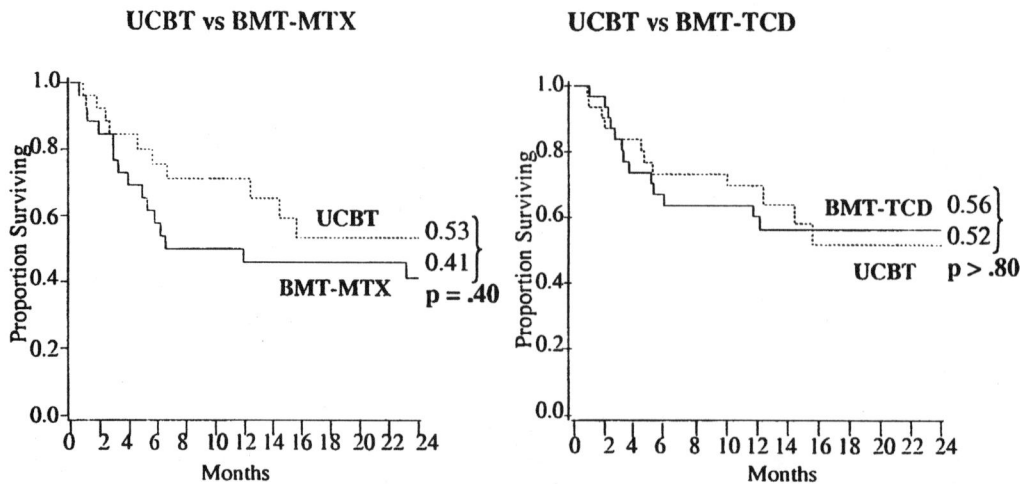

Fig. 4. Survival of pediatric recipients of UCBT vs BMT: results of a matched pair analysis. University of Minnesota.

results are reassuring and indicate that UCB should be considered an acceptable alternative to HLA-matched BM at least for pediatric patients.

6.3. UCBT in Adults

Limitations of cell dose has been the major barrier in the application of UCBT to adult recipients who often weigh ≥70 kg. Laughlin et al. has recently described the first experience of UCBT with adult recipients *(12)*. In this study, 68 patients predominantly with hematological malignancy, at a median age of 31 yr (range 18–58) and weighing a median of 69 kg, from five U.S. institutions were transplanted with unrelated donor UCB between 1995 and 1999. UCB grafts were largely 1–2 HLA-mismatched (6 out of 6 in 2 patients, 5 out of 6 in 18 patients, 4 out of 6 in 37 patients, and 3 out of 6 in 11 patients). The median nucleated cell dose prefreeze was 2.1×10^7/kg.

Of 60 patients surviving beyond d 28, neutrophil engraftment occurred at a median of 27 d (range 13–59) with an estimated probability of 0.90 (95% CI: 0.85–1.0). Chimerism was sustained in long-term survivors with no evidence of late graft failure. Probabilities of grade II–IV and III–IV acute GVHD and chronic GVHD (limited stage in all but one patient) were 0.60 (95% CI: 0.49–0.71), 0.20 (95% CI: 0.11–0.29), and 0.38 (95% CI: 0.23–0.52), respectively, and were not significantly related to HLA disparity. At a follow-up of 22 mo (range 11–51 mo), probability of event-free survival (EFS) was 0.26 (95% CI: 0.18–0.35). The UCB pre-freeze nucleated cell dose and the postthaw CD34 cell dose were significantly related to the myeloid engraftment and the EFS, respectively.

While nonrelapse mortality was high in this study, this may be partially explained by the high risk nature of the patient population. High transplant-related mortalities have also been seen in adult recipients of unrelated donor BM, particularly for indications other than chronic myelogenous leukemia *(5,8)*. How unrelated donor UCBT in adults compares to BMT will need to be studied prospectively. Of significance, rates of GVHD with mismatched unrelated donor UCBT in adults are tolerable and compare favorably to rates in unrelated BMT in adults. Furthermore, as both the neutrophil engraftment and the EFS were predicted by the cell dose of the graft in the Laughlin series *(12)*, future efforts in improving outcomes will need to focus primarily on improving UCB cell dose.

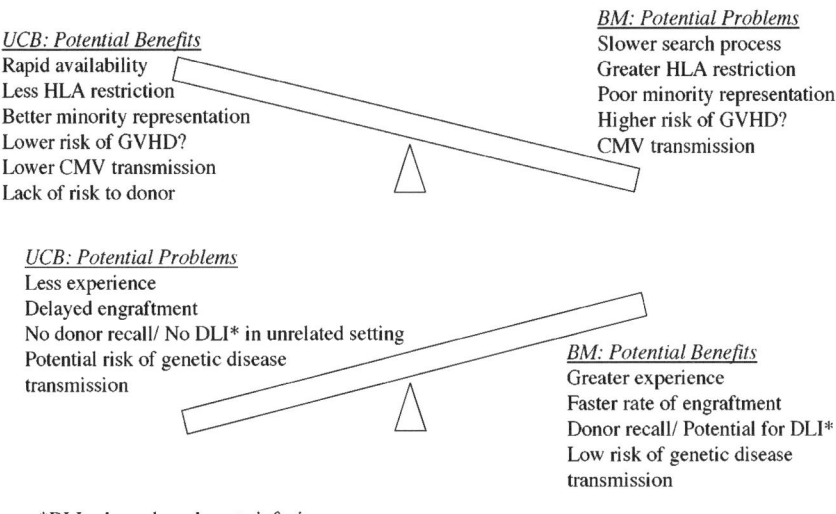

*DLI= donor lymphocyte infusion

Fig. 5. Relative advantages and disadvantages of BM vs UCB as stem cell source for transplantation.

6.4. Summary

The registry results reported by Gluckman et al. *(9)* and Rubinstein et al. *(11)* for unrelated donor UCBT are consistent with the Minnesota series in terms of hematopoietic recovery and risks of grade II–IV acute GVHD, with a survival at 4 yr of 0.40 in the University of Minnesota series comparing favorably to the other reports. The improved survival at the University of Minnesota may be explained by a center effect, likely reflecting greater experience with this relatively new source of HSC. This phenomenon was suggested in the Rubinstein analysis *(11)*.

The EuroCord Registry *(9)* and the University of Minnesota series have shown that the degree of HLA disparity has not impacted upon survival. Although this may reflect limited patient sample sizes with limited numbers of patients receiving 6 out of 6 antigen-matched grafts, it does show that 1–2 HLA-disparate grafts are relatively well-tolerated. This is further supported by the results of the University of Minnesota matched pair analysis, which demonstrated comparable survival in recipients of mismatched UCB vs matched BM. Importantly, the pediatric case series of UCBT have independently documented the importance of cell dose in predicting engraftment and survival, and this is further highlighted by the analysis of adult UCBT outcomes by Laughlin et al. *(12)*. Overall, these results dictate that selection of an unrelated graft should be based primarily on cell dose and secondarily on HLA match, within the confines of 0–2 HLA mismatch.

The relative merits and potential limitations of BM vs UCB are summarized in Fig. 5. In practice, whenever an unrelated donor search is undertaken at the University of Minnesota, we search for both BM donors and UCB. Until randomized studies of BMT vs UCBT can determine the priority for each stem cell source, we have constructed a working algorithm for unrelated donor selection (Fig. 6).

7. UCB BANKING

Documentation of hematological reconstitution after myeloablative therapy and UCBT, and the subsequent recognition of the importance of the UCB cell dose, has resulted in considerable interest in optimizing the collection, storage, and thawing techniques for UCB. As of 2000, it was estimated that >30,000 UCB grafts have been stored in UCB banks around the

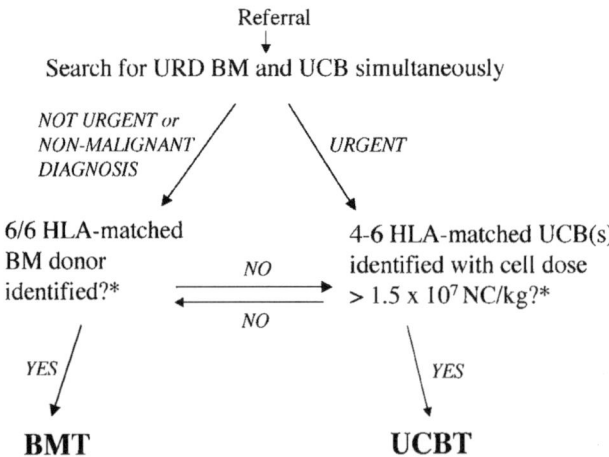

Fig. 6. Algorithm for selection of stem cell source in unrelated donor transplantation.

world (70). It is not known how many UCB units are needed to make a UCB graft available
to all potential recipients. Beatty et al have calculated that as few as 10,000 U may be required
if we accept a 4 out of 6 matched graft or better (2). However, these calculations are based on
HLAs as defined by serology and, therefore, may be an underestimate. Due the tolerance of
HLA disparity, UCB offers the possibility of access to HSC for ethnic minorities not well
represented in unrelated donor BM registries. Notably, Jefferies et al. have indicated that a
problem exists in the targeting of minority groups for UCB collection, as many maternal–
neonatal donor pairs from such groups are ineligible for UCB collection (71). In this study, the
deferral rate, mainly due to factors such as fever at delivery, history of chronic disease, or
history of sexually transmitted diseases, was greater than 50%. Nonetheless, Brown et al have
documented that, in the first 1500 UCB U banked in the London Cord Blood Bank, more than
30% are derived from U.K. ethnic minority groups as compared to only 2% of people from such
groups represented on the British Bone Marrow Registry (72).

Standard operating procedures for UCB banks have been summarized by the Cord Blood
Transplantation Study (COBLT) (73) and can be reviewed at the Web site (www.Emmes.com).
In practice, UCB for public banks is mainly collected at designated centers with specialized
personnel, whereas for private collection, the UCB is collected at the delivery hospital by the
obstetric provider and then shipped to the bank for storage. UCB is most commonly collected
after delivery of the uterus, although collection with the placenta in utero has been investigated
(74). Studies correlating maternal and neonatal characteristics with laboratory UCB parameters, such as cell dose, are currently ongoing so as to determine the best potential donors for
unrelated donor UCB collection (75).

Standardized quality assessment procedures should be the gold standard for all UCB banks,
including total nucleated cell dose, quantification of hematopoietic progenitors by CD34+
count and CFUs, sterility testing, detection for genetic diseases such as hemoglobinopathy, and
transmissible infectious agents including hepatitis B and C, human immunodeficiency virus
(HIV), human T cell lymphotrophic virus (HTLV), CMV, and syphilis. HLA and ABO/Rh
typing must be available as well as samples of donor (baby) plasma, DNA and viable cells, and
maternal plasma, and DNA for additional testing as necessary.

In an attempt to reduce the complication of dimethyl sulfoxide (DMSO) toxicity, reduce
ABO incompatibility reactions, and reduce the volume of the UCB unit, red blood cell (RBC)

depletion of the UCB graft is now routinely performed. Most investigators now thaw UCB after the technique of Rubinstein et al. *(76)*. Whether UCB units will be a viable source of HSC after many decades of storage is not known. Thus far, Broxmeyer et al. indicate high efficiency recovery of primitive progenitors from samples stored for at least 10 yr *(77)*.

7.1. Directed Donation vs Private Company

In contrast to the free donation of UCB to public registries, which make the UCB unit available to anyone, directed donation reserves the UCB unit for the transplantation of the baby's relative when the recipient has a disorder requiring UCBT. In the case when there is not an immediate need for the UCB unit, some parents will still elect to have their child's UCB stored by a private company as "biological insurance". Reimbursement for the cost of UCB collection and storage is usually only available from insurance companies and Medicaid in the case of directed donation (i.e., when there is a medical need within the donor's family). The practice of private UCB collection is not advocated, since the likelihood that a healthy child would subsequently require therapy utilizing HSC is remote, and in this situation, there is no evidence that autologous stem cells would be efficacious. Useful information about details relating to collection of UCB can be found on the Internet by searching under the term "umbilical cord stem cell storage".

8. UNRELATED DONOR UMBILICAL CORD BLOOD SEARCHES

Currently, UCB searches are most commonly accomplished by direct communication of the transplant center (TC) with individual UCB registries such as the New York Blood Center, COBLT, American Red Cross, National Marrow Donor Program (NMDP) or via Netcord (a consortium of banks in Denver, St. Louis, London, Paris, Milano, Dusseldorf, Barcelona, and Tokyo). Ideally, searches would occur through a coordinating center, and the NMDP has recently established relationships with various UCB banks worldwide to potentially serve in this capacity.

Once UCB search requests are submitted, UCB banks will send out reports of units available for the patient ranked by HLA match and size. The TC will then request confirmatory typing on selected UCB units, which is done on small samples of the unit. Based on these results, the TC will then select the unit for transplant, which will be shipped prior to the starting date of the recipient's preparative regimen. This process may be achieved within a few weeks, and this rapid availability represents a major advantage of UCBT over unrelated donor BMT.

9. ETHICAL AND REGULATORY ISSUES

The collection of UCB poses a number of ethical and legal issues *(78)*, many of which are new, complex, and beyond the scope of this chapter. At this time, current practice dictates that written informed consent from the donor's mother should be obtained, ideally prior to labor. Also, linkage (i.e., communication of relevant donor information to the UCB bank) between the donor and recipient should be maintained. Important ethical themes in relation to public UCB registries include issues of recruitment, consent, confidentiality, ownership, and alloca-tion. In addition the marketing and other practices of private commercial banks require close monitoring. These ethical issues are now being reviewed by multidisciplinary teams with representation of the medical specialties, such as pediatric and adult transplanters, obstetri-cians, blood bankers, as well as ethicists, lawyers, social scientists, and others.

With the development of numerous UCB banks around the world, some form of regulation is necessary to ensure optimal quality banking practices at all sites. All banks involved in UCB HSC therapy should be registered with the U.S. Food and Drug Administration (FDA). Key elements of the regulation of UCB include: (i) use of good manufacturing practice; (ii) ad-

Table 8
Future Directions for Unrelated Donor UCBT

Problem	New approach
Lack of HLA-compatible donors in minority groups.	Target UCB collection in these groups.
Engraftment.	Optimize collection techniques. Double UCBT. Ex vivo expansion. New stimulatory cytokines posttransplant. Modified preparative regimen. Ex vivo-expanded mesenchymal stem cells.
High transplant-related mortality.	Improve engraftment. Nonmyeloablative preparative regimens. Improve immune recovery (e.g., IL-7, karatinocyte growth factor [KGF]).
Need for HLA-matched donor.	Deliberate conception and implantation of HLA identical embryo.

equate testing for transmissible diseases; and (iii) development of product standards. At this time, it is recommended by these authors that only banks approved by a recognized regulatory agency be searched.

10. FUTURE DIRECTIONS (TABLE 8)

Currently, a major focus in UCBT is to develop strategies to increase the cell dose of the UCB graft. This could be achieved by the optimizing of UCB collection methods, transplantation of two closely HLA-matched unrelated donor UCB units (79) or by ex vivo expansion. Other approaches that may improve engraftment independent of cell dose may include the use of growth factors other than G-CSF, or an increase in host immunosuppression. The latter may improve the ability of the neonatal immune system to overcome the allogeneic barrier to engraftment. This may be relevant even with myeloablative conditioning, as suggested by the results of UCBT in hemoglobinopathy (66) and could potentially be achieved by the addition of such drugs as fludarabine and mycophenolate mofetil to the transplant regimen. Lastly, the addition of ex vivo-expanded mesenchymal stem cells may facilitate hematopoietic recovery by improving the marrow microenvironment (31). Studies investigating these approaches are underway at the University of Minnesota and elsewhere.

Another area of great interest is the development of nonmyeloablative preparative regimens for the treatment of nonmalignant hematological disorders, such as hemoglobinopathy or aplastic anemia, or for high risk adults. While there are no published series thus far, the addition of fludarabine to nonmyeloablative preparative regimen and mycophenolate mofetil to CSA in the early posttransplant period is being investigated with the aim of allowing UCB engraftment with reduced regimen-related toxicity. Finally, a new area of investigation is the deliberate conception and directed implantation of HLA identical embryo(s) for the purpose of obtaining UCB for a sibling requiring transplantation. This approach, although associated with a number of ethical concerns, has recently been pioneered and accomplished for a patient with Fanconi anemia at the University of Minnesota (80).

11. SUMMARY

Since the first sibling donor UCBT in 1988 *(16)*, the use of HLA-matched sibling donor UCB or 0–2 HLA-mismatched unrelated donor UCB has become an established acceptable alternative to the use of BM as a source for HSC for pediatric allogeneic transplantation. UCBT is associated with durable myeloid and lymphoid engraftment, and the rates of GVHD are relatively low even in the mismatched unrelated donor setting. Clinical experience has documented the importance of graft cell dose in determining engraftment and survival in unrelated UCBT *(9–12)*. Therefore, within the confines of 0–2 HLA-mismatch, the choice of an UCB graft should be based primarily on cell dose.

UCBT is now being investigated in adult recipients *(12)*, and it is hoped that advantages in regard to GVHD in the adult population will offset any adverse impact of reduced cell dose on survival. How UCB compares to BM in terms of immune reconstitution, incidence of relapse, and long-term survival is yet to be determined. Ultimately, prospective randomized studies will be required to establish the relative merits of each stem cell source in the unrelated donor setting. These are currently being considered, although in practice, randomization may be difficult to achieve as UCB can be obtained substantially more quickly than unrelated donor BM.

The immediate availability of this stem cell source is a major advantage of UCB. Furthermore, the ability to tolerate 0–2 HLA mismatch in unrelated UCBT means that the benefits of stem cell transplantation may be extended to those with tissue types poorly represented on the BM registries. The major focus in UCBT is methods to increase cell dose, such as optimization of collection techniques, double UCBT, and ex vivo expansion of UCB. Progress and experience in UCBT is rapidly increasing, making this an exciting new area in HSC transplantation.

REFERENCES

1. Thomas ED, Blume K, Forman S. *Hematopoietic Cell Transplantation.* Blackwell Science, Cambridge, MA, 1999.
2. Beatty PG, Boucher KM, Mori M, Milford EL. Probability of finding HLA-mismatched related or unrelated marrow or cord blood donors. *Hum Immunol* 2000;61:834–940.
3. van Rood JJ, Schipper RF, Bakker JN, van der Zanden HG, Oudshoorn M. Bone marrow donors worldwide and cord blood stem cell transplantation. *Bone Marrow Transplant* 1998;22(Suppl 1):S19–21.
4. Dodson K, Coppo P, Confer D. The National Marrow Donor Program: Improving access to hematopoietic stem cell transplantation. In: Cecka JM, Terasaki PI, eds. *Clinical Transplants.* UCLA Immunogenetics Center, Los Angeles, CA, 1999.
5. Anasetti C, Petersdorf EW, Martin PJ, Woolfrey A, Hansen JA. Improving availability and safety of unrelated donor transplants. *Curr Opin Oncol* 2000;12:121–126.
6. Beatty PG, Mori M, Milford E. Impact of racial genetic polymorphism on the probability of finding an HLA-matched donor. *Transplantation* 1995;60:778–783.
7. Madrigal JA, Scott I, Arguello R, Szydlo R, Little AM, Goldman JM. Factors influencing the outcome of bone marrow transplants using unrelated donors. *Immunol Rev* 1997;157:153–166.
8. Champlin RE, Passweg JR, Zhang MJ, et al. T-cell depletion of bone marrow transplants for leukemia from donors other than HLA-identical siblings: advantage of T-cell antibodies with narrow specificities. *Blood* 2000;95:3996–4003.
9. Gluckman E, Rocha V, Boyer-Chammard A, et al. Outcome of cord-blood transplantation from related and unrelated donors. Eurocord Transplant Group and the European Blood and Marrow Transplantation Group. *N Engl J Med* 1997;337:373–381.
10. Wagner JE, DeFor T, Rubinstein P, Kurtzberg J. Transplantation of unrelated donor umbilical cord blood (UCB): Outcomes and Analysis of Risk Factors. *Blood* 1997;90:398a.
11. Rubinstein P, Carrier C, Scaradavou A, et al. Outcomes among 562 recipients of placental-blood transplants from unrelated donors. *N Engl J Med* 1998;339:1565–1577.
12. Laughlin MJ, Barker J, Bambach B, et al. Hematologic engraftment and survival in adult recipients of umbilical-cord blood from unrelated donors. *N Engl J Med* 2001;24:1815–1822

13. Barker JN, Davies SM, Defor T, Ramsay NKC, Weisdorf DJ, Wagner JE. Survival after transplantation of unrelated donor umbilical cord blood is comparable to that of HLA-matched unrelated donor bone marrow: results of a matched pair analysis. *Blood* 2001;97(10):2957–2961.

14. Broxmeyer HE, Kurtzberg J, Gluckman E, et al. Umbilical cord blood hematopoietic stem and repopulating cells in human clinical transplantation. *Blood Cells* 1991;17:313–329.

15. Broxmeyer HE, Douglas GW, Hangoc G, et al. Human umbilical cord blood as a potential source of transplantable hematopoietic stem/progenitor cells. *Proc Natl Acad Sci USA* 1989;86:3828–3832.

16. Gluckman E, Broxmeyer HA, Auerbach AD, et al. Hematopoietic reconstitution in a patient with Fanconi's anemia by means of umbilical-cord blood from an HLA-identical sibling. *N Engl J Med* 1989;321:1174–1178.

17. Roy V, Verfaillie CM. Expression and function of cell adhesion molecules on fetal liver, cord blood and bone marrow hematopoietic progenitors: implications for anatomical localization and developmental stage specific regulation of hematopoiesis. *Exp Hematol* 1999;27:302–312.

18. Mayani H, Lansdorp PM. Biology of human umbilical cord blood-derived hematopoietic stem/progenitor cells. *Stem Cells* 1998;16:153–165.

19. Wynter EA, Emmerson AJB, Testa NG. Properties of peripheral blood and cord blood stem cells. *Bailliere's Clin Haematol* 1999;1/2:1–17.

20. Leung W, Ramirez M, Novelli EM, Civin CI. In vivo engraftment potential of clinical hematopoietic grafts. *J Invest Med* 1998;46:303–311.

21. Holyoake TL, Nicolini FE, Eaves CJ. Functional differences between transplantable human hematopoietic stem cells from fetal liver, cord blood, and adult marrow. *Exp Hematol* 1999;27:1418–1427.

22. Vaziri H, Dragowska W, Allsopp RC, Thomas TE, Harley CB, Lansdorp PM. Evidence for a mitotic clock in human hematopoietic stem cells: loss of telomeric DNA with age. *Proc Natl Acad Sci USA* 1994;91:9857–9860.

23. Lewis I, Verfaillie CM. Multi-lineage expansion potential of primitive hematopoietic progenitors. Superiority of umbilical cord blood compared to mobilized peripheral blood. *Exp Hematol* 2000;28:1087–1095.

24. Punzel M, Gupta P, Roodell M, Mortari F, Verfaillie CM. Factor(s) secreted by AFT024 fetal liver cells following stimulation with human cytokines are important for human LTC-IC growth. *Leukemia* 1999;13:1079–1084.

25. Gupta P, Oegema TR, Brazil JJ, Dudek AZ, Slungaard A, Verfaillie CM. Human LTC-IC can be maintained for at least 5 weeks in vitro when interleukin-3 and a single chemokine are combined with O-sulfated heparan sulfates: requirement for optimal binding interactions of heparan sulfate with early-acting cytokines and matrix proteins. *Blood* 2000;95:147–155.

26. Theunissen K, Lewis I, Scheller C, Verfaillie C. Ex-vivo expansion of cord blood CD34+ cells in a clinically suitable artificial media that maintains transplantable cells after 14 days in culture. *Blood* 2000;96:775a.

27. Glimm H, Oh IH, Eaves CJ. Human hematopoietic stem cells stimulated to proliferate in vitro lose engraftment potential during their S/G(2)/M transit and do not reenter G(0). *Blood* 2000;96:4185–4193.

28. Shpall E, Quinones R, Giller R, et al. Transplantation of adult and pediatric cancer patients with cord blood progenitors expanded ex vivo. *Blood* 2000;96:207a.

29. Carow CE, Hangoc G, Broxmeyer HE. Human multipotential progenitor cells (CFU-GEMM) have extensive replating capacity for secondary CFU-GEMM: an effect enhanced by cord blood plasma. *Blood* 1993;81:942–949.

30. Kogler G, Nurnberger W, Fischer J, et al. Simultaneous cord blood transplantation of ex vivo expanded together with non-expanded cells for high risk leukemia. *Bone Marrow Transplant* 1999;24:397–403.

31. Almeida-Porada G, Porada CD, Tran N, Zanjani ED. Cotransplantation of human stromal cell progenitors into preimmune fetal sheep results in early appearance of human donor cells in circulation and boosts cell levels in bone marrow at later time points after transplantation. *Blood* 2000;95:3620–3627.

32. Lu L, Xiao M, Clapp DW, Li ZH, Broxmeyer HE. High efficiency retroviral mediated gene transduction into single isolated immature and replatable CD34(3+) hematopoietic stem/progenitor cells from human umbilical cord blood. *J Exp Med* 1993;178:2089–2096.

33. Kohn DB, Weinberg KI, Nolta JA, et al. Engraftment of gene-modified umbilical cord blood cells in neonates with adenosine deaminase deficiency. *Nat Med* 1995;1:1017–1023.

34. Cavazzana-Calvo M, Hacein-Bey S, de Saint Basile G, et al. Gene therapy of human severe combined immunodeficiency (SCID)-X1 disease. *Science* 2000;288:669–672.

35. Theunissen K, Verfaillie CM. Translation of an optimized AFT024 non-contact transduction system into clinically siutable protocols. *Blood* 2000;96:219a.

36. Woods NB, Fahlman C, Mikkola H, et al. Lentiviral gene transfer into primary and secondary NOD/SCID repopulating cells. *Blood* 2000;96:3725–3733.

37. Risdon G, Gaddy J, Stehman FB, Broxmeyer HE. Proliferative and cytotoxic responses of human cord blood T lymphocytes following allogeneic stimulation. *Cell Immunol* 1994;154:14–24.

38. Risdon G, Gaddy J, Horie M, Broxmeyer HE. Alloantigen priming induces a state of unresponsiveness in human umbilical cord blood T cells. *Proc Natl Acad Sci USA* 1995;92:2413–2417.

39. Roncarolo MG, Bigler M, Martino S, Ciuti E, Tovo PA, Wagner J. Immune functions of cord blood cells before and after transplantation. *J Hematother* 1996;5:157–160.

40. Cohen SB, Madrigal JA. Immunological and functional differences between cord and peripheral blood. *Bone Marrow Transplant* 1998;21(Suppl 3):S9–12.
41. Garderet L, Dulphy N, Douay C, et al. The umbilical cord blood alphabeta T-cell repertoire: characteristics of a polyclonal and naive but completely formed repertoire. *Blood* 1998;91:340–346.
42. Leung W, Ramirez M, Mukherjee G, Perlman EJ, Civin CI. Comparisons of alloreactive potential of clinical hematopoietic grafts. *Transplantation* 1999;68:628–635.
43. Kadereit S, Mohammad SF, Miller RE, et al. Reduced NFAT1 protein expression in human umbilical cord blood T lymphocytes. *Blood* 1999;94:3101–3107.
44. Sorg RV, Kogler G, Wernet P. Functional competence of dendritic cells in human umbilical cord blood. *Bone Marrow Transplant* 1998;22(Suppl 1):S52–54.
45. Canque B, Camus S, Dalloul A, et al. Characterization of dendritic cell differentiation pathways from cord blood CD34(+)CD7(+)CD45RA(+) hematopoietic progenitor cells. *Blood* 2000;96:3748–3756.
46. Wagner JE, J. K. Allogeneic Umbilical Cord Blood Transplantation. In: Broxmeyer HE, ed. *Cellular Characteristics of Cord Blood and Cord Blood Transplantation*. AABB Press, Bethesda, MA, 1998, pp. 113–146.
47. van Rood JJ, Loberiza FR, Zhang MJ, et al. Effect of early exposure to non-inherited maternal antigens on outcome of haplo-identical bone marrow transplants. *Blood* 2000;96:840a.
48. Rocha V, Wagner JE, Jr., Sobocinski KA, et al. Graft-versus-host disease in children who have received a cord-blood or bone marrow transplant from an HLA-identical sibling. *N Engl J Med* 2000;342:1846–1854.
49. Giraud P, Thuret I, Reviron D, et al. Immune reconstitution and outcome after unrelated cord blood transplantation: a single paediatric institution experience. *Bone Marrow Transplant* 2000;25:53–57.
50. Abu-Ghosh A, Goldman S, Slone V, et al. Immunological reconstitution and correlation of circulating serum inflammatory mediators/cytokines with the incidence of acute graft-versus-host disease during the first 100 days following unrelated umbilical cord blood transplantation. *Bone Marrow Transplant* 1999;24:535–544.
51. Thomson BG, Robertson KA, Gowan D, et al. Analysis of engraftment, graft-versus-host disease, and immune recovery following unrelated donor cord blood transplantation. *Blood* 2000;96:2703–2711.
52. Talvensaari K, Clave E, Douay C, et al. Immune Reconstitution is improved is improved after 1 year in cord blood compared to HLA-identical sibling bone marrow transplanted patients. *Blood* 2000;96:555a.
53. Demarest JF, Kadereit S, Brenner-Jones S. V Beta Repertoire of t lymphocytes emerging in adults after unrelated umbilical cord blood (UCB) allogeneic transplantation. *Blood* 2000;96:788a.
54. Mackall CL, Fry TJ, Bare C, Morgan P, Galbraith A, Gress RE. IL-7 increases both thymic-dependent and thymic-independent T-cell regeneration after bone marrow transplantation. *Blood* 2001;97:1491–1497.
55. Min D, Taylor P, Chung B, et al. Protection from thymic epithelial cell (TEC) injury by pre-BMT keratinocyte growth factor (KGF): a new approach to speed thymic reconstitution after lethal irradiation. *Blood* 2000;96:474a.
56. Locatelli F, Comoli P, Giorgiani G, et al. Infusion of donor-derived peripheral blood leukocytes after transplantation of cord blood progenitor cells can increase the graft- versus-leukaemia effect. *Leukemia* 1997;11:729–731.
57. Howrey RP, Martin PL, Driscoll T, et al. Graft-versus-leukemia-induced complete remission following unrelated umbilical cord blood transplantation for acute leukemia. *Bone Marrow Transplant* 2000;26:1251–1254.
58. Goldberg SL, Pecora AL, Rosenbluth RJ, Jennis AA, Preti RA. Treatment of leukemic relapse following unrelated umbilical cord blood transplantation with interleukin-2: potential for augmenting graft-versus-leukemia and graft-versus-host effects with cytokines. *Bone Marrow Transplant* 2000;26:353–355.
59. Laws HJ, Nurnberger W, Korholz D, et al. Successful treatment of relapsed CML after cord blood transplantation with donor leukocyte infusion IL-2 and IFNalpha. *Bone Marrow Transplant* 2000;25:219–222.
60. Marshall NA, Howe JG, Formica R, et al. Rapid reconstitution of Epstein-Barr virus-specific T lymphocytes following allogeneic stem cell transplantation. *Blood* 2000;96:2814–2821.
61. Barker JN, Martin PL, Coad J, et al. Low Incidence of Epstein-Barr virus-associated post-transplant lymphoproliferative disorders (EBV-PTLD) in 272 unrelated donor umbilical cord blood transplant recipients. *Biol Blood Marrow Transplant* 2001;7:395–399.
62. Issaragrisil S, Visuthisakchai S, Suvatte V, et al. Brief report: transplantation of cord-blood stem cells into a patient with severe thalassemia [see comments]. *N Engl J Med* 1995;332:367–369.
63. Issaragrisil S, Suvatte V, Visuthisakchai S, et al. Bone marrow and cord blood stem cell transplantation for thalassemia in Thailand. *Bone Marrow Transplant* 1997;19:54,55.
64. Graphacos S, Kitra V, Peristeri J, et al. Haematopoietic transplantation for thalassemic children: the Greek children. *Bone Marrow Transplant* 1997;19:68,69.
65. Li CK, Yen PMP, Shing MK, et al. Stem cell transplant for Thalessemia patients in Hong Kong. *Bone Marrow Transplant* 1997;19:6,69.
66. Miniero R, Rocha V, Saracco P, et al. Cord blood transplantation (CBT) in hemoglobinopathies. Eurocord. *Bone Marrow Transplant* 1998;22(Suppl 1):S78,79.
67. Kurtzberg J, Laughlin M, Graham ML, et al. Placental blood as a source of hematopoietic stem cells for transplantation into unrelated recipients. *N Engl J Med* 1996;335:157–166.

68. Wagner JE, Rosenthal J, Sweetman R, et al. Successful transplantation of HLA-matched and HLA-mismatched umbilical cord blood from unrelated donors: analysis of engraftment and acute graft-versus-host disease. *Blood* 1996;88:795–802.
69. Wagner JE, DeFor T, Barker J, et al. Superior survival in recipients of umbilical cord blood (UCB): results of a case controlled analysis comparing UCB and bone marrow (BM) from unrelated donors. *Blood* 1999;94:711a.
70. Gluckman E. Current status of umbilical cord blood hematopoietic stem cell transplantation. *Exp Hematol* 2000;28:1197–1205.
71. Jefferies LC, Albertus M, Morgan MA, Moolten D. High deferral rate for maternal-neonatal donor pairs for an allogeneic umbilical cord blood bank. *Transfusion* 1999;39:415–419.
72. Brown J, Poles A, Brown CJ, Contreras M, Navarrete CV. HLA-A, -B and -DR antigen frequencies of the London Cord Blood Bank units differ from those found in established bone marrow donor registries. *Bone Marrow Transplant* 2000;25:475–481.
73. Fraser JK, Cairo MS, Wagner EL, et al. Cord Blood Transplantation Study (COBLT): cord blood bank standard operating procedures. *J Hematother* 1998;7:521–561.
74. Surbek DV, Schonfeld B, Tichelli A, Gratwohl A, Holzgreve W. Optimizing cord blood mononuclear cell yield: a randomized comparison of collection before vs after placenta delivery. *Bone Marrow Transplant* 1998;22:311,312.
75. Shlebak AA, Roberts IA, Stevens TA, Syzdlo RM, Goldman JM, Gordon MY. The impact of antenatal and perinatal variables on cord blood haemopoietic stem/progenitor cell yield available for transplantation. *Br J Haematol* 1998;103:1167–1171.
76. Rubinstein P, Dobrila L, Rosenfield RE, et al. Processing and cryopreservation of placental/umbilical cord blood for unrelated bone marrow reconstitution. *Proc Natl Acad Sci USA* 1995;92:10,119–10,122.
77. Broxmeyer HE, Cooper S. High-efficiency recovery of immature haematopoietic progenitor cells with extensive proliferative capacity from human cord blood cryopreserved for 10 years. *Clin Exp Immunol* 1997;107(Suppl 1):45–53.
78. Annas GJ. Waste and longing-the legal status of placental-blood banking. *N Engl J Med* 1999;340:1521–1524.
79. Barker JN, Verfaillie CM, McGlave P, et al. Creation of a double chimera by transplantation of two unrelated donor umbilical cord blood units. *Blood* 2000;96:207a.
80. Wagner JE. Designer babies-are they a reality yet? *RBM Online* 2000;1:77.
81. Locatelli F, Maccario R, Comoli P, et al. Hematopoietic and immune recovery after transplantation of cord blood progenitor cells in children. *Bone Marrow Transplant.* 1996;6:1095–1101.

11

Mesenchymal Stem Cells in Allogeneic Transplantation

Omer N. Koç, MD and Stanton L. Gerson MD

CONTENTS

1. INTRODUCTION

Graft failure and graft-vs-host disease (GVHD) remain significant obstacles to successful outcome in patients undergoing allogeneic hematopoietic stem cell transplantation. This chapter will introduce a novel cellular therapy, which may address these problems, particularly in high risk patients such as those receiving marginal numbers of hematopoietic progenitor cells (i.e., umbilical cord blood [UCB]) and those receiving unrelated donor or related but human leukocyte antigen (HLA)-mismatched donor progenitor cells. Several groups have described nonhematopoietic plastic-adherent progenitor cells derived from human bone marrow aspirates, which are capable of differentiating into mature mesenchymal cells *(1–5)*. It is thought that these progenitors, called mesenchymal stem cells, give rise to adventitial and other mesenchymal cells in the marrow and constitute the microenvironment for hematopoiesis. Such cells fabricate the connective tissue scaffolding and produce cytokines, chemokines, and extracellular matrix proteins that regulate hematopoietic homing and proliferation *(6,7)*. There is growing interest in cotransplantation of allogeneic mesenchymal and hematopoietic progenitors to facilitate hematopoietic engraftment and limit GVHD.

2. MESENCHYMAL STEM CELLS

2.1. Biology

There is increasing evidence that bone marrow contains pluripotential nonhematopoietic progenitors that can differentiate into cells of mesenchymal origin, such as surrounding fibroblasts, osteoblasts, adipocytes, and chondrocytes, as well as cells of distant tissues such as muscle *(8)*, liver *(9,10)*, and brain *(11,12)*. Friedenstein initially reported in 1978 that clonogenic

From: *Current Clinical Oncology: Allogeneic Stem Cell Transplantation*
Edited by: Mary S. Laughlin and Hillard M. Lazarus © Humana Press Inc., Totowa, NJ

stromal cells could be derived from bone marrow (13). Several groups subsequently described nonhematopoietic plastic-adherent progenitor cells derived from human bone marrow aspirates, which were capable of differentiating into mature mesenchymal lineages (1–5). Investigators at Case Western Reserve University (CWRU) described a uniform population of adherent cells with extensive proliferative capacity and the ability to differentiate along the osteogenic, chondrogenic, and adipogenic lineages both in vitro and in vivo. These cells have a high proliferative capacity in vitro without differentiation under normal growth conditions but upon specific stimulation differentiate into various cells of mesenchymal origin (4), including stromal cells of the marrow (14,15), adipocytes (4), osteocytes (16), and chondrocytes (5) and thus have been termed mesenchymal stem cells (MSC) (17). MSCs are likely to represent a restricted progeny of putative pluripotent stem cells selected on the basis of their rapid plastic adherence and high proliferation potential in 10% fetal calf serum. In nonstimulated cultures, MSCs appear as fusiform fibroblasts with expression of unique surface proteins (recognized by monoclonal antibodies SH2 and SH3) (1) not found on hematopoietic precursors. Conversely, MSCs lack expression of hematopoietic markers such as CD45, CD14, CD11, and CD34. MSCs express interleukin (IL)-6, -7, -8, -11, -12, -14, -15, macrophage colony-stimulating factor (M-CSF), flt-3 ligand (FL), and stem cell factor (SCF) in steady state (14,15,18), but not IL-3 and transformation growth factor (TGF)β. Exposure to dexamethasone results in decreased expression of leukemia inhibiting factor (LIF), IL-6, and IL-11. In contrast, IL-1α increases the expression of granulocyte colony-stimulating factor (G-CSF), M-CSF, LIF, IL-1, IL-6, IL-8, and IL-11 and induces expression of granulocyte-macrophage colony-stimulating factor (GM-CSF), but does not alter the expression of IL-7, IL-12, IL-14, IL-15, M-CSF, FL, and SCF. Similar to Dexter type stromal cultures containing a more complex mixture of cells, MSCs can support human long-term culture-initiating cells (LTC-ICs) (14,15). Human MSCs do not express class II antigens and do not present antigen. In preliminary studies, MSCs appear to suppress primary and secondary T lymphocyte proliferation in response to allogeneic stimuli in vitro (19,20), a potential advantage in the setting of allogeneic transplantation and perhaps a therapeutic asset to limit GVHD and organ rejection.

2.2. Preclinical Studies

A number of preclinical animal models of MSC transplantation have been established for purposes of gene delivery, treatment of bone disorders, and support of hematopoietic engraftment. Murine bone marrow stromal cells were successfully transplanted into mice by a number of investigators. Using the *a* and *b* isoenzymes of glucose-6-phosphate isomerase, Anklesaria et al. showed that a bone marrow stromal cell line (GB1/6) could engraft mice pretreated with irradiation (22). Donor stromal cells facilitated hematopoietic recovery from radiation. Host marrow recovery was assessed following 3 Gy total body irradiation (TBI) and 10 Gy unilateral hindleg radiation with or without intravenous infusion of $0.1–1 \times 10^6$ GB1/6 cells 48 h later. GB1/6 cells were identified only in marrow sinusoids of right hindleg (high radiation exposure) 2 mo posttransplant, and up to 80% of the stromal cells established from transplanted mice were of donor origin. Furthermore GB1/6 transplanted mice had significantly higher cell and colony-forming unit (CFU) recovery at 1, 2, and 3 mo posttransplant compared to irradiated but untransplanted mice. Pereira et al. used marrow stromal cells of COL1A1 transgenic mice (human mini-gene for collagen I) to follow their distribution and function in a parental (nontransgenic) inbred strain of mice (22). Transgenic stromal cells (1×10^5) were intravenously co-infused with 6×10^5 nontransgenic bone marrow cells after 9 cGy irradiation. Thirty to 150 d later, COL1A1 positive cells were detected in marrow, spleen, bone, lung, and cartilage and constituted 1.5–12% of the cells. In a murine model of osteogenesis imperfecta (OI), Pereria et al. infused "normal" MSCs expressing wild-type type I collagen to rescue mice from the OI phenotype (23). Although only a small number of donor mesenchymal progenitors and osteoblasts engrafted, there was evidence of normal collagen expression in bone. These studies have been extended to human trials, in which preliminary results indicate a possible therapeutic effect of infused osteoblast precursors on OI (24). Huss et al. showed that following intravenous administration, murine and canine marrow-derived stromal cells could be detected in the marrow cavity and spleens of severe combined immunodeficient (SCID) mice for 21 d (25). Hurwitz et al. transfected canine marrow stromal cells with human growth hormone (hGH) (26). Cells were returned to dogs either intravenously or directly into iliac crest marrow. hGH gene sequences were detected in peripheral blood transiently and in bone marrow for up to 13 wk. Plasma of each dog contained detectable levels of hGH for a mean of 3 d. Green fluorescent protein (GFP)-marked canine MSCs were infused into autologous as well as dog leukemia antigen (DLA)-identical litter-mate dogs following 920 cGy TBI. Polymerase chain reaction (PCR) evidence of GFP-marked canine MSCs was found predominantly in the marrow of sternum, ribs, and limbs at 6 and 14 wk postinfusion (27,28). Human MSCs were also used as bioreactors to synthesize therapeutic proteins in vivo. MSCs were transduced with human erythropoietin using a retroviral vector and delivered into immunodeficient non-obese diabetic-SCID (NOD-SCID) mice within ceramic cubes (29). This resulted in a significantly increased red blood cell counts in all mice up to 90 d of observation. Similarly, baboon MSCs transduced with human erythropoietin gene were delivered to recipient baboons within a TheraCyte immunoisolator device (30). Significant levels of human erythropoietin were detected in vivo starting at d 4 and persisted for the duration of the experiment (70 d). In preclinical efficacy studies Novelli et al. have shown that human MSCs increased engraftment of human CD34+ in NOD-SCID mouse by three- to fourfold (31). These studies point to the feasibility of MSC transplantation for a variety of therapeutic interventions and establish a starting point for human studies. Given the biologic differences between MSCs derived from different species and the differences in the transplant biology among species make it impossible to translate these results to humans without carefully designed clinical trials.

2. 3. Immune Interactions of MSCs

There is experimental evidence that major histocompatibility complex (MHC) mismatch between the donor hematopoietic progenitors and the host bone marrow microenvironment may be disadvantageous to donor cells particularly in the nonmyeloablative setting. Engraftment of hematopoietic cells in a mismatched allogeneic transplant model was shown to be facilitated by MHC-matched bone grafting and the donor engraftment was found predominantly in the donor bone grafts (32). Similarly, MHC-matched osteoblast and CD8+, CD3+, T cell receptor (TCR)[neg] "facilitator cell" cotransplantation was shown to improve engraftment with purified allogeneic hematopoietic progenitors (33,34). These data suggest that stable full or mixed donor hematopoietic chimerism can be supported by cotransplantation of donor bone marrow microenvironment. Mesenchymal stem cells can potentially fulfill this goal either by their direct interaction with the donor immune system or by giving rise to elements of donor bone marrow microenvironment in the host.

Flow cytometry analysis of MSCs indicate that they express a number of molecules appropriate for interaction with T cells including Vascular cell adhesion molecule (VCAM)-1, lymphocyte function-related antigen (LFA)-3, and HLA MHC class I molecules. Upon treatment with interferon (IFN)γ, intercellular adhesion molecule (ICAM)-1 and MHC class II molecules were expressed on MSCs, and the expression of class I molecules could be enhanced. B7-1 and B7-2 co-stimulatory molecules were not detectable on MSCs by flow cytometry. In vitro experiments have shown that MSCs suppress primary and secondary T lymphocyte proliferation in response to allogeneic stimuli (19,20). This effect appears to be maintained in

Table 1
Clinical Trials of Culture-Expanded MSC Transplantation

Phase	MSC source	Setting	Results as of April 2001 (ref.)
I	Autologous	Volunteer patients	Feasible, safe (42)
II		Breast cancer	Safe, rapid hematopoietic recovery (43)
I	Allogeneic	Post-allo BMT genetic disorders	Safe, no Anti-MSC immune response (44)
		Allo BMT or PB HLA-matched sibling	Safe, rapid hematopoietic recovery, GVHD incidence lower than expected (45)
		Osteogenisis imperfecta	Safe, bone growth/endurance (24)
I-II	Allogeneic 3rd party	UCB Tx	Safe
		Lymphoma Auto-PBPC Tx	Ongoing
		MUD-Allo Tx	Ongoing

Tx, Transplantation; PB, peripheral blood; Allo, allogeneic; UCB, umbilical cord blood; MUD, matched unrelated donor.

noncontact culture conditions using a *trans*-well system, leading to a hypothesis that it is due to direct or indirect effect of a soluble protein(s) derived from MSCs. These data support the idea that MSCs not only potentially survive in an allogeneic recipient, but also support survival of allogeneic HSCs by inhibiting immunologic response. It is not yet clear if MSCs are tolerogenic, as they can present class I and II alloantigens in the apparent absence of B7 co-stimulatory signals. Keratinocytes, myoblasts, and T cells have been reported to induce T cell anergy in this manner. Using a baboon skin graft model, Bartholomew and coworkers showed that infusion of ex vivo-expanded donor (baboon) MSCs at a dose of 20×10^6 MSC/kg recipient weight prolonged time to rejection of histoincompatible skin grafts (35). Even "third-party" baboon MSCs, obtained from neither recipient nor skin graft donor, appeared to suppress alloreactivity in vivo.

Based on these observations, a number of clinical transplantation studies with cotransplantation of allogeneic MSCs and hematopoietic stem cells (HSCs) are proposed (Table 1) to improve donor engraftment and limit GVHD.

3. TRANSPLANTATION OF MESENCHYMAL STEM CELLS

The pivotal role of MSCs in the bone marrow microenvironment and their ability to support of hematopoiesis sparked the interest of bone marrow transplant physicians to use MSCs as supportive care for patients undergoing stem cell transplantation. A number of studies have shown that chemotherapy and radiation damage the marrow microenvironment and diminish its hematopoietic support function (36–38). Therefore, it seems logical that if transplanted, MSCs could provide hematopoietic cytokines, help to establish the new bone marrow microenvironment, and support autologous and allogeneic hematopoietic engraftment and regeneration.

Although MSCs can be derived from a bone marrow aspirate, it has been shown that conventional allogeneic bone marrow transplantation (BMT) does not result in transfer of donor MSCs or MSC-derived cells into the recipient (39,40). These results are attributed to the inability of the conditioning regimen to ablate host marrow stroma and/or the inability of stromal progenitors to engraft. In addition, the number of MSCs in an average bone marrow graft is estimated to be too few. For instance, at a frequency of 2–5 MSCs per 1×10^6 mononuclear cells, a bone marrow graft comprised of 2×10^8 mononuclear cells (MNC)/kg would contain only 400–1000 MSCs/kg. On the other hand, a recent report noted that allogeneic osteoblasts could be detected in children with OI after sibling-matched allogeneic BMT *(41)*. It is not clear if this observation indicates that osteoblasts were passively transferred to the recipient or whether MSCs present in the marrow graft were capable of homing to the bone and differentiating into osteoblasts, perhaps because of the growth defects of the host MSCs and osteoblasts. Nevertheless, these data suggest that, under permissive conditions (a loss of endogenous mesenchymal cells or an underlying cell defect), even small number of mesenchymal cells contained in the bone marrow graft may be capable of therapeutic engraftment. It remains unclear how important an underlying defect in MSCs will be in determining the efficacy of donor MSC engraftment.

In an attempt to achieve mesenchymal engraftment, studies were initiated to investigate the transplantation of high numbers of culture-expanded murine and human MSCs. Human MSCs have a high in vitro proliferative potential and can expand their numbers from approx 1500–3500 MSCs/20 mL of bone marrow aspirate at collection to $70–700 \times 10^6$ MSCs (or $1–10 \times 10^6$/kg) at the end of expansion, which is equivalent to the number of MSCs found in >1000 L of fresh bone marrow aspitrate. Although intravenous infusion of MSCs resulted in demonstration of donor MSCs in various tissues of recipient animals, it has not been possible to show donor MSC proliferation and regeneration of tissues, such as bone marrow microenvironment. A major limitation in these applications has been the low level of engraftment that takes place when culture-expanded MSCs are systemically introduced. A number of factors are likely to contribute to poor MSC engraftment. First, the size and surface characteristics of MSCs may not be optimal for homing to tissues in which they can proliferate. There is light microscopy and flow cytometry evidence that culture-expanded adherent MSCs are large ($2–3 \times$ of granulocytes). This is an important issue when cells are given directly into the vasculature. Human MSCs were shown to express $\alpha1–3$ and $\beta1, \beta3, \beta4$ integrins, ICAM-1 and -2, VCAM, L-selectin, and CD44 (hyaluronate), but not $\alpha4$ integrin, E-selectin, P-selectin, ICAM-3, and cadherin-5, important adhesion molecules in hematopoietic stem cell homing. Second, culture-expanded MSCs may have a proliferative defect. Since MSCs are generally subjected to multiple cell divisions during ex vivo expansion, they may approach their proliferative limit and may be unable to expand sufficiently in recipients. Third, the bone marrow and other tissue environments may not attract circulating MSCs through homing peptides and may not provide a survival and proliferation advantage to the transplanted cells. There is ongoing work to understand distribution, homing, and engraftment of intravenously infused MSCs.

4. MSC TRANSPLANTATION IN THE CLINIC

4.1. Autologous MSC Transplantation

Feasibility and safety of clinical scale autologous and allogeneic human MSC expansion and intravenous infusion into adult and pediatric patients have been established *(42–45)*. In a pilot study, our group demonstrated the safety of ex vivo expansion and subsequent infusion of autologous MSCs in 15 patient volunteers *(42)*. These individuals had hematologic malignancies, which were in remission at the time of MSC collection and infusion, and were not given preparative chemotherapy. Only $1–50 \times 10^6$ total autologous MSCs were intravenously infused without any toxicity. In a phase I trial, a total of $1–2.2 \times 10^6$ autologous MSCs/kg were infused into 28 breast cancer patients to augment hematopoietic engraftment after peripheral blood progenitor cell (PBPC) transplantation *(43)*. There was no toxicity related to intravenous MSC infusion. The MSCs were not detected in the blood at baseline in any patient. Clonogenic MSCs were detected in venous blood up to 1 h after infusion of autologous MSCs in 13 out of 21 (62%) patients. Hematopoietic engraftment was prompt in all patients with median neutrophil recovery (>500/μL) of 8 d (range: 6–11) and platelet count recovery >20,000/μL and >50,000 unsupported of 8.5 d (range: 4–19) and 13.5 d (range: 7–44), respectively. Based on these results, a randomized multicenter trial was initiated for patients undergoing PBPC transplantation for breast cancer. Although this trial has not achieved the accrual goal, preliminary results indicate faster recovery of platelet count in patients receiving MSCs (H.M. Lazarus, personal communication).

4.2. Allogeneic MSC Transplantation

Allogeneic bone marrow transplantation has been shown to ameliorate clinical manifestations of selected lysosomal and peroxisomal diseases by providing normal hematopoietic stem cells, which can differentiate into tissue macrophages. Despite the transfer of such cells, some patients have an incomplete correction of their disorder. Our group has shown that normal MSCs express high amounts of α-L-iduronidase (deficient in Hurler disease) and arylsulfatase-A (deficient in metachromatic leukodystrophy [MLD]). In order to provide normal enzyme into tissues of 11 patients with Hurler or MLD, who were previously treated with allogeneic BMT, we infused $2–10 \times 10^6$ normal allogeneic MSCs from the same donor. Toxicity was limited to grade 1 fever in three patients. There was preliminary evidence of clinical benefit in few patients. In this trial, we have analyzed recipient T cell response against donor mesenchymal stem cells. Recipient T cells obtained before and after MSC infusion failed to become activated when mixed with donor MSCs.

These results established the feasibility and safety of allogeneic MSC transplantation and allowed us to propose cotransplantation of MSCs and HSCs during allogeneic transplantation. The objectives of this study are to determine the rate and rapidity of hematopoietic engraftment and the incidence and severity of GVHD. This multi-center clinical trial was open to patients with hematological malignancies who had an HLA identical sibling donor (45). As of January 2002, 31 patients have been given $1–5 \times 10^6$ allogeneic MSCs/kg without any toxicity. All patients engrafted. Both acute and chronic GVHD were less compared to historic controls, and survival was better ($96 \pm 4\%$ vs $68 \pm 8\%$) in patients infused with MSCs. The impact of MSCs on the incidence and severity of GVHD and the graft-vs-leukemia and/ or -tumor effect needs to be tested in a randomized trial. In addition, the effect of MSCs on HSC engraftment should be tested in patients at high risk for engraftment failure such as those receiving UCB or T lymphocyte-depleted donor cells and those undergoing a nonmyeloablative allogeneic transplant. MSCs effect on GVHD and related mortality should be investigated in patients undergoing unrelated or related but non-HLA identical donor transplantation.

UCB represents an attractive alternative source of hematopoietic stem cells for patients who require allogeneic stem cell transplantation. UCB is advantageous compared to other alternative donor sources, since the graft is rapidly available and the potential for GVHD in recipients may be reduced even in the setting of HLA disparity. In adults, however, this approach has been hampered by the small numbers of hematopoietic stem cells available in a single UCB unit. In particular, the time to neutrophil engraftment has been relatively long. Several groups now are exploring ex vivo expansion of cord blood cells in both adults and children using combination of early acting cytokines and adherent MSCs, either autologous or from a third party (e.g., parent or sibling). It will be intriguing to see the effects of such expansion systems, not only on the rate and pace of engraftment, but also on the incidence and severity of GVHD. A phase I trial has been initiated at the University of Minnesota (Minneapolis, MN) in which MSCs are isolated from the parent or sibling and expanded to be infused into the patient at the time of unrelated UCB transplantation. End points of the study are engraftment of nucleated cells and platelets, as well as GVHD incidence and severity.

5. CONCLUSION

Clinical trials with human MSC transplantation are evolving rapidly with the primary objectives of improving hematopoietic engraftment rate and pace, ameliorating or preventing

GVHD, correcting inborn metabolic errors, and delivering a variety of therapeutic genes. In the clinical setting, it remains to be seen whether transplantation of MSCs has significant value, and if preculture of hematopoietic stem cells with MSCs prior to transplantation changes their engraftment and/or immunologic properties. A number of challenging fundamental questions regarding the biology and therapeutic potential of MSCs are simultaneously investigated in preclinical studies. Our ability to culture expand mesenchymal progenitors to high numbers for clinical transplantation purposes and mesenchymal cells' ability to secrete hematopoietic cytokines and recent demonstration of their immunomodulatory effects make this new cellular therapy very promising to improve outcomes of allogeneic stem cell transplants.

REFERENCES

1. Haynesworth S, Baber M, Caplan A. Cell surface antigens on human marrow-derived mesenchymal cells are detected by monoclonal antibodies. *Bone* 1992;13:69–80.
2. Bianco P, Constantini M, Dearden L, Bonucci E. Alkaline phosphatase positive precursors of adipocytes in the human bone marrow. *Br J Haematol* 1988;68:401–411.
3. Prockop DJ. Marrow stromal cells as stem cells for nonhematopoietic tissues. *Science* 1997;276:71–74.
4. Pittinger M, Mackay A, Beck S, Jaiswal R, Douglas R, Mosca J, et.al. Multilineage potential of adult human mesenchymal stem cells. *Science* 1999;284:143–147.
5. Yoo JU, Barthel TS, Nishimura K, Solchaga L, Caplan A, Goldberg VM, et al. The chondrogenic potential of human bone marrow-derived mesenchymal progenitor cells. *J Bone Joint Surg* 1998;80:1745–1757.
6. Toksoz D, Zsebo K, Smith K, Hu S, Brankow D, Suggs S, et al. Support of human hematopoiesis in long term bone marrow cultures by murine stromal cells selectively expressing the membrane bound and secreted forms of the human homologue of the steel gene product, stem cell factor. *Proc Natl Acad Sci USA* 1992;89:7350–7354.
7. Clark B, Keating A. Biology of bone marrow stroma. Ann NY Acad Sci 1995;770:70–88.
8. Ferrari G, Cusella-DeAngelis G, Coletta M, Paolucci E, Stornaiuolo A, Cossu G, et al. Muscle regeneration by bone marrow-derived myogenic progenitors. *Science* 1998;279:1528–1530.
9. Petersen B, Bowen W, Patrene K, Mars W, Sullivan A, Murase N, et al. Bone marrow as a potential source of hepatic oval cells. *Science* 1999;284:1168–1170.
10. Lagasse E, Conners H, Al-Dhalimy M, Reitsma M, Dolhse M, Osbourne L, et al. Purified hematopoietic stem cells can differentiate into hepatocytes in vivo. *Nature Med* 2000;6:1229–1234.
11. Azizi SA, Stokes D, Augelli BJ, DiGirolamo C, Prockop DJ. Engraftment and migration of human bone marrow stromal cells implanted in the brains of albino rats—similarities to astrocyte grafts. *Proc Natl Acad Sci USA* 1998;95:3908–3913.
12. Reyes M, Verfaille C. Turning marrow into brain: generation of glial and neuronal cells from adult bone marrow mesenchymal stem cells. *Blood* 1999;94:377a.
13. Friedenstein A, Ivanov-Smolenski A, Chajlakjan R, Gorskaya U, Kuralesova A, Latzinik N, et al. Origin of bone marrow stromal mechanocytes in radiochimeras and heterotopic transplants. *Exp Hematol* 1978;6:440.
14. Majumdar M, Thiede M, Haynesworth S, Bruder S, Gerson S. Human marrow-derived mesenchymal stem cells express hematopoietic cytokines and support long-term hematopoiesis when differentiated toward stromal and osteogenic lineages. *J Hemathother Stem Cell Res* 2001;9:841–848.
15. Majumdar MK, Thiede MA, Mosca JD, Moorman M, Gerson SL. Phenotypic and functional comparison of cultures of marrow-derived mesenchymal stem cells (MSCs) and stromal cells. *J Cell Physiol* 1998;176:186–192.
16. Haynesworth SE GJ, Goldberg VM, Caplan AI. Characterization of cells with osteogenic potential from human marrow. *Bone* 1992;13:81–88.
17. Caplan A. Mesenchymal stem cells. *J Orthop Res* 1991;9(5):641–650.
18. Haynesworth S, Baber M, Caplan A. Cytokine expression by human marrow derived mesenchymal progenitor cells in vitro: effects of dexamethasone and IL-1a. *J Cell Physiol* 1996;166:585–592.
19. Klyushnenkova E, Mosca J, McIntosh K. Human mesenchymal stem cells suppress allogeneic T cell responses *in vitro*: Implications for allogeneic transplantation. *Blood* 1998;92:642a.
20. McIntosh K, Klyushnenkova E, Shustova V, Moseley A, Deans R. Suppression of alloreactive T cell response by human mesenchymal stem cells involves CD4+ cells. *Blood* 1999;94:133a.
21. Anklesaria P, Kase K, Glowacki J, Holland CA, Sakakeeny MA, Wright JA, et al. Engraftment of a clonal bone marrow stromal cell line *in vivio* stimulates hematopoietic recovery from total body irradiation. *Proc Natl Acad Sci USA* 1987;1987:7681–7685.
22. Pereira RF, Halford KW, O'Hara MD, Leeper DB, Sololov BP, Pollard MD, et al. Cultured adherent cells from marrow can serve as long-lasting precursor cells for bone, cartilage, and lung in irradiated mice. *Proc Natl Acad Sci USA* 1995;92:4857–4861.

23. Pereira RF, O'Hara MD, Laptev AV, Halford AKW, Pollard MD, Class R, et al. Marrow stromal cells as a source of progenitor cells for non-hematopoietic tissue in transgenic mice with a phenotype of osteogenesis imperfecta *Proc Natl Acad Sci USA* 1998;95:1142–1147.

24. Horwitz E, Gordon P, Koo W, Neel M, Brown P, Marx J, et al. Transplanted gene-marked marrow mesenchymal cells engraft and benefit children with severe ostogenesis imperfecta: a pilot trial for cell and gene therapy of mesenchymal disorders. *Mol Ther* 2000;1:S297.

25. Huss R, Smith FO, Myerson DH, Deeg HJ. Homing and immunogenecity of murine stromal cells transfected with xenogeneic MHC class II genes. *Cell Transplant* 1995;4:483–491.

26. Hurwitz D, Krichgesser M, Merrill W, Gellanapoulos T. Systemic delivery of human growth hormone or human factor IX in dogs by reintroduced genetically modified autologous bone marrow stromal cells. *Human Gene Ther* 1997;8:137–156.

27. Mosca J, Buyaner D, Kniley J, Chopra R, Davis-Sproul J, Majumdar M, et al. Biodistribution and bone marrow "homing" of canine mesenchymal stem cells after culture expansion and re-infusion into a canine transplantation model. *Blood* 1998;92:664a.

28. Sandmaier B, Strob R, Kniley J, Hardy W, Black M, Moseley A, et al. Evidence of allogeneic stromal engraftment in bone marrow using canine mesenchymal stem cells. *Blood* 1998;92:116a.

29. Wang G, Liu L, Lee K, Buyaner D, Hendricks K, Hoppa N, et al. Human erythropoietin gene delivery using adult mesenchymal stem cells can prevent drug-induced anemia in NOD/SCID mouse model. *Blood* 1999;94:398a.

30. Bartholomew A, Sturgeon C, Siatskas M, Ferrer K, Hardy W, Moran S, et al. Genetically modified mesenchymal stem cells can effectively deliver bioactive erthropoietin in the baboon. *Blood* 1999;94:378a.

31. Novelli E, Buyaner D, Chopra R, Cheng L, Deans B, McIntosh K, et al. Human mesenchymal stem cells can enhance human CD34+ cell repopulating of NOD/SCID mice. *Blood* 1998;92:117a.

32. Ishida T, Inaba M, Hisha H, Sugiura K, Adachi Y, Nagata N, et al. Requirement of donor-derived stromal cells in the bone marrow for successful allogeneic bone marrow transplantation. *J Immunol* 1994;152:3119–127.

33. El-Badri N, Wang B, Good R. Osteoblasts promote engraftment of allogeneic hematopoietic stem cells. *Exp Hematol* 1998;26:110–116.

34. Kaufman C, Colson Y, Wren S, Watkins S, Simmons R, Ildstad S. Phenotypic characterization of a novel bone marrow-derived cell that facilitates engraftment of allogeneic bone marrow stem cells. *Blood* 1994;84:2436–2446.

35. Bartholomew A, Sturgeon C, Nelson M, McIntosh K, Hardy W, Heckler M, et al. Allogeneic mesenchymal stem cells have significant immunosuppressive activity. *Exp Hematol* 1999;27:123a.

36. Fried W, Kedo A, Barone J. Effects of Cyclophosaphamide and of Busulfan on Spleen Colony-forming Units and on Hematopoietic Stroma. *Cancer Res* 1977;37:1205–1209.

37. McManus PM, Weiss L. Busulfan-Induced Chronic bone marrow failure: changes in cortical bone, marrow stromal cells, and adherent cell colonies. *Blood* 1984;64:1036–1041.

38. Uhlman DL, Verfaillie C, Jones RB, Luikart SD. BCNU treatment of marrow stromal monolayers reversibly alters haematopoiesis. *Br J Haematol* 1991;78:3304–3309.

39. Koç O, Peters C, Raghavan S, DeGasperi R, Kolodny E, BenYoseph Y, et al. Bone marrow derived mesenchymal stem cells of patients with lysosomal and peroxisomal storage diseases remain host type following allogeneic bone marrow transplantation. *Exp Hematol* 1999;27:1675–1681.

40. Simmons PJ, Przepiorka D, Thomas ED, Torok-Storb B. Host origin of marrow stromal cells following allogeneic bone marrow transplantation. *Nature* 1987;328:429–432.

41. Horwitz EM, Prockop DJ, Fitzpatrick LA, Koo WW, Gordon PL, Neel M, et al. Transplantability and therapeutic effects of bone marrow-derived mesenchymal cells in children with osteogenesis imperfecta. *Nat Med* 1999;5(3):309–313.

42. Lazarus H, Haynesworth S, Gerson S, Rosenthal N, Caplan A. *Ex vivo* expansion and subsequent infusion of human bone marrow-derived stromal progenitor cells (mesenchymal progenitor cells): implications for therpeutic use. *Bone Marrow Transplant* 1995;16:557–564.

43. Koç O, Gerson S, Cooper B, Dyhouse S, Haynesworth S, Caplan A, et al. Rapid hematopoietic recovery after co-infusion of autologous culture-expanded human mesenchymal stem cells (hMSCs) and PBPCs in breast cancer patients receiving high dose chemotherapy. *J Clin Oncol* 2000;18:307–316.

44. Koç O, Peters C, Gerson S, Lazarus H, Brewer F, Krivit W. Allogeneic mesenchymal stem cell transplantation in patients with genetic diseases. *Blood* 1999;94:132a.

45. Lazarus H, Curtin P, Devine S, McCarthy P, Holland K, Moseley A, et al. Role of mesenchymal stem cells in allogeneic transplantation: early phase I clinical results. *Blood* 2000;96:392a.

12 Cytokines in Allogeneic Stem Cell Mobilization

Ravi Vij, MD, Randy Brown, MD, and John F. DiPersio, MD, PhD

1. INTRODUCTION

Since the mid-1990s when the first trials of cytokine-mobilized allogeneic peripheral blood stem cell (allo-PBSC) transplants appeared in the literature, there has been a steady increase in the use of allo-PBSC in lieu of bone marrow as a source of stem cells. For normal donors, the collection of PBSC by apheresis techniques is a feasible alternative to undergoing marrow harvest with anesthesia and avoids the potential morbidity associated with marrow collection. This trend has further accelerated with the publication of a randomized trial suggesting a superior survival for patients where peripheral blood was used as a source of stem cells over the use of bone marrow *(1)*.

Currently, two cytokines that effect myeloid development are licensed for use in clinical medicine—granulocyte colony-stimulating factor (G-CSF) and granulocyte-macrophage colony-stimulating factor (GM-CSF). This chapter provides an overview of the biology of hematopoietic stem cell mobilization and the clinical application of these cytokines in the

From: *Current Clinical Oncology: Allogeneic Stem Cell Transplantation*
Edited by: Mary S. Laughlin and Hillard M. Lazarus © Humana Press Inc., Totowa, NJ

mobilization of hematopoietic stem cells from normal donors for allo-PBSC transplantation. We also discuss some of the emerging data on the immunomodulatory effects of G-CSF and GM-CSF on the constitution of the stem cell product and its possible clinical implications.

2. BIOLOGY OF STEM CELL MOBILIZATION

Hematopoietic stem cells are defined functionally by the ability to reconstitute both lymphoid and myeloid hematopoiesis when transplanted into a lethally irradiated recipient. The CD34 molecule is a unique antigen expressed on the surface of hematopoietic stem cells. Putative human hematopoietic stem cells have been purified using expression of the CD34 antigen, lack of HLA-DR expression, and lack of antigens expressed on more lineage-restricted progenitors.

The mechanisms responsible for cytokine-induced egress of stem cells from bone marrow into the circulation are not well understood. Mobilization is thought to be a multistep process and loss of adhesive interactions between hematopoietic stem cells and bone marrow stromal cells and/or its extracellular matrix are thought to be involved. Administration of G-CSF to G-CSF receptor knock-out mice (GCSF-R –/–) results in the mobilization of hematopoietic progenitors, suggesting that G-CSF acts via a different mechanism to mobilize stem cells *(2)*. Optimal mobilization by G-CSF occurs in 4–6 d.

Interaction between the β-1 integrin very late activation antigen-4 (VLA-4) and its ligand, vascular cell adhesion molecule-1 (VCAM-1), is also thought to play an important role in stem cell mobilization. In vivo studies in animal models have shown that the administration of antibodies to VLA-4 and VCAM-1 mobilizes hematopoietic stem cells *(3,4)*. Mobilization by anti-VLA-4 does not depend on a functional G-CSF receptor, interleukin-7 receptor, or interleukin-3 α receptor. By contrast, a functional c-kit receptor is required *(5)*. Recently, it has been proposed that mobilization of progenitor cells is the result of disruption of the VLA-4/VCAM-1 adhesive interaction as a consequence of VCAM-1 cleavage by neutrophil proteases released by neutrophils accumulating in the extravascular compartment of the bone marrow following cytokine administration *(6)*. Administration of anti-VLA-4 results in stem cell mobilization within 24–48 h, which is significantly shorter than with G-CSF.

Interleukin-8 (IL-8) is a CXC chemokine that produces rapid mobilization (30–60 min) of hematopoietic stem cells with radioprotective capacity and long-term myelolymphoid repopulating ability in animal models *(7,8)*. Modulation of the interaction between the β 2-integrin leukocyte function antigen-1 (LFA-1) and intercellular adhesion molecule-1 (ICAM-1) is thought to play a major role in the mobilization of hematopoietic stem cells by IL-8. LFA-1 blocking antibodies prevent the mobilization of hematopoietic progenitor cells induced by IL-8 *(9)*. Using GCSF-R –/–, it has been shown that a functional GCSF-R is required for the mobilization of murine hematopoietic progenitors into peripheral blood by cyclophosphamide and IL-8, but not flt-3 ligand *(10)*. IL-8 induced mobilization in rhesus monkeys can also be inhibited by antibodies to metalloproteinase gelatinase-B (MMP-9) *(11)*. Recent unpublished data suggest that MMP-9 knock-out mice mobilize normally, suggesting that it is not MMP-9 but related MMPs that are the key downstream regulator of IL-8 and G-CSF-induced mobilization.

Sulfated polysaccharides are capable of mobilizing progenitor cells within a few hours posttreatment in a dose dependent manner. Significant increases in the levels of MMP-9 and stromal cell-derived factor (SDF-1), in addition to several circulating cytokines and/or chemokines, are detected within a few hours of treatment with sulfated fucans *(12,13)*.

3. PROGENITOR CELL REQUIREMENTS FOR SUCCESSFUL ALLOENGRAFTMENT

Meaurement of CD34 antigen expression by flow cytometry has become the preferred technique for the enumeration of hematopoietic progenitors. There is an excellent correlation between the number of CD34+ stem cells infused per kg recipient weight and the pace of both neutrophil (> 500/mm^3) and platelet (> 20,000/mm^3) recovery after stem cell infusion. The target CD34+ cell dose for donors varies form center to center. Patients who receive more than 5×10^6 donor CD34+ cells/kg recipient body weight have a 95% likelihood of neutrophil and platelet recovery by d 15 (14). A higher CD34+ cell dose may be necessary for successful engraftment in patients undergoing matched unrelated donor transplants and haploidentical transplants. Also, additional host factors (splenomegaly, marrow fibrosis, disease type, etc.) and transplant factors (type of preparative regimen, etc.) may increase CD34+ requirements.

4. HEMATOPOIETIC PROGENITORS IN THE PERIPHERAL CIRCULATION

CD34+ hematopoietic progenitors constitute, on the average, 0.06% of the peripheral blood of normal individuals (15). This concentration is not sufficient to permit collection of meaningful numbers of CD34+ cells by apheresis. However, building on the experience in stem cell mobilization and collection for autologous transplantation, cytokine priming has proven to be an efficient method for stem cell mobilization in normal donors. Sequential culture assay systems and limiting dilution analysis of long term culture initiating cell (LTC-IC) have revealed a significantly higher clonogenicity and hematopoietic stem cell activity in mobilized apheresis products when compared to bone marrow-derived stem cells (16,17).

5. G-CSF FOR MOBILIZATION OF ALLOGENEIC PERIPHERAL BLOOD STEM CELLS

5.1. Dose

G-CSF has emerged as the cytokine of choice for stem cell mobilization from normal donors. It has been shown that a dose response relationship exists for the mobilization of CD34+ stem cells using G-CSF (18).Most centers use G-CSF at a dose of 10–16 µg/kg/d. However, doses as high as 24 µg/kg/d have been studied. Though such high doses of G-CSF increase the yield of CD34+ cells, side effects like bone pain and headaches are more severe (19). Several investigators have compared schedules of G-CSF 10–12 µg/kg/d to G-CSF 5–10 µg/kg twice daily. Lee et al. reported a higher progenitor cell yield after the administration of split doses of G-CSF, comparing 5 µg/kg administered twice daily vs 10 µg/kg once a day, with apheresis starting on d 5 (20).However, Anderlini et al. reported no benefit comparing G-CSF given 6 µg/kg twice daily vs 12 µg/kg once a day for 3 d (21).

5.2. Kinetics of CD34+ Stem Cell Mobilization

Following treatment with G-CSF 12 µg/kg/d, CD34+ progenitors reach plateau levels (15- to 35-fold increase over baseline levels) from d 4 to 6 (22–24). Most institutions initiate apheresis for stem cell collection at this time point. There is a progressive decline in the mobilization efficiency of CD34+ progenitors when G-CSF is continued for more than 6 d (23). In the setting of autologous transplantation, several institutions measure peripheral blood CD34+ counts after growth factor administration and initiate apheresis once peripheral blood CD34+ cell counts rise above 20/µL. However, normal donors have higher resting CD34+ cell counts, and the peripheral blood CD34+ cell thresholds to initiate apheresis are not well defined.

5.3. Yield of CD34+ Progenitor Cells at Apheresis

PBSCs are collected by single or multiple continuous-flow apheresis. The total blood volume processed per run is usually 2 or 3× the donor's total blood volume (10–15 L). However, large-volume stem cell apheresis processing more than 3× the blood volume (20 L) has also been reported *(25–27)*. Anderlini et al. showed that using a target collection of 4×10^6 C34+ cells/kg recipient body weight, 67% of donors treated with GCSF 12 µg/kg/d for 4 d reached the target in one 10–12 L apheresis procedure. Ninety-four percent of donors reached the target collection after 5 d of G-CSF at the same dose *(28)*. Brown et al. reported that 62% of normal donors reached a target collection of 5×10^6 CD34+ cells/kg recipient body weight following a single 18- to 20-L apheresis procedure after treatment with G-CSF 10 µg/kg/d *(14)*.

5.4. Additional Factors Affecting Collection of CD34+ Progenitor Cells

Anderlini et al. reported that the CD34+ cell yield was significantly lower in donors older than 55 yr *(29)*. They also reported a correlation between CD34+ cell yield and baseline white blood cells (WBC), preapheresis WBC, and preapheresis mononuclear cell count in the blood. Brown et al. reported that donors with low baseline levels of circulating progenitors (<2000 CD34+ cells/mL blood) and those who received lower total doses of G-CSF were less likely to be effectively mobilized *(14)*. Preapheresis peripheral blood CD34+ cell concentration also correlates well with the final CD34+ cell yield *(15)*.

6. GM-CSF FOR MOBILIZATION OF ALLO-PBSCS

Though data are limited, recombinant human GM-CSF appears to be less effective in mobilizing CD34+ progenitors in normal donors. Lane et al. reported on five normal volunteers who received GM-CSF 10 µg/kg/d for 4 d with leukapheresis on d 5. The overall yield of CD34+ mononuclear cells in the leukapheresis product from subjects treated with GM-CSF $(12.6 \pm 6.1 \times 10^6)$ was significantly lower than that from seven subjects treated with G-CSF at the same dose $(119 \pm 65 \times 10^6)$. However, mobilization with GM-CSF yielded a significantly higher percentage of early progenitors (CD34+/human leukocyte antigen [HLA]-DR+/CD38-) *(30)*. Brown et al. reported similar results in a comparison of 10 patients mobilized with the same regimen of GM-CSF. The results were compared to 55 patients mobilized with G-CSF alone at the same dose. The yield of CD34+ stem cells was approximately one-fourth that measured after mobilization with G-CSF (Table 1). Thirty-four of 55 donors (62%) of donors mobilized with G-CSF alone achieved $>5 \times 10^6$ CD 34+ cells/kg recipient weight with a single apheresis compared with 33% of donors mobilized with GM-CSF *(31)*.

7. G-CSF AND GM-CSF COMBINATION FOR MOBILIZATION OF PBSC

Lane et al. reported on five volunteer donors who were mobilized with both G-CSF and GM-CSF each at 5 µg/kg/d. The yield of CD34+ stem cells was similar to eight donors who received G-CSF at 10 µg/kg/d *(30)*. Brown et al. mobilized 25 donors with G-CSF at 10 µg/kg/d and GM-CSF at 5 µg/kg/d in an attempt to increase the probability of collecting $>5 \times 10^6$ CD34+ cells/kg with a single apheresis procedure. Compared with G-CSF alone, mobilization with both G-CSF and GM-CSF resulted in a 28% increase in total CD34+ cells in the first apheresis (Table 1). The likelihood of obtaining over 5×10^6 CD34+ cells/kg in a single collection increased from 62% for G-CSF alone to 84% with the combination of G-CSF and GM-CSF ($p < 0.05$) *(31)*.

8. POOR MOBILIZERS

A review of data from 113 normal donors at our own institution mobilized with GCSF 10 µg/kg/d for 4 d, revealed that four donors (3.5%) failed to mobilize $>1 \times 10^6$ CD34+ cells on the first day of apheresis. Options for optimizing stem cell yield includes the administration of a higher dose of G-CSF, split doses of G-CSF, combination therapy with G-CSF and GM-

Table 1
Effect of Cytokines on Cellular Constitution of ALLO-PBSC Product

PBSC products	G-CSF (N = 55) (mean ± S.D.)	G + GM-CSF (N = 25) (mean ± S.D.)	GM-CSF (N = 10) (mean ± S.D.)
CD34+/kg × 10^6	8.9 ± 7.2	11.0 ± 6.3[a]	2.6 ± 2.1[b]
CD3+/kg × 10^6	3.7 ± 2.5	1.7 ± 1.1[b]	1.2 ± 0.6[b]
CD4+/kg × 10^6	2.8 ± 1.7	1.3 ± 0.8[b]	0.9 ± 0.5[b]
CD8+/kg × 10^6	1.4 ± 1.3	0.3 ± 0.3[b]	0.2 ± 0.2[b]
Dendritic cells (DC) /kg × 10^6	6.6 ± 2.8	15.4 ± 11.8[a]	13.4 ± 18.0
Activated CD80+DC/kg × 10^6	0.16 ± 0.05	5.6 ± 8.3	5.5 ± 6.3

[a]p <0.05 compared with G-CSF alone.
[b]p <0.01 compared with G-CSF alone.

CSF (as discussed above), or, alternatively, proceeding to bone marrow harvest. Despite these measures, in a very small number of normal donors, adequate stem cell numbers may not be achieved. It would be interesting to follow these donors long-term, to see if they develop marrow failure states in the future.

9. IMMUNOMODULATORY EFFECT OF CYTOKINES ON THE COMPOSITION OF THE STEM CELL PRODUCT

Despite an at least a 10-fold greater T cell dose, G-CSF-mobilized PBSC grafts do not cause a higher incidence of acute graft-vs-host disease (GVHD) (1). However, PBSC grafts may be associated with a higher incidence of chronic GVHD (14,32). In an attempt to elucidate the mechanisms responsible for these differences, investigators have looked at the effect of these cytokines on T-cell subsets and dendritic cells (DC). Dendritic cells are the only antigen-presenting cells that can prime naïve T cells to a new antigen. In nature, Th1 cells promote the generation of cytotoxic T-cells and mononuclear cells, which protect against viruses and other intracellular microbes. In contrast, Th2 cells are involved in allergic responses dominated by B-cell production of IgE and the recruitment of eosinophils and basophils. Functional heterogeneity likely accounts for a distinct role of Th1 and Th2 cells in transplantation.

A number of preclinical murine and clinical studies have suggested that G-CSF "polarizes" T cells from the Th1 to the Th2 phenotype (33–35). Arpinate et al. postulate that transplantation of G-CSF-stimulated PBSC did not result in overwhelming acute GVHD because the graft contains predominantly Th2-inducing DC (36). The authors showed that G-CSF treatment increased peripheral blood lymphoid DC (DC2, defined as HLA-DR+/lin-/CD11c-/CD4+/IL-3R α+) counts from a median of $4.9 × 10^6$/L to $24.8 × 10^6$/L whereas myeloid DC (DC1, defined as HLA-DR+/lin-/CD11c+) counts did not change. Activated DC1 induced allogeneic naïve T cells to produce the Th1 cytokine inteferon (IFN)-γ, whereas activated DC2 induced Th2 responses with increase in IL-4 and IL-10. Purified DC1 induced the proliferation of allogeneic naïve T cells, but fresh DC2 were poor stimulators. Also, PBSC transplants were found to contain higher doses of DC2 than marrow transplants (median $2.4 × 10^6$/kg vs $0.5 × 10^6$/kg, $p = 0.006$).

A number of reports have suggested decreased immune function of peripheral blood cells in normal allogeneic allo-PBSC donors mobilized by G-CSF. Miller et al. reported functionally abnormal natural killer (NK) cell function after G-CSF mobilization. It was conjectured that granulocytes may be the source of this NK cell suppressive activity (37). Ageitos et al. have shown that monocytes, which are present in high numbers in PBSC products, may be the source of immune dysfunction (38). Joshi et al. assessed the immunologic function of G-CSF-mobilized PBSC from 104 healthy donors and compared this to 28 steady-state nonmobilized donors. These investigators also saw a significant decrease in NK and lymphokine activated killer (LAK) cell mediated toxicity for G-CSF mobilized effector cells. In addition, they saw a decreased T and B cell mitogenic response when compared with nonmobilized cells. Of interest, these effects were only seen in donors with selected HLA antigens *(39).*

Brown et al., as previously noted, showed that products collected following mobilization with both G-CSF and GM-CSF or GM-CSF alone contained fewer CD3+, CD4+, and CD8+ cells than those collected following mobilization with G-CSF. Mobilization with G-CSF and GM-CSF or GM-CSF alone resulted in an increase in total DC (defined as CD4+, HLA-DR+, lin–ve) and activated (CD 80+) DC (Table 1) *(31).* In a subsequent report comparing results of 77 donors mobilized with G + GM – CSF and 97 donors mobilized with G-CSF alone, the authors reported that there were no significant differences in the rates of Grade II–IV acute GVHD, chronic GVHD, and progression-free survival (PFS) between the two cohorts *(40).*

10. DONOR ELIGIBILITY

There are no known absolute contraindications for the administration of G-CSF to normal donors. There is some evidence that donors with a prior history of inflammatory autoimmune disorders could be at risk for exacerbation or clinical deterioration during or after G-CSF mobilization *(41,42).* Several patients with chronic progressive multiple sclerosis mobilized with G-CSF in preparation for an autologous stem cell transplant developed rapid and significant neurologic deterioration during G-CSF mobilization (R. Nash, personal communication, Fred Hutchinson Cancer Research Institute). Finally, it has been observed that some patients with sickle cell anemia have developed neurologic problems after G-CSF treatment. Donors with specific risk factors (cardiovascular or cerebrovascular disease, pregnancy, thrombocytopenia, splenomegaly, inflammatory or autoimmune disorders) should be deferred or considered only if no other option is available.

11. CLINICAL AND LABORATORY EFFECTS OF CYTOKINE TREATMENT FOR STEM CELL MOBILIZATION IN NORMAL DONORS

The most common adverse events related to administration of G-CSF to normal individuals are bone pain, headache, fatigue, and nausea (Table 2) *(43),* These can usually be controlled with low-potency analgesics and resolve within a few days of discontinuation of the medication. Laboratory abnormalities include transient increases of alkaline phosphatase, lactate dehydrogenase, and less commonly, hypokalemia and hypomagnesemia (due to an intracellular shift of these cations with an increase in circulating mature WBC and progenitor cells) *(44).* After 3 d of G-CSF treatment WBC, neutrophil, and lymphocyte counts increase by 6.4-, 8.0-, and 2.2-fold over baseline values *(15).* WBC may reach $70–80 \times 10^9/L$ by d 5 after G-CSF. Although leukostasis has not been reported, most centers reduce the dose if these levels are attained earlier or if the WBC counts exceed $75 \times 10^9/L$. Transient decreases in donor platelet counts have been observed after G-CSF mobilization, with increasing thrombocytopenia observed after sequential large volume stem cell apheresis *(25,45).* An asymptomatic drop in peripheral blood lymphocyte and granulocyte counts have been reported following completion of stem cell collection after mobilization with G-CSF *(46–48).* Several authors have reported that G-CSF administration induces a transient mild hypercoaguable state. The exact mechanisms responsible for this phenomenon are unclear. However, an increase in fibrinogen and factor VIII levels with a reduction in protein C and S have been observed *(49).* Other authors have reported an increase in the levels of vonWillebrand factor antigen/activity, prothrombin fragment 1, thrombin-antithrombin complex, and in D-dimer levels *(50,51).* There are anec-

Table 2
Common Clinical
and Laboratory Effects
of Cytokines

Bone pain
Headache
Fatigue
Nausea
Leukocytosis
Thrombocytopenia
Increased alkaline phosphatase
Increased lactate dehydrogenase
Hypokalemia
Hypomagnesemia

dotal reports of serious adverse events like anaphylactic reaction, splenic rupture, and unstable angina associated with G-CSF mobilization of normal donors *(52–54)*.

12. LONG-TERM EFFECTS ON DONOR HEALTH

There have been very little data presented relating to this very important area. By 1998, nearly 80% of the allogeneic transplants from HLA identical siblings were performed using cytokine-mobilized PBSC. These trends have continued over the ensuing 3 yr. In contrast, nearly all unrelated allogeneic transplants, up until and including 1998 were performed using bone marrow. More recent data from the National Marrow Donor Program (NMDP) in 2000 and 2001 suggest that nearly 20% of the unrelated stem cell requests to the NMDP are now for cytokine-mobilized PBSC and not bone marrow. The delays in collection centers agreeing to provide allo-PBSC and the delays in transplant centers requesting unrelated allo-PBSC, are probably due to concerns relating to increased GVHD and long-term safety of G-CSF mobilization in volunteer unrelated donors.

Although there is no evidence yet that brief exposure of normal donors to G-CSF results in any long-term risks, young children with congenital neutropenia (Kostmann's Syndrome) who have been exposed to G-CSF for many years have a higher than expected risk of developing acute myeloid leukemia (AML) *(55)*. Many of these cases express a mutated GCSF-R receptors, which may contribute to the development of AML. Also, a study from Japan has reported that 4% of children with aplastic anemia treated with cyclosporine and G-CSF developed AML. However, AML was not observed in 41 children treated with G-CSF alone *(56)*. In addition, several authors have reported normal blood counts in allogeneic PBSC donors many years after mobilization with G-CSF *(57,58)*.

13. SUMMARY

Cytokine-mobilized peripheral blood is being used increasingly as a source of stem cells in lieu of bone marrow for both related and unrelated donor allogeneic transplantation. However, knowledge in the basic science of stem cell mobilization has lagged behind the clinical application of mobilized PBSCs. A vast majority of normal allo-PBSC donors have been mobilized using G-CSF. The use of G-CSF for stem cell mobilization is well tolerated and there is as yet no evidence of any long-term adverse affects. The immunomodulatory effects of G-CSF and GM-CSF on the composition of the stem cell product, on GVHD, and on the outcomes of allogeneic transplantation are the subject of intense investigation.

The future holds the prospect for utilization of novel cytokines for stem cell mobilization. Pegylated G-CSF is a long-acting formulation of G-CSF and is currently being evaluated in clinical trials. In the future, this formulation may be used in stem cell mobilization protocols for normal donors. In addition, Flt-3 ligand combined with G-CSF and GM-CSF is currently being evaluated for the mobilization of stem cells for autologous stem cell transplantation. In the allogeneic transplantation arena, in addition to the potential for increasing the yield of stem cells, Flt-3 ligand has potential to modulate GVHD and graft-vs-tumor responses as it stimulates the production of dendritic cells.

REFERENCES

1. Bensinger WI, Martin PJ, Storer B, et al. Transplantation of bone marrow as compared with peripheral-blood cells from HLA-identical relatives in patients with hematologic cancers. *N Engl J Med* 2001;344:175.
2. Liu F, Poursine-Laurent J, Link DC. Expression of the G-CSF receptor on hematopoietic progenitor cells is not required for their mobilization by G-CSF. *Blood* 2000;95:3025–3031.
3. Papayannopoulou T, Nakamoto B. Peripheralization of hemopoietic progenitors in primates treated with anti-VLA4 integrin. *Proc Natl Acad Sci USA* 1993;90:9374–9378.
4. Papayannopoulou T, Craddock C, Nakamoto B, Priestley GV, Wolf NS. The VLA4/VCAM-1 adhesion pathway defines contrasting mechanisms of lodgement of transplanted murine hemopoietic progenitors between bone marrow and spleen. *Proc Natl Acad Sci USA* 1995;92:9647–9651.
5. Papayannopoulou T, Priestley GV, Nakamoto B. Anti-VLA4/VCAM-1-induced mobilization requires cooperative signaling through the kit/mkit ligand pathway. *Blood* 1998;91:2231–2239.
6. Levesque JP, Takamatsu Y, Nilsson SK, Haylock DN, Simmons PJ. Vascular cell adhesion molecule-1 (CD106) is cleaved by neutrophil proteases in the bone marrow following hematopoietic progenitor cell mobilization by granulocyte colony-stimulating factor. *Blood* 2001;98:1289–1297.
7. Laterveer L, Lindley IJ, Hamilton MS, Willemze R, Fibbe WE. Interleukin-8 induces rapid mobilization of hematopoietic stem cells with radioprotective capacity and long-term myelolymphoid repopulating ability. *Blood* 1995;85:2269–2275.
8. Laterveer L, Lindley IJ, Heemskerk DP, Camps JA, Pauwels EK, Willemze R, Fibbe WE. Rapid mobilization of hematopoietic progenitor cells in rhesus monkeys by a single intravenous injection of interleukin-8. *Blood* 1996;87:781–788.
9. Pruijt JF, van Kooyk Y, Figdor CG, Lindley IJ, Willemze R, Fibbe WE. Anti-LFA-1 blocking antibodies prevent mobilization of hematopoietic progenitor cells induced by interleukin-8. *Blood* 1998;91:4099–4105.
10. Liu F, Poursine-Laurent J, Link DC. The granulocyte colony-stimulating factor receptor is required for the mobilization of murine hematopoietic progenitors into peripheral blood by cyclophosphamide or interleukin-8 but not flt-3 ligand. *Blood* 1997;90:2522–2528.
11. Pruijt JF, Fibbe WE, Laterveer L, et al. Prevention of interleukin-8-induced mobilization of hematopoietic progenitor cells in rhesus monkeys by inhibitory antibodies against the metalloproteinase gelatinase B (MMP-9). *Proc Natl Acad Sci USA* 1999;96:10,863–10,868.
12. Sweeney EA, Priestley GV, Nakamoto B, Collins RG, Beaudet AL, Papayannopoulou T. Mobilization of stem/progenitor cells by sulfated polysaccharides does not require selectin presence. *Proc Natl Acad Sci USA* 2000;97:6544–6549.
13. Sweeney EA, Papayannopoulou T. Increase in circulating SDF-1 after treatment with sulfated glycans. The role of SDF-1 in mobilization. *Ann N Y Acad Sci* 2001;938:48–52.
14. Brown RA, Adkins D, Goodnough LT, et al. Factors that influence the collection and engraftment of allogeneic peripheral-blood stem cells in patients with hematologic malignancies. *J Clin Oncol* 1997;15:3067–3074.
15. Korbling M, Huh YO, Durett A, et al. Allogeneic blood stem cell transplantation: peripheralization and yield of donor-derived primitive hematopoietic progenitor cells (CD34+ Thy- 1dim) and lymphoid subsets, and possible predictors of engraftment and graft-versus-host disease. *Blood* 1995;86:2842–2848.
16. Moore MA. Expansion of myeloid stem cells in culture. *Semin Hematol* 1995;32:183.
17. Pettengell R, Luft T, Henschler R, et al. Direct comparison by limiting dilution analysis of long-term culture-initiating cells in human bone marrow, umbilical cord blood, and blood stem cells. *Blood* 1994;84:3653–3659.
18. Hoglund M, Smedmyr B, Simonsson B, Totterman T, Bengtsson M. Dose-dependent mobilisation of haematopoietic progenitor cells in healthy volunteers receiving glycosylated rHuG-CSF. *Bone Marrow Transplant* 1996;18:19–27.
19. Waller CF, Bertz H, Wenger MK, et al. Mobilization of peripheral blood progenitor cells for allogeneic transplantation: efficacy and toxicity of a high-dose rhG-CSF regimen. *Bone Marrow Transplant* 1996;18:279–283.

20. Lee V, Li CK, Shing MM, et al. Single vs twice daily G-CSF dose for peripheral blood stem cells harvest in normal donors and children with non-malignant diseases. Bone Marrow Transplant 2000;25:931–935.
21. Anderlini P, Donato M, Lauppe MJ, et al. A comparative study of once-daily versus twice-daily filgrastim administration for the mobilization and collection of CD34+ peripheral blood progenitor cells in normal donors. Br J Haematol 2000;109:770–772.
22. Tjonnfjord GE, Steen R, Evensen SA, Thorsby E, Egeland T. Characterization of CD34+ peripheral blood cells from healthy adults mobilized by recombinant human granulocyte colony-stimulating factor. *Blood* 1994;84:2795–2801.
23. Grigg AP, Roberts AW, Raunow H, et al. Optimizing dose and scheduling of filgrastim (granulocyte colony-stimulating factor) for mobilization and collection of peripheral blood progenitor cells in normal volunteers. *Blood* 1995;86:4437–4445.
24. Dreger P, Haferlach T, Eckstein V, et al. G-CSF-mobilized peripheral blood progenitor cells for allogeneic transplantation: safety, kinetics of mobilization, and composition of the graft. *Br J Haematol* 1994;87:609–613.
25. Malachowski ME, Comenzo RL, Hillyer CD, Tiegerman KO, Berkman EM. Large-volume leukapheresis for peripheral blood stem cell collection in patients with hematologic malignancies. *Transfusion* 1992;32:732–735.
26. Comenzo RL, Malachowski ME, Miller KB, et al. Engraftment with peripheral blood stem cells collected by large-volume leukapheresis for patients with lymphoma. *Transfusion* 1992;32:729–731.
27. Passos-Coelho JL, Braine HG, Wright SK, et al. Large-volume leukapheresis using regional citrate anticoagulation to collect peripheral blood progenitor cells. *J Hematother* 1995;4:11–19.
28. Anderlini P, Przepiorka D, Huh Y, et al. Duration of filgrastim mobilization and apheresis yield of CD34+ progenitor cells and lymphoid subsets in normal donors for allogeneic transplantation. *Br J Haematol* 1996;93:940–942.
29. Anderlini P, Przepiorka D, Seong C, et al. Factors affecting mobilization of CD34+ cells in normal donors treated with filgrastim. *Transfusion* 1997;37:507–512.
30. Lane TA, Law P, Maruyama M, et al. Harvesting and enrichment of hematopoietic progenitor cells mobilized into the peripheral blood of normal donors by granulocyte-macrophage colony-stimulating factor (GM-CSF) or G-CSF: potential role in allogeneic marrow transplantation. *Blood* 1995;85:275–282.
31. Vij R, Brown RA, Adkins D, et al. Mobilization of normal donors with G-CSF + GM-CSF is associated with improved yield of hematopoietic progenitors and increased numbers of activated dendritic cells (abstr). *Blood* 1998;92:682a.
32. Storek J, Gooley T, Siadak M, et al. Allogeneic peripheral blood stem cell transplantation may be associated with a high risk of chronic graft-versus-host disease. *Blood* 90:4705–4709.
33. Pan L, Delmonte J, Jr., Jalonen CK, Ferrara JL. Pretreatment of donor mice with granulocyte colony-stimulating factor polarizes donor T lymphocytes toward type-2 cytokine production and reduces severity of experimental graft-versus-host disease. *Blood* 1995;86:4422–4429.
34. Fowler DH, Kurasawa K, Smith R, et al. Donor CD4-enriched cells of Th2 cytokine phenotype regulate graft-versus-host disease without impairing allogeneic engraftment in sublethally irradiated mice. *Blood* 1994;84:3540–3549.
35. Shenoy S, Mohanakumar T, Todd G, et al. Immune reconstitution following allogeneic peripheral blood stem cell transplants. *Bone Marrow Transplant* 1999;23:335–346.
36. Arpinati M, Green CL, Heimfeld S, et al. Granulocyte-colony stimulating factor mobilizes T helper 2-inducing dendritic cells. *Blood* 2000;95:2484–2490.
37. Miller JS, Prosper F, McCullar V. Natural killer (NK) cells are functionally abnormal and NK cell progenitors are diminished in granulocyte colony-stimulating factor-mobilized peripheral blood progenitor cell collections. *Blood* 1997;90:3098–3105.
38. Ageitos AG, Varney ML, Bierman PJ, et al. Comparison of monocyte-dependent T cell inhibitory activity in GM-CSF vs G-CSF mobilized PSC products. *Bone Marrow Transplant* 1999;23:63–69.
39. Joshi SS, Lynch JC, Pavletic SZ, et al. Decreased immune functions of blood cells following mobilization with granulocyte colony-stimulating factor: association with donor characteristics. *Blood* 2001;98:1963–1970.
40. Brown RA AD, Haug J, Pence H, et al. Mobilization of allogeneic peripheral blood stem cell donors with both G and GM-CSF increases progenitor yield without impacting graft-vs-host disease (GVHD), relapse risk or progression free survival (PFS)(abstr). *Blood* 2000;96:181a.
41. Anderlini P, Przepiorka D, Korbling M, et al. Blood stem cell procurement: donor safety issues. *Bone Marrow Transplant* 1998;21(Suppl 3):S35–S39.
42. Parkkali T, Volin L, Siren MK, et al. Acute iritis induced by granulocyte colony-stimulating factor used for mobilization in a volunteer unrelated peripheral blood progenitor cell donor. *Bone Marrow Transplant* 1996;17:433,434.
43. Anderlini P, Przepiorka D, Champlin R, et al. Biologic and clinical effects of granulocyte colony-stimulating factor in normal individuals. *Blood* 1996;88:2819–2825.

44. Anderlini P, Przepiorka D, Seong D, et al. Clinical toxicity and laboratory effects of granulocyte-colony-stimulating factor (filgrastim) mobilization and blood stem cell apheresis from normal donors, and analysis of charges for the procedures. *Transfusion* 1996;36:590–595.

45. Hillyer CD, Tiegerman KO, Berkman EM. Increase in circulating colony-forming units-granulocyte-macrophage during large-volume leukapheresis: evaluation of a new cell separator. *Transfusion* 1991;31:327–332.

46. Anderlini P, Przepiorka D, Seong D, et al. Transient neutropenia in normal donors after G-CSF mobilization and stem cell apheresis. *Br J Haematol* 1996;94:155–158.

47. Korbling M, Anderlini P, Durett A, et al. Delayed effects of rhG-CSF mobilization treatment and apheresis on circulating CD34+ and CD34+ Thy-1dim CD38-progenitor cells, and lymphoid subsets in normal stem cell donors for allogeneic transplantation. *Bone Marrow Transplant* 1996;18:1073–1079.

48. Martinez C, Urbano-Ispizua A, Rozman C, et al. Effects of G-CSF administration and peripheral blood progenitor cell collection in 20 healthy donors. *Ann Hematol* 1996;72:269–272.

49. Sohngen D, Wienen S, Siebler M, et al. Analysis of rhG-CSF-effects on platelets by in vitro bleeding test and transcranial Doppler ultrasound examination. *Bone Marrow Transplant* 1998;22:1087–1090.

50. LeBlanc R, Roy J, Demers C, et al. A prospective study of G-CSF effects on hemostasis in allogeneic blood stem cell donors. *Bone Marrow Transplant* 1999;23:991–996.

51. Falanga A, Marchetti M, Evangelista V, et al. Neutrophil activation and hemostatic changes in healthy donors receiving granulocyte colony-stimulating factor. *Blood* 1999;93:2506–2514.

52. Becker PS, Wagle M, Matous S, et al. Spontaneous splenic rupture following administration of granulocyte colony-stimulating factor (G-CSF): occurrence in an allogeneic donor of peripheral blood stem cells. *Biol Blood Marrow Transplant* 1997;3:45–49.

53. Falzetti F, Aversa F, Minelli O, et al. Spontaneous rupture of spleen during peripheral blood stem-cell mobilisation in a healthy donor. *Lancet* 1999;353:555.

54. Vij R, Adkins DR, Brown RA, et al. Unstable angina in a peripheral blood stem and progenitor cell donor given granulocyte-colony-stimulating factor. *Transfusion* 1999;39:542,543.

55. Freedman MH, Bonilla MA, Fier C, et al. Myelodysplasia syndrome and acute myeloid leukemia in patients with congenital neutropenia receiving G-CSF therapy. *Blood* 2000;96:429–436.

56. Ohara A, Kojima S, Hamajima N, et al. Myelodysplastic syndrome and acute myelogenous leukemia as a late clonal complication in children with acquired aplastic anemia. *Blood* 1997;90:1009–1013.

57. Cavallaro AM, Lilleby K, Majolino I, et al. Three to six year follow-up of normal donors who received recombinant human granulocyte colony-stimulating factor. *Bone Marrow Transplant* 2000;25:85–89.

58. Stroncek DF, Clay ME, Herr G, et al. Blood counts in healthy donors 1 year after the collection of granulocyte-colony-stimulating factor-mobilized progenitor cells and the results of a second mobilization and collection. *Transfusion* 1997;37:304–308.

13 Nonmyeloablative Allogeneic Transplantation

David A. Rizzieri, MD and Nelson J. Chao, MD

CONTENTS

1. INTRODUCTION

High doses of chemotherapy and radiation, combined with a new immune system generated by an allogeneic hematopoietic stem cell transplant, have significant potential benefits for the treatment of multiple types of illnesses, as outlined throughout this text. Unfortunately, the majority of patients are not candidates for this approach. This chapter will discuss a shift in the understanding of the requirements for successful allogeneic hematopoietic transplantation, allowing for less toxic preparative regimens while maintaining reliable donor engraftment. Successful exploitation of this approach will allow older, more debilitated patients to undergo allogeneic immunotherapy in the future. Further, if the risks are truly decreased, the cost–benefit ratio may be sufficiently shifted to allow new diseases to be targeted for therapy, such as patients with hemoglobinopathies, selected genetic deficits, or autoimmune illnesses.

2. RATIONALE FOR THE BENEFIT OF ALLOGENEIC IMMUNOTHERAPY: GRAFT-VS-TUMOR EFFECTS

Standard allogeneic therapy relies on both the benefits of high doses of radiation and/or chemotherapy, as well as the benefits provided by the new immune system. For the potentially

From: *Current Clinical Oncology: Allogeneic Stem Cell Transplantation*
Edited by: Mary S. Laughlin and Hillard M. Lazarus © Humana Press Inc., Totowa, NJ

less toxic, better tolerated, nonmyeloablative approach to have an important impact in the care of patients, further exploitation of the immunotherapeutic benefit of allogeneic transplantation is required. Evidence for the importance of the activity of the new immune system improving outcomes for patients undergoing standard transplantation continues to grow and includes: (i) a temporal relationship between graft-vs-host disease (GVHD) and hematologic remission; (ii) reduced incidence of leukemic relapse after allogeneic bone marrow transplantation (allo-BMT) compared to syngeneic BMT; and (iii) a reduced incidence in leukemic relapse in allogeneic transplant recipients who do develop GVHD compared to those who do not (1–7).

Multiple laboratory studies have been published in support of these clinical data as well. Cytotoxic T cells are known to play an important part in the antitumor effects, though the specific antigenic targets of the immune effector cells are largely uncharacterized. Tumor specific antigens and histocompatibility antigens may play a role and the interactions may be through direct cell contact, activating natural killer (NK) cells, or indirect production of cytotoxic cytokines (interferon [IFN], tumor necrosis factor [TNF]-α, interleukin (IL)-2, IL-12). Tumor-associated antigens recognized by cytotoxic T cells have been found on solid tumor cells (Her-2/neu, mucin [MUC]-1, mutated p53, carcinoembryonic antigen [CEA]) (8) and tumor infiltrating lymphocytes which secrete cytokines toxic to cancer cells have also been identified (9).

Rocha et al. (10) compared graft-vs-leukemia (GVL) and GVH reactions after systemic transfer of allogeneic antitumor immune T lymphocytes from B10.D2 (H-2d; Mls[b]) into DBA/2 (H-2d; Mls[a]) mice. Before immune cell transfer, recipient DBA/2 mice were sublethally irradiated with 5 Gy to prevent host-vs-graft reactivity. Recipients were either bearing syngeneic metastatic ESb lymphomas (GVL system) or were normal nontumor-bearing mice (GVH system). This adoptive immunotherapy (ADI) protocol is known to have pronounced GVL activity from this group's prior work and has led to immune rejection of even advanced metastasized cancer. In this study, monoclonal antibodies were used for immunohistochemical analysis of native frozen tissue sections from either spleen or liver to distinguish donor from host cells, to differentiate between CD4 and CD8 T lymphocytes, and to stain sialoadhesin-positive macrophages at different time points after cell transfer. The kinetics of donor cell infiltration in spleen and liver differed in that the lymphoid organ was infiltrated earlier (d 1–5 after transfer) than the nonlymphoid organ (d 5–20). After reaching a peak, donor cell infiltration decreased gradually and was not detectable in the spleen after d 20 and in the liver after d 30. The organ-infiltrating donor immune cells were mostly T lymphocytes and stained positive for CD4 or CD8 T-cell markers. A remarkable GVL-associated observation was made with regard to a subset of macrophages bearing the adhesion molecule sialoadhesin (SER+ macrophages). In the livers of tumor-bearing mice, their numbers increased between d 1 and 12 after ADI by a factor greater than 30. Double staining for donor cell marker and SER showed that the sialoadhesin-expressing macrophages were of host origin. The SER+ host macrophages from GVL livers were isolated by enzyme perfusion and rosetting 12 d after ADI, when they reached peak values of about 60 cells per liver lobule, and were tested, without further antigen addition, for their capacity to stimulate an antitumor CD8 T-cell response. The results of this immunologic analysis suggest that these cells in the liver function as scavengers of the destroyed metastases and as antigen-processing and antigen-presenting cells for antitumor immune T cells (10).

Recently, important evidence was published to further prove that such an immune mediated antitumor effect has clinical implications for patients with solid tumors, supporting the extension of allogeneic therapy beyond the bounds of hematologic malignancies. A 32-yr-old woman with inflammatory breast cancer received a BMT from her HLA-identical sibling. During GVHD cytotoxic T lymphocytes were grown and tested in a chromium-release assay against

B and T lymphocytes of the patient and donor and against a panel of breast cancer cell lines. Resolution of liver metastases was observed simultaneously with clinical GVHD in the first weeks after transplant. In addition, MiHA-specific and MHC class I antigen-restricted cytotoxic T lymphocytes recognizing breast carcinoma target cells were isolated from the patient simultaneously with clinical GVHD in the first weeks after transplant. In addition, minor histocompatibility antigen (MiHA)-specific and major histocompatibility complex (MHC) class I antigen-restricted cytotoxic T lymphocytes recognizing breast carcinoma target cells were isolated from the blood of the patient. Pretreatment of such target cells with TNF-α, but not with IFN-α or IFN-γ increased susceptibility of these cells to lysis by cytotoxic T lymphocytes. Clinical course and in vitro results suggest that a graft-vs-tumor (GVT) effect existed after allogeneic BMT for breast cancer (11).

These data support the contention that allogeneic transplantation is an effective form of immunotherapy, not just a method to support patients in recovery from aggressive doses of therapy. Optimizing methods for this approach will allow a broadened application of the approach for more patients, with more varied diseases.

3. RATIONALE FOR ALLOGENEIC IMMUNOTHERAPY THERAPY USING NONMYELOABLATIVE INDUCTION REGIMENS

The aggressive induction regimens utilized in standard allogeneic therapy may result in pulmonary or alveolar hemorrhage, venoocclusive disease, or other organ toxicity. In addition, the prolonged time to engraftment and continued use of immunosuppressive agents causes increased and prolonged risks for bacterial, viral, and fungal infections. With advanced age and additional co-morbid conditions in the adult population (i.e., obesity, hypertension, tobacco abuse), patients also have lessened abilities to persevere through pneumonitis, deconditioning, malnutrition, GVHD, or other common complications. Even with the stringent evaluation process patients undergo prior to being offered allogeneic transplantation, nearly 25% die soon after the procedure (12,13).

One approach to decreasing allogeneic treatment-related mortality and morbidity is to use a nonmyeloablative conditioning regimen with lower doses of chemotherapy and/or radiation which is lymphotoxic, but does not induce as much damage to the visceral organs of the body. Through combining agents that target therapy more selectively to the immune system of the patient, with relative sparing of visceral organs of the body, one induces a significant immunosuppressed state. This allows for the patient to accept a donor graft. The more lymphocyte-selective conditioning allows lessened risks of acute therapy-induced damage, shortened time to improved nutritional status and exercise tolerance, and possibly less activation of the mechanisms leading to GVHD.

The terminology in the literature describing this approach is varied. "Mini-Transplant" and "Transplant–Lite," refer to the lessened intensity and improved tolerability of the early post transplant phase of therapy. However, significant infectious and GVHD risks persist, maintaining the high risk nature of the procedure in terms of mortality and morbidity, therefore these terms are misnomers. "Mixed chimeric" transplant denotes the fact that one anticipates both the donor and recipient's hematopoietic systems to be functioning upon recovery. Whether they can continue to co-exist is the subject of continued research. "Nonmyeloablative therapy" seems to be the most accurate term for this process, as it denotes therapy that is specifically not myeloablative, though it is lymphotoxic and does not promise lessened toxicities to the recipient.

Figure 1 depicts the nonmyeloablative approach with both donor and recipient hematopoietic systems likely coexisting following initial recovery. For hemoglobinopathies or autoimmune illnesses, this new blood cell source may be sufficient to mask the phenotype of the

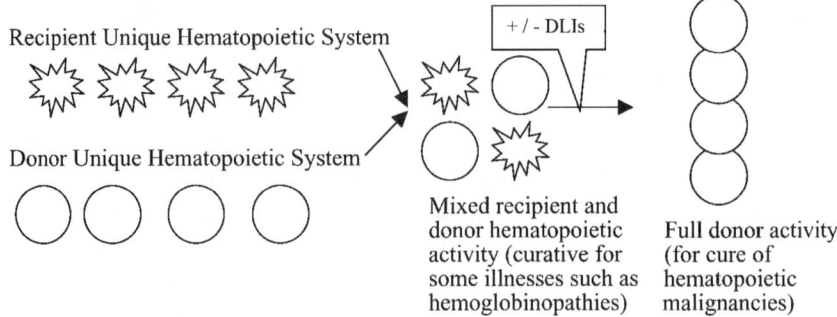

Fig. 1. Schematic of the host donor hematopoietic stem cell and immune competition between the host and donor that occurs during allogeneic therapy. With nonmyeloablative therapy, early hematopoietic recovery typically reveals evidence of both recipient and donor myeloid and lymphoid recovery. Usually, though not always, one system eventually accounts for virtually all of the measurable activity. Tipping the balance in favor of this being the donor system, or improving antitumor efficacy, may rely on the use of DLI as well.

Table 1
Comparison of the Effects of Ablative vs Nonmyeloablative Preparative Regimens

Ablative	*Nonmyeloablative*
No autologous recovery of normal hematopoiesis for 90–120 d.	Autologous recovery may return in 14–21 d.
Severe damage to the skin, liver, and gut with cytokine storms released.	Minimal damage to the skin, liver, and gut may lead to decreased cytokine storm.
Poor nutrition and exercise tolerance is common.	Hastened recovery of nutrition and exercise tolerance.
Increased risk of acute and chronic GVHD.	Possible decreased risk of acute and chronic GVHD.
Increased infectious risks for many months.	Possible decreased risks of severe infections.
Delayed immune recovery.	Immune recovery?

disease. For other illnesses, such as leukemias, progression to full donor hematopoietic function typically occurs in the ensuing months and ensures the donor immune system will be present for surveillance and lysis of the neoplastic recipient clone. This progression may occur naturally over time from initial transplant or with further assistance from infusions of donor lymphocytes to improve donor hematopoietic and immune recovery.

Differing effects of the standard, more intense ablative approaches compared to nonablative approaches are noted in Table 1. Rather than a prolonged cytopenic phase, most patients recover within 10 d with most nonmyeloablative regimens; many never require platelet transfusions during recovery. The immediate risks of damage to the integument, lungs, and liver are significantly decreased, leading to hastened recovery of adequate nutritional intake and exercise tolerance. Further, the decreased damage to the host may relate to lowered infectious and GVHD risks *(14)*.

There are many different specific regimens reported to fall into this nonablative category, though not all are equivalent. Regimens decreasing the intensity of the preparative therapy to about half are more intermediate dose intense regimens, rather than the even less intense and better tolerated regimens referred to as nonmyeloablative for the purposes of this chapter. The intermediate dose regimens typically use half the dose of busulfan, for instance, or substitute an intermediate melphalan dose for other alkylator therapy. The intermediate dosing may well serve an important role in improving the outcomes for patients undergoing allogeneic therapy. Proper utilization of these regimens vs other less toxic nonmyeloablative regimens must await future comparison trials. Immune reconstitution and the rate of recovery after these therapies remains an active area of investigation as manipulation of immune recovery will play a major role in optimizing the success of this approach.

4. LABORATORY EVIDENCE FOR SUCCESSFUL ALLOGENEIC IMMUNOTHERAPY WITHOUT USING MYELOABLATION

4.1. Host–Donor Competition

The theory of the success of the less toxic nonablative hematopoietic transplant is derived from a paradigm shift in the understanding of what is required for successful allogeneic therapy. Rather than aggressive medications used to obliterate the recipient's hematopoietic system and create open space for the donated cells to repopulate, the nonmyeloablative approach relies on successful competitive inhibition of the new immune system versus the endogenous one. Laboratory evidence supportive of the feasibility of this approach is derived from both the rodent and canine models. Storb et al. *(15)* treated canines with successively lower doses of radiotherapy. This group noted that when the dose of radiotherapy was decreased from 920 cGy to 450 cGy (still supralethal, but much less toxic) the rate of successful engraftment from DLA identical littermates decreased from 95 to 41%. The important point was not the decrease, but the fact that engraftment still occurred in a large proportion of canines (41%) *(15)*.

Does this less intense therapy still create space in the marrow or does it assist in the host–donor immune competition for regeneration? Yu et al. *(16)* addressed this question by comparing the effects of radiation to the marrow space vs total lymphoid radiotherapy. Canines were given either local radiotherapy of 1000 cGy at 200 cGy/min to the marrow space or the lower dose of 450 cGy total lymphoid radiation. Though transient donor engraftment was noted in those given marrow radiation, all six of these canines rejected the donated stem cells early in recovery. In contrast, all four canines given only total lymphoid radiation at 450 cGy had sustained donor engraftment *(16)*. These data suggest that immunosuppression may play a larger role than the creation of marrow space in a successful allogeneic transplant.

Another set of experiments addressed the question of the impact of modulation of posttransplant immunotherapy. Table 2 compares the results of dogs treated at 450 cGy at 7 cGy/min and infused with allogeneic grafts from DLA identical littermates, followed by treatment with differing immunotherapy posttransplant. It is noted that those who received cyclosporine after induction therapy had a significantly improved rate of engraftment compared to those who received no posttransplant immunotherapy (100 vs 36%). This is in contrast to those canines that received prednisone following induction having no allogeneic engraftment, suggesting that all post transplant immunomodulation is not created equal *(15,17)*.

Subsequently, the dose of radiotherapy was further decreased to sublethal doses of 100–200 cGy. It was noted that, even with the sublethal conditioning dose, successful engraftment could be maintained with posttransplant immunomodulation. Table 3 shows canines treated at 200 cGy and given differing combinations of cyclosporine, methotrexate, and mycophenylate following induction. A high rate of sustained engraftment is noted in the groups treated with drug combinations for prophylaxis. Again, not all posttransplant immune modulation had the same benefit, as those subjects given only cyclosporine rejected the donor cells with this sublethal dose of radiotherapy. Those receiving methotrexate with cyclosporine had intermediate success, while the best outcome was seen in those who received the combination of mycophenylate and cyclosporine *(18)*. The potential synergy for the combination of cyclosporine and

Table 2
Canines Exposed to 450 cGy and Infused with Stem Cells
from DLA Identical Littermates

Reference	Posttransplant immunotherapy	Proportion engrafting
(15)	None	6 out of 17 (36%)
(17)	Cyclosporine	7 out of 7 (100%)
(17)	Prednisone	0 out of 5 (0%)

Table 3
Canines Exposed to 200 cGy and Infused
with Stem Cells from DLA Identical
Littermates

Posttransplant therapy	Engraftment
CSA	0 out of 5 (0%)
MTX/CSA	3 out of 6 (50%)
MMF/CSA	5 out of 6 (83%)

CSA, cyclosporine 15 mg/kg by mouth 2×/d on d 1–35 MTX, methotrexate 0.4 mg/kg intravenously on d 1, 3, 6, and 11; MMF, mycophenylate 10 mg/kg 2×/d subcutaneously on d 0–27.

mycophenylate supports prior work with this combination, showing improved outcomes in canines undergoing ablative therapy as well (19).

These data support the hypothesis that GVHD and rejection (host-vs-graft [HVG]) reactions are controlled by the same mechanisms of immune competition. Varying immunotherapy may then have a major impact on the success of nonmyeloablative induction regimens as we explore methods of minimizing the toxicity and maximizing the benefits of this approach.

4.2. The Importance Stem Cell Dose

A second piece of the puzzle allowing one to successfully minimize the dose of induction therapy involves understanding the impact of increased doses of hematopoietic stem cells upon donor engraftment. The importance of higher cell dose compensating for less intense induction therapy can be seen from results in rodent models. Balb/c female rodents ablated with 700 cGy of whole animal radiation reliably engraft donor stem cells from Balb/c males at low or high cell doses. In contrast, rodents prepared with a dose of 100 cGy whole animal radiation do not have a high rate of engraftment at low cell doses, but do at higher cell doses (Fig. 2) (20).

5. CLINICAL EVIDENCE IN SUPPORT OF THE FEASIBILITY OF NONMYELOABLATIVE ALLOGENEIC HEMATOPOIETIC TRANSPLANTATION

5.1. Unmanipulated Grafts

Giralt et al. (21) reported on fifteen patients ages 27–71 (median age 59) with aggressive myeloid leukemia. Twelve of the 15 patients had multiple relapses or refractory disease. Therapy included fludarabine 30 mg/m^2/d for 4 d, idarubicin 12 mg/m^2/d for 3 d, and cytarabine 2 g/m^2/d for 4 d (n = 8) (one patient had melphalan 140 mg/m^2 for 1 d substituted). Alternatively, patients received 2-chloro-deoxyadenosine 12 mg/m^2/d for 5 d and cytarabine 1 g/m^2/d for 5 d (n = 7). The median dose of peripheral blood stem cells or marrow infused was

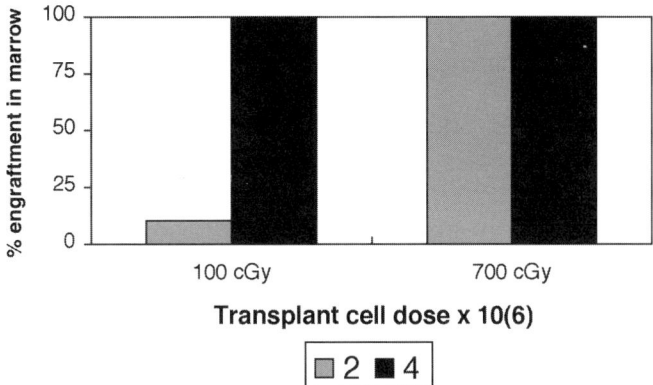

Transplant cell dose x 10(6)

□ 2 ■ 4

Fig. 2. While engraftment is not significantly affected by low numbers of infused stem cells in rodents radioablated with 700 cGy, stem cell dose effects engraftment potential in nonablated rodents (100 cGy), where higher doses of stem cells allows for a significant increase in the rate of engraftment.

4.5×10^6/kg CD34+ cells. GVHD prophylaxis consisted of cyclosporine and prednisone. One patient died during induction therapy, while 13 out of 14 remaining patients had evidence of donor engraftment with 8 out of 14 evaluable patients attaining a remission of their leukemia. Two patients experienced grade 2 GVHD in this small study with 100-d actuarial survival in responding patients of 66% *(21)*. Utilization of single fraction, low dose radiation in preparation has met with similar success. For patients transplanted with a matched donor, preparation with 2 Gy total body irradiation (TBI) resulted in 80% engraftment. The addition of fludarabine to the nonablative preparation increased the engraftment rate to 100% *(22)*. Table 4 summarizes the results as they regard successful engraftment and occurrence of GVHD for recently reported studies using matched siblings and unmanipulated grafts.

The initial clinical results noted those with active progressive disease did not fare as well as others in terms of disease-free survival. This has led to further studies in less aggressive or indolent malignancies. In an early report, 12 patients with less aggressive hematologic malignancies were treated with nonmyeloablative therapy with no prophylaxis for acute GVHD. One patient died of toxicity and six of the remaining nine evaluable patients remained in remission. Two patients died with severe acute GVHD, and therefore, GVHD prophylaxis consisting of tacrolimus ± methotrexate 5 mg on d 1, 3, and 6 was added *(23)*. The use of this more stringent GVH prophylaxis regimen raised the issue of ensuring engraftment with the nonablative preparative regimen, as it remained unclear whether the immunomodulation would impact more on the donor or recipient's immune system in the competition for immune recovery. This concern seems to be manageable, as results with the nonablative transplant experience using fludarabine and cyclophosphamide or cisplatin, fludarabine, and cytarabine, with the posttransplantation prophylaxis for GVHD noted above, are encouraging. Patient age ranged from 45–71 yr. Eight patients had chronic lymphocytic leukemia (CLL) (chemotherapy sensitive, refractory, or Richter's), six patients had low grade or transformed non-Hodgkin's disease, and one patient had mantle cell lymphoma. This approach resulted in engraftment for 11 of 15 patients, one died of liver failure, and other toxicities such as cytomegalovirus (CMV) antigenemia were common but severity was not greater than grade II. One patient had grade II GVHD of the liver and two patients had extensive chronic GVHD. After donor lymphocyte boosts, two other patients developed grade II GVHD, and one patient developed lethal grade IV GVHD. Eight of 11 evaluable patients attained a complete remission of their hematologic malignancy. Those few who did not engraft had autologous hematologic recovery within 2 wk *(24)*. In those with refractory myeloma, similar encouraging results for nonablative therapies

Table 4

Summary Results for Engraftment and GVHD of Studies with Nonmyeloablative Preparative Regimens Using Primarily Unmanipulated Stem Cells from Matched Siblings

Ref.	Regimen	Total patients (early deaths)	Median age (range)	Disease	% Donor engraftment	GVHD prophylaxis	≥ Grade 2 acute GVHD
(21)	F-I-C, F-I-M, CDA-C	15 (1)	59 (27–71)	AML or MDS	13 out of 14 (93%)	CSA, MP	2 out of 14 (14%)
(24)	F-Ctx, F-C-CP	15 (1)	55 (45–71)	Low-grade NHL	11 out of 14	FK506, Mtx	1 out of 14 (7%)
(28)	F-Bu-ATG	26	31 (1–61)	Refractory hematologic malignancies	26 out of 26 (100%)	CSA	6 out of 26 (23%)
(30)	F-Bu-ATG	17	52	Refractory hematologic malignancies	17 out of 17 (100%)	CSA	4 (27%)
(25)	F-M	18 (1)	50	Refractory myeloma	17 out of 17 (100%)	FK506	9 out of 17 (53%)
(29)	F-Bu-ATG	10	52 (45–57)	Refractory myeloma in 90%	10/10 (100%)	CSA	5 out of 10 (50%)
(61)	F-Cyt	19	47 (37–65)	Renal cell	19 out of 19 (100%)	CSA	10 out of 19 (53%)
(31)	F-Cyt	19	–	Resistant HD, NHL	19 out of 19 (100%)	CSA, Mtx	–
(22)	TBI	50	–		– 10 out of 50 (20%)	CSA, MMF	
(22)	TBI- F	28	–		– 28 out of 28 (100%)	CSA, MMF	
(27)	TBI-M	12	49 (40–63)	Myeloma	112 out of 12 (100%)	CSA, MMF	6 out of 12 (50%)
(32)	M	16	57 (42–70)	Myeloma	15 out of 16 (94%)	CSA	10 out of 16
(26)	TBI-ECP-P	10	–	Refractory hematologic malignancies	10 out of 10 (100%)	CSA, MTX	0 out of 10 (0%)

F, fludarabine; I, idarubicin; M, melphalan; C, cytarabine; Cyt, cyclophosphamide; CP, cisplatin; Bu, busulfan; BEAM, BCNU, etoposide, cytarabine, melphalan; ATG, antithymocyte globulin; TBI, total body irradiation; ECP, extracorporeal photopheresis; P, pentostatin; AML, acute myeloid leukemia; NHL, non-Hodgkin's lymphoma; MDS, myelodysplasia; CSA, cyclosporine; MP, methylprednisolone; FK506, tacrolimus; Mtx, methotrexate.

Table 5
Summary of Outcomes for Patients Undergoing
Nonmyeloablative Therapy for Hematologic Disorders

Ref.	Diseases	Complete response	Survival
(21)	AML or MDS	8 out of 14 (57%)	Actuarial 100-d survival: 66%
(24)	Relapsed or refractory low-grade NHL (CLL, mantle cell, Richter's)	8 out of 11 (73%)	Median f/u 8 mo: 50% alive at 1 yr
(28)	CML, AML or MDS, ALL, NHL, MM, Hgb	21 out of 26 (80%)	Median f/u 8 mo: 85% survival
(25)	Refractory myeloma	8 out of 17 (47%)	33% actuarial survival at 1 yr (30% progression-free)
(29)	Refractory myeloma after autologous transplantation	5 out of 10 (50%)	–
(27)	Myeloma	6 out of 12 (50%)	Median f/u 200 d: 10 out of 12 remain alive with response
(32)	Myeloma	7 out of 16 (44%)	Median f/u 11 mo: 69% survival
(47)	Refractory HD, NHL	9 out of 13 (69%)	Median f/u 10 mo: 9 out of 13 (69%) remain alive and disease-free
(57)	HD, NHL, AML, MDS, CML, MM, ALL	21 out of 30 (70%)	71% actuarial survival at 1 yr
(54)	CML	–	Progression-free and overall survival at 3 yr: 6 out of 9 (65%)
(31)	Refractory HD, NHL	6 out of 19 (32%)	Median f/u 1 yr: 1-yr survival of 74%
(50)	AML, NHL, CML, MM, myelofibrosis	10 out of 14 (71%)	–

CML, chronic myeloid leukemia; AML, acute myeloid leukemia; ALL, acute lymphoid leukemia; NHL, non-Hodgkin's lymphoma; MM, multiple myeloma; HGB, hemoglobinopathies; f/u, follow-up.

have been obtained with a progression-free survival at 1 yr of 30% (25). Another approach of interest successfully combines extracorporeal photopheresis with pentostatin and low dose radiation. One group has noted a high rate of engraftment with little severe acute GVHD (26).

Combining nonmyeloablative therapy, as consolidation after aggressive high-dose chemotherapy requiring autologous support, may be another method to exploit the immunotherapeutic benefits of allogeneic therapy with less toxicity. Using this combined approach, one report notes a 30% complete remission and progression-free rate with a median follow-up of 1 yr in those with refractory lymphoma (31). Autologous therapy, followed by a melphalan-TBI nonmyeloablative regimen for those with progressive myeloma, has resulted in a 50% complete response rate as well (27).

As discussed above, not all nonmyeloablative regimens are similar in terms of toxicity or degree of intensity and much remains to be learned concerning the relative strengths and weaknesses of the different approaches. Slavin et al. (28) have reported results from the use of a more intermediate dose nonmyeloablative conditioning regimen for allogeneic stem cell transplant: fludarabine 30 mg/m^2/d for 6 d, busulfan 4 mg/kg/d for 2 d, and ATG 10 mg/kg/d for 4 d. In the first group of 26 patients with primarily hematopoietic malignancies, nine patients engrafted with stable partial chimerism and 17 patients engrafted with complete donor chimerism. Four patients received donor lymphocyte infusions (DLI) for relapsed disease. At a median follow-up of 8 mo, 85% of patients were alive, and 81% are disease-free. There have been no cases of prolonged aplasia (28). Another report concerning patients with myeloma who had failed other aggressive therapies proceeding to nonablative conditioning with fludarabine, busulfan, and ATG notes significant response with 50% complete remission and a 9 out of 10 (90%) overall response rate *(29)*. Others have used a similar regimen with encouraging results in engraftment and response, with approx 28% chance of grade III or IV acute GVHD. Table 5 summarizes some of the early results regarding efficacy of the nonmyeloablative allogeneic transplant in those with varying hematologic malignancies.

Infections, particularly reactivation of CMV, remain a problem as realized in these early trials, underscoring the significant and sometimes prolonged immunosuppression still present with all of the nonmyeloablative approaches *(30)*. The outcomes, in terms of toxicity and efficacy of the various regimens, will likely depend largely on patient selection. Comparing relative benefits must await future comparative studies.

6. IMPROVING OUTCOMES THROUGH MINIMIZING GVHD: ATTENUATED CYTOKINE STORM AND GRAFT MANIPULATION

Evidence is accruing supporting the contention that minimizing the damage from the preparative regimen will decrease GVHD. This is hypothesized to occur through minimizing perturbations in the cytokine storm noted after the preparative regimens for allogeneic transplantation. A comparison of the rates of acute GVHD after allogeneic transplantation with unmanipulated grafts in ablated vs nonmyeloablated patients has shown less overall acute GVHD (28 vs 53%) in the nonmyeloablated group, though severe acute GVHD risks were similar *(33)*. Cytokines are increasingly recognized as important mediators of GVHD. Endogenous serum levels of various cytokines and dependent molecules in sera of 14 patients after T cell depleted BMT were determined and compared with the results of 12 patients undergoing non-T cell-depleted transplantation *(34)*. The effect of various conditioning regimens and of hematopoietic reconstitution on cytokine serum levels was analyzed in detail in these cohorts of patients by measuring IFN-γ, IFN-α, and TFN. Analyses showed that an increase in IFN-γ and neopterin serum levels was a specific feature of cyclophosphamide administration and was not observed after other cytostatic drugs or TBI. In addition, an increase in IFN-α, neopterin, β2-microglobulin, and IFN-α release depends on the presence of T cells in the graft. It was concluded that significant cytokine serum alterations were noted after T cell-depleted allogeneic transplantation as compared with after non-T cell-depleted transplants. Besides depletion of cytotoxic effector cells through the T cell depletion, these alterations might be involved in preventing GVHD after T cell-depleted transplantation *(34)*. These results stress that more attention should be devoted to the cytokine release-inducing capacity of the ablative conditioning regimen as well as the efficacy of the T cell depletion.

There is evidence too that the GVT effects may occur in the absence of GVHD, implying that it may be possible to exert antitumor effects in patients without GVHD *(4)*. Well-established C57BL/6—>BALB/c chimeras that were free of GVHD, reconstituted with T cell-depleted allogeneic bone marrow cells, and inoculated 3 mo after BMT with a high inoculation of murine B cell leukemia (BCL1) showed no evidence of disease. In contrast, all control mice developed leukemia and died within 58 d. Results from adoptive transfer experiments in secondary naive BALB/c recipients indicated that all BCL1 cells were eliminated in the chimeras within 14 d. Hence, all BCL1 cells were eliminated in the chimeras within 14 d. Complete resistance to BCL1 developed in the chimeras despite complete tolerance to host allo-antigens. Administration of immunocompetent allogeneic C57BL/6 spleen cells, low dose rIL-2, or both for 5 d further amplified the GVL effects observed in tolerant chimeras. This datum suggests that GVL effects can develop even after T cell depletion in the absence of clinically overt GVHD and that GVL can be further amplified by rIL-2, either with or without use of additional immuno-competent donor T cells *(35)*. Clinically, this is becoming evident in our work with unrelated cord blood transplantation. We have noted in unrelated adult cord transplants, less than 20% severe GVHD, much less than one would anticipate from adult unrelated bone marrow or peripheral blood stem cell transplants. It is hypothesized that the different T cell subsets and degree of maturity in these subsets relates to this lessened effect. Importantly, we have not seen decreased antitumor effects in the patients transplanted with cord blood, indicating an active antitumor effect with less risk of severe GVHD *(36,37)*.

The lessened toxicity of nonmyeloablative therapies potentially induces a lower cytokine storm, relating to the chance for less GVHD. Further, methods to minimize chances of GVHD have led to attempts at combining nonmyeloablative therapy with stem cell grafts, which have been T cell depleted. Donor peripheral blood progenitor cells are often depleted of T cells with soybean agglutination and e-rosetting, or e-rosetting with positive CD34+ selection One early report of 15 patients treated in this manner with T cell-depleted stem cells noted that 14 patients had evidence for engraftment with some GVHD. Six of 11 evaluable patients achieved a complete response, and two patients had a partial response *(38)*.

Our program has an interest in promoting the potential of T cell depletion targeting the CD52 antigen on lymphocytes using CAMPATH- 1H *(39–41)*. Antibody to CD52 has been used successfully in vitro and in vivo to deplete T lymphocytes, and thereby decrease GVHD and aid engraftment in ablative transplantation *(42,43)*. The CD52 antigen is not highly expressed on NK cells. These cells are, therefore, spared in the purging process and have been implicated as playing a role in surveillance for viral illnesses (i.e., CMV) and expressing antitumor effects *(44)*. The antibody has shown encouraging results in terms of controlling GVHD while simultaneously maintaining a low risk of graft rejection and relapse *(45,46)*. Table 6 summarizes the results with engraftment using T cell-depleted grafts from matched siblings for nonmyeloablative transplantation revealing encouraging engraftment as well as control of acute GVHD.

The lessened GVHD risk with T cell depletion may come at the price of increased infections. The T cell-depleted methods appear to relate to increased time to immune recovery and increased infectious complications. It is further possible that the increased risks may not be due to the T cell depletion alone, but the combination of this with the effective lymphoablation noted with the nonmyeloablative approaches. For instance, comparing similar T cell depletion in patients who have undergone with CAMPATH and posttransplant therapy with that of those treated with cyclosporine reveals that the combination of fludarabine with CAMPATH leads to more frequent reactivation of viral illnesses, which we have noted in our experience with this approach as well *(49,50)*. Further work must be done to optimize the combination of T cell depletion with nonmyeloablative therapies.

Our preliminary results with this approach have yielded encouraging results in terms of engraftment and response (Tables 5 and 6), but more importantly, quality of life may be enhanced as well (Fig. 3). Within 6 wk of transplantation, many patients note the same or improved quality of life compared to the pretransplant state. This rapid recovery is earlier than anticipated and much earlier than one would expect for standard allogeneic therapy. Given the degree of illness of the patients treated, providing a regimen with less toxicity with a potential for immunotherapy and only a brief decrement, in their perceived quality of life is an important step forward. It is likely that the early improvement in performance status is not only due to the gentler doses of chemotherapy used in this procedure compared to historical approaches, but also to the increased cell doses delivered to the patient, resulting in an early recovery of blood cells. In our experience, nearly all patients recover granulocytes and platelets within 2 wk. In fact, eight of the first 21 patients in our trial never had a platelet count <20,000/μL *(50)*.

Table 6
Results of Combining Nonmyeloablative Therapy with T Cell Depletion Using Stem Cells Primarily from HLA-Matched Siblings

Ref.	Regimen	Total patients (early deaths)	Median age (range)	Disease	evaluable patients	% Engraftment with donor cells in prophylaxis	≥ Grade II acute GVHD
(47)	BEAM + CAMPATH 1G	13 (1)	44	Resistant HD, NHL	11/12 (92%)	CSA, Mtx	0 out of 12 (0%)
(50)	F- CYT-CAMPATH 1H	21 (1)	45 (33–62)	Hematologic malignancies, breast cancer	21 out of 21 (100%)	None	2 out of 21 (10%)
(48)	F - T depletion	9	–	Hematologic malignancies	9 out of 9 (100%)	CSA	2 out of 9 (22%)

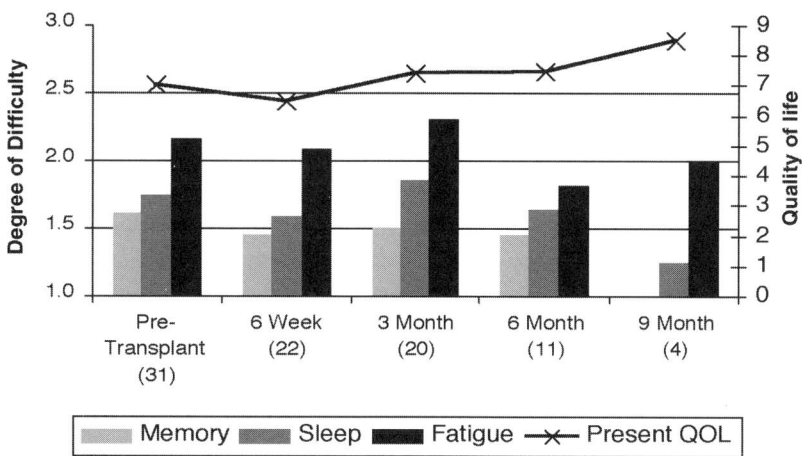

Fig. 3. Summary of the impact on quality of life for patients undergoing nonmyeloablative allogeneic therapy at our institution using a matched or mismatched family member as the stem cell donor. The numbers in parentheses represent the number of patients responding to the assessment questionnaire for the indicated time period. The primary Y axis notes degree of difficulty as reported by the patient on a scale of 1–3 with: 1, not at all; 2, some; 3, quite a bit of difficulty

7. EXPANDING THE AVAILABILITY OF NONMYELOABLATIVE THERAPY USING ALTERNATIVE DONORS

Most patients do not have a matched sibling to allow allogeneic therapy of any sort. For the nonmyeloablative approach to be broadly applicable, success with alternative donor sources must be explored. Transplantation with stem cells from a matched unrelated donor or mismatched family member is known to produce severe GVHD, though it has been improved by using T cell depletion. In one report, no posttransplantation GVHD prophylaxis was otherwise employed, and the difficulty of increased graft rejection associated with severe T cell depletion was overcome by the infusion of megadoses of stem cells, with a mean near 14 ξ 10[6] CD34+ cells/kg of patient weight. Forty-one of 43 patients engrafted, and no GVHD occurred. There was prolonged immunosuppression, however, leading to increased opportunistic infections *(51)*. This technique has also been effectively used in the nonmyeloablative regimens *(38)*. Patients prepared with busulfan (8 mg/kg), fludarabine 30 mg/m[2] for 4 d, and ATG 10 mg/m[2] followed by cyclosporine or cyclosporine and methotrexate engrafted successfully, with four out of six patients being alive and disease-free at a median follow-up of 90 d (52). Some have used CD34+ selection (passive T cell depletion) combined with fludarabine based nonmyeloablative regimens and have noted high rates of engraftment, with <25% incidence of severe acute GVHD *(48)*.

One report with matched unrelated donors (MUD) notes an 87% rate of engraftment in 32 patients who underwent preparation with a single fraction of 2Gy TBI in combination with fludarabine 30 mg/m[2]/d for 3 d. Similar high engraftment rates have been noted with intermediate dose preparative regimens including fludarabine, busulfan, and ATG, followed by cyclosporine with methotrexate or mycophenylate. A 45% complete remission rate in CLL patients was reported *(53)*. Use of matched unrelated donors with T cell-depleted grafts using CAMPATH in vivo has resulted in a nearly 100% engraftment rate with an approx 25% treatment-related mortality and only 5 out of 30 patients with severe acute GVHD. Twenty-one of 30 patients with refractory hematologic malignancies were alive and disease-free at 6 mo median follow-up with 71% actuarial overall 1-yr survival *(54)*. An intermediate intensity regimen of fludarabine, ATG, and busulfan resulted in 7 out of 9 patients infused with MUD stem cells attaining long-term engraftment, with 55% acute GVHD and 65% disease-free survival at 3 yr *(55)*. Table 7 summarizes some of the results using alternative donors.

The use of unmatched unrelated donors for nonmyeloablative allogeneic therapy has met with less encouraging rates of engraftment when compared with the same preparative regimen as for mismatched related donors. This suggests that the increased degree of mismatch noted in secondary targets in unrelated donors must be overcome with still higher cell doses, increased intensity of the preparative regimen, or manipulation of the graft cells *(56)*.

Use of partially matched family members as a donor source is attractive for many reasons. First, the ready availability of at least a haplomatched relative for most patients (parent, sibling or adult child) means most patients will have a donor source. Further, the success of this approach may in large part depend on the care in the peritransplant period. Having a readily available stem cell and T cell source in a family member is a great benefit in deciding on attempts to improve engraftment or with modulation of the immune recovery with donor lymphocyte boosts. We have used a nonmyeloablative approach for patients with mismatched family members with encouraging early results. In our first group of 15 patients with various malignancies, all engrafted with donor cells, most with >80% lymphoid and myeloid donor engraftment by 4 wk after infusion. Viral infections remain a concern with many experiencing reactivation of CMV, though all have been treatable. Combining T cell depletion using CAMPATH 1H with mycophenylate as the sole posttransplant immunomodulation agent, patients have not had grade III–IV acute GVHD, one patient had grade II GVHD of the gut, and a few patients have had grade II skin GVHD, all treated successfully with steroid therapy. Some patients have experienced increased GVHD after receiving donor lymphocyte boosts however, and much work remains to be done concerning the optimal approach for DLI following this approach. Further concern also remains over the risk of chronic GVHD in these patients, and the patients must be followed closely for long-term benefits and complications.

The use of cord blood as a stem cell source for nonmyeloablative therapy remains attractive as well. We have shown that mismatched, unrelated cord blood is a feasible source of stem cells for allogeneic therapy in children and adults *(36,37)*, although the low cell dose remains concerning for extension to nonmyeloablative therapy. For patients without appropriate family members or an identified matched unrelated donor, this may be the only option. In our experience, we have seen successful trilineage engraftment in adult patients using mismatched unrelated cord blood as the stem cell source following nonmyeloablative therapy. To date, three out of four patients have demonstrated donor engraftment, and two patients have sustained full donor engraftment beyond 6 and 12 mo with remission of their hematologic cancer *(57)*.

7.1. Extending Therapy to Those with Solid Tumors

The potential of extending allogeneic therapy to patients with solid tumors is reported in the literature *(58–63)* and is discussed in detail elsewhere in this text. Nonablative conditioning may provide the optimal framework within which to provide this allogeneic immunotherapy and a summary of early results is noted in Table 8. Our group has focused on finding new approaches to the care of patients with breast cancer. We have treated seven patients with advanced rapidly progressive disease noting that many can achieve at least a stable disease state lasting 2–3 mo *(50)*. This may provide a window of opportunity for future advances toward improving the immunotherapy following the transplant, such as with allogeneic vaccines.

7.2. Extending Therapy to Those with Nonmalignant Conditions

Two patients with T cell deficiency received the ultimate in nonmyeloablative therapy, i.e., no preparative therapy, prior to infusion of matched sibling stem cells. Both received

Table 7
Summary of Results Using Nonmyeloablative Therapy with Alternative Donor Stem Cell Sources, with or without T Cell Depletion

Ref.	Regimen	Donor cell source	Total patients (early deaths)	Median age (range)	% Engraftment with donor cells in evaluable patients	GVHD prophylaxis	≥ Grade II acute GVHD
(57)	F-M-CAMPATH 1H	MUD	30 (7)	35 (18–54)	30 out of 30 (100%)	CSA, T cell depleted	5 out of 30 (17%)
(52)	F-BU-ATG	MUD	6 (1)	17 (11–57)	6 out of 6 (100%)	CSA, Mtx	3 out of 6 (50%)
(50)	F-Cyt-CAMPATH 1H	Mismatched family member	8	41 (21–62)	8 out of 8 (100%)	MMF	1 out of 8 (13%)
(22)	TBI-F	MUD	32	–	28 out of 32 (87%)	CSA, MMF	–
(56)	F-Cyt-ATG	Unrelated mismatched cord blood	4	46 (37–62)	3 out of 4 (75%)	CSA, Pred	2 out of 3 (50%)

Table 8
Summary Results for Nonmyeloablative Therapy for Those with Solid Tumors

Ref.	Diseases	Complete response	Survival
(63)	Melanoma	4 out of 15 (27%) Partial responses	–
(61)	Renal cell carcinoma	10 out of 19 (53%)	45% Actuarial 1-yr survival
(50)	Breast cancer	4 out of 7 (50%) Partial responses	–

cyclosporine and mycophenylate after donor stem cell infusion and engrafted (64). These approaches with lessened toxicities allow patients with deficient immune systems, such as combined immunodeficiencies and adenosine deaminase deficiency, an opportunity to undergo allogeneic therapy with less initial risk.

Hemoglobinopathies represent a special challenge and potential area of opportunity. For reasons that are not completely understood, there may be an increase in graft rejection using standard, ablative, allogeneic therapy (65,66). We are concerned that this risk may be further augmented using a less intense, nonmyeloablative regimen. Further, results in adult patients with ablative therapy for these illnesses have not been encouraging due to significant complications from toxicity as a result of the procedure. However, given the lack of a neoplastic process, the establishment of even a partial mixed chimeric state by this approach may be sufficient to mask the abnormal phenotype of diseases in this category. The nonmyeloablative approaches are currently being extended to this group with mixed results. One encouraging report has used fludarabine, busulfan, ATG, and lymphoid radiation in three patients, followed by cyclosporine and mycophenylate. Two of three have evidence of donor engraftment over 100 d following infusion (67). This approach is being explored in multicenter trials in both adult and pediatric populations at this time.

7.3. Allogeneic Immunotherapy and the Future

Evidence is mounting in patients that undergo nonmyeloablative therapy that immune recovery may occur with antitumor efficacy separate from GVHD (68). Recovery after intermediate dose preparative regimens has been noted in those who receive unmanipulated grafts in which T cell recovery is rapid and diverse within 2 mo of transplantation, as compared with slower recovery after infusion with T depleted grafts with DLIs following recovery (69). There appears to be rapid lymphoid engraftment following infusion of unmanipulated stem cells with normal CD8 T cell phenotypes and significant reactions to third party stimuli noted within the first 2 mo in many patients, except following GVHD or in using T cell-depleted grafts. The blunted measured third party response in this situation may be due to the immunosuppressive therapies employed (70). The kinetics of recovery in these situations will be important to understand as we move forward. Further, the impact of utilizing donor lymphocyte boosts must be explored. Strong published evidence suggests that the infusion of donor lymphocytes may be suffiecient to induce durable remissions in patients who have relapsed disease after allogeneic transplantation (71,72). This immune effect will be important to exploit in optimizing the use of nonmyeloablative therapy. However more questions than answers exist as to the optimal use of this modality. Presently, our group begins DLI approx 4–6 wk after allogeneic stem cell infusion if the patient does not have active GVHD. A second or third infusion may be used at 8-wk intervals depending on patient and disease status. We are presently performing a trial accessing the impact of the number of infusions (1, 2 , or 3) on toxicity and efficacy. We typically infuse 1×10^7 CD3+ cells/kg patient weight, though in a non-T cell-depleted nonmyeloablative setting many groups infuse 1×10^8 CD3+ cells/kg. In the mismatched setting, we use a log lower of CD3+ stem cells given the increased risk of inducing severe acute GVHD. What is the proper timing of lymphocyte infusions in terms of when to start after transplantation, and how long should one wait before deciding on delivering subsequent infusions? What is the proper cell dose? Should one infuse a bulk dose or escalated doses based on tolerance? Can infusing only certain T cell subsets allow an effective antitumor response without increasing the occurrence of severe acute GVHD? These and other issues await further testing in comparative trials.

Our experience with T cell depletion, using CAMPATH, notes a relative sparing of the NK cell population, which may be particularly important for antitumor efficacy. Further, to date we have not noted a change in the rate of lymphoid versus myeloid recovery *(50)*. It is important to recognize that all regimens are not equal, and immune recovery and antitumor responses must be individually investigated for each of the approaches to T depletion employed.

The use of mismatched donors expands the pool of donors and significantly increases the chance for allogeneic therapy for many. Further, we are learning that it may allow one to exploit the anti-tumor effect beyond that seen with HLA-matched situations. Donor NK cells are potent antitumor agents. In situations in which HLA class I allele matching at the C locus is present, both the donor and the patient express the same inhibitory receptors (killing inhibitory receptors [KIR] epitope) and no antidonor effect occurs. However, in mismatched situations, in which the patient does not express the same KIR epitope as the donor cells, the donor NK cells are able to recognize this difference and lyse the patient's cells. This does not appear to relate to the incidence of GVHD either. This relationship must be explored in detail, as the use of mismatched donor–recipient pairs increases and immune activity and antitumor function is explored.

The field of nonmyeloablative allogeneic immunotherapy has really just begun. Early results noted above confirm the feasibility of extending this less intense approach to older more debilitated patients. Our enthusiasm must be tempered with the realization that the standard concerns of GVHD and infections remain limiting for many patients. This is particularly so, considering that those who are more debilitated are less likely to have the reserve to tolerate such complications. Further, we are still exploring our limits with this approach: What is the risk of severe morbidity and mortality? How much time do we need for the antitumor effects to activate? How can we manipulate immune function to make the antitumor effect more robust?

These initial studies will form the basis for the future improvements in minimizing toxicity and GVHD while maximizing engraftment and antitumor effects to improve long term outcomes.

REFERENCES

1. Keil F, Kalhs P, Haas O, et al. Relapse of Philadelphia chromosome positive acute lymphoblastic leukemia after marrow transplantation: sustained molecular remission after early and dose- escalating infusion of donor leukocytes. *Br J Haematol* 1997;97:161–164.
2. Gurman G, Arslan O, Koc H, et al. Donor leukocyte infusion for relapsed ANLL after allogeneic BMT and the use of interferon alpha to induce graft versus leukemia effect. Bone Marrow Transplant 1996;18:825,826.
3. Odom L, August C, Githens J, et al. Remission of relapsed leukemia during a graft versus host reaction. *Lancet* 1978;2:537–540.
4. Drobyski W, Keever C, Roth M, et al. Salvage immunotherapy using donor leukocyte infusions as treatment for relapsed chronic myelogenous leukemia after allogeneic bone marrow transplantation: effficacy and toxicity of a defined T cell dose. *Blood* 1993;82:2310–2318 .
5. Weiden P, Flournoy N, Thomas E, et al. Antileukemic effect of graft versus host disease in human recipients of allogeneic marrow grafts. *N Engl J Med* 1979;300:1068–1073 .
6. Sullivan K, Weiden P, Storb R, et al. Influence of acute and chronic graft versus host disease on relapse and survival after bone marrow transplantation from HLA identical siblings as treatment of acute and chronic leukemia. *Blood* 1989;73:1720–1728.

7. Horowitz M, Gale R, Sondel P, et al. Graft versus leukemia reactions after bone marrow transplantation. *Blood* 1990;75:555–562.
8. Anichini A, Mortarini R, Maccalli C, et al. Cytotoxic T cells directed to tumor antigens not expressed on normal melanocytes dominate HLA-A2.1- restricted immune repertoire to melanoma. *J Immunol* 1996;156:208–217.
9. Dadmarz R, Sgagias N, Rosenberg S, et al. CD4+ T lymphocytes infiltrating human breast cancer recognise autologous tumor in an MHC class II restricted fashion. *Cancer Immunol Immunother* 1995;40:1–9.
10. Rocha M, Umansky V, Lee KH, et al. Differences between graft-versus-leukemia and graft-versus-host reactivity. I. Interaction of donor immune T cells with tumor and/or host cells. *Blood* 1997;89:2189–2202.
11. Eibl B, Schwaighofer H, Nachbaur D, et al. Petersen F, Niederwieser D. Evidence for a graft versus tumor effect in a patient treated with marrow ablative chemotherapy and allogeneic bone marrow transplantation for breast cancer. *Blood* 1996;88:1501–1508.
12. Mehta J, Powles R, Treleaven J, et al. Long term follow up of patients undergoing allogeneic transplantation for acute myeloid leukemia in first remission after cyclophosphamide-total body irradiation and cyclosporine. *Bone Marrow Transplant* 1996;18:741–746,.
13. Bradley J, Reft C, Goldman S, Rubin C, Nachman J, Larson R, Hallahan DE. High energy total body irradiation as preparation for bone marrow transplantation in leukemia patients: treatment technique and related complication.s *Int J Radiat Oncol Biol Phys* 1998;40:391–396.
14. Reddy V, Pollock BH, Sharda A, et al. GVHD and CMV antigenemia after allogeneic peripheral blood stem cell transplantation: comparison between myeloablative and nonmyeloablative conditioning regimens. *Blood* 2000;96(Suppl 1):817.
15. Storb R, Raff RF, Appelbaum FR, et al. Comparison of fractionated to single-dose total body irradiation in conditioning canine littermates for DLA-identical marrow grafts. *Blood* 1989;74:1139–1143.
16. Yu C, Sandmaier BM, Deeg HJ, Storb R. What role for radiation in novel nonmyeloablative transplant regimen for DLA-identical marrow grafts: Immunosuppression versus 'creation' of marrow space? *Blood* 1997;90(Suppl 1):1608.
17. Yu C, Storb R, Mathey B, et al. DLA identical bone marrow grafts after low dose total body irradiation effects of high dose corticosteroids and cyclosporine on engraftment. *Blood* 1995;86:4376–4381.
18. Storb R, Yu Cong , Wagner J, et al. Stable mixed hematopoietic chimerism in DLA Identical littermate dogs given sublethal total body irradiation before pharmacological immunosuppression after marrow transplantation. *Blood* 1997;89:3048–3054.
19. Yu C, Seidel K, Nash RA, et al. Synergism between mycophenylate mofetil and cyclosporine in preventing graft vrsus host disease among lethally irradiated dogs given DLA-non identical unrelated marrow grafts. *Blood* 1998;91:2581–2587.
20. Stewart FM, Zhong S, Wuu J, et al. Lymphohematopoietic engraftment in minimally myeloablated hosts. *Blood* 1998;91:3681–3687.
21. Giralt S, Estey E, Albitar M, et al. Engraftment of allogeneic porgenitor cells with purine analog-containing chemotherapy: harnessing graft versus leukemia without myeloablative therapy. *Blood* 1997;89:4531–4536.
22. Maris MB, Sandmaier BM, Niederwieser D, et al. Comparisons of donor chimerism, graft rejection, and GVHD after hematopoietic stem cell transplants from HLA matched siblings and unrelated donors using conditioning with 2 Gy TBI with and without fludarabine. *Blood* 2000;96(Suppl 1):2239.
23. Khouri I, Keating MJ, Przepiorka D, et al. Engraftment and induction of GVL with fludarabine (FAMP)-based non-ablative preparative regimen in patients with chronic lymphocytic leukemia (CLL) and lymphoma. *Proc ASH Blood* 1996;301A:1194.
24. Khouri IF, Keating M, Korbling M, et al. Transplant lite: induction of graft versus malignancy using fludarabine-based nonablative chemotherapy and allogeneic blood progenitor cell transplantation as treatment for lymphoid malignancies. *J Clin Oncol* 1998;16:2817–2824.
25. Giralt S, Weber D, Aleman A, et al. Non-myeloablative conditioning with fludarabine/melphalan for patients with multiple myeloma. *Blood* 1999;94(Suppl 1):1549.
26. Alcindor T, Chan G, Al-Olama A, et al. Engraftment and immunologic effects of a novel less myeloablative allogeneic transplant conditioning regimen of continuous infusion pentostatin, photopheresis, and low dose TBI. *Blood* 2000;96(Suppl 1):5160.
27. Molina A, Sahebi F, Maloney DG, et al. Nonmyeloablative peripheral blood stem cell allografts following cytoreductive autotransplants for the treatment of multiple myeloma. *Blood* 2000;96(Suppl 1):2063.
28. Slavin S., Nagler A, Naparstek E., et al. Nonmyeloablative stem cell transplantation and cell therapy as an alternative to conventional bone marrow transplantation with lethal cytoreduction for the treatment of malignant and non-malignant hematologic diseases. *Blood* 1998;91:756–763.
29. Garban F, Attal M, Rossi JF, Sotto JJ. High efficiency of non myeloablative allogeneic stem cell transplantation in poor prognosis myeloma patients. *Blood* 1999;94(Suppl 1):1550.
30. Faucher C, Mohty M, Vey N, et al. Allogeneic BMT with nonmyeloablative regimen: early full donor chimerism and increased rate of infections. *Blood* 1999;94(Suppl 1):654.

31. Carella AM, Corsetti MT, Lerma E, Cavaliere M. Auologous transplants followed by mini allografts for hodgkin's disease and non hodgkin's lymphoma. *Blood* 2000;96(Suppl 1):1752.
32. Badros A, Tricot G, Morris C, et al. Significant graft versus myeloma effect after nonmyeloablative allogeneic transplantation in multiple myeloma. *Blood* 2000;96(Suppl 1):5273.
33. Couriel D, Giralt S, De Lima M, et al. Graft versus host disease after non-myeloablative versus ablative conditioning regimens in fully matched sibling donor hematopoietic stem cell transplants. *Blood* 2000;96(Suppl 1):1758.
34. Schwaighofer H, Kernan NA, O'Reilly RJ, et al. Serum levels of cytokines and secondary messages after T-cell-depleted and non-T-cell-depleted bone marrow transplantation: influence of conditioning and hematopoietic reconstitution. *Transplantation* 1996;62:947–953.
35. Weiss L, Lubin I, Factorowich I, et al. Effective graft-versus-leukemia effects independent of graft-versus-host disease after T cell-depleted allogeneic bone marrow transplantation in a murine model of B cell leukemia/lymphoma. Role of cell therapy and recombinant IL-2. *J Immunol* 1994;153:2562–2567, 1994.
36. Long GW, Laughlin MJ, Madan B, et al. Unrelated umbilical cord blood transplantation in adult patients. *Blood* 2001; accepted.
37. Laughlin MJ, Barker J, Bambach B, et al. Hematopoietic engraftment ans survival after unrelated donor umbilical cord blood transplant in adult recipients. *N Engl J Med* 2001;344(24):1815–1822, 2001.
38. Spitzer TR, McAfee SL, Sackstein R, et al. Induction of mixed chimerism and potent anti-tumor responses following mon-myeloablative conditioning therapy and HLA-matched and mismatched donor bone marrow transplantation for refractory hematologic malignancies. *Blood* 1998;92:519a.
39. Osterborg A, Fassas A, Anagostopoulos A, et al. Humanized CD52 monoclonal antibody Campath-1H as frontline treatment in chronic lymphocytic leukemia. *Br J Hematol* 1996;93;151–153.
40. Dyer M, Kelsey S, Mackey H, et al. In vivo 'purging' of residual disease in CLL with Campath-1H. *Br J Heamtol* 1997;97:669–672.
41. Osterborg A, Dyer M, Bunjes D, et al. Phase II multicenter study of human CD52 antibody in previously treated chronic lymphocyte leukemia. *J Clin Oncol* 1997;15:1567–1574.
42. Hale G, Waldmann H. Control of graft-versus-host disease and graft rejection by T-cell depletion of donor and recipient with Campath-1H antibodies. Results of matched sibling transplants for malignant diseases. *Bone Marrow Transplant* 1994;13:597–611.
43. Hertenstein B, Arseniev L, Bötel V, Hale J. Abstract. 2d International Symposium on Allogeneic Peripheral Blood and Cord Blood Transplantation. Geneva, Switzerland. October 30–November 1997, p. 36.
44. Hale G, Waldmann H. CAMPATH User's Group. Risks of developing EBV-related lymphoproliferative disorders following T cell depleted marrow transplants. *Blood* 1998;91:3079–3083.
45. Hale G, Zhang MJ, Bunjes D, et al. Improving the outcome of bone marrow transplantation by using CD52 monoclonal antibodies to prevent graft versus host disease and graft rejection. *Blood* 1998;92:4581–4590.
46. Reittie J, Gottlieb D, Heslop H, et al. Brenner MK. Endogenously generated activated killer cells circulate after autologous and allogeneic transplantation but not after chemotherapy. *Blood* 1989;73:1351–1358.
47. Russell NH, Cull G, Byrne JL, et al. Evaluation of non-myeloablative conditioning combining BEAM with in vivo pre-transplant CAMPATH 1G for allogeneic transplantation in patients with lymphoma. *Blood* 1999;94(Suppl 1):1554.
48. Craddock C, Hughes T, Johnston R, et al. Engraftment of T depleted allogeneic peripheral blood stem cells using a non myeloablative conditioning regimen. *Blood* 1999;94(Suppl 1):1746.
49. Chakrabarti S, Steven N, Collingham K, et al. Viral reactivation and immune reconstitution following CAMPATH 1H and fludarabine based non-myeloablative conditioning for allogeneic stem cell transplantation compared to CAMPATH bsed T cell depletion regimens: a preliminary report. *Blood* 1999;94(Suppl 1):668.
50. Rizzieri DA, Long GD, Vredenburgh J, et al. Chimerism mediated immunotherapy using CAMPATH T cell depleted peripheral blood ptogenitor cells with nonablative therapy provides reliable, durable, allogeneic engraftment. *Blood* 2000;96(Suppl 1):2241.
51. Aversa F, Tabilio A, Velardi A, et al. Treatment of high risk acute leukemia with T cell depleted stem cells from related donors with one fully mismatched HLA haplotype. *N Engl J Med* 1998;339:1186–1193.
52. Bornhauser M, Neubauer A, Thiede C, et al. Allogeneic blood stem cell transplants from unrelated donors after nonablative conditioning therapy. *Blood* 1998;92(Suppl 1):4530.
53. Schetelig J, Held T, Bornhauser M, et al. Nonmyeloablative allogeneic stem cell transplantation in chronic lymphocytic leukemia from related and unrelated donors. *Blood* 2000;96(Suppl 1):857.
54. Peggs KS, Mahendra P, Milligan DW, et al. Non myeloablatvie transplantation using matche dunrelated donors-in vivo campath 1H limits graft versus host disease.
55. Nagler A, Or R, Varadi g, Shapira M, Slavin S. Fludarabine based low intensity conditioning protocol for unrelated matched stem cell transplantation in chronic myelogenous leukemia. *Blood* 2000;96(Suppl 1):5322.
56. Nagler A, Or R, Naparstek E, et al. A non-myeloablative regimen may suffice for engraftment of allogeneic mismatched related stem cell transplantation but not of unrelated bone marrow transplantation with a similar degree of HLA mismatch. *Blood* 1998;92(Suppl 1):2815.

57. Rizzieri DA, Long GD, Vredenburgh JJ, et al. Successful allogeneic engraftment of mismatched unrelated cord blood following a non-myeloablative preparative regimen. *Blood* 2001;98:3486–3488.

58. Ueno N, Rondon G, Mirza N, et al. Allogeneic peripheral blood progenitor cell transplantation for poor risk patients with metastatic breast cancer. *J Clin Oncol* 1998;16:986–993 .

59. Childs RW, Clave E, Tisdale J, et al. Successful treatment of metastatic renal cell carcinoma with a nonmyeloablative allogeneic peripheral blood progenitor cell transplant: evidence for a graft versus tumor effect. *J Clin Oncol* 1999;17:2044–2049.

60. Childs R, Bahceci E, Clave E, et al. Non-myeloablative peripheral blood stem cell transplants for malignant disease reduces transplant related mortality. *Blood* 1998;92(Supp 1):552.

61. Childs R, Chernoff A, Contentin N, et al. Regression of metastatic renal cell carcinoma after nonmyeloablative allogeneic peripheral blood stem cell transplantation. *N Engl J Med* 2000;343:750–758.

62. Seong C, Lee S, Im S, et al. HLA identical peripheral blood progrenitor cells transplantation for metastatic gastric carcinoma using non-myeloablative conditioning regimen. *Blood* 1998;92(Suppl 1):4270.

63. Childs RW, Bradstock KF, Gottlieb D, et al. Non-myeloablative allogeneic stem cell transplantation as immunotherapy for metastatic melanoma: results of a pilot study. *Blood* 2000;96(Suppl 1):5277.

64. Woolfrey A, Nash R, Frangoul H, et al. Non-myeloablative transplant regimen used for induction of multi lineage allogeneic hematopoietic mixed donor-host chimerism in patients with T cell immunodeficiency. *Blood* 1998;92(Suppl 1):2135.

65. Walters MC, Patience M, Leisenring W, et al. Collaborative multicenter investigation of marrow transplantation for sickle cell disease: current results and future directions. *Biol Blood Marrow Transplant* 1997;3:310–315.

66. Lucarelli G, Clift RA, Galimberti M, et al. Marrow transplantation for patients with thalassemia: results in class 3 patients. *Blood* 1996;87:2082–2088.

67. Krishnamurti L, Blazer B, Grossi M, et al. Successful use of non-myeloablative therapy in the treatment of severe hemoglobinopathies: proof of principle. *Blood* 2000;96(Suppl 1):3734.

68. Toh HC, Preffer F, Spitzer TR, et al. Characterization of phenotypic and functional lymphocyte reconstitution in adult patients with chemoradiorefractory hematologic malignancies receiving a non-myeloablative conditioning therapy and HLA matched and mismatched donor bone marrow transplantation. *Blood* 1998;92(Suppl 1):2818.

69. Bahceci E, Epperson D, Patibandla A, et al. Rapid reconstitution of T cell compartment after non-myeloablative allogeneic stem cell transplantation. *Blood* 1999;94(Suppl 1):590.

70. Childs R, Clave E, Contentin N, et al. Engraftment kinetics after nonmyeloablative allogeneic peripheral blood stem cell transplantation: full donor T cell chimerism preceded alloimmune responses. *Blood* 1999;94:3234–3241.

71. Keil F, Kalhs P, Haas O, et al. Relapse of Philadelphia chromosome positive acute lymphoblastic leukemia after marrow transplantation: sustained molecular remission after early and dose- escalating infusion of donor leukocytes. *Br J Haematol* 1997;97:161–164.

72. Ruggeri L, Capanni M, Urbani E, et al. KIR epitope incompatibility in th eGvH direction predicts control of leukemia relapse after mismatched hematopoietic transplantation. *Blood* 2000;96(Suppl 1):2059.

IV   SUPPORTIVE CARE
IN ALLOGENEIC TRANSPLANTATION

14

Recent Developments in Epidemiology and Management of Invasive Fungal Infections

Andreas H. Groll and Thomas J. Walsh

1. INTRODUCTION

Invasive fungal infections (IFIs) have emerged as important causes of morbidity and mortality following allogeneic hematopoietic stem cell transplantation (HSCT). Depending on the institution and the transplantation protocol, the overall frequency of IFIs in this setting ranges from 10–25%, and crude mortality exceeds 70% and is close to 100% in patients with disseminated disease or persistent deficiencies in host defenses *(1,2)*. Coinciding with the rapid evolution of HSCT and supportive care, the epidemiology of IFIs continues to evolve and considerable progress has been made in the development of novel therapeutics and strategies for antifungal prevention and treatment.

2. EVOLUTION OF RISK FACTORS AND HOST SUSCEPTIBILITY

The vast majority of invasive mycoses in allogeneic HSCT recipients are caused by opportunistic fungi. *Candida* species and *Aspergillus* species are the most commonly isolated pathogens *(3)*. Invasive *Candida* infections can be classified as candidemia or acute disseminated candidiasis with or without fungemia, and arise by the entry of the organism into the bloodstream from colonized mucosal surfaces or catheters. In contrast, invasive infections by *Aspergillus* spp. primarily affect the paranasal sinuses and the lungs and are initiated by

From: *Current Clinical Oncology: Allogeneic Stem Cell Transplantation*
Edited by: Mary S. Laughlin and Hillard M. Lazarus © Humana Press Inc., Totowa, NJ

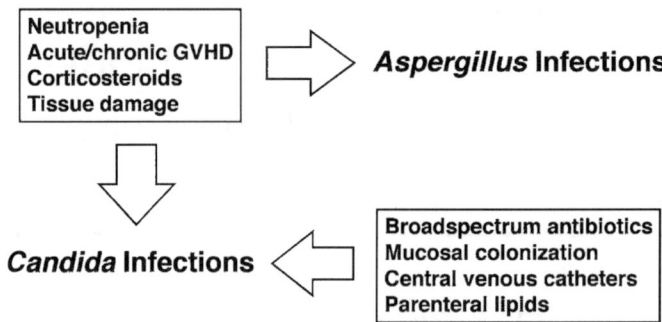

Fig. 1. Overview of established risk factors for invasive fungal infections by *Aspergillus* spp. and *Candida* spp. in the setting of allogeneic hematopoietic. Specific risk factors for emerging pathogens have not been formally defined. As a general rule, however, risk factors for infections by yeast-like organisms appear similar to those known from *Candida* spp., and risk factors for infections by emerging filamentous fungi resemble those of *Aspergillus* spp.

exposure to airborne conidia of the organism *(4)*. Despite differences in biology, mode of acquisition, and disease pattern, the most important clinical risk factors for these two groups of fungal pathogens following allogeneic are prolonged and profound granulocytopenia and use of corticosteroids in pharmacological dosages (Fig. 1). This is reflected in the classical bimodal risk distribution pattern of allogeneic bone marrow transplant patients with an early peak during the pre-engraftment phase that is characterized by granulocytopenia and mucosal damage and a late peak early post-engraftment that corresponds to the onset of acute graft-vs-host disease (GVHD) and its treatment with corticosteroids *(3)*. While little more than a decade ago, the overwhelming majority of IFIs in allogeneic stem cell recipients used to occur in temporal association with the pre-engraftment period *(5)*, most infections now are diagnosed late and even very late, i.e., more than 6 mo after transplantation *(6–8)*. This shift coincided with the advent of effective approaches to decrease early *Candida*-related and cytomegalovirus (CMV)-related morbidity and mortality, but may also be related to a shortening of the pre-engraftment phase through the introduction of hematopoetic growth factors, the increased stem cell content of peripheral allogeneic grafts, and more recently, the introduction of nonmyeloablative HSCT. On the other hand, transplantation of T cell-depleted or CD34+ selected grafts, the increasing utilization of alternate donors, and potent T cell-specific immunosuppression with antithymocyte globulin (ATG), monoclonal antibodies, or fludarabine-based regimens has led to a growing subset of patients with profound and prolonged deficits of T cell function *(9)*. While mono- and polymorphonuclear phagocytes are crucial effectors, a quantitatively and qualitatively intact production of T helper cell cytokines may contribute substantially to host defenses against invasive infections by *Candida* spp. and *Aspergillus* spp. In support of this notion are earlier observations of an increased risk for invasive candidiasis in T cell-depleted allogeneic bone marrow transplant recipients *(5)* and, later on, the occurrence of invasive *Aspergillus* infections in patients with advanced human immunodeficiency virus (HIV)-infection *(10,11)*. Indeed, recent experimental investigations, in murine models of disseminated candidiasis and disseminated and pulmonary aspergillosis collectively, suggest that a Th1-type cytokine response is critical to mobilize and activate fungicidal phagocytes, whereas a predominantly Th2-type cytokine pattern deactivates phagocytic effector cells and leads to progressive disease *(12–14)*. Non-neutropenic patients with chronic disseminated candidiasis *(15)* and invasive aspergillosis *(16)* have been shown to have significantly higher plasma levels of interleukin (IL)-10 as compared to controls or patients with other infections, which suggests that Th1-Th2 imbalances may play a pathogenetic role in this setting. These new insights not only help to explain the association of GVHD and T cell depletion and dysfunction, respectively, with the occurrence of IFIs in allogeneic stem cell recipients, but also provide potential avenues for novel preventive and adjuvant immunotherapies.

3. SHIFTS IN FUNGAL PATHOGENS

The last decade has witnessed striking shifts in the microbiological etiology of IFIs in the setting of allogeneic HSCT (Table 1). Most notable is the overall decrease in invasive candidiasis *(7,17–19)*, which traditionally accounted for the majority of invasive mycoses in the 1980s *(5)*. However, this decrease has been counterbalanced by a steady increase in invasive *Aspergillus* infections *(8,20)*, the emergence of non-*albicans Candida* spp. *(7,21)* and previously uncommon fungal pathogens (22), and an increasing number of patients with chronic mold infections *(23,24)*. In comparison, the frequency of endemic mycoses *(25–27)* is overall low and appears unchanged in patients who live in endemic areas.

An increase of *Aspergillus* spp., predominantly late after transplantation, has been observed in centers around the globe *(8,20,28)*. In some centers, the organism has become the most common cause of pneumonic death in allogeneic stem cell recipients *(29)*. This shift is epidemiologically associated with the introduction of fluconazole prophylaxis and effective prevention of CMV disease, which led to a significant decrease in early infectious morbidity and mortality and an increasing pool of severely immunocompromised patients at high risk. As exemplified for *A. terreus (30,31)*, non-*fumigatus Aspergillus* spp. may be less susceptible to amphotericin B, underscoring the need for a microbiological diagnosis and development of predictive in vitro testing methods.

In addition to the expanding frequency of invasive aspergillosis, previously uncommon opportunistic fungi are increasingly encountered in allogeneic HSCT recipients *(22,32)*. These emerging pathogens include, among others, yeast-like pathogens (such as *Trichosporon* spp. and *Blastoschizomyces capitatus*), hyaline filamentous fungi (such as *Paecilomyces* spp., *Fusarium* spp., *Pseudallescheria boydii*, and *Scedosporium prolificans*), a large variety of dematiaceous molds (such as *Bipolaris* spp., *Exophiala* spp., and *Alternaria* spp.), and the Zygomycetes *(22,32–34)*. While the yeast-like organisms follow the pattern of fungemia and dissemination known from *Candida* spp., the emerging filamentous fungi cause infections that are virtually indistinguishable from those of *Aspergillus* spp. *(22)*. However, some of the hyaline molds, including *Fusarium* spp., *Paecilomyces* spp., and *Acremonium* spp., disseminate via the bloodstream, which often allows for the detection of the organism in blood culture systems and embolic skin lesions. Infections by the emerging fungal pathogens display exceedingly high case fatality rates; several of these organisms, in *particular Trichosporon beigelii (35,36)*, *Paecilomyces lilacinus (37,38)*, *Fusarium* spp. *(39,40)*, *Pseudallescheria boydii (41,42)*, and *Scedosporium prolificans (43,44)* are not inherently susceptible to amphotericin B and may require therapies with alternative agents *(22)* (Tables 2, 3, and 4), underscoring again the importance of microbiological identification and development of in vitro testing methods that predict resistance.

Approximately 50% of allogeneic stem cell recipients are colonized with *Candida* spp. prior to conditioning. Without chemoprophylaxis, proven invasive candidiasis develops in up to 15% and is associated with a crude mortality of 40–50% and close to 100% with documented involvement of deep tissue sites *(2,45)*. The introduction of fluconazole prophylaxis in the early 1990s had a major impact on the epidemiology of IFIs after allogeneic marrow transplantation. A randomized double-blind placebo-controlled clinical trial conducted at the Fred Hutchinson Cancer Research Center demonstrated that prophylaxis with fluconazole 400 mg/d administered from the start of the conditioning regimen until d 75 may reduce the frequency

Table 1
Spectrum of fungal pathogens in the setting of allogeneic SCT[a]

| Yeasts | Molds | | | | |
| | Septate hyphae | | | | Aseptate hyphae |
	Hyaline molds	Pigmented molds	Dimorphic molds		Zygomycetes
Candida albicans	**Aspergillus spp.**	Bipolaris spp.	Histoplasma capsulatum		Rhizopus spp.
Non-albicans Candida spp.	Fusarium spp.	Exophiala spp.	Coccidioidesimmitis		Mucor spp.
Cryptococcus neoformans	Pseudallescheria boydii	Alternaria spp.	Blastomycesdermatidis		Rhizomucor spp.
Trichosporonbeigelii	Scedosporium prolificans				Absidia spp.
Blastoschizomyces capitatus	Paecilomyces spp. and				
	Acremonium spp.				

[a]Most frequently encountered pathogens are depicted in bold face.

Table 2
Antifungal Agents for Prevention and Treatment of Invasive Fungal Infections

Class and compounds	Mechanism of action	Comment
Polyene antibiotics Amphotericin B deoxycholate Amphotericin B colloidal dispersion Amphotericin B lipid complex Liposomal amphotericin Liposomal nystatin[a]	Intercalation with ergosterol in fungal cell membranes, leading to the formation of ion-channels and concentration-dependent cell death.	Broad-spectrum rapid mostly cidal antifungal activity. Primary resistance uncommon except for some of the emerging pathogens; secondary resistance virtually nonexistent. Clinical utility compromised by renal toxicity and unfusion-related reactions; both are reduced to a variable degree with the lipid formulations.
Antifungal triazoles Fluconazole Itraconazole Posaconazole[a] Ravuconazole[a] Voriconazole[a]	Inhibition of ergosterol biosynthesis, leading to ergosterol depletion and accumulation of potentially toxic alternative sterols in the fungal cell membrane.	With exception of fluconazole, broad-spectrum antifungal activity; generally static against yeast-like organisms and cidal against filamentous molds. Primary resistance common in C. krusei; secondary resistance observed after long-term exposure. Usually well-tolerated. Clinical utility somewhat compromised by interference with CYP450-mediated oxidative metabolism (all), the possibility of primary and secondary resistance (all), and variations in plasma pharmacokinetics (itraconazole, voriconazole).
Echinocandin lipopeptides Anidulofungin[a] Caspofungin Micafungin[a]	Inhibition of glucan biosynthesis, leading to disruption of the fungal cell wall, osmotic instability, and, organism-dependent cell death.	Broad-spectrum and mostly cidal antifungal activity against Candida spp.; not entirely cidal activity against Aspergillus spp.; well-tolerated and devoid of significant CYP450-mediated oxidative metabolism. Spectrum appears limited to Candida spp. and Aspergillus spp.
Nucleoside analogs 5-Flucytosine	Intracellular deamination to 5-fluorouracil; interference with both DNA and RNA synthesis–function.	Broad-spectrum mostly static activity against yeast-like pathogens and certain dematiaceous molds; favorable pharmacokinetics. High propensity for secondary resistance; indications therefore restricted to combination therapy of cerebral crytococcosis and complicated Candida spp. infections.

[a]Investigational.

Table 3
Chemotherapy of Invasive Infections by Opportunistic Yeasts

Fungal disease	Chemotherapy
Invasive Candidiasis	
Uncomplicated fungemia	D-AmB (0.5–1.0 mg/kg/d)
Fluconazole[a,b] (400–800 mg/d)	
Acute single site or disseminated	D-AmB (0.5–1.0 mg/kg/d) ± 5-FC[c] (100 mg/kg/d)
candidiasis ± fungemia	Fluconazole[a,b] (400–800 mg/d)
	AmB lipid formulations[d] (5 mg/kg/d starting dose)
	Echinocandin-lipopeptides (investigational)
	2nd generation triazoles (investigational)
Trichosporon and Blastoschizomyces	Fluconazole[a] (400–800 mg/d) ± D-AmB (≥1.0 mg/kg/d)
infection	2nd generation triazoles (investigational)
Cryptococcosis	D-AmB (0.7 mg/kg/d) plus 5-FC[c] (100 mg/kg/d) for a
	minimum of 2 wk (induction), followed instable
	patients by fluconazole[a] (400 mg/d) for consolidation
	and maintenance.
	L-AmB (AmBisome™; 5 mg/kg/d)[d]
Other rare yeast infections	D-AmB (0.5–1.0 mg/kg/d) ± 5-FC[c] (100 mg/kg/d)
(Rhodotorula rubra, Hansenula anomala,	Fluconazole[a,b] (400–800 mg/d)
Saccharomyces cerevisiae, others)	

[a]Loading dose: twice the target dose on the first day of treatment. Dose adjustment may be required with reduced creatinine clearance and high dosages.

[b]Only for identified and in vitro susceptible isolates.

[c]Monitoring of serum levels required (<100 µg/mL; target: 40–60 µg/mL). Dose adjustment with reduced creatinine clearance.

[d]In patients intolerant or refractory to amphotericin B deoxycholate (D-AmB).

of invasive *Candida* infections and lower both attributable and overall mortality at d 110 *(18)*. Even more striking, the recently published follow-up at 8 yr after completion of the study showed a persistent protection against invasive candidiasis and *Candida*-related death, a decreased frequency of severe gut-related GVHD, and an overall survival benefit of 17% that was independent of the underlying condition and the occurrence of relapses *(46)*. The impact of fluconazole prophylaxis also is reflected in autopsy data from the same institution that document a lower prevalence of invasive candidiasis in patients who had received ≥5 doses of fluconazole as compared to patients that had not received prophylaxis with fluconazole *(19)*. These data are corroborated by a multivariant analysis of allogeneic stem cell recipients with chronic myeloic leukemia and unrelated donors that showed fluconazole prophylaxis as independently predictive of survival *(47)*.

A potential drawback of fluconazole prophylaxis may be the selection of resistant *Candida* spp. in patients receiving the drug and, more generally, the generation of selective antifungal pressure in the nosocomial environment. During the past decade, non-*albicans Candida* spp. have assumed increasing importance as causes of nosocomial infections in immunocompromised patients *(21,48–51)*. According to an international prospective survey of invasive candidiasis in cancer patients, antifungal prophylaxis with azoles and hematological malignancy were significantly associated with infections by non-*albicans Candida* spp. *(21)*, and the emergence of *C. glabrata* and *C. krusei* infections in association with fluconazole prophylaxis has been reported from individual centers *(52–54)*. A recently published study from Seattle in 585 patients with allogeneic HSCT and fluconazole prophylaxis (400 mg/d until d 75), however, showed a low incidence of breakthrough candidemia (i.e., 4.6%; in two-

Table 4
Chemotherapy of Invasive Infections by Opportunistic Molds

Fungal disease	Chemotherapy
Aspergillus infections	
A.fumigatus	D-AmB (1.0–1.5 mg/kg/d)
A.flavus	Voriconazole[a] (4 mg/kg BID)
A.niger	AmB lipid formulations[b] (5 mg/kg/d starting dose)
A. terreus	Itraconazole[c,d] (200–600 mg/d)
	Caspofungin[e] (50 mg/d)
	2nd generation antifungal triazoles (investigational)
Fusarium infections	
F. solani	D-AmB (1.0–1.5 mg/kg/d)
F. oxysporon	AmB lipid formulations[b] (5 mg/kg/d starting dose)
. *F. moniliforme*	Itraconazole*d* (200–600 mg/d; only for 2nd line therapy
Acremonium infections	of *P. variotii, Ps. boydii,* and *S. apiospermum* infections)
Paecilomyces infections	2nd generation antifungal triazoles (investigational)
P. lilacinus	*S. prolificans*: consider high-dose lipid-based AmB or
P. variotii	combination of itraconazole and terbinafine.
Pseudallescheria infections	
Pseudallescheria boydii	
Scedosporium apiospermum	
Scedosporium prolificans	
Infections by pigmented molds	
Bipolaris	D-AmB (1.0–1.5 mg/kg/d) ± 5-FC[f] (100 mg/kg/d)
Exophiala	or Lipid formulations of AmB[b] (5 mg/kg/d starting
Alternaria and other	dose) or Itraconazole*d* (200–600 mg/d) or 2nd
	generation antifungal triazoles (investigational)
Zygomycetes infections	
Rhizopus spp.	D-AmB (1.0–1.5 mg/kg/d)
Mucor spp.	Lipid formulations of AmB[b] (5 mg/kg/d starting dose)
Absidia spp.	
Infections by endemic molds	
H. capsulatum	D-AmB (0.5–1.0 mg/kg/d)
B. dermatidis	Itraconazole[c,d] (200–400 mg/d; *Histoplasma* and *Blastomyces*)
C. immitis	Fluconazole*g* (400–800 mg/d; *Coccidioides immitis*)

[a]A recently published open randomized trial has demonstrated superior response rates and improved survival at wk 12 of voriconazole (6 mg/kg iv for two doses, followed by 4 mg/kg iv every 12 h with option to switch to 200 mg PO BID) in comparison to amphotericin B deoxycholate (D-AmB) (1 mg/kg/d). Approval of this indication by the Food and Drug Administration (FDA) was pending at the time of the preparation of this manuscript.

[b]In patients intolerant or refractory to D-AmB.

[c]For maintenance in stable patients.

[d]Monitoring of serum levels recommended (>0.5 μg/mL (HPLC) or >2.0 μg/mL (bio-assay) at trough. Loading dose: 200 mg tid over 3 d. Maximum: 600 mg/d. IV therapy: 200 mg BID over 2 d, followed by 200 mg QD (maximum: 14 d).

[e]In patients intolerant of or refractory to standard therapy; loading dose: 70 mg on d 1 of therapy.

*f*Monitoring of serum levels required (<100 μg/mL; target: 40–60 μg/mL). Dose adjustment with reduced creatinine clearance.

[g]Loading dose: twice the target dose on the first day of treatment. Dose adjustment may be required with reduced creatinine clearance and high dosages.

Abbreviations: BID, twice daily; PO, orally; HPLC, high-pressure liquid chromatography; TID, 3× daily; QD, 4× daily.

thirds caused by *C. glabrata* or *C. krusei*) and a low attributable mortality (i.e., 20%) despite frequent colonization with fluconazole-resistant *Candida* spp. *(7)*. Nevertheless, selection and nosocomial spread of azole-resistant *Candida* isolates appear inevitable and remain a matter of continued concern.

4. EXPANSION OF THERAPEUTIC OPTIONS

For more than three decades, the treatment of IFIs was essentially limited to amphotericin B deoxycholate (D-AmB) with or without 5-fluorocytosine (5-FC). Therapeutic options only emerged with the clinical development of fluconazole and itraconazole in the late 1980s. The past 10 yr, however, have witnessed a major expansion in antifungal drug research, reflected by the introduction of the lipid formulations of amphotericin B and the development of novel echinocandin derivatives and improved antifungal triazoles *(55)* (Table 2). Considerable progress also has been achieved in harmonizing disease definitions, in defining paradigms for antifungal interventions (Table 5), and in designing and implementing clinical trials *(56–58)*. A standardized method for testing the in vitro susceptibility of yeasts to current antifungal agents has become available *(59)*, and a similar method has been proposed for filamentous fungi *(60)*. However, mainly due to ongoing methodological problems and the pivotal role of host- and disease-related factors for outcome, prediction of antifungal efficacy or failure from in vitro susceptibility data remains difficult and has not been incorporated in clinical practice *(61)*.

D-AmB historically has been the standard treatment of most invasive opportunistic fungal infections in immunocompromised patients (Tables 2, 3, and 4). The recommended dosages of D-AmB range from 0.5 to 1.0 mg/kg/d for candidemia to 1.0 to 1.5 mg/kg for acute disseminated candidiasis and suspected or proven invasive aspergillosis *(4)*. Apart from infusion-related reactions, however, treatment with high dosages of D-AmB is associated with significant nephrotoxicity. A recent multicenter retrospective analysis of more than 200 immunocompromised patients receiving D-AmB for suspected or proven aspergillosis revealed that the serum creatinine level doubled in 53% of patients and exceeded 2.5 mg/dL in 29%; 14.5% of the patients underwent dialysis. Patients whose creatinine level exceeded 2.5 mg/dL and allogeneic marrow recipients were at greatest risk for requiring hemodialysis; use of hemodialysis, duration of therapy with D-AmB, and use of nephrotoxic agents such as cyclosporine A were associated with greater risk of death *(62)*.

The advent of the lipid formulations of AmB (AmB colloidal dispersion, ABCD, Amphotec™; AmB lipid complex, ABLC, Abelcet™; and liposomal AmB, L-AmB, AmBisome™) represents a major advance in the management of life-threatening invasive opportunistic mycoses, particularly on allogeneic stem cell transplant recipients. Open label clinical trials have demonstrated that the lipid formulations of AmB are, overall, less nephrotoxic but at least as effective as D-AmB *(63–70)*. The lipid formulations may thus be indicated when preexisting or arising nephrotoxicity or concomitant nephrotoxic agents precludes the delivery of therapeutically effective dosages of D-AmB or when treatment with D-AmB fails to induce a response to an otherwise susceptible organism (Tables 3 and 4) *(71–73)*. The frequency of infusion-related reactions varies among the different compounds *(74–76)*; with AmB colloidal dispersion, frequency and severity of infusion-related reactions may exceed those associated with D-AmB *(74)*. While the optimal dosages of the lipid formulations for most therapeutic indications remain to be defined, there is considerable uncertainty among physicians regarding dose along with a tendency to compensate for high acquisition cost by cutting dosages. However, based on the concentration- and dosage-dependent activity of AmB in vitro and in animal models *(77)*, and the few randomized studies that have used D-AmB for comparison *(64,66,78)*, we strongly advocate the use of the highest approved dosages of the lipid formulations for treatment of suspected or documented infections.

The introduction of fluconazole clearly has had major impact on the management of fungal infections, largely due to its exceptionally favorable pharmacokinetic and toxicological pro-

Table 5
Paradigms of Antifungal Interventions in Patients with Cancer

Intervention	Basis
Primary prophylaxis	High-risk (>10%) and high mortality.
Empirical therapy	Neutropenia and fever not responding to broad spectrum antibacterial agents.
Preemptive therapy of probable infections	Clinical, radiographic, or serological findings indicative of an invasive fungal infection.

Therapy of proven infections
  Induction
  Consolidation
  Maintenance
	Microbiologically and/or microscopically proven invasive fungal infection.

Secondary prophylaxis	High risk of exacerbation and/or recurrence of documented infections during continued immunosuppression.

file. The drug is active against most pathogenic *Candida* spp. and several other yeast-like fungi *(55)*. Despite its apparently fungistatic activity *(77)*, experimental *(79)*, and clinical *(80,81)* data support the usefulness of fluconazole (400–800 mg/kg/d intravenously [iv]) for treatment of uncomplicated candidemia in neutropenic patients who are hemodynamically stable; the use of fluconazole in neutropenic patients with acute disseminated candidiasis is controversial and warrants further investigation *(4)*. Nevertheless, in allogeneic stem cell recipients, the role of fluconazole as a therapeutic agent is very limited by its widespread use for antifungal prophylaxis. Breakthrough infections in this setting are highly likely to be caused by fluconazole-resistant *Candida* species, including *C. glabrata*, *C. krusei* and fluconazole-resistant *C. albicans* isolates *(7)*. Therefore, AmB remains the current agent of choice for most allogeneic HSCT recipients with positive blood cultures for a yeast-like organism (Table 3). For the near future, however, the echinocandins hold great promise to provide a valid alternative to treatment of invasive candidiasis with AmB *(82,83)*.

Itraconazole has become an important therapeutic option for the treatment of IFIs caused by *Aspergillus* spp., *Ps. boydii*, and many dematiaceous molds (Table 4). While itraconazole has potent activity against *Candida* spp. in vitro, no clinical data exists on its efficacy for treatment of invasive *Candida* infections *(55)*. Besides clinically relevant drug–drug interactions, including but not limited to cyclosporine A, the therapeutic usefulness of itraconazole was for long curtailed by the lack of an iv formulation and erratic absorption from the gastrointestinal tract. Oral bioavailability has been considerably improved with the novel suspension in cyclodextrin *(84)*, and an iv formulation that uses the same principle as carrier has recently been approved in the U.S. However, despite response rates that overall are similar to those of D-AmB, the reported clinical experience with itraconazole in either formulation for induction therapy of suspected or proven invasive aspergillosis, particularly in profoundly neutropenic patients, is still limited *(85–87)*. Nevertheless, itraconazole has an important role for consolidation therapy of patients with invasive aspergillosis *(4)* and for therapy of certain infections caused by dematiaceous molds *(22)*.

The ongoing development of echinocandin lipopeptides and novel antifungal triazoles has already opened new horizons for the treatment of invasive aspergillosis. Based on a complete or partial response in 41% of 63 patients enrolled on a clinical phase II trial for invasive aspergillosis *(88)*, the echinocandin caspofungin was approved in early 2001 for treatment of invasive aspergillosis refractory of or intolerant to AmB formulations or antifungal triazoles (Table 4). Because of mild and transient hepatic transaminase elevations in single-dose interaction studies, however, the concomitant use of caspofungin and cyclosporin (but not tacrolimus) is currently not recommended. More recently, a multinational open randomized comparison of the second-generation triazole voriconazole and D-AmB, followed by other licensed antifungal therapy for primary therapy, of invasive aspergillosis has been completed *(89)*. Therapy with voriconazole resulted in superior antifungal efficacy and improved survival at wk 12. Approval by the regulatory authorities was provided, and the results of this pivotal study suggest that voriconazole will replace D-AmB as the standard agent for induction therapy of invasive aspergillosis (Table 4).

5. REFINED ANTIFUNGAL PREVENTION AND EMPIRICAL THERAPY

The high morbidity and mortality from invasive opportunistic fungal infections following allogeneic HSCT provide the rationale for preventive approaches. Apart from nosocomial infection control measures, current paradigms for prevention include primary chemoprophylaxis, empirical antifungal therapy, and secondary chemoprophylaxis for HSCT candidates with a preexisting deep-seated fungal infection (Table 5).

As discussed earlier in greater detail, effective primary chemoprophylaxis of IFIs has been demonstrated for *Candida* species and has had a major impact on the epidemiology of IFIs in allogeneic patients. Fluconazole, given at 400 mg/d administered from the start of the conditioning regimen until d 75, may reduce the frequency of invasive *Candida* infections, lower overall mortality at d 110 *(18)*, and may have a significant impact on long-term survival, independent of the underlying condition and the occurrence of relapses *(46)*. Considering this substantial benefit and the overall minor risk of prolonged therapy with this agent, there is little to argue against the routine use of this prophylactic regimen in the setting of allogeneic HSCT. Nevertheless, selection and spread of resistant *Candida* spp. and the compound's ineffectiveness against filamentous fungi remain important drawbacks of antifungal prophylaxis with fluconazole. Thus, investigations of the utility of agents with a broader spectrum are clearly warranted. Of note, no clinical trials have been published on the use of itraconazole as antifungal prophylaxis following allogeneic HSCT. The drug has been shown to be effective in preventing candidemia and death due to candidemia in patients with hematological malignancies undergoing remission induction chemotherapy *(90)*; effective chemoprophylaxis against infections by *Aspergillus* spp., however, has not been demonstrated thus far *(91–93)*. Apart from studies that compare prophylaxis with itraconazole *(94)* or current investigational agents to fluconazole as the standard of antifungal prophylaxis during the first 75–100 d posttransplantation, clinical trials are under way that investigate preventive approaches targeted for patients requiring aggressive immunosuppression for acute or chronic GVHD. Given the high risk of infections by filamentous molds in these situations, participation in one of these trials or administration of an approved agent with documented efficacy against these organism should be offered for the time of increased immunosuppression.

Hematopoietic stem cell recipients who have persistent or recurrent fever despite treatment with broad-spectrum antibacterial agents are considered to be at high risk for developing an IFIs. In this setting, broad spectrum empirical antifungal therapy provides effective antifungal prophylaxis and early therapy for clinically occult infections *(95–97)* that may arise despite prophylaxis with fluconazole. Agents approved for this indication in the U.S. include D-AmB (Fungizone™; 0.6 mg/kg/d) and L-AmB (AmBisome™; 3 mg/kg/d). Two large randomized multicenter trials, one of which included patients after allogeneic HSCT, have shown that L-AmB is as effective as D-AmB while being associated with less infusion-related toxicity, less nephrotoxicity *(75,98)*, and fewer proven breakthrough fungal infections *(75)*. Efficacy equivalent to D-AmB has also been demonstrated for itraconazole (administered iv for a minimum of 6 d and a maximum of 14 d, followed by oral suspension) *(99)* and iv fluconazole *(100)* in patients with hematological malignancies not receiving allogeneic grafts. Very recently, a large randomized multicenter trial has been completed that compared voriconazole, an investigational broad-spectrum triazole, with L-AmB for empirical antifungal therapy *(101)*. The preliminary results of this study, which included a large number of recipients of allogeneic HSCT recipients, showed comparable composite success rates but less proven and probable breakthrough infections, infusion-related toxicity, and nephrotoxicity in the voriconazole-treated cohort. However, patients receiving voriconazole had significantly more frequent episodes of transient visual disturbances and hallucination. Trials are currently under way that investigate the role of other novel triazoles and of antifungal echinocandins for this indication.

The presence of a deeply invasive fungal infection is no longer considered an absolute contraindication for allogeneic *(102)*. Two small observational studies indicate that the majority of patients with at least stable chronic disseminated candidiasis continue to improve with continuing antifungal chemotherapy *(23,103,104)*. Similarly, patients with invasive aspergillosis, who had at least a partial response, can be successfully transplanted provided that they receive continuing antifungal chemotherapy with agents that are effective against *Aspergillus* spp. *(24,105)*. A recent retrospective analysis suggests that the type of antifungal therapy, surgical resection of residual lesions, and the achievement of a complete response to antifungal therapy prior to transplantation had no predictive importance *(24)*.

6. ADVANCES IN EARLY DIAGNOSIS AND PREEMPTIVE THERAPY

Successful management of IFIs relies on an early diagnosis with prompt institution of effective antifungal chemotherapy. Improved blood culture detection techniques such as the lysis-centrifugation and the BacTec Alert system are able to detect candidemia earlier and more frequently than conventional systems *(4)*. However, it must be emphasized that candidemia is only one manifestation of invasive candidiasis and that single-organ or early-disseminated candidiasis are not reliably detected by blood culture techniques and may, therefore, require more invasive diagnostic procedures *(106)*. For such tissue-invasive *Candidia* infections, ultrasound, high-resolution computed tomography (HRCT), and magnetic resonance imaging (MRI) have become indispensable tools for detection, monitoring, and guidance of diagnostic procedures *(107–110)*. In the future, nonculture techniques—particularly nucleic acid amplification-based systems—may complement existing blood culture systems not only for early detection purposes, but also for determining resistance patterns to antifungal agents *(111)*.

Apart from improved detection of invasive mold infections of the paranasal sinuses *(112)*, the advent of modern imaging techniques has also permitted earlier detection of pulmonary infiltrates consistent with invasive pulmonary aspergillosis and early preemptive treatment *(113–115)*. However, although peripheral nodules, the halo-sign, and cavitation are all characteristic of pulmonary aspergillosis, these radiological criteria are not entirely specific, and nonspecific air space consolidation is common in early phases *(116)*. Accordingly, a microbiological diagnosis by fiberoptic bronchoscopy with bronchoalveolar lavage or bioptic measures, if feasible, is encouraged to the greatest extent possible. Serial monitoring of galactomannan antigen and *Aspergillus*-specific nucleic acid sequences in blood *(117–120)* may also contribute substantially to the detection of invasive pulmonary aspergillosis, particularly in the neutropenic host, and warrants further investigation.

Current approaches to prophylactic and empirical antifungal therapy treat more patients than those that would ultimately develop IFIs. Fever refractory to broad-spectrum antibacterial agents in the setting of profound neutropenia currently serves as the more sensitive, albeit less specific, surrogate for treating patients at high risk. Similar to the setting of CMV disease, nonculture detection systems, such as the galactomannan antigen assay and polymerase chain reaction (PCR)-based techniques, may permit further narrowing of the population at highest risk. Carefully-designed clinical trials will be needed to determine the role of these preemptive strategies in comparison to fever-based empirical antifungal therapy and primary chemoprevention.

7. THE EVOLVING ROLE OF SURGERY

Surgical interventions are important therapeutic options in the management of fungal endocarditis, endopthalmitis, central nervous system (CNS) lesions, progressive sinusitis, infections of bones and joints, skin and soft tissue lesions, and other focal processes amenable to a surgical procedure *(4,121,122)*. Surgery can also be an important consideration in the management of patients with invasive pulmonary aspergillosis, although its exact role has not been defined. Surgery may prevent local extension and hematogenous dissemination and may be curative *(123)*. Several case series suggest that surgery can be safely and effectively performed in patients who have localized infection *(115,123–127)*, even during neutropenia *(115,125)*. In a recent series of 36 patients with hematological malignancies and proven or probable invasive pulmonary aspergillosis, surgery combined with medical treatment was successful in 15 out of 16 patients. In four cases, the intervention was performed for diagnostic purposes, and in 12 cases, intervention was performed for therapeutic purposes. In eight of the latter cases, surgery was an emergency procedure based on observations by repeat chest CT scans that showed contact of lesions with larger pulmonary arteries; six of these patients were neutropenic. Surgery was uneventful in all cases. Serial CT scans were an important part of this novel approach, and altogether, 72% of 36 patients responded to medical or combined medical and surgical treatment *(115)*. Indeed, the risk of exsanguination from the erosion of a major pulmonary artery ought not be underestimated. Panos et al. found that pulmonary aspergillosis was the most common treatable cause of hemoptysis in patients with hematological malignancies *(128)*, and in a retrospective analysis of 116 patients with acute leukemia and invasive infections by filamentous fungi reported by the Italian GIMEMA group, major hemoptysis was the cause of death in 10% of these patients *(129)*. Of note, similar to the series of *Albelda* and coworkers *(130)*, massive hemoptysis occurred exclusively within 7 d after the granulocyte count exceeded 500/µL, underscoring the pivotal role of neutrophils in pathogenesis and the recognition of neutrophil recovery as a risk period for massive pulmonary hemorrhage *(129,130)*. Nevertheless, hemoptysis may also occur in neutropenic patients with invasive aspergillosis as the result of hemorrhagic infarction *(128)*.

8. NEW ANTIFUNGAL DRUGS UNDER CLINICAL DEVELOPMENT

Further insights into the structure–activity relationship have led to the development of a new generation of systemic antifungal triazoles that includes posaconazole (SCH 56592; Schering-Plough, Kenilworth, NJ), ravuconazole (Bristol-Myers Squibb, Wallingford, CT), and voriconazole (Pfizer, Sandwich, UK) (Table 2 and Fig. 2). Ravuconazole and voriconazole are structurally related to fluconazole, whereas the structure of posaconazole is very similar to that of itraconazole. These new agents are characterized by enhanced potency and broad-spectrum antifungal activity, including *Candida* spp., *Trichosporon beigelii*, *Cryptococcus neoformans*, *Aspergillus* spp., *Fusarium* spp., dematiaceous as well as dimorphic molds, and, perhaps, the zygomycetes *(82)*. While all three agents display some nonlinearity in their disposition, undergo hepatic metabolism and have the potential for significant drug–drug interactions through handling by the CYP450 enzyme system, key pharmacokinetic parameters (oral bioavailability, protein binding, plasma clearance, and volume of distribution) vary. However, no fundamental

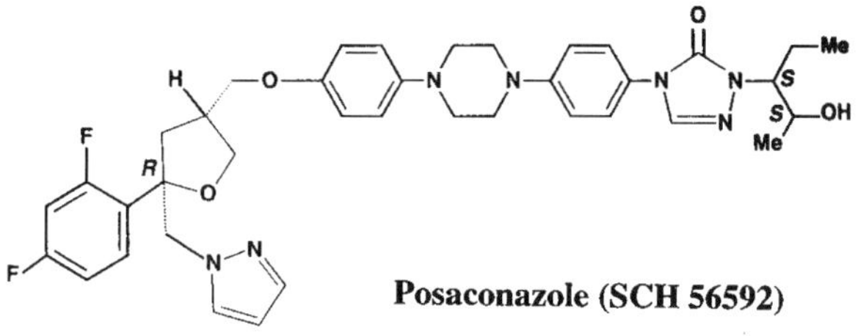

Posaconazole (SCH 56592)

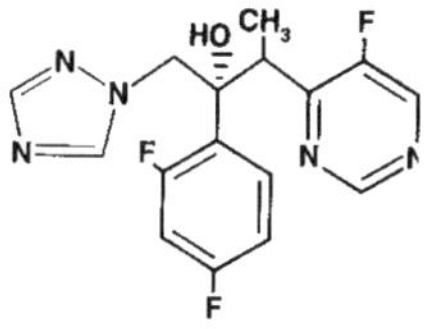

Voriconazole (UK 109496) 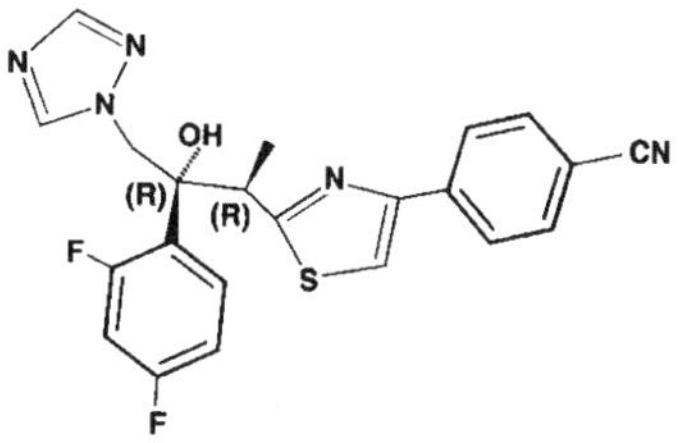   **Ravuconazole (BMS 207147)**

Fig. 2. Structural formulas of second generation antifungal triazoles.

differences between the three compounds in potency, spectrum, and antifungal efficacy have been noted thus far *(82,83,131)*.

Posaconazole, ravuconazole, and voriconazole have demonstrated therapeutic efficacy in a number of experimental immunocompromised animal models of fungal infections, including oropharyngeal and disseminated candidiasis and invasive pulmonary aspergillosis *(82,83)*. Currently, preliminary data from phase II and phase III clinical trials indicate highly promising clinical efficacy of these agents against oropharyngeal and esophageal candidiasis *(134–140)* and invasive aspergillosis *(89,132–134)*. Indeed, as noted earlier, recently published results from randomized phase III trials have demonstrated that voriconazole is superior to D-AmB as the standard agent for primary therapy of invasive aspergillosis, and that it is an appropriate alternative to AmB for empirical antifungal therapy in persistently febrile neutropenic patients *(89,101)*. A number of case reports also suggest the potential usefulness of these novel triazoles for treatment of unsusual hyaline and dematiaceous fungi *(141–144)*.

The echinocandins are an entirely novel class of antifungal lipopeptides. The echinocandins inhibit the synthesis of 1,3-β-glucan, which is a polysacharide in the cell wall of many pathogenic fungi. In concert with chitin, the rope-like glucan fibrils are responsible for the cell wall's strength and shape and play an important role in cell division and cell growth *(145–148)*. Three echinocandin compounds are in advanced stages of clinical development: Caspofungin (MK-0991; Merck, Rahway, NJ), micafungin (FK463; Fujisawa, Deerfield, ILL), and anidulafungin (VER-002; formerly LY303366; Versicor, Freemont, CA) (Table 2 and Fig. 3). Current knowledge indicates that these agents possess similar pharmacological properties. All three compounds have potent and broad-spectrum cidal in vitro activity against *Candida* species and potent inhibitory activity against *Aspergillus* spp. They are not metabolized through the CYP450 enzyme system and are generally well-tolerated due to the lack of mechanism-based toxicity. Although presently only available in parenteral formulations, the echinocandins possess favorable pharmacokinetic properties and are targeted for once-daily dosing *(149–151)*.

The antifungal efficacy of the current echinocandins has been demonstrated in several immunocompromised animal models of superficial and disseminated candidiasis and invasive pulmonary aspergillosis *(82,83)*. Phase II clinical trials of all three echinocandins, performed

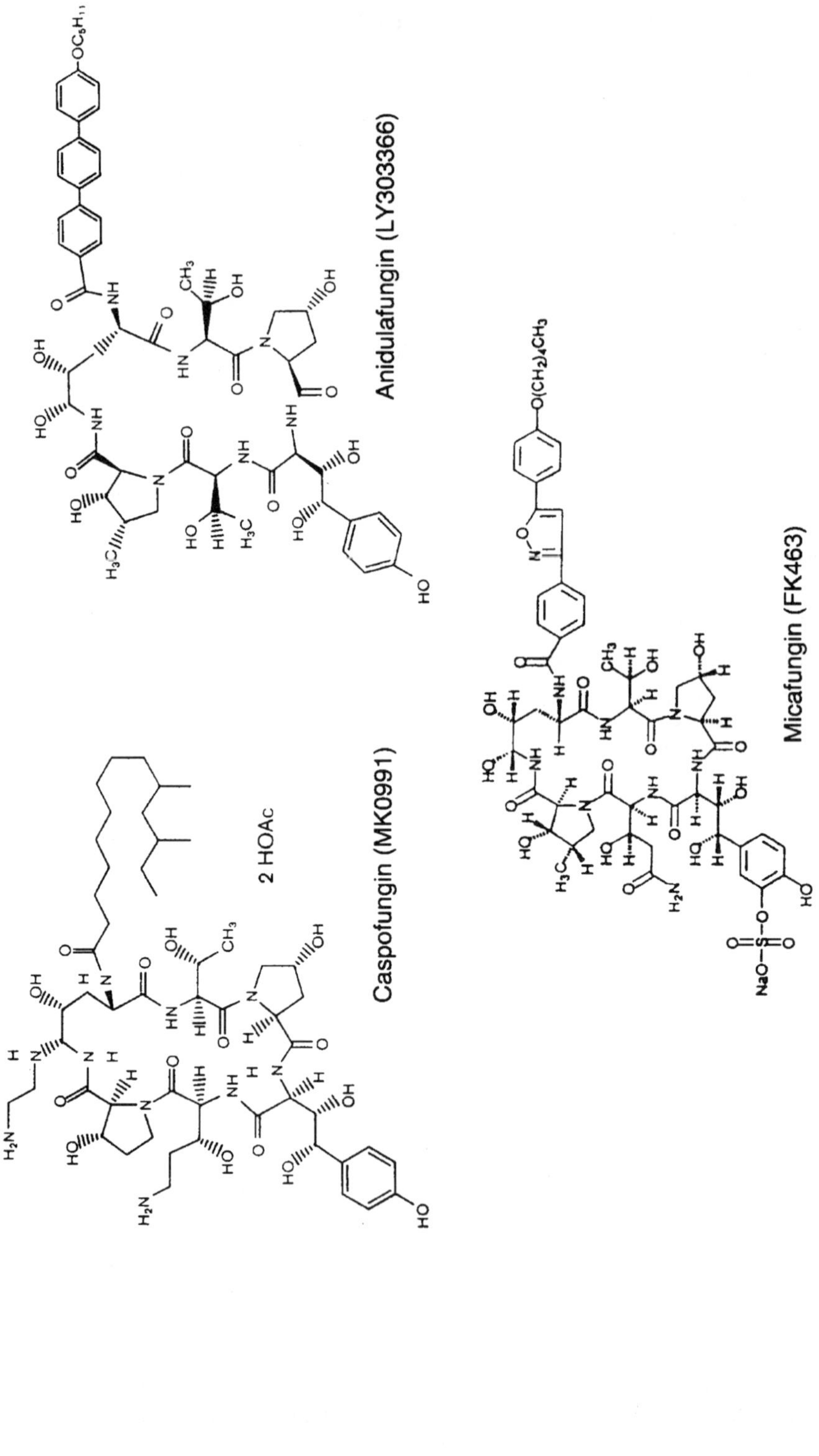

Fig. 3. Structural formulas of echinocandin lipopeptides.

in patients with esophageal candidiasis, have demonstrated potent clinical efficacy in conjunction with an excellent safety profile *(152–154)*. Published data on the clinical efficacy of the echinocandins in the treatment of more invasive infections are currently limited to caspofungin *(87)* and micafungin *(155,156)*. Caspofungin was recently approved for treatment of invasive aspergillosis refractory of or intolerant to AmB formulations or antifungal triazoles *(88)*. Because of mild and transient hepatic transaminase elevations in single-dose interaction studies, however, the concomitant use of caspofungin and cyclosporine (but not tacrolimus) is presently not recommended.

A multilamellar liposomal formulation of nystatin (Nyotran™; formerly Aronex Pharmaceuticals, The Woodlands, TX, now Antigenics, New York, NY) has been developed. The compound displayed promising activity in neutropenic animal models of invasive candidiasis and pulmonary aspergillosis *(157,158)*. The plasma pharmacokinetics of this novel polyene formulation are markedly different from those of all four AmB formulations. After achievement of comparatively high peak plasma concentrations, the drug is rapidly eliminated from plasma with an elimination half-life of ≤6 h *(159,160)*. Clinical phase II trials have documented the clinical efficacy and safety of liposomal nystatin in the treatment of invasive candidiasis and aspergillosis *(161–163)*. However, it is unclear at present whether the clinical development of this compound will be further pursued.

9. PROSPECTS FOR IMMUNOTHERAPIES

Restoration or amelioration of host defenses is paramount to the successful management of opportunistic fungal infections and, at present, may include dose-reduction or discontinuation of corticosteroids, the administration of recombinant cytokines if feasible, and donor-elicited granulocyte transfusions for profoundly neutropenic patients *(4,14,164)*.

The prognostic importance of corticosteroids is emphasized by a recent retrospective study of allogeneic patients with invasive aspergillosis, which showed a direct relationship of high cumulative corticosteroid dosages prior to diagnosis with dismal outcome *(28)*. Similarly, in a discriminative animal model of invasive pulmonary aspergillosis, methylprednisolone was the major immunosuppressive drug in animals treated with the combination of cyclosporine and methylprednisolone. Cyclosporin A alone did not increase the progression of pulmonary aspergillosis and did so only when used chronically with methylprednisolone *(165)*.

Recombinant hematopoietic cytokines, such as granulocyte colony-stimulating factor (G-CSF) and granulocyte-macrophage colony-stimulating factor (GM-CSF), shorten the duration of neutropenia and reduce the period of greatest risk for developing IFIs. While the full impact of this potentially preventive modality on the incidence of IFIs is unclear, a considerable body of preclinical in vitro and in vivo data has now accumulated that shows that recombinant cytokines (i.e., G-CSF, GM-CSF, M-CSF, interferon γ), effector cells, and antifungal drugs can work synergistically to oppose fungal growth *(164)*. Beyond the direct effects of G-CSF and GM-CSF on phagocytic effector cells, there is growing experimental evidence that Th 1-dependent immunity plays an important role in successful host defenses against invasive candidiasis and aspergillosis. Cytokines and anti-cytokines that promote this pathway (i.e., interferon γ, IL-12, and anti-IL-4) may be protective in vivo and act in cooperation with antifungal drugs *(166–171)*.

The administration of G-CSF to healthy donors prior to leukapheresis, improvements in collection techniques, and cytokine exposure to harvested and irradiated granulocytes are able to increase both dose and function of transfused granulocytes *(172)* and are currently investigated as adjunctive therapy for refractory fungal infections in patients with persistent neutropenia *(173)*. Novel avenues to cellular immunotherapy and prevention may include the cotransplantation of novel granulocyte–monocyte progenitors that give rise to granulocytes and monocytes *(174)*, the adoptive transfer of immunocompetent T cells *(175)*, and perhaps, the development of T cell vaccines *(176)*.

10. CONCLUSIONS

Cognizant of past and present epidemiological trends, IFIs are likely to remain a frequent and important complication of allogeneic patients. Indeed, the successful induction of graft-vs-tumor effects in patients with high risk solid tumors by means of nonmyeloablative alloge-neic *(177,178)* suggests that the number of patients at risk is only too likely to expand. Improved diagnostic tools, an expanded and refined antifungal armamentarium, further elucidation of antifungal resistance, incorporation of pharmacodynamics, as well as combination and immu-notherapies offer hope for substantial progress. Rationally-designed clinical trials are needed more than ever to translate this progress into clinical practice.

REFERENCES

1. Denning DW, Stevens DA. Antifungal and surgical treatment of invasive aspergillosis: review of 2,121 published cases. *Rev Infect Dis* 1990;12:1147–201.
2. Goodrich JM, Reed EC, Mori M, et al. Clinical features and analysis of risk factors for invasive Candidal infection after marrow transplantation. *J Infect Dis* 1991;164:731–740.
3. Bowden RA. Fungal infections after hematopoietic cell transplantation. In: Bowden R, Ljungman P, Paya CV (eds). *Transplant Infections*. Lippincott-Raven, Philadelphia, PA, 1998, pp. 550–559.
4. Walsh TJ, Hiemenz JW, Anaissie E. Recent progress and current problems in treatment of invasive fungal infections in neutropenic patients. *Infect Dis Clin N Am* 1996;10:365–400.
5. Meyers JD. Fungal infections in bone marrow transplant patients. *Sem Oncol* 1990;17(Suppl.6): S10–13.
6. Baddley JW, Stroud T, Salsman D, Pappas PG. Invasive mould infections in bone marrow transplant recipients: etiology, risk factors, and outcome. In: *Abstracts of the 39th International Conference on Antimicrobial Agents and Chemotherapy*. American Society for Microbiology, Washington, D.C., 2000, abstract 960, p. 557.
7. Marr KA, Seidel K, White TC, Bowden RA. Candidemia in allogeneic blood and marrow transplant recipi-ents: evolution of risk factors after the adoption of prophylactic fluconazole. *J Infect Dis* 2000;181:309–316.
8. Wald A, Leichsenring W, van Burik JA, Bowden RA. Epidemiology of Asper-gillus infections in a large cohort of patients undergoing bone marrow transplantation. *J Infect Dis* 1997;175:1459–1466.
9. Wingard JR. Fungal infections after bone marrow transplant. *Biol Blood Marrow Transplant* 1999;5:55–68.
10. Denning DW, Follansbee SE, Scolaro M, et al. Pulmonary aspergillosis in the acquired immunodeficiency syndrome. *N Engl J Med* 1991;324:654–662.
11. Groll AH, Shah PM, Mentzel C, et al. Trends in the postmortem epidemiology of invasive fungal infections at a university hospital. *J Infect* 1996;33:23–32.
12. Cenci E, Mencacci A, Fe d'Ostiani C, et al. Cytokine- and T-helper-dependent immunity in murine aspergillo-sis. *Res Immunol* 1998;149:445–454.
13. Romani L. Innate and adaptive immunity in *Candida albicans* infections and saprophytism. *J Leukoc Biol* 2000;68:175–179.
14. Stevens DA, Walsh TJ, Bistoni F, et al. Cytokines and mycoses. *Med Mycol* 1998;36(Suppl 1):174–182.
15. Roilides E, Sein T, Schaufele R, et al. Increased serum concentrations of interleukin-10 in patients with hepatosplenic candidiasis. *J Infect Dis* 1998;178:589–592.
16. Roilides E, Sein T, Roden M, Set al. Elevated serum concentrations of interleukin-10 in nonneutropenic patients with invasive aspergillosis. *J Infect Dis* 2001;183:518–520.
17. Goodman JL Winston DJ, Greenfield RA, et al. A controlled trial of fluconazole to prevent fungal infections in patients undergoing bone marrow transplantation. *N Engl J Med* 1992;326:845–851.
18. Slavin MA, Osborne B, Adams R,et al. Efficacy and safety of fluconazole prophylaxis for fungal infections after marrow transplantation—a prospective, randomized, double-blind study. *J Infect Dis* 1995;171:1545–1552.
19. van Burik JH, Leisenring W, Myerson D, et al. The effect of prophylactic fluconazole on the clinical spectrum of fungal diseases in bone marrow transplant recipients with special attention to hepatic candidiasis. An autopsy study of 355 patients. *Medicine* (Baltimore) 1998;77:246–254.
20. Jantunen E, Ruutu P, Niskanen L, et al. Incidence and risk factors for invasive fungal infections in allogeneic BMT recipients. *Bone Marrow Transplant* 1997;19:801–808.

21. Viscoli C, Girmenia C, Marinus A, et al. Candidemia in cancer patients: a prospective, multicenter surveillance study by the Invasive Fungal Infection Group (IFIG) of the European Organization for Research and Treatment of Cancer (EORTC). *Clin Infect Dis* 1999;28:1071–1079.

22. Groll AH, Walsh TJ. Uncommon opportunistic fungi: new nosocomial threats. *Clin Microbiol Infect* 2001;7(Suppl2):8–24. Review.

23. Bjerke JW, Meyers JD, Bowden RA. Hepatosplenic candidiasis—a contraindication to marrow transplantation? *Blood* 1994; 84:2811–2814.

24. Offner F, Cordonnier C, Ljungman P, et al. Impact of previous aspergillosis on the outcome of bone marrow transplantation. *Clin Infect Dis* 1998;26:1098–1103.

25. Walsh TJ, Catchatourian R, Cohen H. Disseminated histoplasmosis complicating bone marrow transplantation. *Am J Clin Pathol* 1983;79:509–511.

26. Riley DK, Galgiani JN, O'Donnell MR, et al. Coccidioidomycosis in bone marrow transplant recipients. *Transplantation* 1993;56:1531–1533.

27. Serody JS, Mill MR, Detterbeck FC, et al. Blastomycosis in transplant recipients: report of a case and review. *Clin Infect Dis* 1993;16:54–58.

28. Ribaud P, Chastang C, Latge JP, et al. Survival and prognostic factors of invasive aspergillosis after allogeneic bone marrow transplantation. *Clin Infect Dis* 1999;28:322–330.

29. Pannuti C, Gingrich R, Pfaller MA, et al. Nosocomial pneumonia in patients having bone marrow transplant. Attributable mortality and risk factors. *Cancer* 1992:69:2653–2662.

30. Sutton DA, Sanche SE, Revankar SG, et al. In vitro amphotericin B resistance in clinical isolates of *Aspergillus* terreus, with a head-to-head comparison to voriconazole. *J Clin Microbiol* 1999;37:2343–2345.

31. Iwen PC, Rupp ME, Langnas AN, et al. Invasive pulmonary aspergillosis due to *Aspergillus* terreus: 12-year experienc and review of the literature. *Clin Infect Dis* 1998;26:1092–1097.

32. Walsh TJ, Groll AH. Emerging fungal pathogens: evolving challenges to immunocompromised patients for the twenty-first century. *Transplant Infect Dis* 1999;1:247–261.

33. Perfect JR, Schell WA. The new fungal opportunists are coming. *Clin Infect Dis* 1996;22(Suppl 2):S112–118.

34. Vartivarian SE, Anaissie EJ, Bodey GP. Emerging fungal pathogens in immunocompromised patients: classification, diagnosis, and management. *Clin Infect Dis* 1993;17(Suppl 2):S487–491.

35. Walsh TJ, Melcher GP, Rinaldi MG, et al. Trichosporon beigelii, an emerging pathogen resistant to amphotericin B. *J Clin Microbiol* 1990;28:1616–1622.

36. Anaissie E, Gokoslan A, Hachem R, Rubin R. Azole therapy for trichosporonosis: clinical evaluation of eight patients, experimental therapy for murine infection, and review. *Clin Infect Dis* 1992;15:781–787.

37. Aguilar C, Pujol I, Sala J, Guarro J. Antifungal susceptibilities of Paecilomyces species. *Antimicrob Agents Chemother* 1998;42:1601–1604.

38. Chan-Tack KM, Thio CL, Miller NS, et al. Paecilomyces lilacinus fungemia in an adult bone marrow transplant recipient. *Med Mycol* 1999;37:57–60.

39. Reuben A, Anaissie E, Nelson PE, et al. Antifungal susceptibility of 44 clinical isolates of Fusarium species determined by using a broth microdilution method. *Antimicrob Agents Chemother* 1989;33:1647–1649.

40. Boutati EI, Anaissie EJ. Fusarium, a significant emerging pathogen in patients with hematologic malignancy: ten years' experience at a cancer center and implications for management. *Blood* 1997; 90:999–1008.

41. Travis LB, Roberts GD, Wilson WR. Clinical significance of Pseudallescheria boydii: a review of 10 years' experience. *Mayo Clinic Proc* 1985;60:531–537.

42. Walsh TJ, Peter J, McGough DA, et al. Activities of amphotericin B and antifungal azoles alone and in combination against Pseudallescheria boydii. *Antimicrob Agents Chemother* 1995;39:1361–1364.

43. Berenguer J, Rodriguez-Tudela JL, et al. Deep infections caused by Scedosporium prolificans. A report on 16 cases in Spain and a review of the literature. Scedosporium Prolificans Spanish Study Group. *Medicine (Baltimore)* 1997;76:256–265.

44. Maertens J, Lagrou K, Deweerdt H, et al. Disseminated infection by Scedosporium prolificans: an emerging fatality among haematology patients. Case report and review. *Ann Hematol* 2000;79:340–344.

45. Groll AH, Just-Nuebling G, Kurz M, et al. Fluconazole versus nystatin in the prevention of *Candida* infections in children and adolescents undergoing remission induction or consolidation chemotherapy for cancer. *J Antimicrob Chemother* 1997;40:855–862.

46. Marr KA, Seidel K, Slavin MA, et al. Prolonged fluconazole prophylaxis is associated with persistent protection against candidiasis-related death in allogeneic marrow transplant recipients: long-term follow-up of a randomized, placebo-controlled trial. *Blood* 2000;96:2055–2061.

47. Hansen JA, Gooley TA, Martin PJ, et al. Bone marrow transplants from unrelated donors for patients with chronic myeloid leukemia. *N Engl J Med* 1998;338:962–968.

48. Anaissie E. Opportunistic mycoses in the immunocompromised host: Experience at a cancer center and review. *Clin Infect Dis* 1992;14(Suppl 1):S43–53.

49. Wingard JR. Importance of *Candida* species other than *C. albicans* as pathogens in oncology patients. *Clin Infect Dis* 1995;20:115–125.
50. Nguyen MH, Peacock JE, Jr, Morris AJ, et al. The changing face of candidemia: emergence of non-*Candida albicans* species and antifungal resistance. *Am J Med* 1996;100: 617–623.
51. Abi-Said D, Anaissie E, Uzun O, et al. The epidemiology of hematogenous candidiasis caused by different *Candida* species. *Clin Infect Dis* 1997;24:1122–1128.
52. Wingard JR, Merz WG, Rinaldi MG, Jet al. Increase in *Candida krusei* infection among patients with bone marrow transplantation and neutropenia treated prophylactically with fluconazole. *N Engl J Med* 1991;325:1274–1277.
53. Wingard JR, Merz WG, Rinaldi MG, et al. Association of *Torulopsis glabrata* infections with fluconazole prophylaxis in neutropenic bone marrow transplant patients. *Antimicrob Agents Chemother* 1993;37:1847–1849.
54. Jarque I, Saavedra S, Martin G, et al. Delay of onset of candidemia and emergence of *Candida krusei* fungemia in hematologic patients receiving prophylactic fluconazole. *Haematologica* 2000;85:441–443.
55. Groll AH, Piscitelli SC, Walsh TJ. Clinical pharmacology of systemic antifungal agents: a comprehensive review of agents in clinical use, current investigational compounds, and putative targets for antifungal drug development. *Adv Pharmacol* 1998;44:343–500.
56. Ascioglu S, de Pauw B, Bennet JE, et al. Analysis of definitions used in clinical research on invasive fungal infections: consensus proposal for new, standardized definitions. In *Abstracts of the 39th International Conference on Antimicrobial Agents and Chemotherapy*. American Society for Microbiology, Washington, D.C., 1999, abstract 1639, p. 573.
57. Walsh TJ, Roden M, Roilides E, et al. Concepts in design of comparative clinical trials of antifungal therapy in neutropenic patients. *Int J Antimicrob Agents* 2000;16:151–156.
58. Rex JR, Walsh TJ, Nettleman M, et al. Need for alternative trial designs and evaluation strategies for therapeutic studies of invasive mycoses. *Clin Infect Dis* 2001;35:95–106.
59. NCCLS. Reference method for broth dilution antifungal susceptibility testing of yeasts; approved standard. NCCLS document M27A. NCCLS, Wayne, PA, 1997.
60. NCCLS. Proposed reference method for broth dilution antifungal susceptibility testing of filamentous fungi. NCCLS document M28-P. NCCLS, Wayne, PA, 1998.
61. Rex JH, Pfaller MA, Galgiani JN, et al. Development of interpretive breakpoints for antifungal susceptibility testing: conceptual framework and analysis of in vitro-in vivo correlation data for fluconazole, itraconazole, and *Candida* infections. *Clin Infect Dis* 1997;24:235–247.
62. Wingard JR, Kubilis P, Lee L, et al. Clinical significance of nephrotoxicity in patients treated with amphotericin B for suspected or proven aspergillosis. *Clin Infect Dis* 1999;29:1402–1407.
63. Ringden O, Meunier F, Tollemar J, et al. Efficacy of amphotericin B encapsulated in liposomes (AmBisome) in the treatment of invasive fungal infections in immunocompromised patients. *J Antimicrob Chemother* 1991;28(Suppl B):73–82.
64. Anaissie EJ, White M, Uzun O, et al. Amphotenin B lipid complex (ABLC) versus amphotericin B (AMB) for treatment of hematogenous and invasive candidiasis: a prospective, randomized, multicenter trial. In: *Abstracts of the 35th Interscience Conference on Antimicrobial Agents and Chemotherapy*. American Society for Microbiology, Washington, D.C., 1995, abstract LM 21, p. 330.
65. Oppenheim BA, Herbrecht R, Kusne S. The safety and efficacy of amphotericin B colloidal dispersion in the treatment of invasive mycoses. *Clin Infect Dis* 1995;21:1145–1153.
66. White MH, Anaissie EJ, Kusne S, et al. Amphotericin B colloidal dispersion vs. amphotericin B as therapy for invasive aspergillosis. *Clin Infect Dis* 1997;24:635–642.
67. Wingard JR. Efficacy of amphotericin B lipid complex injection (ABLC) in bone marrow transplant recipients with life-threatening systemic mycoses. *Bone Marrow Transplant* 1997;19:343–347.
68. Noskin GA, Pietrelli L, Coffey G, et al. Amphotericin B colloidal dispersion for treatment of candidemia in immunocompromised patients. *Clin Infect Dis* 1998;26:461–467.
69. Walsh TJ, Hiemenz JW, Seibel NL, et al. Amphotericin B lipid complex for invasive fungal infections: analysis of safety and efficacy in 556 cases. *Clin Infect Dis* 1998;26:1383–1396.
70. Noskin G, Pietrelli L, Gurwith M, et al. Treatment of invasive fungal infections with amphotericin B colloidal dispersion in bone marrow transplant recipients. *Bone Marrow Transplant* 1999;23 697–703.
71. Hiemenz JW, Walsh TJ. Lipid formulations of amphotericin B: recent progress and future directions. *Clin Infect Dis* 1996;22(Suppl 2): S133–S144.
72. Groll AH, Mueller FMC, Piscitelli SC, et al. Lipid formulations of Amphotericin B: clinical perspectives for the management of invasive fungal infections in children with cancer. *Klin Padiatr* 1998;210:264–273.
73. Wong-Beringer A, Jacobs RA, Guglielmo BJ. Lipid formulations of amphotericin B: clinical efficacy and toxicities. *Clin Infect Dis* 1998;27:603–618.
74. White MH, Bowden RA, Sandler ES, et al. Randomized, double-blind clinical trial of amphotericin B colloidal dispersion vs. amphotericin B in the empirical treatment of fever and neutropenia. *Clin Infect Dis* 1998;27:296–302.

75. Walsh TJ, Finberg RW, Arndt C, et al. Liposomal amphotericin B for empirical therapy in patients with persistent fever and neutropenia. National Institute of Allergy and Infectious Diseases Mycoses Study Group. *N Engl J Med* 1999;340:764–771.

76. Wingard JR, White MH, Anaissie E, et al. A randomized, double-blind comparative trial evaluating the safety of liposomal amphotericin B versus amphotericin B lipid complex in the empirical treatment of febrile neutropenia. L Amph/ABLC Collaborative Study Group. *Clin Infect Dis* 2000;31:1155–1163.

77. Groll AH, Piscitelli SC, Walsh TJ. Antifungal pharmacodynamics. Concentration-effect relationships in vitro and in vivo. *Pharmacotherapy* 2001;21:133S–148S.

78. Leenders AC, Daenen S, Jansen RL, et al. Liposomal amphotericin B compared with amphotericin B deoxycholate in the treatment of documented and suspected neutropenia-associated invasive fungal infections. *Br J Haematol* 1998;103:205–212.

79. Walsh TJ, Aoki S, Mechinaud F, et al. Effects of preventive, early, and late antifungal chemotherapy with fluconazole in different granulocytopenic models of experimental disseminated candidiasis. *J Infect Dis* 1990;161:755–760.

80. Anaissie EJ, Darouiche RO, Abi-Said D, et al. Management of invasive candidal infections: results of a prospective, randomized, multicenter study of fluconazole versus amphotericin B and review of the literature. *Clin Infect Dis* 1996;23:964–972.

81. Anaissie EJ, Vartivarian SE, Abi-Said D, et al. Fluconazole versus amphotericin B in the treatment of hematogenous candidiasis: a matched cohort study. *Am J Med* 1996;101:170–176.

82. Groll AH Walsh TJ. Potential new antifungal agents. *Curr Opin Infect Dis* 1997;10:449–458.

83. Chiou CC, Groll AH, Walsh TJ. New drugs and novel targets for treatment of invasive fungal infections in patients with cancer. *Oncologist* 2000;5:120–135.

84. Barone JA, Moskovitz BL, Guarnieri J, et al. Enhanced bioavailability of itraconazole in hydroxypropyl-beta-cyclodextrin solution versus capsules in healthy volunteers. *Antimicrob Agents Chemother* 1998;42:1862–1865.

85. Denning DW, Lee JY, Hostetler JS, et al. NIAID Mycoses Study Group multicenter trial of oral itraconazole therapy for invasive aspergillosis. *Am J Med* 1994;97:135–144.

86. Stevens DA, Lee JY. Analysis of compassionate use itraconazole therapy for invasive aspergillosis by the NIAID Mycoses Study Group criteria. *Arch Intern Med* 1997;157:1857–1862.

87. Caillot D, Bassaris H, Seifert WF, et al. Efficacy, safety, and pharmacokinetics of intravenous followed by oral itraconazole in patients with invasive pulmonary aspergillosis. In *Abstracts of the 39th International Conference on Antimicrobial Agents and Chemotherapy.* American Society for Microbiology, Washington, D.C., 1999, abstract 1646, p. 575.

88. Maertens J, Raad I, Sable CA, et al. Multicenter, noncomparative study to evaluate safety and efficacy of caspofungin in adults with invasive aspergillosis refractory or intolerant to amphotericin B, amphotericin B lipid formulations, or azoles. In *Abstracts of the 40th International Conference on Antimicrobial Agents and Chemotherapy.* American Society for Microbiology, Washington, D.C., 2000, abstract 1103, p. 371.

89. Herbrecht R, Denning DW, Patterson TF, et al. Open, randomized comparison of voriconazole (VRC) and amphotericin B (AmB) followed by other licensed antifungal therapy (OLAT) for primary therapy of invasive aspergillosis (IA). In *Abstracts of the 41th International Conference on Antimicrobial Agents and Chemotherapy.* American Society for Microbiology, Washington, D.C., 2001, abstract J-680, p. 378.

90. Menichetti F, Del Favero A, Martino P, et al. Itraconazole oral solution as prophylaxis for fungal infections in neutropenic patients with hematologic malignancies: a randomized, placebo-controlled, double-blind, multicenter trial. GIMEMA Infection Program. Gruppo Italiano Malattie Ematologiche dell' Adulto. *Clin Infect Dis* 1999;28:250–255.

91. Gubbins PO, Bowman JL, Penzak SR. Antifungal prophylaxis to prevent invasive mycoses among bone marrow transplantation recipients. *Pharmacotherapy* 1998;18:549–564.

92. Uzun O, Anaissie EJ. Antifungal prophylaxis in patients with hematologic malignancies: a reappraisal. *Blood* 1995;86:2063–2072.

93. Lortholary O, Dupont B. Antifungal prophylaxis during neutropenia and immunodeficiency. *Clin Microbiol Rev.* 1997;10:477–504.

94. Crippa F, Corey L, Leichsenring Q, et al. Administration of itraconazole for antifungal prophylaxis in stem cell transplant recipients: levels and drug interactions. In *Abstracts of the 40th Interscience Conference on Antimicrobial Agents and Chemotherapy.* American Society for Microbiology, Washington, D.C., 2000, abstract 850, p. 25.

95. Pizzo PA, Robichaud KJ, Gill FA, et al. Empiric antibiotic and antifungal therapy for cancer patients with prolonged fever and granulocytopenia. *Am J Med* 1982;72:101–111.

96. EORTC. Empiric antifungal therapy in febrile granulocytopenic patients. EORTC International Antimicrobial Therapy Cooperative Group. *Am J Med* 1989;86:668–672.

97. Cornely OA, Hiddemann W, Link H, et al. Interventional antimicrobial therapy in febrile neutropenic patients: Paul Ehrlich Society for Chemotherapy (PEG) Study II. *Ann Hematol* 1997;74(Suppl 1):A51

98. Prentice HG, Hann IM, Herbrecht R, et al. A randomized comparison of liposomal versus conventional amphotericin B for treatment of pyrexia of unknown origin in neutropenic patients. *Br J Haematol* 1997;98:711–718.

99. Boogaerts M, Winston DJ, Bow EJ, et al. Intravenous and oral itraconazole versus intravenous amphotericin B as empirical antifungal therapy for persistent fever in neutropenic patients with cancer who are receiving broad-spectrum antibacterial therapy. *Ann Intern Med* 2001;135:412–422.

100. Winston DJ, Hathorn JW, Schuster MG, et al. A multicentre, randomized trial of fluconazole vs. amphotericin B for empiric antifungal therapy of febrile neutropenic patients with cancer. *Am J Med* 2000;108:282–289.

101. Walsh TJ, Pappas P, Winston D, et al. Voriconazole versus liposomal amphotericin B for empirical antifungal therapy of persistently febrile neutropenic patients: a randomized, international multicenter trial. In *Abstract Addendum of the 40th International Conference on Antimicrobial Agents and Chemotherapy*. American Society for Microbiology, Washington, D.C., 2000, abstract L-1, p. 20.

102. Centers for Disease Control and Prevention. Guidelines for preventing opportunistic infections among hematopoietic stem cell transplant recipients. *MMWR Morb Mortal Wkly Rep* 2000;49(RR-10):1–95.

103. Walsh TJ, Whitcomb PO, Revankar SG, et al. Successful treatment of hepatosplenic candidiasis through repeated cycles of chemotherapy and neutropenia. *Cancer* 1995;76:2357–2362.

104. Walsh TJ, Whitcomb P, Piscitelli S, et al. Safety, tolerance, and pharmacokinetics of amphotericin B lipid complex in children with hepatosplenic candidiasis. *Antimicrob Agents Chemother* 1997;41:1944–1948.

105. Martino R, Lopez R, Sureda A, et al. Risk of reactivation of a recent invasive fungal infection in patients with hematological malignancies undergoing further intensive chemo-radiotherapy. A single-center experience and review of the literature. *Haematologica* 1997;82:297–304.

106. Berenguer J, Buck M, Witebsky F, et al. Lysis-centrifugation blood cultures in the detection of tissue-proven invasive candidiasis. Disseminated versus single-organ infection. *Diag Microbiol Infect Dis* 1993;17:103–109.

107. Pastakia B, Shawker TH, Thaler M, et al. Hepatosplenic candidiasis: wheels within wheels. *Radiology* 1988;166:417–421.

108. Semelka RC, Shoenut JP, Greenberg HM, et al. Detection of acute and treated lesions of hepatosplenic candidiasis: comparison of dynamic contrast-enhanced CT and MR imaging. *J Magn Reson Imaging* 1992;2:341–345.

109. Wheeler JH, Fishman EK. Computed tomography in the management of chest infections: current status. *Clin Infect Dis* 1996;23:232–240.

110. Sallah S, Semelka R, Kelekis N, et al. Diagnosis and monitoring response to treatment of hepatosplenic candidiasis in patients with acute leukemia using magnetic resonance imaging. *Acta Haematol* 1998;100:77–81.

111. Walsh TJ, Chanock SJ. Diagnosis of invasive fungal infections: advances in nonculture systems. *Curr Clin Top Infect Dis* 1998;18:101–153.

112. Savage DG, Taylor P, Blackwell J, et al. Paranasal sinusitis following allogeneic bone marrow transplant. *Bone Marrow Transplant* 1997;19:55–59.

113. Kuhlman JE, Fishman EK, Burch PA, et al. Invasive pulmonary aspergillosis in acute leukemia: the contribution of CT to early diagnosis and aggressive management. *Chest* 1987;92:95–99.

114. von Eiff M, Zuehlsdorf M, Roos N, et al. Pulmonary fungal infections in patients with hematological malignancies -diagnostic approaches. *Ann Hematol* 1995;70:135–141.

115. Caillot D, Casasnovas O, Bernard A, et al. Improved management of invasive pulmonary aspergillosis in neutropenic patients using early thoracic computed tomography scan and surgery. *J Clin Oncol* 1997;15:139–147.

116. Caillot D, Couaillier JF, Bernard A, et al. Increasing volume and changing characteristics of invasive pulmonary aspergillosis on sequential thoracic computed tomography scans in patients with neutropenia. *J Clin Oncol* 2001;19:253–259.

117. Einsele H, Hebart H, Roller G, et al. Detection and identification of fungal pathogens in blood by using molecular probes. *J Clin Microbiol* 1997;35:1353–1360.

118. Maertens J, Verhaegen J, Demuynck H, et al. Autopsy-controlled prospective evaluation of serial screening for circulating galactomannan by a sandwich enzyme-linked immunosorbent assay for hematological patients at risk for invasive Aspergillosis. *J Clin Microbiol* 1999;37:3223–3228.

119. Hebart H, Loffler J, Meisner C, et al. Early detection of *Aspergillus* infection after allogeneic stem cell transplantation by polymerase chain reaction screening. *J Infect Dis* 2000;181:1713–1719.

120. Maertens J, Verhaegen J, Lagrou K, et al. Screening for circulating galactomannan as a noninvasive diagnostic tool for invasive aspergillosis in prolonged neutropenic patients and stem cell transplantation recipients: a prospective validation. *Blood* 2001;97:1604–1610.

121. Bodey GP, Vartivarian S. Aspergillosis. *Eur J Clin Microbiol Infect Dis* 1989;8:413–437.

122. Denning DW. Invasive aspergillosis. *Clin Infect Dis* 1998;26:781–805.

123. Shamberger RC, Weinstein HJ, Grier HE, et al. The surgical management of fungal pulmonary infections in children with acute myelogenous leukemia. *J Pediatr Surg* 1985;20:840–844.

124. Lupinetti FM, Behrendt DM, Giller RH, et al. Pulmonary resection for fungal infection in children undergoing bone marrow transplantation. *J Thorax Surg* 1992;104:684–687.

125. Wong K, Waters CM, Walesby RK. Surgical management of invasive pulmonary aspergillosis in immunocompromised patients. *Eur J Cardiothorac Surg* 1992;6:138–142.

126. Young VC, Maghur HA, Luke DA, et al. Operation for cavitating invasive pulmonary aspergillosis in immunocompromised patients. *Ann Thorac Surg* 1992;53:621–624.

127. Yeghen T, Kibbler CC, Prentice HG, et al. Management of invasive pulmonary aspergillosis in hematology patients: a review of 87 consecutive cases at a single institution. *Clin Infect Dis* 2000;31:859–868.

128. Panos RJ, Barr LF, Walsh TJ, et al. Factors associated with fatal hemoptysis in cancer patients. *Chest* 1988;94:1008–1013.

129. Pagano L, Ricci P, Nosari A, et al. Fatal haemoptysis in pulmonary filamentous mycosis: an underevaluated cause of death in patients with acute leukaemia in haematological complete remission. A retrospective study and review of the literature. Gimema Infection Program (Gruppo Italiano Malattie Ematologiche dell'Adulto) *Br J Haematol* 1995;89:500–505.

130. Albelda SM, Talbot GH, Gerson SL, et al. Pulmonary cavitation and massive hemoptysis in invasive pulmonary aspergillosis. Influence of bone marrow recovery in patients with acute leukemia. *Am Rev Respir Dis* 1985;131:115–120

131. Hoffman HL, Ernst EJ, Klepser ME. Novel triazole antifungal agents. *Expert Opin Investig Drugs* 2000;9:593–605.

132. Denning D, de Favero A, Gluckman E, et al. UK-109,496, a Novel, wide-spectrum triazole derivative for the treatment of fungal infections: clinical efficacy in invasive aspergillosis. In: *Program and Abstracts of the 35th Interscience Conference on Antimicrobial Agents and Chemotherapy.* American Society for Microbiology, Washington, D.C., 1995, abstract F80, p. 126.

133. Dupont B, Denning D, Lode H, et al. UK-109,496, a Novel, wide-spectrum 'triazole derivative for the treatment of fungal infections: clinical efficacy in chronic invasive aspergillosis. In: *Program and Abstracts of the 35th Interscience Conference on Antimicrobial Agents and Chemotherapy.* American Society for Microbiology, Washington, D.C., 1995, abstract F81, p. 126.

134. Hegener P, Troke PF, Fakenheuer G, et al. Treatment of Fluconazole-Resistant Candidiasis with Voriconazole in Patients with AIDS. *AIDS* 1998;12:2227,2228.

135. Dupont B, Ally R, Burke J, et al. A double-blind, randomized, multicenter trial of voriconazole vs. fluconazole in the treatment of esophageal candidiasis in immunocompromised adults. In: *Abstracts of the 40th Interscience Conference on Antimicrobial Agents and Chemotherapy.* American Society for Microbiology, Washington, D.C., 2000, abstract 706, p. 365.

136. Walsh TJ, Gharamani P, Hodges MR, et al. Efficacy and safety of voriconazole in the treatment of invasive fungal infections in children. In: *Abstracts of the 40th Interscience Conference on Antimicrobial Agents and Chemotherapy.* American Society for Microbiology, Washington, D.C., 2000, abstract 1100, p. 372.

137. Vazquez JA, Northland R, Miller S, et al. Posaconazole compared to fluconazole for oral candidiasis in HIV-positive patients. In: *Abstracts of the 40th Interscience Conference on Antimicrobial Agents and Chemotherapy.* American Society for Microbiology, Washington, D.C., 2000, abstract 1107, p. 370.

138. Hachem RY, Raad II, Afif CM, et al. An open, non-comparative multicenter study to evaluate efficacy and safety of posaconazole (SCH 56592) in the treatment of invasive fungal infections refractory to or intolerant to standard therapy. In: *Abstracts of the 40th International Conference on Antimicrobial Agents and Chemotherapy.* American Society for Microbiology, Washington, D.C., 2000, abstract 1109, p. 372.

139. Nieto L, Northland R, Pittisuttithum P, et al. Posaconazole equivalent to fluconazole in the treatment of oropharyngeal candidiasis. In: *Abstracts of the 40th Interscience Conference on Antimicrobial Agents and Chemotherapy.* American Society for Microbiology, Washington, D.C., 2000, abstract 1108, p. 372.

140. Beale M, Queiroz-Telles F, Banhegyi D, et al. Randomized, double-blind study of the safety and antifungal efficacy of ravuconazole relative to fluconazole in esophageal candidiasis. In: *Abstracts of the 41th Interscience Conference on Antimicrobial Agents and Chemotherapy.* American Society for Microbiology, Washington, D.C., 2001, abstract J-1621, p. 392.

141. Munoz P, Marin M, Tornero P, et al. Successful Outcome of scedosporium apiospermum disseminated infection treated with voriconazole in a patient receiving corticosteroid therapy. *Clin Infect Dis* 2000;31:1499–1501.

142. Nesky MA, McDougal EC, Peacock JE, Jr. Pseudallescheria boydii brain abscess successfully treated with voriconazole and surgical drainage: case report and literature review of central nervous system pseudallescheriasis. *Clin Infect Dis* 2000;31:673–677.

143. Reis A, Sundmacher R, Tintelnot K, et al. Successful treatment of ocular invasive mould infection (fusariosis) with the new antifungal agent voriconazole. *Br J Ophthalmol* 2000;84:932,933.

144. Hilmarsdottir I, Thorsteinsson SB, Asmundsson P, et al. Cutaneous infection caused by Paecilomyces lilacinus in a renal transplant patient: treatment with voriconazole. *Scand J Infect Dis* 2000;32:331,332.

145. Hector, RF. Compounds active against cell walls of medically important fungi. *Clin Microbiol Rev* 1993;6:1–21.

146. Debono M, Gordee RS. Antibiotics that inhibit fungal cell wall development. *Ann Rev Microbiol* 1994;48:471–497.

147. Denning DW. Echinocandins and pneumocandins- a new antifungal class with a novel mode of action. *J Antimicrob Chemother* 1997;40:611–614.

148. Kurtz MB, Douglas CM. Lipopeptide inhibitors of fungal glucan synthase. *J Med Vet Mycol* 1997;35:79–86.

149. Groll AH, Walsh TJ. MK-0991. *Curr Opin Anti-Infect Invest Drugs* 1999;1:334–345.

150. Groll AH, Walsh TJ. FK-463. *Curr Opin Anti-Infect Invest Drugs* 2000;2:405–412.

151. Hawser S. LY-303366. *Curr Opin Anti-Infect Invest Drugs* 1999;1:353–360.

152. Sable CA, Villanueva, Arathon E, et al. A randomized, double-blind, multicenter trial of MK-0991 (L-743,872) vs amphotericin B (AmB) in the treatment of *Candida* esophagitis in adults. In *Abstracts of the 37 th Interscience Conference on Antimicrobial Agents and Chemotherapy.* American Society for Microbiology, Washington, D.C., 1997:

153. Brown GL, White RJ, Turik M. Phase II, randomized, open label study of two intravenous dosing regimens of V-echinocandin in the treatment of esophageal candidiasis. In: *Abstracts of the 40th Interscience Conference on Antimicrobial Agents and Chemotherapy.* American Society for Microbiology, Washington, D.C., 2000, abstract 1106, p. 371.

154. Pettengell K, Mynhardt J, Kluyts T, et al. A multicenter study of the echinocandin antifungal FK463 for the treatment of esophageal candidiasis in HIV positive patients. In: *Abstracts of the 40th Interscience Conference on Antimicrobial Agents and Chemotherapy.* American Society for Microbiology, Washington, D.C., 2000, abstract 1104, p. 371.

155. Kohno S, Masaoka T, Yamaguchi H. A multicentre, open-label clinical study of FK463 in patients with deep mycoses in Japan. In: *Abstracts of the 41th Interscience Conference on Antimicrobial Agents and Chemotherapy.* American Society for Microbiology, Washington, D.C., 2001, abstract J-834, p. 384.

156. Kontoyiannis DP, Buell D, Frisbee-Hume S, et al. Initial experience with FK463 for the treatment of candidemia in cancer patients. In: *Abstracts of the 41th Interscience Conference on Antimicrobial Agents and Chemotherapy.* American Society for Microbiology, Washington, D.C., 2001,abstract J-1629, p. 394.

157. Groll AH, Gonzalez CE, Giri N, et al. Liposomal nystatin against experimental pulmonary aspergillosis in persistently neutropenic rabbits: efficacy, safety and non-compartmental pharmacokinetics. *J Antimicrob Chemother* 1999;43:95–103.

158. Groll AH, Petraitis V, Petraitiene R, et al. Antifungal efficacy and safety of multilamellar liposomal nystatin against disseminated candidiasis in persistently neutropenic rabbits. *Antimicrob Agents Chemother* 1999;43:2463–2467.

159. Cossum PA, Wyse J, Simmons Y, et al. Pharmacokinetics of Nyotran (liposomal nystatin) in human patients. In: *Program and Abstracts of the 36th Interscience Conference on Antimicrobial Agents and Chemotherapy,* American Society for Microbiology, Washington, D.C., 1996, abstract A88, p. 17.

160. Groll AH, Mickiene D, Werner K, et al. Compartmental pharmacokinetics and tissue distribution of multilamellar liposomal nystatin in rabbits. *Antimicrob Agents Chemother* 2000;44:950–957.

161. Boutati E, Maltezou HC, Lopez-Berestein G, et al. Phase I study of maximum tolerated dose of intravenous liposomal nystatin for the treatment of refractory febrile neutropenia in patients with haematological malignancies. In: *Program and Abstracts of the 35th Interscience Conference on Antimicrobial Agents and Chemotherapy.* American Society for Microbiology, Washington, D.C., 1995, abstract LM 22, p. 330.

162. Offner FCJ, Herbrecht R, Engelhard D, et al. EORTC-IFCG phase II study on liposomal nystatin in patients with invasive aspergillosis refractory or intolerant to conventional/lipid amphotericin B. In: *Abstracts of the 40th Interscience Conference on Antimicrobial Agents and Chemotherapy.* American Society for Microbiology, Washington, D.C., 2000, abstract 1102, p. 372.

163. Rolston K, Baird I, Graham DR, et al. Treatment of refractory candidemia in non-neutropenic patients with liposomal nystatin (Nyotran™). In: *Program and Abstracts of the 38h Interscience Conference on Antimicrobial Agents and Chemotherapy.* American Society for Microbiology, Washington, D.C., 1998, abstract LB-1, p. 24.

164. Roilides E, Dignani MC, Anaissie EJ, et al. The role of immunoreconstitution in the management of refractory opportunistic fungal infections. *Med Mycol* 1998;36(Suppl 1):12–25.

165. Berenguer J, Allende MC, Lee JW,et al. Pathogenesis of pulmonary aspergillosis. Granulocytopenia versus cyclosporine and methylprednisolone-induced immunosuppression. *Am J Respir Crit Care Med* 1995;152:1079–1086.

166. Romani L, Mencacci A, Grohmann U, et al. Neutralizing antibody to interleukin-4 induces systemic protection and T helper type I-associated immunity in murine candidiasis. *J Exp Med* 1992;176:19–25.

167. Romani L, Pucetti P, Mencacci A, et al. Neutralization of IL-10 up-regulates nitric-oxide production and protects susceptible mice from challenge with *Candida albicans. J Immunol* 1994;152:3514–3521.

168. Puccetti P, Mencacci A, Cenci E, et al. Cure of murine candidiasis by recombinant soluble interleukin-4 receptor. *J Infect Dis* 1994;169:1325–1331.

169. Tonnetti L, Spaccapelo R, Cenci R, et al. Interleukin 4 and 10 exacerbate candidiasis in mice. *Eur J Immunol* 1995;25:1559–1565.

170. Cenci E, Perito S, Enssle KH, et al. Th1 and Th2 cytokines in mice with invasive aspergillosis. *Infect Immun* 1997;65:564–570.
171. Cenci E, Mencacci A, Fe d'Ostiani C, et al. Cytokine- and T helper-dependent lung mucosal immunity in mice with invasive pulmonary aspergillosis. *J Infect Dis* 1998;178:1750–1760.
172. Chanock SJ, Gorlin JB. Granulocyte transfusions. Time for a second look. *Infect Dis Clin N Am* 1996;10:327–343.
173. Dignani MC, Anaissie EJ, Hester JP, et al. Treatment of neutropenia-related fungal infections with granulocyte colony-stimulating factor-elicited white blood cell transfusions: a pilot study. *Leukemia* 1997;11:1621–1630.
174. Akashi K, Traver D, Miyamoto T, et al. A clonogenic common myeloid progenitor that gives rise to all myeloid lineages. *Nature* 2000;404:193–197.
175. BitMansur AA, Weissman LL, Brown JM. Non-myelocytic immune response to invasive aspergillosis following lethal irradiation and hematopoietic stem cell transplantation. *Biol Blood Marrow Transplant* 2000;6:132.
176. Cenci E, Mencacci A, Bacci A, et al. T cell vaccination in mice with invasive pulmonary aspergillosis. *J Immunol* 2000;165:381–388.
177. Childs R, Chernoff A, Contentin N, et al. Regression of metastatic renal-cell carcinoma after nonmyeloablative allogeneic peripheral-blood stem-cell transplantation. *N Engl J Med* 2000;343:750–758.
178. Bishop MR. Non-myeloablative allogeneic hematopoietic stem cell transplantation as adoptive cellular therapy. In: Rosenberg SA (ed): *Principles and Practice of Biologic Therapy of Cancer Updates*, vol. 2, no. 1, 2001, pp. 1–9.

15

Immune Recovery Following Allogeneic Blood Transplantation

Mechanisms of Immune Dysfunction

James E. Talmadge, PhD

1. INTRODUCTION

High-dose chemotherapy (HDT) followed by stem cell transplantation (SCT), using mobilized blood stem cell product (BSCP), cord blood, or bone marrow (BM), is used to treat a variety of advanced malignancies, as well as congenital and autoimmune conditions. In the last decade, it has become apparent that following HDT with an SCT, using either an allogeneic or autologous BSCP, causes more rapid neutrophil, platelet, and immune recoveries to be observed in comparison to an SCT with a BM product. We and others have observed an immune dysfunction in the peripheral blood (PB) of patients following HDT and SCT despite restoration of total T cell numbers. This immunologic dysfunction includes an inversion in the CD4:CD8 T cell ratio and a depression of T cell function. Mechanistic studies have demonstrated a cell-mediated suppression of T cell function in mobilized BSCP and the PB of allogeneic and autologous SCT patients. This loss of function has been associated with increased T cell apoptosis, which occurs predominantly within CD4+ T cell subpopulations. The induction of apoptosis is mediated, at least in part, by Fas Ligand (FasL) expression on monocytes, which are found in significantly higher numbers in mobilized BSCP and in the PB following SCT. In addition, high levels of type 2 cytokines are found in the infused T cells and monocytes as well as in the PB post-transplantation. These defects in immune function may be clinically relevant, as the tolerance induced following HDT and SCT may limit the acute graft-vs-host disease (GVHD) that occurs following the infusion of 10- to 100-fold greater numbers of T cells by an allogeneic mobilized BSCP, as compared to bone marrow transplant

From: *Current Clinical Oncology: Allogeneic Stem Cell Transplantation*
Edited by: Mary S. Laughlin and Hillard M. Lazarus © Humana Press Inc., Totowa, NJ

(BMT). It should be noted that a significant increase in chronic GVHD does occur post-SCT compared to post-BMT. Graft manipulation to reduce T cell contamination is currently being used with increased frequency to reduce GVHD. However, if the graft contains less than 2×10^5 $CD3^+$ T cells, an increased risk of graft failure is observed, concomitant with an increase in the relapse rate. These observations and results suggest that graft manipulation and the cytokine used for mobilization and/or acceleration of hematopoietic recovery may have the potential to induce peripheral tolerance and reduce GVHD while retaining graft-versus-tumor (GVT) activity.

2. COMPARISON OF IMMUNE RECOVERY FOLLOWING PERIPHERAL BLOOD STEM CELL TRANSPLANTATION VS BONE MARROW TRANSPLANTATION

At present, most autologous transplants use mobilized BSCP for transplant, and there is a clear trend for this to occur with allogeneic transplants, although some pediatric donors will likely continue to require the use of BM products. Hematopoietic cells are found predominantly in the BM, but are mobilized in substantiated numbers to the PB by the administration of recombinant granulocyte-macrophage colony-stimulating factor (GM-CSF), granulocyte colony-stimulating factor (G-CSF), Flt3 Ligand (Flt3L), stem cell factor (SCF), and interleukin (IL)-3. Apheresis products containing G-CSF-mobilized cells are now widely used instead of BM for autologous and allogeneic transplantation (1). Transplantation with a mobilized BSCP results in a more rapid hematopoietic and hematologic recovery compared to that observed following bone marrow transplantation (BMT) (2–7). The initial favorable results with autologous mobilized BSCP prompted the evaluations of allogeneic BSCP for hematopoietic rescue (8–10). The results of these studies, which used historical controls, suggested that the recovery of neutrophils, red blood cells, and platelets was faster with the use of mobilized BSCP than steady state BM products, with no apparent increase in the incidence of acute GVHD (11–13). However, in the initial retrospective analyses, the relapse and survival outcomes were conflicting (14–20). Several randomized studies, each involving 37–100 patients, have been reported (21–23). The initial trials found that engraftment with mobilized BSCP was more rapid. However, because of the size and design of the trials, questions remained about the effects of mobilized BSCP vs steady state BM products on the incidence of chronic GVHD, relapse, and survival.

Bensinger et al. (24). recently reported a large multicenter randomized trial that compared the use of allogeneic BM to mobilized BSCP from human leukocyte antigen (HLA) identical and related donors with respect to the incidence of acute and chronic GVHD and hematopoietic engraftment. In this study, patients were randomly assigned to receive either BM or filgrastim-mobilized BSCP from HLA identical relatives for hematopoietic rescue after HDT, with or without radiation. It was found that the recovery of both neutrophils and platelets was significantly faster following transplantation with mobilized BSCP than with BM. The cumulative incidence of grade I, II, III, or IV acute GVHD at 100 d was similar, with 64% following transplantation with mobilized BSCP and 57% with BM. The cumulative incidence of chronic GVHD, following allogeneic transplantation, was 46% with a mobilized BSCP and 35% with a BM product. The overall survival at 2 yr was 66% with BSCP and 54% with BMT, and the rate of disease-free survival (DFS) was significantly extended at 2 yr to 65% following transplantation with BSCP and to 45% following BMT. As part of this study, a comparison was also undertaken on immune recovery, which showed a more rapid T cell reconstitution following transplant with a BSCP. In contrast, despite the infusion of 12-fold more $CD3^+$ cells (i.e., T cells) in the mobilized BSCP than in the BM product, the rates of acute and chronic GVHD were not significantly higher. They concluded that the transplantation of mobilized BSCP might offer advantages over BM in terms of overall survival (OS) and DFS. Further, patients with advanced disease may have a lower risk of interstitial pneumonia and recurrent disease following SCT with a BSCP, due to the more rapid immunologic recovery. Similar results were reported earlier from a retrospective registry analysis in which the rate of survival was higher among patients with advanced disease who received a mobilized BSCP compared to a BMT *(20)*.

In four smaller randomized studies that compared SCT using mobilized BSCP to BMT after HDT *(21–23)*, it was found that platelet recovery occurred earlier following an SCT, and in three of the four studies, neutrophil recovery also occurred earlier. In addition, the risk of acute GVHD was similar in recipients of mobilized BSCP compared to recipients of steady state BM products. However, in two of the four studies, the risk of chronic GVHD was higher in the patients who received a mobilized BSCP. These disparities in chronic GVHD might be due to the small numbers of patients in each study, differences among the studies in the length of follow-up, the type of prophylaxis against GVHD, or the G-CSF regimen used for mobilization. The GVHD prophylaxis may have been critical, because in the two studies that reported a higher incidence of chronic GVHD following SCT as compared to BMT, methotrexate was not given on d 11 after SCT. Significantly, patients who received an allogeneic BM graft and did not receive methotrexate on d 11 also had an increased risk of acute GVHD *(25)*. Although this does not directly explain the higher incidence of chronic GVHD in patients who receive mobilized BSCP, acute GVHD predisposes patients to the development of chronic GVHD. The registry analysis *(20)* also reported a significantly higher incidence of chronic GVHD among recipients of mobilized BSCP (65 vs 53% among BM recipients), which was similar to that observed in the Bensinger study *(24)*.

Another difference found in these four randomized studies was the use of G-CSF at 10 μg/kg/d for mobilization, which was lower than the 16 μg/kg/d dose used in the Bensinger study *(24)*. The latter regimen of G-CSF was based on data indicating that the yield of $CD34^+$ cells is better with higher doses of G-CSF. Another possible reason for similar levels of GVHD following infusion of a higher number of T cells with an SCT is the finding in animal and clinical studies that G-CSF induces type 2 T cells, which produce IL-4 and IL-10 *(26–30)*. IL-4 and IL-10 (type 2 T cells) downregulate inflammatory responses, including those involved in GVHD *(31)*. In addition, G-CSF mobilizes greater numbers of $CD14^+$ monocytes with suppressor-cell function *(32)* and greater numbers of dendritic cells (DCs) that can induce a type 2 helper T cell response *(28)* Thus, the use of G-CSF and potentially the dose administered may reduce the risk of chronic GVHD by inducing qualitative or quantitative changes in the cytokines produced by T cells, monocyte,s and DCs.

Furthermore, the results of one randomized and one retrospective study suggest that allogeneic SCT, as compared to BMT, may be associated with a lower risk of relapse *(33,34)*. Bensinger et al. found a similar trend, although in their original study the subgroups of patients with specific cancers were too small for individual analysis *(11)*. This study also suggested that the graft-vs-leukemia (GVL) effect of allogeneic T cells may be greater in patients with chronic myeloid leukemia (CML) and less obvious in other types of leukemia. Further studies are needed to answer questions about the antileukemic potency of mobilized BSCP as compared to BM products.

Recently, Shenoy et al. reported results from an in-depth study of immune reconstitution and cytokine expression in SCT recipients in the first year posttransplantation *(35)*. Engraftment of neutrophils and monocytes stabilized early, but natural killer (NK) cells, B cells, and $CD4^+$ T cell numbers were significantly depressed, with an inversed CD4:CD8 ratio. In this study, NK function remained low throughout the first year, as did T cell proliferative responses to mitogens and alloantigens. Furthermore, a third of SCT recipients developed acute GVHD (grades II–IV) and 72% of those patients went on to develop extensive chronic GVHD. Clinically, over half of the patients developed cytomegalovirus (CMV) viremia, including some with overt CMV disease in the first year post-SCT (PSCT). The authors concluded that the balance between lymphocyte reconstitution and function, as well as changes in lymphocyte patterns, influenced both infection rates and GVHD.

The lymphocyte and monocyte composition of cytokine-mobilized BSCP, as well as their cellular function, is different from BM and resting PB (31,36–38). Differences in immune reconstitution by BM and BSCP may be due to the product characteristics, which include a fourfold monocyte increase in the PB of normal allogeneic donors mobilized with G-CSF (38,39). In addition, CD19+ B cells are increased about threefold, and CD3+ T cells are increased around twofold. The increase in CD3+ cells is reflected as a proportionate increase in CD4+ and CD8+ T cell subsets, thus maintaining a normal CD4:CD8 ratio (39,40). In addition to increases in the absolute numbers of B and T cells, NK cells are increased 150% from baseline after G-CSF mobilization. Several recent studies have confirmed the observations that growth factors promote the mobilization of lymphocytes and NK cells in allogeneic donors. Korbling et al. (41) described a 16-fold increase in CD3+ cells and a 13-fold increase in CD4+ T cells, and Mills et al. (38) described an increase in CD4RO+ memory cells and γδ cells. Korbling et al. also observed a 27.4-fold increase in CD8+ T cells after PB growth factor mobilization compared to BM harvests. An 11-fold increase in CD19+ B cells and a 19.4-fold increase in CD56+ NK cells was also noted (41).

Numerous studies have now shown that an autologous SCT results in a significantly more rapid recovery of monocytes, NK cells, and naïve CD4+ T lymphocytes, which translates into rapid recovery of immune function compared to the delayed reconstitution of naïve CD4+ T lymphocytes after conventional BMT (42,43). Therefore, it is conceivable that the infusion of stem cell products with altered numbers of lymphocytes, monocytes, and NK cells in an allogeneic setting could affect posttransplant immune reconstitution, as well as the extent and severity of GVHD. Conversely, immune reconstitution, which is crucial following transplantation, is linked to the development and treatment of GVHD, and influences infectious complications (44–47).

Pavletic et al. examined lymphocyte recovery in 41 patients after allogeneic SCT (48). BSCP were mobilized with G-CSF from HLA-matched related donors and cryopreserved, and G-CSF was administered posttransplant. Median time to an absolute lymphocyte count (ALC) ≥500/μL was 17 d vs 41 d for a cohort of historical allogeneic BMT patients. In these studies, the CD4:CD8 ratio was 1.9 on d 28 after SCT, which gradually declined to 0.8 at 1 yr, due to a rapid CD8+ cell recovery. T cell function, as measured by phytohemagglutinin antigen (PHA) mitogen, was lower than normal on d 28 but returned to normal values by 6 mo. In contrast, NK cell function was depressed from d 28 to 1 yr post-allogeneic SCT. In these studies, faster lymphocyte recovery correlated with better survival (median follow-up 287 d), and it was suggested that ALC recovery was not affected by acute GVHD, CMV infections, or the number of infused cells. In contrast, ALC recovery did not correlate with survival in the historical allogeneic BMT group. These data suggest that lymphocyte reconstitution is faster following allogeneic SCT than following BMT and that quicker lymphocyte recovery may be associated with better survival, in SCT, but not BMT, patients.

In contrast to the study reported by Pavletic et al., patients generally demonstrate a varying period of immune incompetence following allogeneic BMT that can last for several years after transplantation and may cause significant morbidity and mortality (49–52), in association with acute and chronic GVHD (49,53). Immune reconstitution after allogeneic BMT has been studied extensively in adults (43,49,51,54), and the innate immune system, i.e., the function of phagocytes, recovers in the first weeks to months after BMT, whereas complete reconstitution of the adaptive immune system, i.e., B and T lymphocytes, takes longer. As a result, a risk of infectious complications often exists for a prolonged period after allogeneic BMT *(55)*.

3. MECHANISMS OF IMMUNE SUPPRESSION

A number of studies have examined the origin of the immune dysfunction that occurs following SCT, using both allogeneic and autologous stem cell products. Immune dysfunction, at least T cell abnormalities, appears to be associated with the induction of tolerance. Central tolerance occurs in the thymus and is triggered by the recognition of "self" antigens (Ags), providing a mechanism to eliminate autoreactive T cells *(56,57)*. In contrast, mature T cells may undergo activation-induced cell death (AICD) following Ag stimulation, thereby providing another mechanism of homeostasis *(58–60)*. During allogeneic SCT, donor T cells, which are alloreactive, can cause GVHD, resulting in significant morbidity and mortality. In addition, a prolonged immune deficiency can occur, which is characterized by lymphopenia and susceptibility to infection *(61–64)*. In adults, the prolonged lymphopenia is characterized by a delay in the recovery of naïve $CD4^+$ T cells, presumably due to age-related loss of thymus function, although a more active loss of CD4 cellularity appears to occur as described below *(43,65,66)*.

Apoptosis provides one mechanism for the regulation of peripheral $CD4^+$ T cell homeostasis. It is a highly regulated process that is dependent upon the expression of a family of death-inducing ligands, including tumor necrosis factor (TNF), Fas ligand (FasL), TNF-related apoptosis-inducing ligand (TRAIL), and their receptors *(67–74)*. Initial studies demonstrated monocyte-dependent $CD4^+$ T cell apoptosis, which is postulated to contribute to $CD4^+$ T cell depletion in HIV-infected individuals and an inverted CD4:CD8 T cell ratio *(75–79)*. We have shown that cancer patients undergoing HDT and SCT, like human immunodeficiency virus (HIV)-infected individuals, have a prolonged immune dysfunction, an inverted CD4:CD8 ratio, and may appear to have peripheral tolerance *(31,42,80–83)*. This profile of immune dysregulation following HDT and SCT provides a potential prophylactic and/or therapeutic mechanism for autoimmune and inflammatory diseases, as well as a strategy to reduce GVHD.

Recently, Li et al. *(84)* demonstrated that treatments which enhance the induction of apoptosis in activated T cells, such as a co-stimulator blockade administered together with Rapamycin, could promote allograft tolerance in model systems. However, it is not clear why newly maturing T cells did not replace the apoptotic cells that were lost to AICD, resulting in the elimination of an allograft or continuation of an autoimmune or inflammatory disease process *(85)*. These studies suggest that in addition to clonal deletion, apoptotic T cells trigger an immunoregulatory effect that serves to maintain tolerance. An alternative explanation, based on studies that we and others have undertaken, suggests that a type 2 cytokine profile is induced following transplantation, perhaps in association with the high levels and/or multiple cycles of chemotherapy, which may be critical to the maintenance of tolerance *(86,87)*. Thus, the mechanisms of immunoregulation following SCT and BMT may be multifactorial, including clonal deletion via AICD as well as regulation via type 2 cytokines. The finding of prognostic significance for IL-10 production in patients prior to an allogeneic BMT provides support for the roles of a type 2 response in tolerance *(88)*. In these studies, high spontaneous IL-10 production was correlated with low incidence of GVHD and transplant-related mortality as compared to patients with low or intermediate levels of IL-10 *(88)*. Support for the role of IL-10 is also provided by the observation that increased IL-10 production by mononuclear cells is associated with tolerance in severe combined immunodeficiency disease (SCID) patients following haplotype identical BMT *(89)*. Recently, the injection of mononuclear cells, i.e., ex vivo-expanded and mature DCs, was shown to prolong haplotype-specific cardiac allograft survival when administered prior to transplantation *(90)*. It is likely that this is due to DC expression of FasL as well as secretion of IL-10; thus they may be key mediators of tolerance *(90)*.

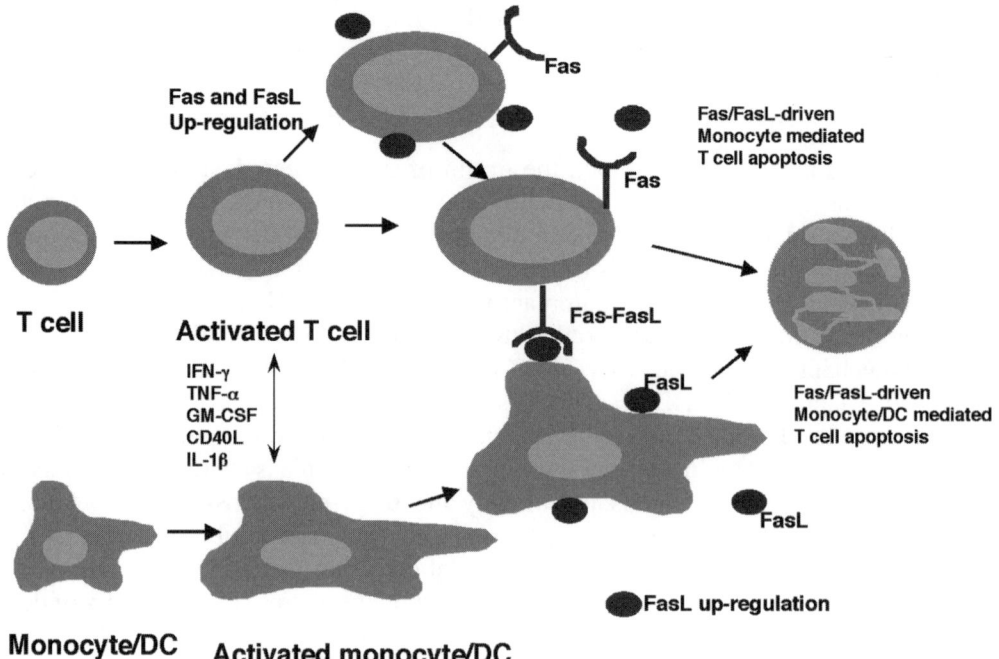

Fig. 1. This represents one hypothetical mechanism for the peripheral tolerance that is observed following SCT. This multi-stepped process involves activated T cells secreting interferon (IFN)-γ, as well as other cytokines, which activate monocytes and DCs. These activated mononuclear cells express FasL on their membrane as well as release soluble FasL into the serum, which can then induce the apoptosis of Fas-expressing (activated) T cells.

The selective depletion of CD4+ T cells is one mechanism associated with the peripheral tolerance observed following HDT and SCT. This selective depletion is associated not only with peripheral tolerance, but also with immune dysfunction and a depressed CD4:CD8 T cell ratio, which are all observed following HDT and SCT *(31,42,91)*. In our published studies, we associated the loss of T cell function in the PB with both frequency of monocytes and monocytes expressing FasL *(92)*. We suggest that the preferential deletion of CD4+ T cells is due to their increased expression of Fas, as compared to CD8+ T cells, which have a normal frequency of Fas expression and a high frequency of monocytes expressing FasL in the PB. Further, we have observed high levels of mRNA for monocyte-activating cytokines in T cells following transplantation, which may upregulate FasL expression by the monocytes *(87)*. We have shown that monocytes in mobilized PSC products, as well as in PB following transplantation, inhibit T cell function *(31,42,83,93)* by inducing T cell apoptosis *(93)*. While these studies do not prove a cause-and-effect relationship, the high frequency of apoptotic CD4+ T cells in the PB of patients following HDT and SCT might contribute to clonal deletion and a loss of T cell receptor (TCR) diversity *(92)*. Please see Fig. 1, which provides an overview of this process. Reports by Donnenberg et al. *(94,95)* suggest that T cell apoptosis parallels lymphopoiesis in patients who have had BMTs. In vitro, it appears that T cell apoptosis *(96–99)* is associated with T cell activation by either CD3+ crosslinking, phorbol myristate acetate (PMA), or PHA *(31,38,42,83,93,100,101)*. The requirement for T cell activation appears to be a common feature of monocyte-dependent T cell apoptosis mediated by Fas–FasL interaction *(71,78,79)*. Our previous results suggest that the T cells and monocytes in the PB of HDT and SCT patients are highly activated based on the expression of immunoregulatory cytokines *(86,87)*. The circulating T lymphocytes from HIV-infected individuals are activated *(97)*, and the CD4+ T cells have an increased expression of Fas on their membranes *(98,99)*, resulting in an increased susceptibility to FasL-mediated killing *(99)*. Thus, we suggest that activated CD4$^+$ T cells in the PB of HDT and SCT patients undergo apoptosis after encountering monocytes expressing FasL. However, the circumstance and site(s) whereby a susceptible CD4$^+$ T cell encounters an apoptosis-inducing ligand are unknown.

During normal T cell maturation, BM-derived T cell precursors home to the thymus, where they are subjected to positive and negative selection processes upon interaction with major histocompatibility complex (MHC) class I and II molecules expressed on thymic epithelial cells and DC *(102–104)*. These selection processes ensure a nonautoreactive peripheral T cell repertoire. MHC class II-mediated interactions result primarily in CD4$^+$ T cell development, whereas MHC class I-mediated interactions direct CD8$^+$ T cell development. During T cell selection in normal individuals, TCR genes are sequentially and randomly spliced together in a diverse TCR repertoire *(105–108)*. Complementarity determining region 3 (CDR3) β chain size heterogeneity arises during developmental DNA rearrangement when a consistent segment is joined with 1 of 22 variable segments via a diversity (D) and a joining (J) segment to give rise to a complete gene. During this process, random numbers of nucleotides are inserted and deleted at the junctions between the gene segments *(109)*. Successful rearrangements differ in size, and any other rearrangements would be out of frame and are rarely detected in PB T cells *(110)*. As the ratio of transcripts per cell is fairly constant *(111)*, the amount of polymerase chain reaction (PCR) product in each size class gives an indication of the number of clonotypes and thus T cell repertoire diversity. Predominance of only a few size classes in a spectratype would indicate oligoclonality. Gaps in a spectratype indicate a lack of T cells expressing a certain CDR3 size class.

The loss of mature T cells following myeloablative conditioning protocols in preparation for SCT allows regeneration of the T cell population via at least two pathways. First, there is a transfer of graft-derived mature donor T cells to the periphery followed by Ag-driven expansion. This process, which represents a thymus-independent pathway of reconstitution, may provide the first wave of T cells *(112–114)*. It should be noted, however, that T cell recovery occurs only slightly less rapidly following infusion of T cell-depleted autografts *(115)*. These mature T cells have a limited TCR diversity *(116)* and can be maintained in the periphery for 10–20 yr *(117)*, provided appropriate TCR-peptide/MHC interactions occur *(118,119)*. The second mechanism involves selection of graft-derived precursor cells in the thymus *(120-122)* and/or other peripheral selection sites *(123,124)*. The process of thymic T cell selection probably accounts for a durable reconstitution of the T cell compartment and a potentially more diverse TCR repertoire. Because thymic functions decrease with age *(52,114)*, this selection mechanism is most effective in young SCT recipients and may contribute to the delayed recovery of T cells in adults *(43,51,54)*.

The role of T cell selection in the thymus and/or periphery during T cell recovery after allogeneic SCT has been analyzed based on overall and Ag-specific T cell repertoires in pediatric SCT recipients treated for leukemia. A lack of TCR diversity occurs in the repopulating T cells at 3 mo after SCT, based on CDR3 size distribution patterns displaying reduced complexity. This is increasing in recipients of a T cell-depleted (TCD) graft and, to a lesser extent, in recipients of unmanipulated grafts. One year after allogeneic SCT, normalization occurs in the TCR, CDR3 size complexity in almost all recipients. Further, an analysis of an Ag-specific T cell repertoire at 1 yr after SCT showed that the T cells responding to tetanus toxoid differed in TCR gene segment usage and in amino acid composition of the CDR3 region as compared to the donor *(125)*. Further, the tetanus toxoid-specific TCR repertoire is stable within an SCT recipient because tetanus toxoid-specific T cells with identical TCRs have been observed over 3 consecutive years after transplantation *(125)*.

Other studies have used CDR3 size spectratyping to study TCR reconstitution after BMT. Gorski et al. *(110)* suggested that T cell repertoire complexity in BMT recipients was associated with their state of immune function. Similarly, Dietrich et al. *(126)* examined T cell spectratypes in GVHD skin lesions, and Akatsuka et al. *(127)* and Roux et al. *(64,116)* examined differences in T cell repertoire reconstitution in patients who received TCD BM as compared to ones who received an undepleted BM. Lastly, Claret et al. *(128)* characterized T cell repertoires in BMT recipients with GVL responses following donor leukocyte infusion (DLI). However, these studies were limited by the small number of patients and a short follow-up.

Recently Verfuerth, O'Reilly, et al. *(129)* examined immune reconstitution following allogeneic SCT with TCD BMT, based on CDR3 size spectratyping to monitor TCR reconstitution. The study included 19 patients over approx 2 yr who received a transplant for the treatment of CML. In addition, they examined the effect of DLI on CDR3 spectratyping. In these studies, all patients had irregular spectratypes in the first 3–6 mo after transplantation, which evolved over the next 6 mo to express more normal patterns. In approximately one-third of the patients, 2–3 yr were required for the spectratypes to normalize and some patients had abnormal spectratypes even at 3 yr. DLI, which was used for the treatment of relapse in 18 of the 19 patients, had varying effects on CDR3 size profiles. In 9 out of 18 patients, there was no change in CDR3 size profiles, whereas in six patients, the spectratypes became more restricted and irregular. Overall, it appears that T cell spectratypes in BMT patients demonstrated instability over time and in patients with GVHD, this instability is exaggerated. In addition, as a conditioning regimen, T cell depletion, loss or reduction in thymic function, exposure to infectious agents, GVHD, and immunosuppressive treatments are also likely to contribute to the TCR expression abnormalities and delay in T cell repertoire reconstitution.

In one recent study *(91)*, investigators reached an additional conclusion regarding the T cell apoptosis that occurs following allogeneic SCT. This study demonstrated a significant increase in the apoptosis of CD3$^+$ T cells obtained from patients 19–23 d following transplantation, as well as 1 yr posttransplantation, compared to healthy individuals. The increase in apoptosis occurred preferentially in HLA-DR$^+$ cells and in both CD4$^+$ and CD8$^+$ T cell subsets. CD4$^+$ T cell apoptosis was greater in patients with extensive acute GVHD and was increased in patients who received HLA-mismatched donors or matched unrelated donors compared with patients who received transplants from HLA identical siblings. There also was a significant correlation between the apoptosis of CD4$^+$ T cells and decreased CD4$^+$ T cell count.

This mechanism of apoptosis occurs by AICD in which a key role is played by CD95/Fas, which is a molecule expressed by the majority of CD45RO$^+$T cells, and by a much smaller number of CD45RA$^+$ cells.(130) Crosslinking of CD95 causes cell death of sensitive cells *(131,132)* and the susceptibility to CD95-induced AICD is a function of the activation of CD45RO$^+$ T cells *(133,134)*. Peripheral T cell repopulation after BMT has a characteristic CD45RO$^+$ activated phenotype *(43,135–138)* and defective production of IL-2 *(139)*. In one study *(140)*, regeneration of naïve (CD4$^+$CD45RA$^+$) T cells correlated with the recovery of mitogen-induced proliferative responses. This occurs in the few months posttransplantation in association with a mature or CD45RO$^+$ CD4+ cell phenotype.

Additional studies have suggested that posttransplantation increased cell death occurs as a consequence of the defective production of IL-2 and down-regulation of basic cycle length (BCL)-2, resulting in an increased susceptibility to AICD following mitogen stimulation. This observation suggests a role for CD95, which is supported by the observation of high levels of CD95 expression on CD4$^+$ cells. Thus, a decrease in lymphocyte activation may contribute to recovery from the apoptosis and lymphopenia that occurs post-HDT and SCT. Similar results were reported by Hebib et al. *(141)* who examined T cell reconstitution following allogeneic BMT. In these studies, for at least 1 yr posttransplantation, there was an expansion of T cells with a memory phenotype (CD45RO) and a CD4:CD8 ratio inversion. Their studies revealed an increased susceptibility to apoptosis via anti-Fas triggering in vitro *(141)*. Apoptosis was reduced over time and appeared to occur when the absolute numbers of naïve T cells (CD45RA$^+$/ CD62-L$^+$) increased. In addition, in vivo apoptosis was significantly correlated with lower levels of BCL-2 expression as assessed by cytofluorometry and Western Blot analysis. In contrast, the levels of Bax protein remained unchanged, resulting in a dysregulated BCL-2/Bax ratio. Overall, these studies are consistent with murine models, in which small numbers of mature T cells are coinjected with BM cells into thymectomized and lethally irradiated mice. In these models, T cell regeneration occurs via the expansion of the injected T cells *(142,143)*. This suggests that adult BMT patients (with an aged and/or irradiated thymus) develop T cell populations, following SCT, from thymus-independent expansion of mature T cells from within the BM graft *(142,144)*. Further, the peripheral expansion of donor T cells may be driven by host histocompatibility Ags *(145)* and viral Ags *(146,147)*, resulting in a restricted T cell repertoire *(145)*, and occasionally oligoclonality *(148)*. T cell regeneration may also be driven by an Ag-independent homeostatic process controlling the size of the T cell compartment *(113)*.

4. TCD OF STEM CELL PRODUCTS

Allogeneic BMT or SCT from HLA-matched donors can provide a curative therapy for CML *(149)* and other hematologic disorders. However, the immune suppression associated with SCT is a significant cause of morbidity and mortality. T cell immunity is primarily affected because T cells are eliminated by the pretransplant conditioning regimen and thymic output is limited in adults *(66,150)*. Thus, the T cell immunodeficiency that occurs in SCT recipients can result in a life-threatening, opportunistic infection *(49,63)*. Depletion of T cells from the donor BSCP reduces the risk of GVHD by limiting the number of alloreactive T cells. However, this results in an increased risk of relapse and is compared with unmanipulated SCT because T cells, which are critical to GVL responses, are also removed *(151,152)*. Further, the reduced number of CD3$^+$ cells can inhibit myeloid and platelet recovery if depleted to $\leq 0.54 \times 10^5$. Indeed, a recent study revealed that a depletion of CD3$^+$ cells to below 0.2×10^6/kg significantly increased the risk of graft failure *(153)*.

Several studies have directly compared immune recovery after transplantation with TCD and unselected progenitor cell populations. In one study *(154)*, which used CD34$^+$ stem cell selection to deplete T cells, the number of CD3$^+$ lymphocytes posttransplantation was found to be below the normal range in both groups. In contrast, the absolute number of CD19$^+$ B lymphocytes after transplantation with a TCD product were within the normal range. In contrast, CD4$^+$ lymphocyte recovery was depressed, while CD8$^+$ lymphocyte recovery was increased in eight patients transplanted with TCD products and within the normal range for patients transplanted with an intact product. As a result, an inversion in the CD4:CD8 ratio was found in both groups. Activated T lymphocytes and NK cells were also increased in both groups. Godthelp et al. *(125)* also examined CDR3 usage by T cells responding to tetanus toxoid. They found, in this direct comparative study, a lack of overall TCR diversity in the repopulating T cells at 3 mo after allogeneic SCT based on CDR3 size distribution. This was particularly noted in those patients who received a TCD graft, and to a lesser extent, in recipients of unmanipulated grafts. At 1 yr following allogeneic BMT, normalization was observed in the CDR3 size complexity in almost all recipients. An analysis of the Ag-specific T cell repertoire 1 yr after allogeneic BMT showed that the T cells responding to tetanus toxoid differed in TCR gene segment usage and amino acid composition of the CDR3 region as compared to the donor. Further, the tetanus toxoid-specific T cell repertoire was found to be stable within each allogeneic BMT recipient because tetanus toxic-specific T cells with identical TCRs were found 3 yr after transplantation. In a more extensive study by Martinez et al. *(155)*, it was found that CD4+ T cell counts were significantly lower in patients receiving a TCD transplant as compared to ones receiving an intact transplant. In these studies, CD4+ T cell counts were lower in the TCD patient as compared to patients transplanted with an intact product 0.5, 1, 2, 3, and 6 mo posttransplantation. In contrast, there was no difference between the two groups at eight months posttransplantation and thereafter. Normal levels of CD8+ T cells were achieved 1 mo posttransplantation in both groups, and increased numbers of NK cells (CD3-CD56+) were observed in both groups. These results suggested that during the first 6 mo following allogeneic SCT with TCD allografts, as compared to intact allografts, the number of CD4+, CD4+CD45RA+, and TCR-γδ+ cells were significantly lower than following transplantation with an unmanipulated allogeneic BSCP. The number of naïve (CD45RA+) CD4+ cells was also low throughout the study period in both groups, although it was significantly lower in the TCD group as compared to the patients transplanted with an intact stem cell product, especially during the first 3 mo following transplantation. In contrast and consistent with other allogeneic and autologous transplant studies, normal levels of CD8 cells were achieved one month posttransplantation in both groups. Consistent with previous studies discussed above, TCR-γδ+ cells were lower in the TCD group than in the intact stem cell product group during the first 4 mo posttransplantation. Normalization of NK cells (CD3-CD56+) was achieved 1 mo posttransplantation in both groups, an observation consistent with prior studies of autologous and allogeneic SCT. In contrast, B lymphocytes (CD19+ cells) were undetectable throughout the first 4 mo in both groups and reached normal levels 8 mo posttransplantation.

In summary, studies that directly compare transplantation with TCD to intact allogeneic stem cell products suggest that a significantly longer time period is needed for the recovery of CD4+, CD4+CD45RA+, and TCR-γδ+ cells when using TCD products. In contrast, there appears to be no differences in the immunologic recovery of CD56+, CD8+, and CD19+ lymphocytes, although the CD4:CD8 ratio, in many instances, is significantly reduced following transplantation with a TCD product. This conclusion was first reached and is largely similar to those reported by Roux et al. *(64)* in 1996.

As discussed herein, the majority of TCD studies have utilized positive selection of CD34+ cells, which results in a 2- to 3-log depletion of T cells. However, other studies have used CAMPATH-1M to deplete the T cell allogeneic stem cell products and have shown that this mechanism of T cell purging also results in significant immunosuppression *(156)*. Thus, the poor recovery of T cells following TCD is independent of the TCD technique used. One of the most important clinical sequelae to the use of TCD stem cell grafts, in addition to loss of graft function and tumor relapse, is an increased incidence of viral, bacterial, and parasitic infections. Many of these infections are of an "exotic" nature and represent ones typically associated with patients who have an HIV infection or an organ transplant. In a recent study by Small et al. *(157)*, they discussed 10 patients who developed disseminated toxoplasmosis following a TCD BMT. Of the patients who developed toxoplasmosis infections, only one survived, and this patient was treated empirically on the day of presentation for fever and headache *(157)*. This suggested that early empirical treatment, even before the results of a sensitivity test are obtained, may help improve survival. Other studies have included the examination of CD4+ T cell recovery. And several of these studies have established a correlation between the rate of CD4+ T cell recovery and the risk of developing a post-transplant opportunistic infection *(158–160)*. These "exotic" infections include not only toxoplasmosis, but also CMV *(158,161)* and herpes virus *(162)*.

Autologous BSCP obtained following mobilization and apheresis contain significant numbers of T cells, which are reinfused into the patient. Presumably, these infused T cells include immunoreactive cells, which can contribute to the autoimmune–inflammatory conditions. Hence, reinfusion of autologous T cells may inhibit the efforts to control or eliminate autoreactive T cell clones. An initial report by Euler *(163)* demonstrated an early recurrence–persistence of autoimmune disease following transplantation with unmanipulated autologous stem cell products. Since that time, several techniques have been employed to reduce the infusion of T cells. These strategies have included depletion of T cells (negative selection) or positive selection of the hematopoietic (CD34$^+$) stem cells. Given the rigor of both techniques, questions remain regarding the level of T cell depletion that should be targeted. Prior studies have shown that allograft patients who receive less than 10^5 T cells/kg body weight develop no GVHD *(164)*. In contrast, four out of seven patients who received between 1 and 4.4 × 10^5 T cells/kg developed dermatologic GVHD *(163)*. These results suggest that the infusion of less than 1 × 10^5 T cells/kg may be a reasonable target dose.

4.1. Infectious Complications of the Immune Dysfunction following HDT and SCT

Within the first year following HDT and SCT, recipients follow a relatively predictable pattern of immunologic reconstitution and develop associated systemic immunodeficiency. In addition to the hypothetical impact that this may have on tumor growth, there is also a significant risk of infectious complications associated with the immunodeficiency (Table 1) caused in part by the chemotherapy or radiation therapy administered just prior to SCT to treat the primary disease. Unfortunately, this conditioning regimen also significantly impacts normal hematopoiesis and hematologic parameters, in addition to damaging mucosal progenitor cells and introducing a temporary loss of the mucosal barrier integrity. Thus, the gastrointestinal tract, which normally contains bacteria and commensal fungi, and other bacteria-carrying sources (e.g., skin or mucosa) become reservoirs of potential pathogens. In the immediate posttransplant period (1–30 d), SCT recipients have two critical risk factors for infection. These include prolonged neutropenia, which occurs most markedly in adult transplant patients receiving isolated CD34 stem cell products, and breaks in the mucocutaneous barrier, which occur in association with the HDT preparative regimens. Further, the need for frequent vascular access results in the induction of oral, gastrointestinal, and skin flora as sources of infection at the site of central-line catheters. Resolution of these infections generally occurs in association with neutrophil recovery (within 30 d). Reactivations of herpes virus infections are also commonly observed during this period. Typically, an SCT recipient's initial fever is caused by a bacterial pathogen, although the causative organism is rarely identified. Such infections are usually treated preemptively or empirically *(165)* until the resolution of neutropenia *(166)*. In addition, growth factors are commonly administered during this period to accelerate neutrophil reconstitution and limit the complications associated with the neutropenia, including febrile neutropenia *(167)*.

Following hematopoietic engraftment (30–100 d), patients remain at a heightened risk of infection from a wide variety of pathogens, including bacterial, viral, and fungal origins. In addition to those listed above, CMV reactivity or infections are commonly observed, as are respiratory syncytial virus (RSV), and influenza infections, all of which may contribute to morbidity and mortality *(168,169)*. Primary infections by and reactivation of varicella zoster infections are also observed following transplantation *(170–173)*.

Bacterial infections are also a significant cause of morbidity and mortality in patients during the late posttransplantation period (100 d–1 yr), particularly those adult patients with chronic GVHD *(44,174–177)*. There is also a strong association between the development of pneumococcal infections and a decrease in circulating levels of IgG and IgM type specific antibody levels and antibody-mediated opsonic activity *(178)*. During the postengraftment phase (30–100 d), this is typically characterized by an impairment in cell-mediated immunity and may be

Table 1
Kinetics of Infections Occurring in Allogeneic SCT Recipients

Preiengraftment (1–30 d)	Postengraftment (30–100 d)	Late phase (100 d–1 yr)
Neutrophils, mucositis, and acute GVHD.	Impaired cellular immunity and acute and chronic GVHD.	Impaired cellular and humoral immunity and chronic GVHD.
Respiratory and enteric viruses	Cytomegalovirus	Varicella-zoster virus
Herpes simplex virus	Epstein-Barr virus lymphoproliferative disease	Encapsulated bacteria
Faculative Gram-negative bacilli	*Toxoplasma gondii*	*Pneumocystitis carinii*
Staphylococcus epidermidis	*Strongyloides stercoralis*	*Mycobacterium* species
Gastrointestinal tract *Streptococci* species		
All *Candida* species		
Aspergillus species		

associated with the presence of GVHD and immunosuppressive therapy. Following engraftment, human herpes virus type 6, CMV, and other herpes viruses are also critical pathogens.

During the late phases of immunologic recovery, there continue to be defects in humoral- and cell-mediated immunity, in addition to impaired reticular endothelial system (RES) system function. Because of these cell-mediated and humoral defects and impaired RES function, patients with chronic GVHD and/or who are recipients of donor allogeneic SCT are at risk for numerous infections. Patients receiving mismatched allogeneic transplants have a higher rate and severity of GVHD, therefore, they also have an increased risk of opportunistic infections than do patients receiving matched allogeneic hematopoietic stem cells (HSC). Losses of antibody titers increase the risk of infection and poor titers to vaccination have been documented in many patients following hemtopoietic cell transplantation (HCT) and SCT. In one study of 40 patients posttransplant, only three patients maintained protective antibody levels to Hib. This response could be increased with the use of a tetanus toxoid conjugate, particularly in those patients who have pronounced immunoglobulin deficiency *(179,180)*. The late immunosuppression is associated with a significant frequency of CMV conversion and frank CMV infections. It is recommended by the Centers for Disease Control that those recipients who receive a product from a CMV seropositive donor should be placed on a CMV prevention program from the time of engraftment until 100 d following SCT. Prophylactic strategies commonly incorporate the administration of ganciclovir. In addition, intravenous immunoglobulin (IVIG) may be used as well as appropriate vaccines. The infusion of donor-derived CMV-specific clones of CD8[+] T cells into the transplant recipient has also been utilized to treat or prevent CMV infection *(181)*, as has high dose acyclovir, but its utility is limited *(182)*. Similar to CMV in an allotransplant setting, Epstein-Barr virus (EBV) is also a significant concern *(183)* and again the infusion of donor-derived EBV-specific cytotoxic T lymphocytes (CTL) has shown highly significant promise in the prophylaxis of EBV-associated lymphomas amont recipients of TCD, unrelated or mismatched allogeneic recipients *(184–189)*. Because this chapter is directed at the immunologic aspects of SCT, questions focused on antibiotic therapy of infectious referred are directed to the excellent review of treatment prophylaxis for infections following SCT found in ref. *190*.

Acute viral infections in normal hosts are controlled by the induction and expansion of antigen-specific, MHC-restricted T cells. As suggested above, human CMV and EBV are ubiquitous pathogens and can utilize a variety of novel strategies to evade immunologic control. CD4[+] and CD8[+] T cells have been shown to have a pivotal role in controlling the initial infection and maintaining CMV and EBV in a latent state. EBV causes potentially lethal immunoblastic lymphomas in approx 25% of SCT recipients receiving a stem cell product from unrelated or HLA-mismatched donors. Risk factors, which include TCD, major MHC-mismatched transplants, and intensity of immunosuppression, support the role of T cell immune surveillance in the control of EBV *(188)* and CMV infections. CMV pneumonitis *(191)*, despite ganciclovir and specific immunoglobulin therapy, has a poor outcome with a mortality rate of 30–70% *(192)*. Thus, strategies involving the adoptive transfer of CMV- or EBV-specific CTL clones or boosting of donor or patient immunity using CMV or EBV vaccines are encouraging. If the allo-donor is vaccinated, the T cells contained within the stem cell product include, in theory, viral-specific CTL. Alternatively, CTL may be derived following ex vivo-expansion of virus-specific CTL using donor leukocytes. In either case, the leukocytes or isolated T cells can be given either prophylactically or therapeutically for the treatment of CMV and EBV infections. The EBV-specific CTL are readily stimulated and expanded using EBV-immortalized B lymphoblastoid cell lines as stimulators. Current protocols for CMV-specific CTL use transfection of PP65, an immunodominant CMV antigen into CMV-infected fibroblasts, DCs or EBV-transformed B lymphoblastic cell lines and used for antigen stimulation *(186)*. Thus, graft manipulation via antigen-specific T cell augmentation, either ex vivo or by donor vaccination, has significant potential as a strategy to affect infection. Further, the utilization of DLI from vaccinated donors or ex vivo-stimulated and expanded viral-specific CTLs provides an exciting new strategy for the control of these life-threatening viral infections *(186)*. Regardless of the strategy used to prevent or treat infections, the marked and prolonged cellular immunodeficiency that is observed following SCT—especially following transplantation with positively selected stem cells—results in an increased incidence of infections, including rare and unusual infections, such as *Pneumocystis carinii*, toxoplasmosism and *Mycobacterium species*.

5. SUMMARY

In summary, we suggest that "primed" or activated Fas[+] CD4[+] T lymphocytes interact with activated monocytes that express FasL, resulting in apoptosis, which leads to the deletion of clonal populations of CD4[+] T cells. Further, manipulation of the stem cell product or cytokine support posttransplantation may provide a strategy to control GVHD. One such manipulation includes the removal of T cells from the product with the retention of monocytes/DCs. If used with a G-CSF-mobilized product, which biases to a DC2 and type 2 response, this technique might help induce tolerance. Indeed, additional knowledge on mobilization, graft processing, conditioning, and manipulation of the product may be necessary to achieve additional clinical benefit. In addition to maximal protocols, objective criteria for treatment responses as well as analysis of nonspecific and specific immunologic reconstitution is needed to help determine strategies for future trials, including low dose conditioning, use of monoclonal antibodies for the depletion of lymphocyte subsets, and blockade of co-stimulatory factors. It appears, as discussed herein, that manipulation of the stem cell product has the potential to control immunologic reconstitution. Further, both the conditioning regimen and the actual transplantation product have immunosuppressive characteristics, and it is likely that these can be taken advantage of to induce peripheral tolerance.

REFERENCES

1. Bensinger W, Appelbaum F, Rowley S, et al. Factors that influence collection and engraftment of autologous peripheral-blood stem cells. *J Clin Oncol* 1995;13(10):2547–2555.

2. Langenmayer I, Weaver C, Buckner CD, et al. Engraftment of patients with lymphoid malignancies transplanted with autologous bone marrow, peripheral blood stem cells or both. *Bone Marrow Transplant* 1995;15(2):241–246.

3. Pavletic ZS, Bishop MR, Tarantolo SR, et al. Hematopoietic recovery after allogeneic blood stem-cell transplantation compared with bone marrow transplantation in patients with hematologic malignancies. *J Clin Oncol* 1997;15(4):1608–1616.

4. Kessinger A, Bierman PJ, Vose JM, et al. High-dose cyclophosphamide, carmustine, and etoposide followed by autologous peripheral stem cell transplantation for patients with relapsed Hodgkin's disease [published erratum appears in Blood 1991 Dec 15;78(12):3330]. B*lood* 1991;77(11):2322–2325.

5. Vose JM, Anderson JR, Kessinger A, et al. High-dose chemotherapy and autologous hematopoietic stem-cell transplantation for aggressive non-Hodgkin's lymphoma. *J Clin Oncol* 1993;11(10):1846–1851.

6. Appelbaum FR. The use of bone marrow and peripheral blood stem cell transplantation in the treatment of cancer [see comments]. *CA Cancer J Clin* 1996;46(3):142–164.

7. Korbling M, Fliedner TM. The evolution of clinical peripheral blood stem cell transplantation. *Bone Marrow Transplant* 1996;17(5):675–678.

8. Bensinger WI, Weaver CH, Appelbaum FR, Rowley S, Demirer T, Sanders J et al. Transplantation of allogeneic peripheral blood stem cells mobilized by recombinant human granulocyte colony-stimulating factor [see comments]. *Blood* 1995;85(6):1655–1658.

9. Korbling M, Przepiorka D, Huh YO, Engel H, van Besien K, Giralt S et al. Allogeneic blood stem cell transplantation for refractory leukemia and lymphoma: potential advantage of blood over marrow allografts. *Blood* 1995;85(6):1659–1665.

10. Schmitz N, Dreger P, Suttorp M, et al. Primary transplantation of allogeneic peripheral blood progenitor cells mobilized by filgrastim (granulocyte colony-stimulating factor). *Blood* 1995;85(6):1666–1672.

11. Bensinger WI, Clift R, Martin P, et al. Allogeneic peripheral blood stem cell transplantation in patients with advanced hematologic malignancies: a retrospective comparison with marrow transplantation. *Blood* 1996;88(7):2794–2800.

12. Przepiorka D, Anderlini P, Ippoliti C, et al. Allogeneic blood stem cell transplantation in advanced hematologic cancers. *Bone Marrow Transplant* 1997;19(5):455–460.

13. Schmitz N, Bacigalupo A, Labopin M, et al. Transplantation of peripheral blood progenitor cells from HLA-identical sibling donors. European Group for Blood and Marrow Transplantation (EBMT). *Br J Haematol* 1996;95(4):715–723.

14. Storek J, Gooley T, Siadak M, et al. Allogeneic peripheral blood stem cell transplantation may be associated with a high risk of chronic graft-versus-host disease. *Blood* 1997;90(12):4705–4709.

15. Solano C, Martinez C, Brunet S, et al. Chronic graft-versus-host disease after allogeneic peripheral blood progenitor cell or bone marrow transplantation from matched related donors. A case-control study. Spanish Group of Allo-PBT. *Bone Marrow Transplant* 1998;22(12):1129–1135.

16. Miflin G, Russell NH, Hutchinson RM, et al. Allogeneic peripheral blood stem cell transplantation for haematological malignancies—an analysis of kinetics of engraftment and GVHD risk. *Bone Marrow Transplant* 1997;19(1):9–13.

17. Majolino I, Saglio G, Scime R, et al. High incidence of chronic GVHD after primary allogeneic peripheral blood stem cell transplantation in patients with hematologic malignancies. *Bone Marrow Transplant* 1996;17(4):555–560.

18. Urbano-Ispizua A, Solano C, et al. Allogeneic peripheral blood progenitor cell transplantation: analysis of short-term engraftment and acute GVHD incidence in 33 cases. allo-PBPCT Spanish Group. *Bone Marrow Transplant* 1996;18(1):35–40.

19. Brown RA, Adkins D, Khoury H, et al. Long-term follow-up of high-risk allogeneic peripheral-blood stem-cell transplant recipients: graft-versus-host disease and transplant-related mortality. *J Clin Oncol* 1999;17(3):806–812.

20. Champlin RE, Schmitz N, Horowitz MM, et al. Blood stem cells compared with bone marrow as a source of hematopoietic cells for allogeneic transplantation [in process citation]. *Blood* 2000;95(12):3702–3709.

21. Vigorito AC, Azevedo WM, Marques JF, et al. A randomised, prospective comparison of allogeneic bone marrow and peripheral blood progenitor cell transplantation in the treatment of haematological malignancies. *Bone Marrow Transplant* 1998;22(12):1145–1151.

22. Schmitz N, Bacigalupo A, Hasenclever D, et al. Allogeneic bone marrow transplantation vs filgrastim-mobilised peripheral blood progenitor cell transplantation in patients with early leukaemia: first results of a randomised multicentre trial of the European Group for Blood and Marrow Transplantation. *Bone Marrow Transplant* 1998;21(10):995–1003.

23. Blaise D, Kuentz M, Fortanier C, et al. Randomized trial of bone marrow versus lenograstim-primed blood cell allogeneic transplantation in patients with early-stage leukemia: a report from the Societe Francaise de Greffe de Moelle. *J Clin Oncol* 2000;18(3):537–546.

24. Bensinger WI, Martin PJ, Storer B, et al. Transplantation of bone marrow as compared with peripheral-blood cells from HLA-identical relatives in patients with hematologic cancers. *N Engl J Med* 2001;344(3):175–181.

25. Nash RA, Pepe MS, Storb R, et al. Acute graft-versus-host disease: analysis of risk factors after allogeneic marrow transplantation and prophylaxis with cyclosporine and methotrexate. *Blood* 1992;80(7):1838–1845.

26. Vasconcelos ZF, Diamond HR, Tabak DG, et al. Th1/Th2 lymphokine profile of T cells present in the blood of granulocyte-colony stimulating factor-treated stem-cell donors: up or down modulation. *Blood* 2001;97(1):333–335.

27. Sivakumaran M. Modulation of Th1/Th2 subsets by granulocyte-colony stimulating factor. *Blood* 2001;97(1):333.

28. Arpinati M, Green CL, Heimfeld S, et al. Granulocyte-colony stimulating factor mobilizes T helper 2-inducing dendritic cells. *Blood* 2000;95(8):2484–2490.

29. Sloand EM, Kim S, Maciejewski JP, et al. Pharmacologic doses of granulocyte colony-stimulating factor affect cytokine production by lymphocytes in vitro and in vivo. *Blood* 2000;95(7):2269–2274.

30. Pan L, Delmonte J, Jr., Jalonen CK, et al. Pretreatment of donor mice with granulocyte colony-stimulating factor polarizes donor T lymphocytes toward type-2 cytokine production and reduces severity of experimental graft-versus-host disease. *Blood* 1995;86(12):4422–4429.

31. Talmadge JE, Reed EC, Kessinger A, et al. Immunologic attributes of cytokine mobilized peripheral blood stem cells and recovery following transplantation. *Bone Marrow Transplant* 1996;17(1):101–109.

32. Mielcarek M, Roecklein BA, Torok-Storb B. CD14+ cells in granulocyte colony-stimulating factor (G-CSF) mobilized peripheral blood mononuclear cells induce secretion of interleukin-6 and G-CSF by marrow stroma. *Blood* 1996;87(2):574–580.

33. Powles R, Mehta J, Kulkarni S, et al. Allogeneic blood and bone-marrow stem-cell transplantation in haematological malignant diseases: a randomised trial. *Lancet* 2000;355(9211):1231–1237.

34. Elmaagacli AH, Beelen DW, Opalka B, Set al. The risk of residual molecular and cytogenetic disease in patients with Philadelphia-chromosome positive first chronic phase chronic myelogenous leukemia is reduced after transplantation of allogeneic peripheral blood stem cells compared with bone marrow. *Blood* 1999;94(2):384–389.

35. Shenoy S, Mohanakumar T, Todd G, et al. Immune reconstitution following allogeneic peripheral blood stem cell transplants. *Bone Marrow Transplant* 1999;23(4):335–346.

36. Tjonnfjord GE, Steen R, Evensen SA, et al. Characterization of CD34+ peripheral blood cells from healthy adults mobilized by recombinant human granulocyte colony-stimulating factor. *Blood* 1994;84(8):2795–2801.

37. Weaver CH, Longin K, Buckner CD, et al. Lymphocyte content in peripheral blood mononuclear cells collected after the administration of recombinant human granulocyte colony-stimulating factor. *Bone Marrow Transplant* 1994;13:411–415.

38. Mills KC, Gross TG, Varney ML, et al. Immunologic phenotype and function in human bone marrow, blood stem cells and umbilical cord blood. *Bone Marrow Transplant* 1996;18(1):53–61.

39. Todd G, Hang JS, Brown R, et al. The effect of G-CSF mobilization on lymphocyte subsets, monocytes, NK cells, RBCs, platelets and CD34+/LIN- progenitors in normal allogeneic PBSC donors. *Blood* 2001;88:679a.

40. Hassan HT, Stockschlader M, Schleimer B, et al. Comparison of the content and subpopulations of CD3 and CD34 positive cells in bone marrow harvests and G-CSF-mobilized peripheral blood leukapheresis products from healthy adult donors. *Transplant Immunol* 1996;4(4):319–323.

41. Korbling M, Huh YO, Durett A, et al. Allogeneic blood stem cell transplantation: peripheralization and yield of donor-derived primitive hematopoietic progenitor cells (CD34+ Thy-1dim) and lymphoid subsets, and possible predictors of engraftment and graft-versus-host disease. *Blood* 1995;86(7):2842–2848.

42. Talmadge JE, Reed E, Ino K, et al. Rapid immunologic reconstitution following transplantation with mobilized peripheral blood stem cells as compared to bone marrow. *Bone Marrow Transplant* 1997;19(2):161–172.

43. Storek J, Witherspoon RP, Storb R. T cell reconstitution after bone marrow transplantation into adult patients does not resemble T cell development in early life. *Bone Marrow Transplant* 1995;16(3):413–425.

44. Atkinson K, Storb R, Prentice RL, et al. Analysis of late infections in 89 long-term survivors of bone marrow transplantation. *Blood* 1979;53(4):720–731.

45. Meyers JD. Infection in bone marrow transplant recipients. *Am J Med* 1986;81(1A):27–38.

46. Paulin T, Ringden O, Nilsson B, et al. Variables predicting bacterial and fungal infections after allogeneic marrow engraftment. *Transplantation* 1987;43(3):393–398.

47. Wingard JR. Infections in allogeneic bone marrow transplant recipients. *Semin Oncol* 1993;20(Suppl 6):80–87.

48. Pavletic ZS, Joshi SS, Pirruccello SJ, et al. Lymphocyte reconstitution after allogeneic blood stem cell transplantation for hematologic malignancies. *Bone Marrow Transplant* 1998;21(1):33–41.

49. Lum LG. The kinetics of immune reconstitution after human marrow transplantation. *Blood* 1987;69(2):369–380.

50. Storb R, Thomas ED. Allogeneic bone-marrow transplantation. *Immunol Rev* 1983;71:77–102.

51. Forman SJ, Nocker P, Gallagher M, et al. Pattern of T cell reconstitution following allogeneic bone marrow transplantation for acute hematological malignancy. *Transplantation* 1982;34(2):96–98.

52. Parkman R, Weinberg KI. Immunological reconstitution following bone marrow transplantation. *Immunol Rev* 1997;157:73–78.
53. Noel DR, Witherspoon RP, Storb R, et al. Does graft-versus-host disease influence the tempo of immunologic recovery after allogeneic human marrow transplantation? An observation on 56 long-term survivors. *Blood* 1978;51(6):1087–1105.
54. Keever CA, Small TN, Flomenberg N, et al. Immune reconstitution following bone marrow transplantation: Comparison of recipients of T-cell depleted marrow with recipients of conventional marrow grafts. *Blood* 1989;73(5):1340–1350.
55. Storek J, Gooley T, Witherspoon RP, et al. Infectious morbidity in long-term survivors of allogeneic marrow transplantation is associated with low CD4 T cell counts. *Am J Hematol* 1997;54(2):131–138.
56. Ramsdell F, Fowlkes BJ. Clonal deletion versus clonal anergy: the role of the thymus in inducing self tolerance. *Science* 1990;248(4961):1342–1348.
57. Penninger JM, Kroemer G. Molecular and cellular mechanisms of T lymphocyte apoptosis. *Adv Immunol* 1998;68:51–144.
58. Gunthert U, Hofmann M, Rudy W, et al. A new variant of glycoprotein CD44 confers metastatic potential to rat carcinoma cells. *Cell* 1991;65(1):13–24.
59. Cerra RF, Nathanson SD. Organ-specific chemotactic factors present in lung extracellular matrix. *J Surg Res* 1989;46(5):422–426.
60. Orr FW, Sanchez-Sweatman OH, Kostenuik P, et al. Tumor-bone interactions in skeletal metastasis. *Clin Orthop* 1995;(312):19–33.
61. Mackall CL, Fleisher TA, Brown MR, et al. Lymphocyte depletion during treatment with intensive chemotherapy for cancer. *Blood* 1994;84(7):2221–2228.
62. Witherspoon RP, Kopecky K, Storb RF, et al. Immunological recovery in 48 patients following syngeneic marrow transplantation or hematological malignancy. *Transplantation* 1982;33(2):143.
63. Atkinson K. Reconstitution of the hematopoietic and immune recovery systems after human marrow transplantation. *Bone Marrow Transplant* 1990;5(4):209–226.
64. Roux E, Helg C, Dumont-Girard F, Chapuis B, Jet al. Analysis of T-cell repopulation after allogeneic bone marrow transplantation: significant differences between recipients of T-cell depleted and unmanipulated grafts. *Blood* 1996;87(9):3984–3992.
65. Weinberg K, Annett G, Kashyap A, et al. The effect of thymic function on immunocompetence following bone marrow transplantation. *Biol Blood Marrow Transplant* 1995;1(1):18–23.
66. Mackall CL, Fleisher TA, Brown MR, et al. Age, thymopoiesis, and CD4+ T-lymphocyte regeneration after intensive chemotherapy. *N Eng J Med* 1995;332(3):143–149.
67. Dhein J, Walczak H, Baumler C, et al. Autocrine T-cell suicide mediated by APO-1/(Fas/CD95). *Nature* 1995;373(6513):438–441.
68. Brunner T, Mogil RJ, LaFace D, et al. Cell-autonomous Fas (CD95)/Fas-ligand interaction mediates activation induced apoptosis in T cell hybridomas. *Nature* 1995;373(6513):441–444.
69. Ju ST, Panka DJ, Cui H, et al. Fas (CD95)/FasL interactions required for programmed cell death after T-cell activation. *Nature* 1995;373(6513):444–448.
70. Ettinger R, Panka DJ, Wang JK, et al. Fas ligand mediated cytotoxicity is directly responsible for apoptosis of normal CD4+ T cells responding to bacterial superantigens. *J Immunol* 1995;154(9):4302–4308.
71. Badley AD, Dockrell D, Simpson M, et al. Macrophage-dependent apoptosis of CD4+ T lymphocytes from HIV-infected individuals is mediated by FasL and tumor necrosis factor. *J Exp Med* 1997;185(1):55–64.
72. Krammer PH, Behrmann I, Daniel P, et al. Regulation of apoptosis in the immune system. *Curr Opin Immunol* 1994;6(2):279–289.
73. Alderson MR, Tough TW, Braddy S, et al. Regulation of apoptosis and T cell activation by Fas-specific mAb. *Int Immunol* 1994;6(11):1799–1806.
74. Smith CA, Farrah T, Goodwin RG. The TNF receptor superfamily of cellular and viral proteins: activation, costimulation, and death. *Cell* 1994;76(6):959–962.
75. Badley AD, McElhinny JA, Leibson PJ, et al. Upregulation of Fas ligand expression by human immunodeficiency virus in human macrophages mediated apoptosis of uninfected T lymphocytes. *J Virol* 1996;70(1):199–206.
76. Mosier D, Sieburg H. Macrophage-tropic HIV: critical for AIDS pathogenesis? *Immunol Today* 1994;15(7):332–339.
77. Schuitemaker H, Meyaard L, Kootstra NA, et al. Lack of T cell dysfunction and programmed cell death in human immunodeficiency virus type 1-infected chimpanzees correlates with absence of monocytotropic variants. *J Infect Dis* 1993;168(6):1140–1147.
78. Groux H, Torpier G, Monte D, et al. Activation-induced death by apoptosis in CD4+ T cells from human immunodeficiency virus infected asymptomatic individuals. *J Exp Med* 1992;175(2):331–340.
79. Wu MX, Daley JF, Rasmussen RA, et al. Monocytes are required to prime peripheral blood T cells to undergo apoptosis. *Proc Natl Acad Sci USA* 1995;92(5):1525–1529.

80. Mackall CL, Stein D, Fleisher TA, et al. Prolonged CD4 depletion after sequential autologous peripheral blood progenitor cell infusions in children and young adults. *Blood* 2000;96(2):754–762.

81. Small TN, Papadopoulos EB, Boulad F, et al. Comparison of immune reconstitution after unrelated and related T-cell- depleted bone marrow transplantation: effect of patient age and donor leukocyte infusions. *Blood* 1999;93(2):467–480.

82. Small TN, Avigan D, Dupont B, et al. Immune reconstitution following T-cell depleted bone marrow transplantation: effect of age and posttransplant graft rejection prophylaxis. *Biol Blood Marrow Transplant* 1997;3(2):65–75.

83. Ino K, Singh RK, Talmadge JE. Monocytes from mobilized stem cells inhibit T cell function. *J Leuko Biol* 1997;61(5):583–591.

84. Li Y, Li XC, Zheng XX, Wells AD, Tet al. Blocking both signal 1 and signal 2 of T-cell activation prevents apoptosis of alloreactive T cells and induction of peripheral allograft tolerance. *Nat Med* 1999;5(11):1298–1302.

85. Ferguson TA, Green DR. T cells are just dying to accept grafts [news]. *Nat Med* 1999;5(11):1231,1232.

86. Varney ML, Ino K, Ageitos AG, et al. Expression of interleukin-10 in isolated CD8+ T cells and monocytes from growth factor-mobilized peripheral blood stem cell products: a mechanism of immune dysfunction. *J Interferon Cytokine Res* 1999;19(4):351–360.

87. Singh RK, Ino K, Varney ML, et al. Immunoregulatory cytokines in bone marrow and peripheral blood stem cell products. *Bone Marrow Transplant* 1999;23(1):53–62.

88. Holler E, Roncarolo MG, Hintermeier-Knabe R, et al. Prognostic significance of increased IL-10 production in patients prior to allogeneic bone marrow transplantation. *Bone Marrow Transplant* 2000;25(3):237–241.

89. Bacchetta R, Bigler M, Touraine JL, et al. High levels of interleukin 10 production in vivo are associated with tolerance in SCID patients transplanted with HLA mismatched hematopoietic stem cells. *J Exp Med* 1994;179(2):493–502.

90. Lutz MB, Sure RM, Niimi M, et al. Immature dendritic cells generated with low doses of GM-CSF in the absence of IL-4 are maturation resistant and prolong allograft survival in vivo. *Eur J Immunol* 2000;30:1813–1822.

91. Lin MT, Tseng LH, Frangoul H, et al. Increased apoptosis of peripheral blood T cells following allogeneic hematopoietic cell transplantation. *Blood* 2000;95(12):3832–3839.

92. Singh RK, Varney ML, Buyukberber S, et al. Fas-FasL-mediated CD4+ T-cell apoptosis following stem cell transplantation. *Cancer Res* 1999;59(13):3107–3111.

93. Ageitos AG, Varney ML, Bierman PJ, et al. Comparison of monocyte-dependent T cell inhibitory activity in GM-CSF vs G-CSF mobilized PSC products. *Bone Marrow Transplant* 1999;23(1):63–69.

94. Donnenberg AD, Margolick JB, Beltz LA, et al. Apoptosis parallels lymphopoiesis in bone marrow transplantation and HIV disease. *Res Immunol* 1995;146(1):11–21.

95. Donnenberg AD, Margolick JB, Donnenberg VS. Lymphopoiesis, apoptosis, and immune amnesia. *Ann NY Acad Sci* 1995;770:213–226.

96. Finkel TH, Tudor-Williams G, Banda NK, et al. Apoptosis occurs predominantly in bystander cells and not in productively infected cells of HIV- and SIV-infected lymph nodes. *Nat Med* 1995;1(2):129–134.

97. Giorgi JV, Detels R. T-cell subset alterations in HIV-infected homosexual men: NIAID Multicenter AIDS cohort study. *Clin Immunol Immunopathol* 1989;52(1):10–18.

98. Debatin KM, Fahrig-Faissner A, Enenkel-Stoodt S, et al. High expression of APO-1 (CD95) on T lymphocytes from human immunodeficiency virus-1-infected children. *Blood* 1994;83(10):3101–3103.

99. Katsikis PD, Wunderlich ES, Smith CA, et al. Fas antigen stimulation induces marked apoptosis of T lymphocytes in human immunodeficiency virus-infected individuals. *J Exp Med* 1995;181(6):2029–2036.

100. Tanaka J, Mielcarek M, Torok-Storb B. Impaired induction of the CD28-responsive complex in granulocyte colony-stimulating factor mobilized CD4 T cells. *Blood* 1998;91(1):347–352.

101. Mielcarek M, Martin PJ, Torok-Storb B. Suppression of alloantigen-induced T-cell proliferation by CD14+ cells derived from granulocyte colony-stimulating factor-mobilized peripheral blood mononuclear cells. *Blood* 1997;89(5):1629–1634.

102. Von Boehmer H. Thymic selection: a matter of life and death. *Immunol Today* 1992;13(11):454–458.

103. Lucas B, Germain RN. Unexpectedly complex regulation of CD4/CD8 coreceptor expression supports a revised model for CD4+CD8+ thymocyte differentiation. *Immunity* 1996;5(5):461–477.

104. Bevan MJ. In thymic selection, peptide diversity gives and takes away. *Immunity* 1997;7(2):175–178.

105. Hunkapillar T, Hood L. Diversity of the immunoglobulin gene superfamily. *Adv Immunol* 1989;44:1–63.

106. Wilson RK, Lai E, Concannon P, et al. Structure, organization and polymorphism of murine and human T-cell receptor alpha and beta chain gene families. *Immunol Rev* 1988;101:149–172.

107. Chothia C, Boswell DR, Lesk AM. The outline structure of the T-cell alpha beta receptor. *EMBO J* 1988;7(12):3745–3755.

108. Hawes GE, Struyk L, van den Elsen PJ. Differential usage of T cell receptor V gene segments in CD4+ and CD8+ subsets of T lymphocytes in monozygotic twins. *J Immunol* 1993;150(5):2033–2045.

109. Siu G, Kronenberg M, Strauss E, et al. The structure, rearrangement and expression of D beta gene segments of the murine T-cell antigen receptor. *Nature* 1984;311(5984):344–350.

110. Gorski J, Yassai M, Zhu X, et al. Circulating T cell repertoire complexity in normal individuals and bone marrow recipients analyzed by CDR3 size spectratyping. Correlation with immune status. *J Immunol* 1994;152(10):5109–5119.

111. Naumov YN, Naumova EN, Gorski J. CD4+ and CD8+ circulating alpha/beta T-cell repertoires are equally complex and are characterized by different levels of steady-state TCR expression. *Hum Immunol* 1996;48(1–2):52–62.

112. Mackall CL, Bare CV, Granger LA, et al. Thymic-independent T cell regeneration occurs via antigen-driven expansion of peripheral T cells resulting in a repertoire that is limited in diversity and prone to skewing. *J Immunol* 1996;156(12):4609–4616.

113. Tanchot C, Rocha B. The peripheral T cell repertoire: independent homeostatic regulation of virgin and activated CD8+ T cell pools. *Eur J Immunol* 1995;25(8):2127–2136.

114. Mackall CL, Hakim FT, Gress RE. T-cell regeneration: all repertoires are not created equal. *Immunol Today* 1997;18(5):245–251.

115. Nachbaur D, Kropshofer G, Heitger A, et al. Phenotypic and functional lymphocyte recovery after CD34+-enriched versus non-T cell-depleted autologous peripheral blood stem cell transplantation. *J Hematother Stem Cell Res* 2000;9(5):727–736.

116. Roux E, Helg C, Chapuis B, et al. T-cell repertoire complexity after allogeneic bone marrow transplantation. *Hum Immunol* 1996;48(1–2):135–138.

117. Pawelec G. Molecular and cell biological studies of ageing and their application to considerations of T lymphocyte immunosenescence. *Mech Ageing Dev* 1995;79(1):1–32.

118. Brocker T. Survival of mature CD4 T lymphocytes is dependent on major histocompatibility complex class II-expressing dendritic cells. *J Exp Med* 1997;186(8):1223–1232.

119. Tanchot C, Rocha B. The organization of mature T-cell pools. *Immunol Today* 1998;19(12):575–579.

120. Peault B, Weissman IL, Baum C, et al. Lymphoid reconstitution of the human fetal thymus in SCID mice with CD34+ precursor cells. *J Exp Med* 1991;174(5):1283–1286.

121. Vandekerckhove BA, Baccala R, Jones D, et al. Thymic selection of the human T cell receptor V beta repertoire in SCID- hu mice. *J Exp Med* 1992;176(6):1619–1624.

122. Muller-Hermelink HK, Sale GE, Borisch B, et al. Pathology of the thymus after allogeneic bone marrow transplantation in man. A histologic immunohistochemical study of 36 patients. *Am J Pathol* 1987;129 (2):242–256.

123. Lundqvist C, Baranov V, Hammarstrom S, et al. Intra-epithelial lymphocytes. Evidence for regional special-ization and extrathymic T cell maturation in the human gut epithelium. *Int Immunol* 1995;7(9):1473–1487.

124. Collins C, Norris S, McEntee G, et al. RAG1, RAG2 and pre-T cell receptor alpha chain expression by adult human hepatic T cells: evidence for extrathymic T cell maturation. *Eur J Immunol* 1996;26(12):3114–3118.

125. Godthelp BC, Van Tol MJ, Vossen JM, et al. T-Cell immune reconstitution in pediatric leukemia patients after allogeneic bone marrow transplantation with T-cell-depleted or unmanipulated grafts: evaluation of overall and antigen-specific T-cell repertoires. *Blood* 1999;94(12):4358–4369.

126. Dietrich PY, Caignard A, Lim A, et al. In vivo T-cell clonal amplification at time of acute graft-versus-host disease. *Blood* 1994;84(8):2815–2820.

127. Akatsuka Y, Cerveny C, Hansen JA. T cell receptor clonal diversity following allogeneic marrow grafting. *Hum Immunol* 1996;48(1-2):125–134.

128. Claret EJ, Alyea EP, Orsini E, et al. Characterization of T cell repertoire in patients with graft-versus- leukemia after donor lymphocyte infusion. *J Clin Invest* 1997;100(4):855–866.

129. Verfuerth S, Peggs K, Vyas P, et al. Longitudinal monitoring of immune reconstitution by CDR3 size spectratyping after T-cell-depleted allogeneic bone marrow transplant and the effect of donor lymphocyte infusions on T-cell repertoire. *Blood* 2000;95(12):3990–3995.

130. Miyawaki T, Uehara T, Nibu R, et al. Differential expression of apoptosis-related Fas antigen on lymphocyte subpopulations in human peripheral blood. *J Immunol* 1992;149(11):3753–3758.

131. Dhein J, Daniel PT, Trauth BC, et al. Induction of apoptosis by monoclonal antibody anti-APO-1 class switch variants is dependent on cross-linking of APO-1 cell surface antigens. *J Immunol* 1992;149(10):3166–3173.

132. Suda T, Nagata S. Purification and characterization of the Fas-ligand that induces apoptosis. *J Exp Med* 1994;179(3):873–879.

133. Owen-Schaub LB, Yonehara S, et al. DNA fragmentation and cell death is selectively triggered in activated human lymphocytes by Fas antigen engagement. *Cell Immunol* 1992;140(1):197–205.

134. Wesselborg S, Janssen O, Kabelitz D. Induction of activation-driven death (apoptosis) in activated but not resting peripheral blood T cells. *J Immunol* 1993;150(10):4338–4345.

135. Atkinson K. T cell subpopulations defined by monoclonal antibodies after HLA- identical sibling marrow transplantation. II. Activated and functional subsets of helper-inducer and cytotoxic-suppressor subpopula-tions defined by two-colour fluorescence flow cytometry. *Bone Marrow Transplant* 1986;1(2):121–132.

136. Leino L, Lilius EM, Nikoskelainen J, et al. The reappearance of 10 differentiation antigens on peripheral blood lymphocytes after allogeneic bone marrow transplantation. *Bone Marrow Transplant* 1991;8(5):339–344.

137. Gorla R, Airo P, Ferremi-Leali P, et al. Predominance of 'memory' phenotype within CD4+ and CD8+ lymphocyte subsets after allogeneic BMT. *Bone Marrow Transplant* 1993;11(4):346–347.

138. Heitger A, Neu N, Kern H, et al. Essential role of the thymus to reconstitute naive (CD45RA+) T-helper cells after human allogeneic bone marrow transplantation. *Blood* 1997;90(2):850–857.

139. Cooley MA, McLachlan K, Atkinson K. Cytokine activity after human bone marrow transplantation. III. Defect in IL2 production by peripheral blood mononuclear cells is not corrected by stimulation with Ca++ ionophore plus phorbol ester. *Br J Haematol* 1989;73(3):341–347.

140. Brugnoni D, Airo P, Pennacchio M, et al. Immune reconstitution after bone marrow transplantation for combined immunodeficiencies: down-modulation of Bcl-2 and high expression of CD95/Fas account for increased susceptibility to spontaneous and activation-induced lymphocyte cell death. *Bone Marrow Transplant* 1999;23(5):451–457.

141. Hebib NC, Deas O, Rouleau M, et al. Peripheral blood T cells generated after allogeneic bone marrow transplantation: lower levels of bcl-2 protein and enhanced sensitivity to spontaneous and CD95-mediated apoptosis in vitro. Abrogation of the apoptotic phenotype coincides with the recovery of normal naive/primed T-cell profiles. *Blood* 1999;94(5):1803–1813.

142. Rocha B, Dautigny N, Pereira P. Peripheral T lymphocytes: expansion potential and homeostatic regulation of pool sizes and CD4/CD8 ratios in vivo. *Eur J Immunol* 1989;19(5):905–911.

143. Mackall CL, Granger L, Sheard MA, et al. T-cell regeneration after bone marrow transplantation: differential CD45 isoform expression on thymic-derived versus thymic-independent progeny. *Blood* 1993;82(8):2585–2594.

144. Mackall CL, Gress RE. Pathways of T-cell regeneration in mice and humans: implications for bone marrow transplantation and immunotherapy. *Immunol Rev* 1997;157:61–72.

145. Gaschet J, Denis C, Milpied N, et al. Alterations of T cell repertoire after bone marrow transplantation: Characterization of over-represented subsets. *Bone Marrow Transplant* 1995;19(3):427–435.

146. de Gast GC, Verdonck LF, Middeldorp JM, et al. Recovery of T-cell subsets after autologous BMT is mainly due to porliferation of mature T cells in the graft. *Blood* 1985;66(2):428.

147. Dolstra H, Van de Wiel-van Kemenade, de Witte T, et al. Clonal predominance of cytomegalovirus-specific CD8+ cytotoxic T lymphocytes in bone marrow recipients. *Bone Marrow Transplant* 1996;18(2):339–345.

148. Masuko K, Kato S, Hagihara M, et al. Stable clonal expansion of T cells induced by bone marrow transplantation. *Blood* 1996;87(2):789–799.

149. Goldman JM, Apperley JF, Jones L, et al. Bone marrow transplantation for patients with chronic myeloid leukemia. *N Engl J Med* 1986;314(4):202–207.

150. Douek DC, McFarland RD, Keiser PH, et al. Changes in thymic function with age and during the treatment of HIV infection. *Nature* 1998;396(6712):690–695.

151. Goldman JM, Gale RP, Horowitz MM, et al. Bone marrow transplantation for chronic myelogenous leukemia in chronic phase. Increased risk for relapse associated with T-cell depletion. *Ann Intern Med* 1988;108(6):806–814.

152. Apperley JF, Mauro FR, Goldman JM, et al. Bone marrow transplantation for chronic myeloid leukaemia in first chronic phase: importance of a graft-versus-leukaemia effect. *Br J Haematol* 1988;69(2):239–245.

153. Urbano-Ispizua A, Rozman C, Pimentel P, et al. The number of donor CD3(+) cells is the most important factor for graft failure after allogeneic transplantation of CD34(+) selected cells from peripheral blood from HLA-identical siblings. *Blood* 2001;97(2):383–387.

154. Laurenti L, Sica S, Sora F, et al. Long-term immune recovery after CD34+ immunoselected and unselected peripheral blood progenitor cell transplantation: a case-control study. *Haematologica* 1999;84(12):1100–1103.

155. Martinez C, Urbano IA, Rozman C, et al. Immune reconstitution following allogeneic peripheral blood progenitor cell transplantation: comparison of recipients of positive CD34+ selected grafts with recipients of unmanipulated grafts. *Exp Hematol* 1999;27(3):561–568.

156. Lowdell MW, Craston R, Ray N, et al. The effect of T cell depletion with Campath-1M on immune reconstitution after chemotherapy and allogeneic bone marrow transplant as treatment for leukaemia. *Bone Marrow Transplant* 1998;21(7):679–686.

157. Small TN, Leung L, Stiles J, et al. Disseminated toxoplasmosis following T cell-depleted related and unrelated bone marrow transplantation. *Bone Marrow Transplant* 2000;25(9):969–973.

158. Holmberg LA, Boeckh M, Hooper H, et al. Increased incidence of cytomegalovirus disease after autologous CD34- selected peripheral blood stem cell transplantation. *Blood* 1999;94(12):4029–4035.

159. Rutella S, Rumi C, Laurenti L, et al. Immune reconstitution after transplantation of autologous peripheral CD34+ cells: analysis of predictive factors and comparison with unselected progenitor transplants. *Br J Haematol* 2000;108(1):105–115.

160. Sica S, Salutari P, La Barbera EO, et al. Infectious complications after CD34-selected autologous peripheral blood stem cell transplantation. *Br J Haematol* 1998;101(3):592–593.

161. Eckle T, Prix L, Jahn G, et al. Drug-resistant human cytomegalovirus infection in children after allogeneic stem cell transplantation may have different clinical outcomes. Blood 2000;96(9):3286-3289.
162. Tiacci E, Luppi M, Barozzi P, Get al. Fatal herpesvirus-6 encephalitis in a recipient of a T-cell-depleted peripheral blood stem cell transplant from a 3-loci mismatched related donor. Haematologica 2000;85(1):94-97.
163. Euler HH, Marmont AM, Bacigalupo A, et al. Early recurrence or persistence of autoimmune diseases after unmanipulated autologous stem cell transplantation. Blood 1996;88(9):3621-3625.
164. Kernan NA, Collins NH, Juliano L, et al. Clonable T lymphocytes in T cell-depleted bone marrow transplants correlate with development of graft-v-host disease. Blood 1986;68(3):770-773.
165. Hughes WT, Armstrong D, Bodey GP, et al. 1997 guidelines for the use of antimicrobial agents in neutropenic patients with unexplained fever. Infectious Diseases Society of America. Clin Infect Dis 1997;25(3):551-573.
166. Pizzo PA, Hathorn JW, Hiemenz J, et al. A randomized trial comparing ceftazidime alone with combination antibiotic therapy in cancer patients with fever and neutropenia. N Engl J Med 1986;315(9):552-558.
167. Amgen I. Filgrastim. In: *Physician's Desk Reference*. Medical Economics Company, Montvale, NJ, 2000, pp. 528–533.
168. Peterson PK, McGlave P, Ramsay NK, et al. A prospective study of infectious diseases following bone marrow transplantation: emergence of Aspergillus and Cytomegalovirus as the major causes of mortality. *Infect Control* 1983;4(2):81–89.
169. Meyers JD, Flournoy N, Thomas ED. Nonbacterial pneumonia after allogeneic marrow transplantation: a review of ten years' experience. *Rev Infect Dis* 1982;4(6):1119–1132.
170. Leung TF, Chik KW, Li CK, et al. Incidence, risk factors and outcome of varicella-zoster virus infection in children after haematopoietic stem cell transplantation. *Bone Marrow Transplant* 2000;25(2):167–172.
171. Koc Y, Miller KB, Schenkein DP, et al. Varicella zoster virus infections following allogeneic bone marrow transplantation: frequency, risk factors, and clinical outcome. *Biol Blood Marrow Transplant* 2000;6(1):44–49.
172. Schuchter LM, Wingard JR, Piantadosi S, et al. Herpes zoster infection after autologous bone marrow transplantation. *Blood* 1989;74(4):1424–1427.
173. Han CS, Miller W, Haake R, et al. Varicella zoster infection after bone marrow transplantation: incidence, risk factors and complications. *Bone Marrow Transplant* 1994;13(3):277 283.
174. Ochs L, Shu XO, Miller J, et al. Late infections after allogeneic bone marrow transplantations: comparison of incidence in related and unrelated donor transplant recipients. *Blood* 1995;86(10):3979–3986.
175. Ambrosino DM, Molrine DC. Critical appraisal of immunization strategies for prevention of infection in the compromised host. *Hematol Oncol Clin N Am* 1993;7(5):1027–1050.
176. Winston DJ, Ho WG, Champlin RE, et al. Infectious complications of bone marrow transplantation. *Exp Hematol* 1984;12(3):205-215.
177. Wingard J. Bacterial infections. In: Thomas ED, Blume K, Forman SJ (eds.) *Hematopoietic Cell Transplantation*. Blackwell Science, Malden, MA, 1999, pp. 537-554.
178. Rege K, Mehta J, Treleaven J, et al. Fatal pneumococcal infections following allogeneic bone marrow transplant. *Bone Marrow Transplant* 1994;14(6):903–906.
179. Avanzini MA, Carra AM, Maccario R, et al. Immunization with Haemophilus influenzae type b conjugate vaccine in children given bone marrow transplantation: comparison with healthy age- matched controls. *J Clin Immunol* 1998;18(3):193–201.
180. Parkkali T, Kayhty H, Ruutu T, et al. A comparison of early and late vaccination with Haemophilus influenzae type b conjugate and pneumococcal polysaccharide vaccines after allogeneic BMT. *Bone Marrow Transplant* 1996;18(5):961–967.
181. Prentice HG, Gluckman E, Powles RL, et al. Impact of long-term acyclovir on cytomegalovirus infection and survival after allogeneic bone marrow transplantation. European Acyclovir for CMV Prophylaxis Study Group. *Lancet* 1994;343(8900):749–753.
182. Boeckh M, Gooley TA, Reusser P, et al. Failure of high-dose acyclovir to prevent cytomegalovirus disease after autologous marrow transplantation. *J Infect Dis* 1995;172(4):939–943.
183. American Public Health Association. Mononucleosis, infectious. In: Chin J (ed.) *Control of Communicable Diseases Manual*. American Public Health Association, Washington, D.C., 2001, pp. 350–352.
184. Papadopoulos EB, Ladanyi M, Emanuel D, et al. Infusions of donor leukocytes to treat Epstein-Barr virus-associated lymphoproliferative disorders after allogeneic bone marrow transplantation. *N Engl J Med* 1994;330(17):1185–1191.
185. Rooney CM, Smith CA, Ng CY, et al. Infusion of cytotoxic T cells for the prevention and treatment of Epstein-Barr virus-induced lymphoma in allogeneic transplant recipients. *Blood* 1998;92(5):1549–1555.
186. Riddell SR, Greenberg PD. T cell therapy of human CMV and EBV infection in immunocompromised hosts. *Rev Med Virol* 1997;7(3):181–192.
187. Heslop HE, Perez M, Benaim E, et al. Transfer of EBV-specific CTL to prevent EBV lymphoma post bone marrow transplant. *J Clin Apheresis* 1999;14(3):154–156.

188. Aguilar LK, Rooney CM, Heslop HE. Lymphoproliferative disorders involving Epstein-Barr virus after hemopoietic stem cell transplantation. *Curr Opin Oncol* 1999;11(2):96–101.

189. Heslop HE, Ng CY, Li C, et al. Long-term restoration of immunity against Epstein-Barr virus infection by adoptive transfer of gene-modified virus-specific T lymphocytes. *Nat Med* 1996;2(5):551–555.

190. Dykewicz CA, Jaffe HW, Kaplan JE. Guidelines for preventing opportunistic infections among hematopoietic stem cell transplant recipients: recommendations of CDC, the Infectious Disease Society of America, and the American Society of Blood and Morrow Transplantations. 49(RR10), 1–128. 10-20-2000.

191. Walter EA, Greenberg PD, Gilbert MJ, et al. Reconstitution of cellular immunity against cytomegalovirus in recipients of allogeneic bone marrow by transfer of T-cell clones from the donor. *N Engl J Med* 1995;333(16):1038–1044.

192. Stocchi R, Ward KN, Fanin R, et al. Management of human cytomegalovirus infection and disease after allogeneic bone marrow transplantation. *Haematologica* 1999;84(1):71–79.

16

Grading and Management of Graft-vs-Host Disease

Donna Przepiorka, MD, PhD

1. INTRODUCTION

Clinical graft-vs-host disease (GVHD) is a challenging area of study. Objective documentation of organ involvement is frequently not available, there is considerable interobserver variability in staging, and response criteria used are inconsistent between studies. Despite these shortcomings, there has been a clear trend of progress in the field, and patient survival has improved. Herein, we discuss recent developments in grading and analysis, and review the outcomes using new approaches to prevention or treatment of GVHD.

2. GRADING OF GVHD

2.1. Acute GVHD

Staging and grading acute GVHD provide transplant physicians with two important tools: (i) a simplified way to communicate GVHD-related risks, and (ii) a relatively objective means to compare the effectiveness of different therapeutic strategies in the setting of competing risks. The importance of assessing GVHD-related risk is based on the observation that severe acute GVHD is a surrogate for death. An accurate grading system would enable physicians to provide patients with a meaningful assessment of the risk-benefit ratio of a specific treatment strategy, aid in the appropriate choice of risk-stratified therapies, direct new methods for risk factor modification in an effort to reduce treatment-related morbidity and mortality, and accelerate development of new therapies in a field.

The Seattle GVHD grading system as modified by Thomas et al. was established as a simple descriptive system of the degree of rash, hyperbilirubinemia, and diarrhea due to GVHD *(1,2)*. Subsequent studies by both the International Blood and Marrow Transplantation Registry (IBMTR) and the European Cooperative Group for Blood and Marrow Transplantation

From: *Current Clinical Oncology: Allogeneic Stem Cell Transplantation*
Edited by: Mary S. Laughlin and Hillard M. Lazarus © Humana Press Inc., Totowa, NJ

(EBMT) demonstrated the prognostic value of this grading system; there was an incremental increase in treatment-related mortality associated with increasing GVHD grade *(3,4)*. In addition, others reported that the applicability of the grading system was independent of the degree of donor histoincompatibility, recipient age, or method of GVHD prophylaxis *(5)*.

Martin et al. *(6)* reported a lack of concurrence between observers in grading GVHD in an individual patient. The difficulties contributing to this problem include accurate establishment of the diagnosis of GVHD within an organ, the contribution of concurrent etiologies to organ dysfunction, and the subjective assessment of performance status as part of the grading criteria. The former is especially problematic, even with histologic assessment. GVHD may not be uniformly present throughout an organ, and physicians can be tragically misled by false negative biopsies *(7)*. Therefore, in the setting of typical rash or diarrhea with bowel wall edema on imaging studies, some have applied negative biopsies as support for exclusion of alternate diagnoses rather than to exclude GVHD.

The consensus criteria for grading acute GVHD *(5)* attempted to address some of these issues. These criteria (Table 1) are a minor modification of the criteria proposed by Thomas et al. *(2)*. The modifications include the recognition of nausea as a manifestation of upper gastrointestinal GVHD and use of downstaging if additional causes of organ dysfunction have been documented. Participants in the conference had no data to support elimination of performance status from the grading system, so this was not eliminated. It was clarified, however, that poor performance be defined by standardized scales. Commonly used criteria include Karnofsky performance status <50, Lansky performance status <40, and Zubrod or Eastern Cooperative Oncology Group (ECOG) performance status 3–4.

The IBMTR Severity Index (Table 2) is the first grading system based on objective criteria alone *(4)*. To develop this grading system, human leukocyte antigen (HLA)-identical marrow transplant recipients receiving a uniform GVHD prophylaxis regimen were assigned a three-part designation based on the maximal degree of organ involvement; then, treatment-related mortality was determined for patients within each three-part designation, and those cohorts with similar outcomes were combined. The results demonstrated that treatment-related mortality depended on the maximal degree of organ involvement in any of the three organ systems. The homogeneity of outcome for patients within an index was verified in a testing set of patients receiving T cell-depleted transplants, and the prognostic value of the system has been validated in two prospective studies *(8,9)*.

2.2. Chronic GVHD

Shulman et al., who first described clinical chronic GVHD in 1980, proposed a classification scheme based on limited vs extensive organ involvement that was predictive of prognosis *(10)*. In this system, the extensive grade required that patients have (i) generalized skin involvement or (ii) localized skin disease or hepatopathy in addition to advanced hepatic histology, sicca manifestations, or other organ involvement. An international survey later found that this scheme for grading was highly reproducible *(11)*, and it has been widely adopted. As more patients with chronic GVHD have been assessed, however, it is apparent that this system may not be applicable to all circumstances encountered. An alternative system defines limited as localized skin or single organ involvement not requiring systemic therapy, and extensive disease includes generalized skin rash or advanced organ involvement requirng systemic therapy (Table 3). This modification can thus be applied to patients without skin or liver disease who may have mild oral mucosal abnormalities that resolve spontaneously (limited) or severe ocular inflammation requiring systemic therapy (extensive).

Sullivan et al. were the first to note that thrombocytopenia was an adverse prognostic factor for survival from diagnosis of chronic GVHD *(12)*. It is less well-appreciated that the throm-

Table 1
Consensus Criteria for Grading of Acute GVHD

	Skin		Liver		Gut
Stage					
1	Rash <25%[a]		Bilirubin 2-3 mg/dL[b]		Diarrhea >500 mL/d[c] or persistent nausea[d]
2	Rash 25–50%		Bilirubin 3–6 mg/dL		Diarrhea >1000 mL/d
3	Rash >50%		Bilirubin 6–15 mg/dL		Diarrhea >1500 mL/d
4	Generalized erythroderma with bullae		Bilirubin >15 mg/dL		Severe abdominal pain with or without ileus
Grade[e]					
I	Stage 1-2		None		None
II	Stage 3	or	Stage 1	or	Stage 1
III	—		Stage 2–3	or	Stage 2–4
IV	Stage 4	or	Stage 4	or	Stage 4[f]

[a]Use "Rule of Nines" or burn chart to determine extent of rash.

[b]Range given as total bilirubin. Downgrade one stage if an additional cause of elevated bilirubin has been documented.

[c]Volume of diarrhea applies to adults. For pediatric patients, the volume of diarrhea should be based on body surface area. Downgrade one stage if an additional cause of diarrhea has been documented.

[d]Persistent nausea with histologic evidence of GVHD in the stomach or duodenum.

[e]Criteria for grading given as degree of organ involvement required to confer that grade.

[f]Grade IV may also include lesser organ involvement when the Karnofsky performance status is <50%, so patients with Stage 4 gut GVHD are usually grade IV.

Table 2
Criteria for IBMTR Severity Index for Acute GVHD

Index[a]	Extent of rash		Total bilirubin		Volume of diarrhea
A	<25%	or	<2.0 mg/dL	or	<500 mL/d
B	25–50%	or	2.0–6.0 mg/dL	or	500–1500 mL/d
C	>50%	or	6.1–15.0 mg/dL	or	>1500 mL/d
D	Bullae	or	>15 mg/dL	or	Severe pain or ileus

[a]Index assignment is based on maximal involvement in any single organ system.

Table 3
Criteria for Classification of Chronic GVHD

Classification	Criteria
Subclinical	Histologic evidence on screening biopsies without clinical signs or symptoms.
Limited	Localized skin or single organ involvement not requiring systemic therapy.
Extensive low risk	Platelet count >100,000 and extensive skin disease or other organ involvement requiring systemic therapy.
Extensive high risk	Platelet count <100,000 and extensive skin disease or other organ involvement requiring systemic therapy.

bocytopenic patients also have a substantially worse survival from the time of transplantation, since time of onset of their disease is earlier than that for nonthrombocytopenic patients with chronic GVHD *(12,13)*. Consequently, thrombocytopenia has become a common method for risk stratification of patients with chronic GVHD (Table 3). In multivariate analyses of patients with chronic GVHD, other risk factors for mortality identified include progressive onset, lichenoid type skin rash, elevated total bilirubin, poor performance status, alternative donorm and sex-mismatched donor *(14–18)*. Many of these analyses were performed in heterogeneous populations, and it is not clear that prognostic factors are uniform across patient groups *(15)*. Prospective study of more complex risk stratification systems are lacking.

3. ASSESSMENT OF GVHD CLINICAL TRIALS

3.1. Acute GVHD Prophylaxis Trials

All of the acute GVHD grading systems have demonstrated a correlation between maximal grade and treatment-related mortality. Grades II–IV acute GVHD, which require systemic therapy, are considered clinically significant and used as outcomes in clinical trials of GVHD prophylaxis. Grades III–IV acute GVHD are associated with a substantial increase in mortality and, therefore, are reported separately. Maximal grade, however, can be impacted by a number of factors, including patient age, degree of donor histoincompatibility, inclusion of persisting anti-T cell antibodies in the preparative regimen, T cell depletion of the allograft, criteria for initiating therapeutic measures, the drugs used as the initial treatment of acute GVHD, and incomplete chimerism. Nonrandomized comparisons of preventive regimens are highly misleading when these parameters are inconsistent between groups. The recommendations for uniform assessment of GVHD prophylaxis trials from the consensus conference *(5)* are listed in Table 4.

The optimal method for estimating GVHD risk would (i) provide consistent results independent of the proportion of patients censored for lack of follow-up, and (ii) provide an accurate representation of the clinical reality. The Kaplan-Meier product-limit estimate *(19)* has long been used as the preferred means for reporting GVHD risks for populations of patients. Incorporating the consensus recommendations, patients are censored at the time of last follow-up alive, treatment-related death, relapse, or graft failure. The estimate of GVHD is reported as 1 minus the Kaplan-Meier estimate of no GVHD occuring (Table 5). This method assumes that the risk of GVHD would be the same in patients censored as in those who were not censored, so the estimate would clearly be inaccurate if GVHD and the competing risks were mutually exclusive. In addition, the calculation of the estimate of the risk of GVHD is 1 minus a product of probabilities, which is not a mathematically logical way of calculating a risk.

Two alternative methods for reporting GVHD risk have been promoted recently. One alternative is the cumulative incidence. This method is based on the simple proportion without censoring (Table 5). The assumption made is that those not followed for any reason through the longest time on study would not have developed GVHD if longer follow-up were available; if this assumption were incorrect, then the cumulative risk would be an underestimate of the GVHD rate.

Gooley et al. *(20)* demonstrated how the method of calculating the risk of GVHD affects the results reported. The authors generated three sets of outcome data by varying the rate of the competing risk. The hazard rate of the Outcome Risk (e.g., GVHD) was set to be the same in all three data sets, but that of the the Competing Risk (e.g., relapse) was varied from 0 to 0.99, such as occurs clinically in different studies. The authors reported that the Kaplan-Meier estimates of the Outcome Risk were the same for all three data sets; that is, the estimate calculated was independent of the variation in competing risk. In contrast, the cumulative incidences of the Outcome Risk varied from 0.18 to 0.40, depending on the rate of the competing risk. The authors then used both methods to calculate the probability of chronic GVHD in a cohort of adult unrelated donor marrow transplant recipients who received standard GVHD prophylaxis without T cell depletion *(20)*. The Kaplan-Meier estimate of chronic GVHD was

Table 4
Recommendations for Assessment of GVHD Prophylaxis Regimens

1. A specific grading system should referenced or described in detail if not published previously.
2. Criteria (grade) for initiation of treatment of acute GVHD and the drugs used for first-line therapy of acute GVHD should be provided.
3. The incidence or risk of grades II–IV and grades III–IV GVHD should be provided.
4. When calculating the risk of acute GVHD, patients should be censored at:
    a. The time of graft failure.
    b. The time GVHD prophylaxis is discontinued when relapse occurs.
    c. The time of initiation of treatment of relapse if the patient is off prophylaxis.
5. When evaluating acute GVHD as the end-point, data should be reported separately and/or stratified for groups with known differences in risk of GVHD (e.g., pediatric vs adult patients, T cell-depleted vs unmanipulated allograft recipients, HLA identical vs alternative donor allgraft recipients).
6. When evaluating survival as the end-point, data should be reported separately for groups with known differences in risk of treatment-failure (e.g., pediatric vs adult patients, HLA identical vs alternative donor allograft recipients, early vs advanced disease).

Table 5
Methods for Calculation of the Rate of GVHD

Method	Calculation	Assumption
Kaplan-Meier	$P_k = 1 - [\prod_{i \le k}(s/r)]$ P_k is the estimate of GVHD at time k, $\prod$ indicated the cumulative product, s is the number of patients surviving without GVHD or a competing risk at time k, r is the number of patients at risk in the interval.	The risk of GVHD is the same in the censored and the noncensored patients.
Cumulative incidence	$CI_k = g/n$ CI_k is the cumulative incidence of GVHD at time k, g is the number of patients who developed GVHD up to that time, n is the total number of patients.	GVHD does not occur in patients without follow-up throught the end of a defined perioud or who were lost to a competing risk.
Conditional probability	$CP_k = g/(n\text{-}d)$ CP_k is the conditional probability of GVHD at time k, g is the number of patients who developed GVHD up to that time, n is the total number of patients, d is the number of patients with competing risks.	GVHD does not occur in patients without follow-up through the end of a defined period.

0.60, while the cumulative incidence was only 0.28, the latter being a rate clearly not consistent with clinical experience. In this example, the Kaplan-Meier estimate appeared to be the more accurate probability.

The second alternative method for calculating GVHD risk is the conditional probability *(21)*. This method provides a rate of GVHD in those patients without the competing outcomes (early death, relapse, or graft failure) (Table 5). The assumption made is that GVHD would not occur in the patients without competing outcomes who were still early in their follow-up. When the rate of the competing risks is high, however, the conditional probability might overestimate the GVHD rate. When no patients have competing risks and follow-up is complete to the end of the observation period, the rate of GVHD would be nearly the same by all three methods.

3.2. GVHD Treatment Trials

The primary outcome parameter in acute GVHD treatment trials is complete response, the resolution of all signs and symptoms of acute GVHD. A complete response is not only a measure of the biologic activity of the drug under study, but also a surrogate for survival *(22)*. However, the time point at which outcome is evaluated is not standardized. Early acute GVHD treatment studies assessed patients immediately at the end of a short treatment course, while more recent trials included a specified duration of response and survival in the criteria. Criteria for partial response have not been validated; whether partial response as defined in various studies impacts treatment-related mortality and survival in a clinically meaningful way is questionable *(22–25)*.

The lack of validated response criteria is also problematic in chronic GVHD treatment trials. For most, the clinical complete response remains the cornerstone in the assessment of efficacy. More recently, quality of life indicators and time for discontinuation of all immunosuppressive therapy have been used as additional outcome parameters *(26)*.

4. RECENT ADVANCES IN THE MANAGEMENT OF GVHD

4.1. CD34-Selection

It is well accepted that T cell depletion of marrow or blood stem cells is an effective means for prevention of acute and chronic GVHD. Wide adoption of T cell depletion has been prohibited by a number of obstacles, the most important of which are the lack of approved reagents and problems with reproducibility in the depletion procedures. A number of devices are now available commercially for selection of CD34+ cells from marrow or peripheral blood; all are affinity methods using monoclonal antibodies directed against CD34. The Ceprate system uses a biotin-avidin-based approach, while the Isolex and MACS systems utilize immunomagnetic beads. The latter have the advantage of largely being automated, which in theory should maximize reproducibility.

Investigators have reported substantial differences between the CD34 selection devices in CD34+ cell recovery and purity *(27–29)*. These differences have been attributed by some to the devices themselves. It is less well-appreciated that characteristics of the starting component also contributes to the efficiency of the selection procedure. Each device has a maximum capacity for CD34+ cells, and when components have high numbers of CD34+ cells, the capacity may be exceeded, resulting in poor recovery. In addition, contamination of components by granulocytes and other mature cells adversely affects purity and recovery. Thus, for CD34 selection procedures, the advantages of high volume leukapheresis to increase CD34+ cell collection may be outweighed by the reduction in postselection recovery due to the granulocyte contamination in these components.

There have been a number of studies evaluating transplantation of CD34-selected marrow or blood stem cells from HLA identical related donors (Table 6) *(30–44)*. The only obvious advantage for use of blood stem cells over marrow for these procedures is the higher dose of CD34+ cells in blood stem cell components. Independent of the source of stem cells, however, the risk of graft failure varies widely between studies. In a multivariate analysis, Urbano-Ispuzua et al. *(45)* reported that the risk of graft failure was associated with the CD3+ cell dose rather than the CD34+ cell dose. Patients who received a CD3+ cell dose $\leq 2 \times 10^5$/kg had a 17-fold

Table 6
CD34-Selection for Prevention of GVHD

Ref.	Method	Cells	Age group	No.	CD34 dose (× 10^6/kg)	CD3 dose (× 10^4/kg)	Graft failure	GVHD prophylaxis	Acute GVHD[a]	Chronic GVHD
HLA identical sibling										
30	Ceprate	BM	Adult	12	1.7	23.0	4/12	CSA	3/12	—
31	Isolex	BM	Adult	14	1.2	9.4	0/14	None	4/14	—
32	—	BM	Adult	27	1.5	3.0	2/27	Mixed	—	—
33	Ceprate	PB	Adult	10	7.4	110.0	0/10	CSA ± MTX	6/10	5/10
34	Ceprate	PB	Adult	16	9.0	73.0	0/16	CSA/MTX	86%	75%
35	Ceprate	PB	Adult	20	2.9	42.0	0/20	CSA/MP	0/20	0/20
36	Ceprate	PB	Adult	10	4.1	42.0	0/10	CSA	3/10	—
37	Mixed	PB	Adult	62	3.5	40.0	2/62	CSA/MP+	5/60	6/43
38	Mixed	PB	Adult	10	3.1	30.0	0/10	Mixed	—	10%
39	Isolex	PB	Adult	12	4.6	17.0	4/12	Mixed	4/12	—
40	Isolex	PB	Adult	17	5.3	16.0	0/17	CSA/MP	—	—
41	Isolex	PB	—	82	5.7	13.0	0/82	CSA	—	—
42	MACS	PB	Adult	11	10.5	10.0	0/11	—	1/11	—
43	Isolex	PB	Adult	10	6.3	4.4	0/10	CSA	3/10	—
44	MACS	PB	Adult	10	9.7	1.0	1/10	None	2/10	—
Haploidentical donor										
49	Isolex	PB	Pediatric	13	7.7	10.0	6/11	Mixed	2/8	—
50	Isolex	PB	Mixed	10	12.9	4.1	3/10	CSA	3/7	—
51	Mixed	PB	Adult	10	8.3	3.0	1/10	None	0/9	6/9
52	MACS	PB	Pediatric	39	20.7	1.6	3/39	None	1/36	—
53	MACS	PB	Adult	9	10.7	0.3	0/9	None	0/9	—
54	Ceprate	PB + BM	Adult	10	5.7	55.0	0/10	CSA	8/10	—
55	Isolex	PB ± BM	Mixed	135	3.2–5.5	6–12	27/128	Mixed	29/118	20/57
56[b]	MACS	—	Pediatric	17	8.0–28.0	0.9	3/17	None	1/17	1/17

Abbreviations: —, not stated; BM, bone marrow; PB, peripheral blood stem cells; CSA, cyclosporine; MTX, methotrexate; MP, prednisone or equivalent corticosteroid.
[a] Grades II–IV.
[b] Includes some patients with unrelated donors.

increased risk of graft failure. In addition, patients with chronic myeloid leukemia (CML) conditioned without total body irradiation (TBI) had a 4.8-fold increase in graft failure.

The rates of acute and chronic GVHD after HLA identical CD34-selected blood stem cell transplantation are also highly variable (Table 6). With other types of T cell depletion, the CD3+ cell dose is strongly predictive of acute GVHD. With CD34-selected HLA identical allografts, the highest rates of GVHD occurred in the two studies having median CD3+ cell doses >5 × 10^5/kg $(33,34)$, and with very low CD3+ cell doses, the risk of GVHD appeared to be acceptable even with no additional immunosuppressive drugs given posttransplant (44). Interestingly, however, in a preliminary report of a multivariate analysis of risk factors for GVHD after CD34-selected blood stem cell transplantation, the CD3+ cell dose was predictive of chronic but not acute GVHD (46). However, in this series, the range of CD3+ cell doses was narrow, and the risk of acute GVHD overall was low, so the analysis may have lacked to power to detect a significant association between CD3+ cell dose and risk of acute GVHD.

Following the initial publications by Aversa et al. reporting that high doses of CD34+ cells can overcome resistance to engraftment across major histocompatibility barriers in humans $(47,48)$, a number of studies were performed using CD34-selection of blood stem cells from haploidentical donors (Table 6) $(49–56)$. These studies targeted higher CD34+ cell doses and much lower CD3+ cell doses than used with HLA identical sibling donors. In the largest retrospective analysis to date, Kato et al. (55) reported that 21% of CD34-selected haploidentical blood stem cell transplant recipients had graft failure; the risk of graft failure in these patients did not vary with the CD34+ cell dose, and the effect of CD3+ cell dose on graft failure was not assessed. In this report, however, CD34+ cell dose was the only factor predictive of time to neutrophil and platelet recovery. Others have reported that the risk of graft failure was lower when TBI or ATG was included in the conditioning regimen $(49,50)$. Kato et al. (55) also indicated that use of antithymocyte globulin (ATG) in the conditioning regimen for haploidentical allograft recipients was associated with a lower risk of acute or chronic GVHD, but CD3+ cell dose had no impact.

Most patients appear to have achieved complete chimerism after transplantation of HLA identical CD34-selected blood stem cells with CD3+ cell doses exceeding 1 × 10^5/kg $(33,34,36,39,40,42)$, but substantial mixed chimerism was reported with lower CD3+ cell doses (57). In addition, high rates of mixed chimerism (70–83%) were reported in recipients of CD34 selected marrow transplants from matched unrelated donors when using a conditioning regimen with reduced intensity $(58,59)$.

Severe infections have emerged as the major complication in recipients of CD34 selected allografts. In studies of immune reconstitution in these patients, T and B cell recovery appears to be comparable to that in recipients of unmanipulated grafts when assessed at 1 yr after transplantation, but immune reconstitution, and especially CD4+ cell recovery, appears to be delayed when measured at earlier timepoints $(60,61)$. In one study, CD34+ cell doses >20 × 10^6/kg resulted in more rapid recovery of T cells (52). To hasten immune reconstitution and prevent relapse, some have administered unselected donor lymphocytes posttranplant. This, however, has resulted in substantial GVHD $(40,43,49,62)$. Infusion of donor lymphocytes depleted of recipient-reactive cells (63) appears more promising for this setting.

It is clear that CD34-selection of allografts results in a lower incidence of GVHD in high-risk populations. Amelioration of other transplant-related complcations has been reported as well (64). However, published studies may be biased toward positive results (39), and follow-up is too short to determine the full impact of this procedure on long-term outcome. Thus, while individual institutions may have ascertained empirically how to apply this technology to achieve "acceptable" patient outcomes, the optimal methodology has not yet been determined.

Table 7
Common GVHD Prophylaxis Regimens

Regimen	Drug	Dose schedule
CSA/MTX	CSA[a]	iv 1.5 mg/kg BID from d –1, taper 5% weekly starting d 60.
	MTX	iv 15 mg/m^2 d 1, 10 mg/m^2 d 3, 6, and 11.
TAC/MiniMTX	TAC[a]	iv 0.03 mg/kg/d CI from d –2, taper 20% every 2 wk from d 180.
	MTX	iv 5 mg/m^2 d 1, 3, 6, and 11.

Abbreviations: MTX, methotrexate; CSA, cyclosporine; TAC, tacrolimus; iv, intravenously; BID, twice daily; CI, cumulative incidence.

[a]Tacrolimus and cyclosporine have been used interchangeably with this methotrexate dose-schedule. Tacrolimus dosing is based on ideal body weight, and doses are modified for blood levels outside the target concentration range and for toxicities.

4.2. Pharmacologic Management of GVHD

A number of newly approved immunosuppressive drugs have been evaluated for the prevention or treatment of GVHD (Tables 7–10) *(65–111)*. These can be broadly grouped as T cell activation inhibitors, antimetabolites, interleukin (IL)-2 receptor antagonists, tumor necrosis factor (TNF) antagonists, anti-T cell antibodies, and inhibitors of antigen processing or presentation.

4.3. T Cell Activation Inhibitors

4.3.1. Tacrolimus

Tacrolimus is a calcineurin inhibitor that prevents early T cell activation. Its mechanism of action, pharmacology, drug interactions and toxicities are similar to those of cyclosporine. Three randomized studies have demonstrated that tacrolimus is superior to cyclosporine for prevention of acute GVHD when used in combination with methotrexate after HLA-identical or unrelated donor marrow transplantation *(112–114)*. Tacrolimus has also been evaluated for prevention of acute GVHD in recipients of HLA-identical donor blood stem cells, HLA partially matched related donor marrow, and HLA partially matched unrelated donor cord blood (reviewed in ref. *115*), and a consensus conference in 1998 concluded that there was no population in which tacrolimus was contraindicated for use in prevention of GVHD *(116)*. The most common dosing regimens are shown in Table 7. Therapeutic drug monitoring is recommended when using tacrolimus *(116)*.

Whether tacrolimus can be used as prophylaxis in patients suffering complications from cyclosporine was evaluated retrospectively by Furlong et al. *(77)*. In their experience, 8 of 11 patients with cyclosporine-associated neurotoxicity had resolution of symptoms when converted to tacrolimus, and 3 others improved. In contrast, only 1 of 11 patients with cyclosporine-associated hemolytic uremic syndrome improved when converted to tacrolimus.

For treatment of acute GVHD, tacrolimus has been used for patients who had steroid refractory disease while on cyclosporine prophylaxis (Table 8). Due to the high incidence of renal failure reported in solid organ transplant, recipients converted immediately from cyclosporine to tacrolimus, we first used ATG as a bridge until cyclosporine blood levels were undetectable before administering tacrolimus. In a series of 14 patients, only two patients achieved a complete response, and survival was only 7%. Others have now reported institution of tacrolimus safely after only 1–2 d off cyclosporine *(76,78,79)*. Complete response rates were only 10–17% using tacrolimus alone. The complete response was higher, 40%, when tacrolimus and ATG were used in combination for treatment of steroid-refractory GVHD *(76)*, but in the absence of a randomized trial, it is unclear if tacrolimus added any benefit over ATG alone in these patients. Topical tacrolimus has been applied for treatment of limited skin rash with some

Table 8
New Regimens for Prevention of Acute GVHD

Ref.	Preparative regimen	Donor	Drug	Regimen	Patients	Gr 2-4 GVHD	Gr 3-4 GVHD	Chronic GVHD
65	Nonmyelo	Sib-PBSC	MMF 15 mg/kg PO BID	CSA/MMF d 0-27	36	7%[a]	11%[a]	74%[a]
66	Nonmyelo	Sib-PBSC	MMF	CSA/MMF d 0-27	88	47%	17%	65%
67	Nonmyelo	Sib-PBSC	MMF 15 mg/kg PO BID	CSA/MMF (days not stated)	15	38%	—	—
68	Ablative	Sib-PBSC/BM	MMF 1 g PO BID	CSA/MMF d 1-14	14	47%	7%	56%
69	—	Mixed	MMF 1 g IV BID	CSA/MP/MMF (days not stated)	16	—	19%	—
70	Ablative	Alt-PBSC/BM	MMF 1 p PO daily	CSA/MTX/MP/MMF d 10-100	13	23%	15%	—
71	Ablative	Sib-PBSC	CP1H 10-60 mg ITB	CP1H +/- CSA/MTX	107	4%	1%	22%
72	Nonmyelo	Sib-PBSC	CP1H 20 mg IV	CP1H d –8 to –4/CSA+/-MTX	36	6%	0%	3%
73	Nonmyelo	MUD-BM	CP1H 20 mg IV	CP1H d –8 to –4/CSA	30	7%	0%	—
74	Nonmyelo	Sib-PBSC	CP1H ITB + 20 mg IV	CP1H +/- MMF	14	14%	0%	—
75	Mixed	Mixed	CP1H (mixed schedules)	CP1H +/- CSA	28	47%	0%	14%

Abbreviations: —, not stated; nonmyelo, nonmyeloablative or reduced intensity; sib, HLA identical sibling; alt, alternative donor; PBSC, peripheral blood stem cell; BM, bone marrow; MMF, mycophenolate mofetil; CP1H, Campath-1H, Alemtuzumab; PO, orally; BID, twice daily; IV intravenously; ITB, in the bag (ex vivo incubation prior to infusion of allograft); CSA, cyclosporine; MP, methylprednisolone; MTX methotrexate.

[a] Actuarial estimate, cumulative incidence or proportion, depending on the result reported.

Table 9
New Regimens for Treatment of Acute GVHD

Ref.	Indication	Drug	Regimen	Response assessed	Patients	CR	CR + PR
—[a]	Refractory	Tacrolimus	0.03 mg/kg/d iv after ATG	2 wk	14	14%	14%
76	Refractory	Tacrolimus	0.03 mg/kg/d iv + ATG	d 28	20	40%	14%
77	Refractory	Tacrolimus	0.03 mg/kg/d iv	6 wk	20	10%	10%
78	Refractory	Tacrolimus	0.03 mg/kg/d iv	—	6	17%	50%
79	Refractory	Tacrolimus	0.03 mg/kg/d iv	18 d	13	—	(54%)[b]
80	Refractory	MMF	1 g po daily	—	2	*[c]	*
81	Refractory	MMF	1 g po BID	—	7	—	29%
82	Refractory	MMF	1 g po BID + CSA/MP daily × 27	—	36	—	72%
83	Primary	Anti-CD25		—	1	*	*
84	Refractory Gr IV	Daclizumab	1 mg/kg iv weekly × 5	d 43	24	29%	33%
84	Refractory	Daclizumab	1 mg/kg iv d 1, 4, 8, 15, and 21	d 43	19	47%	74%
85	Refractory	Daclizumab	1 mg/kg iv d 1–5, 7, 14, and 21	d 28	12	8%	67%
86	Refractory Gr III–IV	Basiliximab	10–20 mg iv weekly × 4	—	12	25%	58%
87	Refractory Gr III–IV	Infliximab	10 mg/kg weekly	—	4	*	*
88	Refractory	Etanercept	0.4 mg/kg sc twice weekly for 2 mo	—	1	*	*
89	Primary	Thalidomide	400–800 mg po daily	—	1	0%	*
90	Refractory	Thalidomide	200–1000 mg po daily	—	3	0%	0%
91	Refractory	Thalidomide	200–400 mg po daily	—	3	0%	0%
92	Refractory	Thalidomide	12.5–25 mg/kg po daily	—	2	0%	50%

Abbreviations: —, not stated; CR, complete response; PR, partial response; ATG, antithymocyte globulin; MMF, mycophenolate mofetil.
[a]Unpublished data.
[b]Response rates in parentheses were reported as "improved."
[c]Case report of responsive disease indicated by *.

Table 10
New Regimens for Treatment of Chronic GVHD

Ref.	Drug	Indication	Regimen	Response assessed	Patients	CR	CR + PR
93	Tacrolimus	Refractory liver	4–20 mg po daily	—	15	33%	(60%)[b]
—[a]	Tacrolimus	Refractory/dependent	0.06 mg/kg po BID	2 mo	32	13%	50%
79	Tacrolimus	Refractory	0.075 mg/kg po BID	48 d	26	—	(67%)
82	MMF	Primary	1 g po BID+CSA/MP	—	12	—	(50%)
94	MMF	Intolerant	1 g po BID	—	5	—	(80%)
95	MMF	Refractory liver	1 g po BID	—	11	—	(100%)
80	MMF	Refractory	1 g po daily	—	6	—	(33%)
94	MMF	Refractory	1 g po BID	—	9	—	(55%)
81	MMF	Refractory	1 g po BID	—	12	—	33%
96	MMF	Refractory	10 mg/kg po daily	6 wk	12	17%	83%
97	MMF	Refractory	15–40 mg/kg po daily	—	15	—	60%
98	MMF	Refractory	1 g po BID + tacrolimus	3 mo	26	8%	46%
85	Daclizumab	Refractory	1 mg/kg iv d 1–5, 7, 14, and 21	28 d	4	25%	(75%)
99	Rituximab	Refractory	375 mg/m^2 iv weekly × 4	—	1	*[c]	*
100	Rituximab	Refractory	375 mg/m^2 iv weekly × 4	—	1	*	*
101	Thalidomide	Primary	200–800 mg po daily + CSA/MP	2 mo	24	8%	83%
102	Thalidomide	High risk	By blood levels	6 mo	21	33%	38%
103	Thalidomide	Dependent	12–25 mg/kg po daily	—	5	*	*
104	Thalidomide	Refractory	300 mg po daily	—	1	0%	*
91	Thalidomide	Refractory	200–400 mg po daily	—	3	0%	*
105	Thalidomide	Refractory	100–200 mg po daily	—	2	0%	*
106	Thalidomide	Refractory		—	6	—	(83%)
102	Thalidomide	Refractory	By blood levels	6 mo	23	30%	78%
107	Thalidomide	Refractory	100–300 mg po QID	3 mo	80	11%	20%
108	Thalidomide	Refractory	3–12 mg/kg po daily	—	13	28%	69%
92	Thalidomide	Refractory	12.5–25 mg/kg po daily	1–3 mo	4	25%	25%
109	Thalidomide	Refractory	50–200 mg po QID	—	37	3%	38%
110	Thalidomide	Refractory	200–1000 mg po daily	—	12	33%	75%
111	Plaquenil	Dependent	12 mg/kg po daily	1 mo	12	25%	50%
111	Plaquenil	Refractory	12 mg/kg po daily	1 mo	20	0%	35%

Abbreviations: —, not stated; CR, complete response; PR, partial response; CSA, cyclosporine; MP, methylprednisolone; MMF, mycophenolate mofetil; po, orally; BID, twice daily; iv, intravenously.

[a] Unpublished data.

[b] Response rates in parentheses were reported as "improved."

[c] Case report of responsive disease indicated by *.

success; although at least one patient had substantial transcutaneous absorption when using tacrolimus in this fashion *(117)*.

For patients with steroid refractory chronic GVHD, response rates for tacrolimus as first or second salvage have been only 13–33%, but a substantial proportion of patients experienced clinically meaningful improvement (Table 10). We have also found tacrolimus to be useful in patients with steroid-dependent chronic GVHD, allowing for a reduction in steroid dose and steroid-related complications. Long-term use of tacrolimus in this setting, however, was complicated by tacrolimus-related side effects, most notably renal insufficiency *(118)*.

4.3.2. SIROLIMUS

Sirolimus is an inhibitor of late T cell activation, blocking the calcium-independent signal transduction pathway used by growth factors, such as IL-2. Use in prevention or treatment of GVHD has not been reported. Side effects noted in solid organ transplant recipients include hyperlipidemia, myelosuppression, and capillary leak syndrome. Therapeutic drug monitoring has been recommended for safe use in solid organ transplant recipients.

4.4. Antimetabolites

4.4.1. MYCOPHENOLATE MOFETIL

Mycophenolate mofetil (MMF), a prodrug of mycophenolic acid (MPA), inhibits inosine monophosphate dehydrogenase (IMPDH). IMPDH is a key enzyme in the *de novo* pathway of purine synthesis, which is the major pathway utilized by cycling T lymphocytes. As a result, inhibition of IMPDH is thought to be selectively toxic for proliferating but not resting T cells, a paradigm similar to that for low dose methotrexate. Common side effects of MMF include nausea, vomiting, diarrhea, and myelosuppression. The active drug is eliminated renally. MMF is generally administered orally at a dose of 15 mg/kg or 1 g 2× daily. Targeted dosing based on blood levels has been suggested for solid organ transplant recipients, but this approach has not been evaluated fully in hematopoietic stem cell recipients.

A short course of MMF orally (d 0–27) has been studied most extensively in combination with cyclosporine for prevention of GVHD when using a nonmyeloablative preparative regimen (Table 8). Canine studies demonstrated that graft rejection was less in HLA identical littermate allograft recipients using MMF rather than methotrexate with cyclosporine after sublethal TBI was given *(119)*. In clinical studies of HLA identical allografts, the risk of graft rejection was 20% in patients receiving MMF rather than methotrexate when only 2 Gy TBI was used for conditioning, but most patients achieved stable mixed chimerism when conditioned with TBI and fludarabine *(66,67)*. At 38–47%, the risk of acute GVHD was considerable, and usually occurred following discontinuation of MMF at d 27.

Bornhauser et al. performed a retrospective comparison of cyclosporine with MMF vs methotrexate as prophylaxis for HLA-identical stem cell recipients using a myeloabative preparative regimen *(68)*. All patients on MMF achieved neutrophil recovery, and the time to neutrophil recovery was significantly shorter than in the group receiving methotrexate (11 vs 17 d, $p = 0.02$). There were no differences between the groups in the incidence of moderate or severe GVHD. Some have suggested that a longer course of MMF might be useful in achieving greater control of GVHD. Basara et al. have in fact reported a strikingly low incidence of GVHD—23%, in HLA-mismatched marrow transplant recipients when MMF was given d 10–100 *(70)*—however, this was in combination with cyclosporine, methotrexate, and prednisolone, so it is not clear how much the long course of MMF contributed to the control of GVHD in these patients.

In a phase I study of MMF and cyclosporine for GVHD prevention, Jenke et al. found higher MPA trough levels in patients with less severe GVHD *(120)*, indicating perhaps that a threshold drug exposure would be needed for adequate control of GVHD. MMF is generally well-absorbed (>90%), but the bioavailability appeared to be reduced in the stem cell transplant recipients *(68)*, suggesting that the intravenous route may be preferable early after transplantation. However, low MPA trough levels were found even with intravenous dosing *(120)*. This may be explained in part by loss of enterohepatic recirculation as a result of toxicity of the preparative regimen or altered bowel flora *(68,120)*. Clearly, the optimal dose-schedule of MMF for prevention of GVHD is not established.

The potential selective action of MMF on proliferating lymphocytes has been cited as an advantage for use of this drug in the treatment of GVHD. As primary treatment, the combination of MMF and prednisone induced improvement by at least one grade in 72% of patients *(82)*. Several case series suggest that MMF is active for treatment of steroid-refractory acute GVHD as well (Table 9) *(80,81)*, but prospective studies are lacking. Drug exposure appears to play an important role in treatment of acute GVHD; Kiehl et al. reported higher trough MPA levels in responders than in nonresponders *(121)*. The need for adequate drug exposure may prove problematic in patients with gut GVHD, where MPA concentrations were significantly lower than in those without gut involvement *(121)*.

There are several reports of small numbers of patients treated with MMF for chronic GVHD (Table 10). Although the documented complete-response rate is low *(96,98)*, the major benefit of therapy with MMF is sufficient control or resolution of symptoms to allow tapering of steroids without a flare *(94,95,97)*. Long-term use of MMF in clinically stable patients has also allowed for a greater appreciation of the toxicities of the drug. Cytopenias remain the most common problem, with mild leukopenia in as much as 42% of patients *(81,82,94)*. Diarrhea and elevations of liver enzymes were also noted in a small percentage of patients, but drug toxicities accounted for only a few discontinuations.

4.4.2. Leflunomide

Leflunomide is an inhibitor of dihydroorotate dehydrogenase, an enzyme involved in *de novo* pyrimidine synthesis. As such, its major activity is inhibition of proliferating lymphocytes. In vitro, high concentrations of leflunomide also inhibit the tyrosine kinases involved in T and B cell activation. The drug is administered orally, and elimination of the active metabolite is by both renal and hepatic clearance. Common side effects include elevated liver enzymes, diarrhea, alopecia and rash. Leflunomide has been shown to be effective in the treatment of rheumatoid arthritis, but it has not been tested in patients with GVHD.

4.5. IL-2 Receptor Antagonists

4.5.1. Daclizumab

Daclizumab is a humanized monoclonal antibody directed against CD25, the α chain of the IL-2 receptor. Expression of the IL-2 receptor α chain is up-regulated in activated T lymphocytes, and blockade of the receptor by the antibody is thought to result in activation-induced cell death (AICD) by inhibiting the effect of IL-2. Thus, treatment with daclizumab during clinical or subclinical GVHD would potentially eliminate alloreactive T cells specifically. Few side effects have been reported with use of daclizumab; it does not induce a first-dose reaction or a cytokine-release syndrome. The drug is administered intravenously at a dose of 1 mg/kg. In marrow transplant recipients with acute GVHD, daclizumab has a half-life of 3.5 d, considerably shorter than that seen in solid organ transplant recipients *(122)*. Despite the long half-life, frequent dosing may be required in patients with acute GVHD, since circulating soluble IL-2 receptor in these patients neutralizes the activity of the drug.

For prevention of GVHD, Anasetti et al. performed a randomized study of placebo vs one of two dose levels of daclizumab given weekly for five doses from d –1 for unrelated donor marrow transplantation *(123)*. Although the time to onset of GVHD was delayed in the patients who received daclizumab, there was no significant difference between arms in the incidence of GVHD, relapse, or survival. The lack of elimination of alloreactive cells in these patients may have been due to the early administration of the drug; blockade from the day of transplantation may have inhibited activation, an absolute requirement for AICD.

For treatment of steroid refractory acute GVHD, complete response rates have varied from 8 to 47% (Table 9) *(84,85,122)*. Response may vary with dose-schedule, grade and organ involvement. Frequent dosing was used during the first week of therapy in an effort to saturate circulating soluble IL-2 receptors. Best responses were seen in patients with skin GVHD. Willenbacher et al. also reported that patients with refractory chronic GVHD may respond to treatment with daclizumab *(85)*. Infectious complications, however, were substantial.

4.5.2. BASILIXIMAB

Basiliximab is a chimeric anti-CD25 antibody. The half-life of basiliximab is shorter than that of daclizumab, and the drug has no substantial side effects. Basiliximab has been studied only for treatment of grades III–IV steroid refractory acute GVHD. Pasquini et al. administered the drug at a dose of 20 mg intravenously every 2 wk. They reported a complete response rate of 25%, although overall, 58% of the patients treated improved *(86)*.

4.5.3. DENILEUKIN DIFTITOX

Denileukin diftitox is a diphtheria toxin-IL-2 fusion protein. Its mechanism of action is to inhibit protein synthesis and induce cytotoxicity in cells binding IL-2. Like IL-2, denileukin diftitox has a short half-life, with distribution occurring within minutes. The side effect profile is similar to that of IL-2, and includes flu-like symptoms, hypotension, edema, and renal insufficiency. As a result of its high incidence of toxicity and the partial agonistic effects, denileukin diftitox does not appear to be a suitable drug for elimination of activated T cells in patients with GVHD.

4.6. TNF Antagonists

4.6.1. INFLIXIMAB

Infliximab is a chimeric monoclonal antibody directed against TNF-α. Its main effect is neutralization of the soluble cytokine, but the antibody can also mediate antibody-dependent cellular cytotoxicity (ADCC) of cells bearing surface TNF. Infliximab has a half-life of about 1 wk. Hypersensitivity reactions have been reported with its administration. Kobbe et al treated four patients with grade IV refractory acute GVHD using infliximab at 10 mg/kg intravenously weekly for 1–3 wk *(87)*. Three of the four patients achieved a complete response, including resolution of severe diarrhea.

4.6.2. ETANERCEPT

Etanercept is a TNF receptor p75-IgG Fc fusion protein. Like infliximab, etanercept neutralizes soluble and membrane-bound TNF, but it binds both the α and β forms of TNF. When administered subcutaneously, etanercept has a slow uptake with a time to Cmax of about 3 d and median half-life of 5 d in patients with autoimmune diseases. Injection site reactions are generally mild, and few other side effects have been noted. Andolina et al. treated one patient with refractory intestinal acute GVHD using etanercept 0.4 mg/kg weekly *(88)*. The diarrhea resolved slowly. The symptoms returned approx 3 wk after the drug was discontinued, and a second remission was induced by retreatment.

4.7. Anti-T Cell Antibodies

4.7.1. ALEMTUZUMAB

Alemtuzumab (CAMPATH-1H) is a humanized monoclonal antibody against CD52, a glycoprotein expressed on lymphocytes, mature phagocytes, and some CD34+ cells. The antibody is complement-fixing and eliminates CD52-positive cells by inducing cytotoxicity or by opsonization. The half-life following intravenous administration is approx 12 d in patients with lymphoid malignancies; there is a high degree of interpatient variability in the pharmacokinetics of the drug due to differences in the number of CD52-bearing cells that form the major portion of the volume of distribution. The most common side effect is an anaphylactoid reaction that occurs with infusion; the reaction can be ameliorated partially by slowing the infusion or by starting a treatment course with a small dose. Myelosuppression has been reported infrequently, but ex vivo incubation of marrow with alemtuzumab did not have any significant effect on in vitro growth of committed progenitors (124).

For prevention of GVHD, alemtuzumab has been administered in two ways, following incubation of the allograft ("in the bag") or intravenously pretransplant (Table 8). Hale et al. reported a retrospective analysis of 107 patients who received HLA identical blood stem cells treated ex vivo with 10–60 mg alemtuzumab (71). The cells and drug were infused after a 30-min incubation without further manipulation. Some patients also received cyclosporine and methotrexate after transplantation. The incidence of grades II–IV GVHD was quite low, at 4%. Graft rejection occurred in only 2% of the patients, but results of chimerism studies were not reported.

A number of investigators have evaluated alemtuzumab given pretransplant with nonmyeloablative preparative regimens (Table 8). The prolonged half-life results in immunosuppressive activity extending into the posttransplant period, but cyclosporine was administered to most patients as well. The risk of GVHD was exceedingly low, but mixed chimerism occurred in several patients in each series (72–75). Immune reconstitution occurs slowly in patients treated with alemtuzumab, and a high incidence of ctomegalovirus (CMV) infections early after transplantation has been reported in this group (125).

These studies clearly demonstrate that GVHD can be prevented effectively using alemtuzumab either in the bag or administered intravenously during the peritransplant period. Appropriate dosing, however, is unclear in the absence of well-designed Phase Ib studies, and long-term outcome for these patients is still unclear.

4.7.2. ATG

ATG consists of serum from horses or rabbits immunized with human lymphocytes or thymocytes. Preparations are highly heterogeneous with regard to titers against specific epitopes (126,127). In solid organ transplantation, outcomes vary with the type of ATG used (128–130), but this has not been studied in hematopoietic stem cell transplantation. Following administration of standard doses, ATG was detected in the serum for 1–2 mo, and serum levels were proportional to the dose adminstered (131,132). The half-life of free anti-T cell antibody was reported to be 4 d (132), although lymphocytes coated with ATG were found in the circulation as late as 100 d after treatment (131). Side effects include fever, chills, bronchspasm, anaphylactoid reactions, serum sickness, hypertension, interstitial pneumonitis, arthralgias, platelet consumption, and myelosuppression. In patients who received ATG as part of the preparative regimen, elevations of bilirubin and transaminases were also noted (133). In a retrospective comparison, fewer side effects were reported with Frensenius-S[ATG] (ATG-F) than with thymoglobulin (R-ATG) or OKT3 (134). A higher level of type 2 cytokines was induced by OKT3, but differences between ATG-F and R-ATG were not commented upon (134).

Although ATG was introduced as part of the preparative regimen in order to reduce graft rejection (135), its use in this fashion was also associated with a reduction in GVHD. For unrelated donor marrow transplant patients, the risk of grades II–IV GVHD was 12–25% using ATG-F or R-ATG, significantly less than in patients who received OKT3 in the preparative regimen (134). To determine if dose was important, Holler et al. conducted a phase I study of ATG-F; they reported that unrelated donor marrow transplant recipients who received doses of 20–30 mg/kg in the preparative regimen had less grades III–IV acute GVHD than those receiving doses of 5–10 mg/kg (8–10% vs 27–28%) *(136)*. Control of GVHD was also associated with a reduction in treatment-related mortality in these patients. How dose affects outcome for other types of ATG has not been evaluated.

Lymphocyte recovery was reported to be delayed in patients receiving ATG as part of the preparative regimen *(131)*. This raised a concern regarding the potential for increased relapse *(136)*. Relapse has not been assessed comparing cohorts with or without ATG pretreatment. Remberger et al. *(131)*, however, did find that the risk of relapse for patients with CML was significantly higher when using R-ATG rather than ATG-F or OKT3 (61 vs 0%). Delayed immune recovery in this setting was also associated with an increase in CMV infection and an impairment in overall survival for those who were CMV-seropositive *(137,138)*.

ATG has been used extensively for treatment of steroid-refractory acute GVHD. In a recent survey *(139)*, horse ATG was used by 50% of transplant centers and rabbit ATG by 24%, but the response rates to different preparations of ATG have not been compared in a randomized trial. Dose schedules vary widely *(139)*, and the optimal dose and target population have not been determined.

4.8. Anti-B Cell Antibodies

4.8.1. Rituximab

Rituximab is a chimeric anti-CD20 antibody that eliminates B cells by complement-mediated and opsonic mechanisms. Infusion-related adverse events are severe, but the drug has few other toxicities. There are two case reports of rituximab 375 mg/m^2/wk as treatment of patients with refractory chronic GVHD having manifestations associated with autoimmune antibodies *(99,100)*. Whether rituximab will be active in patients with other manifestations of chronic GVHD has not been evaluated.

4.9. Other Agents

4.9.1. Thalidomide

Thalidomide is an organic small molecule. The drug binds to GC-rich nucleotides, but how this effects its ultimate actions is unclear. Thalidomide's best known activities include inhibition of angiogenesis and inhibition of production of TNF-α in monocytes and T cells. The drug is absorbed poorly with great interpatient variability in bioavailability *(109)*, but its pharmacokinetics are otherwise not well-studied in marrow transplant recipients. Some have recommended monitoring blood concentrations to avoid levels associated with irreversible toxicity *(102,140)*. Common side effects include sedation, peripheral neuropathy, rash, and teratogenicity. In one case, a patient developed severe skin ulcers thought to be due to the antiangiogenic properties of thalidomide *(141)*. Unexpectedly, neutropenia was also noted with long-term use *(26,104)*. In prospective studies, thalidomide was discontinued in 10–92% of patients due to toxicities, with the lowest rate of discontinuation in the protocol that monitored blood levels of the drug.

There are few case series of thalidomide for treatment of refractory acute GVHD (Table 9). It does not appear to be active in this setting. It also does not appear to be effective for prevention of chronic GVHD. In a randomized study comparing placebo to thalidomide starting d 80 after transplantation, there was a high rate of chronic GVHD with thalidomide, and better survival with placebo *(142)*.

Use of thalidomide for treatment of chronic GVHD appears more promising. In the initial case reports, no patient with refractory chronic GVHD had a clear complete response to thalidomide alone, but there was substantial improvement in signs and symptoms *(91,103–106)*. In larger series and prospective studies, complete responses were reported in 3–38%, and combined complete and partial responses were reported in 20–78% (Table 10). In an uncontrolled study, clinical improvement occurred more frequently in patients with refractory rather than untreated high risk chronic GVHD (78 vs 38%) (102). In addition, in a randomized study of patients with untreated GVHD, the addition of thalidomide to the combination of cyclosporine and prednisone did not improve response or short-term survival (101). Whether disease-free survival might be impacted by the antitumor effects of thalidomide will require longer follow-up.

4.9.2. HYDROXYCHLOROQUINE

Hydroxychloroquine is a lysosomotropic amine that affects acidity of cytoplasmic vacuoles. This action has been associated with interference in antigen processing and loading major histocompatibility complex (MHC) molecules. Hydroxychloroquine has also been found to inhibit mitogen-induced TNF-α production and calcium-dependent signaling in T and B cells during activation. Gilman et al. evaluated the activity of hydroxychloroquine for treatment of chronic GVHD (111). No patient with chronic GVHD had a complete response, but clinical improvement was enough to allow for a decrease in steroids in 35% with refractory disease and 50% with steroid-dependent disease. Retinopathy and myelosuppression were not noted in these patients, and few had gastrointestinal problems. However, neuropathy or myopathy were reported in three patients, all of whom had renal insufficiency.

5. CONCLUSIONS

For prevention of acute GVHD, CD34 selection appears to be a promising technology, especially for haploidentical blood stem cell transplantation. Use of alemtuzumab pretransplant also appears to be an effective strategy, although the optimal dose schedule is still unclear. Development of the means to hasten immune reconstitution in these patients in order to reduce treatment-related mortality from opportunitistic infections is badly needed. For pharmacologic prophylaxis, tacrolimus has been the major advance in the last decade. Use of MMF to replace methotrexate is a logical step to reduce mucositis. However, current data do not demonstrate that MMF is any better than methotrexate in combination with cyclosporine for prevention of acute GVHD, so whether the cost of the drug and toxicities of extended use are warranted should be considered carefully.

For treatment of acute GVHD, there has been little progress. The IL-2 receptor antagonists appear to be most active of the drugs currently available, but randomized studies have yet to demonstrate efficacy. There have been two major obstacles to progress in this area. One is the lack of patients. With improvements in GVHD prophylaxis, there are fewer patients with steroid-refractory disease. The other obstacle is the heterogeneity of the patient population. Current staging and grading systems for acute GVHD have not been validated as predictive of response or prognosis in treatment trials. Once a staging system has been validated in this setting, it is likely that well-powered studies will require cooperation of multiple institutions to be completed within a meaningful period of time.

Treatment of chronic GVHD has been a very active area of study. Although investigators report that the newer immunosuppressive drugs are active for treatment of chronic GVHD, complete response rates have not been very high. Several of the drugs, notably MMF and thalidomide, have a steroid-sparing effect, which in itself can be of considerable benefit to the patient. It has also been noted that a response may take more than 2–3 mo to occur (100). Using the current strategy of declaring failure at an early time point in the absence of progressive disease may result in changing patients from a potentially effective therapy to one of unknown activity or no benefit at all. In addition, design of randomized studies for treatment of chronic GVHD first requires validation of response criteria.

REFERENCES

1. Glucksberg H, Storb R, Fefer A, et al. Clinical manifestations of graft-versus-host disease in human recipients of marrow from HLA-matched sibling donors. *Transplantation* 1974;18:295–304.
2. Thomas ED, Storb R, Clift RA, et al. Bone marrow transplantation. *N Engl J Med* 1975;292:895–902.
3. Gratwohl A, Hermans J, Apperley J, et al. Acute graft-versus-host disease: grade and outcome in patients with chronic myelogenous leukemia. *Blood* 1995;86:813–818.
4. Rowlings PA, Przepiorka D, Klein JP, et al. IBMTR Severity Index for grading acute graft-versus-host disease: retrospective comparison with Glucksberg grade. *Br J Haematol* 1997;97:855–864.
5. Przepiorka D, Weisdorf D, Martin P, et al. Consensus conference on acute GVHD grading. *Bone Marrow Transplant* 1995;15:825–828.
6. Martin P, Nash R, Sanders J, et al. Reproducibility in retrospective grading of acute graft-versus-host disease after allogeneic marrow transplantation. *Bone Marrow Transplant* 1998;21:273–279.
7. Elliott CJ, Sloane JP, Sanderson KV, et al. The histological diagnosis of cutaneous graft-verus-host disease: relationship of skin changes to marrow purging and other clinical variables. *Histopathology* 1987;11:145–155.
8. Martino R, Romero P, Subira M, et al. Comparison of the classic Glucksberg criteria and the IBMTR Severity Index for grading acute graft-versus-host disease following HLA-identical sibling stem cell transplantation. *Bone Marrow Transplant* 1999;24:283–287.
9. Cahn JY, Cordonnier JM, Lee S, et al. Societe Francaise de Greffe de Moelle (SFGM) and Dana Farber Cancer Institute (DFCI) prospective multicenter evaluation of two acute graft versus host disease grading systems: a preliminary analysis of 607 patients. *Blood* 2000;96:397a.
10. Shulman HM, Sullivan KM, Weiden PL, et al. Chronic graft-versus-host syndrome in man. A long-term clinicopathologic study of 20 Seattle patients. *Am J Med* 1980;69:204–217.
11. Atkinson K, Horowitz MM, Gale RP, et al. Consensus among bone marrow transplanters for diagnosis, grading and treatment of chronic graft-versus-host disease. *Bone Marrow Transplant* 1989;4:247–254.
12. Sullivan KM, Witherspoon RP, Storb R, et al. Prednisone and azathioprine compared with prednisone and placebo for treatment of chronic graft-v-host disease: prognsotic influence of prolonged thrombocytopenia after allogeneic marrow transplantation. *Blood* 1988;72:546–554.
13. Przepiorka D, Anderlini P, Saliba R, et al. Chronic graft-versus-host disease after allogeneic blood stem cell transplantation. *Blood* 2001;6:1695–1700.
14. Wingard JR, Piantadosi S, Vogelsang GB, et al. Predictors of death from chronic graft-versus-host disease after bone marrow transplantation. *Blood* 1989;74:1428–1435.
15. Pavletic S, Tarantolo S, Lynch J, et al. Chronic graft-versus-host disease after allogeneic blood stem cell or bone marrow transplantation: factors determining onset and survival. *Proc Am Soc Clin Oncol* 1999:18:A201.
16. Lee SJ, Klein JP, Barrett J, et al. Chornic graft-vs-host disease (cGVHD) severity score: effects on leukemia-free survival. *Blood* 2000;96:556a.
17. Akpek G, Zahurak ML, Piantadosi S, et al. Development of a prognostic model for grading chronic graft-versus-host disease. *Blood* 2001;97:1219–1226.
18. Arora M, Wagner JE, Davies SM, et al. Randomized clinical trial of thalidomide, cyclosporine, and prednisone versus cyclosporine and prednisone as initial therapy for chornic graft-versus-host disease. *Biol Blood Marrow Transplant* 2001;7:265–273.
19. Kaplan EL, Meier P. Nonparametric estimation from incomplete observations. *J Am Stat Assoc* 1958;53:457–481.
20. Pepe MS, Longton G, Pettinger M, Mori M, Fisher LD, Storb R. Summarizing data on survival, relapse, and chronic graft-versus-host disease after bone marrow transplantation: motivation for and description of new methods. *Br J Haematol* 1993;83:602–607.
21. Gooley TA, Leisenring W, Crowley J, Storer BE. Estimation of failure probabilities in the presence of competing risks: new representations of old estimators. *Stat Med* 1999;18:695–705.
22. Weisdorf D, Haake R, Blazar B, et al. Treatment of moderate/severe acute graft-verusu-host disease after allogeneic bone marrow transplantation: an analysis of clinical risk features and outcome. *Blood* 1990;75:1024–1030.
23. Martin PJ, Schoch G, Fisher L, et al. A retrospective analysis of therapy for acute graft-versus-host disease: initial treatment. *Blood* 1990;76:1464–1472.
24. Martin PJ, Schoch G, Fisher L, et al. A retrospective analysis of therapy for acute graft-versus-host disease: secondary treatment. *Blood* 1991;77:1821–1828.
25. Aschan J. Treatment of moderate to severe acute graft-versus-host diseae: a retrospective analysis. *Bone Marrow Transplant* 1994;14:601–607.

26. Koc S, Leisenring W, Flowers ME, et al. Thalidomide for treatment of patients with chronic graft-versus-host disease. *Blood* 2000;96:3995–3996.

27. Dreger P, Viehmann K, Steinmann J, et al. G-CSF-mobilized peripheral blood progenitor cells for allogeneic transplantation: comparison of T cell depletion strategies using different CD34+ selection systems or CAMPATH-1. *Exp Hematol* 1995;23:147–154.

28. Stainer CJ, Miflin G, Anderson S, Davy B, McQuaker IG, Russell NH. A comparison of two different systems for CD34+ selection of autologous or allogeneic PBSC collections. *J Hematother* 1998;7:375–383.

29. Fritsch G, Scharner D, Froschl G, et al. Selection of CD34-positive blood cells for allogeneic transplantation: approaches to optimize CD34-cell recovery, purity, viability and T-cell depletion. *Onkologie* 2000;23:449–456.

30. Mavroudis DA, Read EJ, Molldrem J, et al. T cell-depleted granulocyte colony-stimulating factor (G-CSF) modified allogeneic bone marrow transplantation for hematological malignancy improves graft CD34+ cell content but is associated with delayed pancytopenia. *Bone Marrow Transplant* 1998;21:431–440.

31. Cornetta K Gharpure V, Mills B, et al. Rapid engraftment after allogeneic transplantation using CD34-enriched marrow cells. *Bone Marrow Transplant* 1998;21:65–71.

32. Stoppa AM, Chabannon C, Faucher C, et al. Feasibility of CD34 selected allogeneic bone marrow transplantation (ABMT) followed after 3 months by prophylactic donor lymphocyte infusion (DLI) in hematologic malignancies. *Blood* 2000;96:790a.

33. Link H, Arseniev L, Bahre O, Kadar JG, Diedrich H, Poliwoda H. Transplantation of allogeneic CD34+ blood cells. *Blood* 1996;87:4903–4909.

34. Bensinger WI, Buckner CD, Shannon-Dorcy K, et al. Transplantation of allogeneic CD34+ peripheral blood stem cells in patients with advanced hematologic malignancy. *Blood* 1996;88:4132–4138.

35. Urbano-Ispizua A, Rozman C, Martinez C, et al. Rapid engraftment without significant graft-versus-host disease after allogeneic transplantation of CD34+ selected cells from peripheral blood. *Blood* 1997;89:3967–3973.

36 Finke J, Brugger W, Bertz H, et al. Allogeneic transplantation of positively selected peripheral blood CD34+ progenitor cells from matched related donors. *Bone Marrow Transplant* 1996;18:1081–1086.

37. Urbano-Ispizua A, Solano C, Brunet S, et al. Allogeneic transplantation of selected CD34+ cells from peripheral blood: experience of 62 cases using immunoadsorption or immunomagnetic techniques. Apanish Group of Allo-PBT. *Bone Marrow Transplant* 1998;22:519–525.

38. Alegre A, Arranz R, Granda A, et al. Allogeneic peripheral blood stem cell transplantation (allo-PBSCT) with CD34 positive selection for advanced hemopathies. *Blood* 2000;96:336b.

39. Viret F, Chabannon C, Aurran-Schleinitz T, et al. Transplantation of allogeneic CD34+ blood cells in leukemia or lymphoma patients at high risk of GVHD. *Bone Marrow Transplant* 1999;24:225–227.

40. Waller EK, Langston AA, Bucur S, et al. Sequential CD34+ and CD3+ allogeneic cell transplants in patients with poor risk hematologic malignancies. *Blood* 2000;96:359b.

41. Bensinger W, Cornetta K, Carabasi M, et al. T cell depleted allogeneic PBSC transplantation using CD34+ cell selection. *Blood* 2000;96:199a.

42. Haddad N, Zuckerman T, Katz T, et al. Allogeneic BMT for CML using T-cell depletion and megadoses of CD34 cells; potential for reduced toxicity without loss of efficacy? *Blood* 2000;96:142a.

43. Martino R, Martin-Henao G, Sureda A, et al. Allogeneic peripheral blood stem cell transplantation with CD34+-cell selection and delayed T-cell add-back in adults. Results of a single center pilot study. *Haematology* 2000;85:1165–1171.

44. Beelen DW, Peceny R, Elmaagacli A, et al. Transplantation of highly purified HLA-identical sibling donor peripheral blood CD34+ cells without prophylactic post-transplant immunosuppression in adult patients with first chronic phase chronic myeloid leukemia: results of a phase II study. *Bone Marrow Transplant* 2000;26:823–829.

45. Urbano-Ispizua A, Rozman C, Pimentel P, et al. The number of donor CD3+ cells is the most important factor for graft failure after allogeneic transplantation of CD34+ selected cells from peripheral blood from HLA-identical siblings. *Blood* 2001;97:383–387.

46. Urbano-Ipsizua A, Pimental P, Solano C, et al. Predictive factors for graft versus host disease after allogeneic transplantation of CD34+ selected cells from peripheral blood (allo-PBT/CD34+) from HLA-identical siblings. *Blood* 2000;96:396a.

47. Aversa F, Tabilio A, Terenzi A, et al. Successful engraftment of T-cell-depleted haploidentical "three-loci" incompatible transplants in leukemia patients by addition of recombinant human granulocyte colony-stimulating factor-mobilized peripheral blood progenitor cells to bone marrow inoculum. *Blood* 1994;84:3948–3955.

48. Aversa F, Tabilio A, Velardi A, et al. Treatment of high-risk acute leukemia with T-cell-depleted stem cells from related donors with one fully mismatched HLA haplotype. *N Engl J Med* 1998;339:1186–1193.

49. Kawano Y, Takaue Y, Watanabe A, et al. Partially mismatched pediatric transplants with allogeneic CD34+ blood cells from a related donor. *Blood* 1998;92:2123–3130.

50. Passweg JR, Kuhne T, Gregor M, et al. Increased stem cell dose, as obtained using currently available technology, may not be sufficient for engraftment of haploidentical stem cell transplants. *Bone Marrow Transplant* 2000;26:1033–1036.

51. Bunjes D, Duncker C, Wiesneth M, et al. CD34+ selected cells in mismatched stem cell transplantation: a single centre experience of haploidentical peripheral blood stem cell transplantation. *Bone Marrow Transplant* 2000;26(suppl 2):S9–S11.

52. Handgretinger R, Klingebiel T, Lang P, et al. Megadose transplantation of purified peripheral blood CD34+ progenitor cells from HLA-mismatched parental donors in children. *Bone Marrow Transplant* 2001;27:777–783.

53. McGuirk JP, Dix SP, Greenfield RJ, et al. Ex vivo T-cell depletion for graft versus host disease prophylaxis in related haplo-identical allogeneic stem cell transplant recipients. *Blood* 2000;96:362b.

54. Bacigalupo A, Mordini N, Pitto A, et al. Transplantation of HLA-mismatched CD34+ selected cells in patients with advanced malignancies: severe immunodeficiency and related complications. *Br J Haematol* 1997;98:760–766.

55. Kato S, Yabe H, Yasui M, et al. Allogeneic hematopoietic transplantation of CD34+ selected cells from an HLA haplo-identical related donor. A long-term follow-up of 135 patients and a comparison of stem cell source between the bone marrow and the peripheral blood. *Bone Marrow Transplant* 2000;26:1281–1290.

56. Lang P, Handgretinger R, Schlegel PG, et al. Transplantation of allogeneic purified peripheral CD34+ stem cells for nonmalignant diseases in children. *Blood* 2000;96:418a.

57. Briones J, Urbano-Ispizua A, Lawler M, et al. High frequency of donor chimerism after allogeneic transplantation of CD34+-selected peripheral blood cells. *Exp Hematol* 1998;26:415–420.

58. Socie G, Cayuela JM, Raynal B, et al. Influence of CD34 cell selection on the incidence of mixed chimaerism and minimal residual disease after allgoeneic unrelated donor transplantation. *Leukemia* 1998;12:1440–1446.

59. Craddock C, Bardy P, Kreiter S, et al. Engraftment of T-cell-depleted allogeneic haematopoietic stem cells using a reduced intensity conditioning regimen. *Br J Haematol* 2000;111:797–800.

60. Martinez C, Urbano-Ispizua A, Rozman C, et al. Immune reconstitution following allogeneic peripheral blood progenitor cell transplantation: comparison of recipients of positive CD34+ selected grafts with recipients of unmanipulated grafts. *Exp Hematol* 1999;27:561–568.

61. Behringer D, Bertz H, Schmoor C, Berger C, Dwenger A, Finke J. Quantitative lymphocyte subset reconstitution after allogeneic hematopoietic transplantation from amtched related donors with CD34+ selected PBPC grafts unselected PBPC grafts or BM grafts. *Bone Marrow Transplant* 1999;24:295–302.

62. Knauf W, Fietz T, Schrezenmeier H, Thiel E. CD34 selected alloPBSCT and adoptive immunotherapy. *Bone Marrow Transplant* 2000;26(Suppl 2):S2–S5.

63. Cavazzana-Calvo M, Hacein-Bey S, Schindler J, et al. Donor T lymphocyte infusion following ex vivo depletion of donor anti-host reactivity by an anti-CD25 immunotoxin(IT). Preliminary results of a Phase I/II trial. *Blood* 2000;96:477a.

64. Moscardo F, Sanz GF, de la Rubia J, et al. Marked reduction in the incidence of hepatic veno-occlusive disease after allogeneic hematopoietic stem cell transplantation with CD34+ positive selection. *Bone Marrow Transplant* 2001;27:983–988.

65. McSweeney PA, Niederweiser D, Shizuru JA, et al. Hematopoietic cell transplantation in older patietns with hematologic malignancies: replacing high-dose cytotoxic therapy with graft-versus-tumor effects. *Blood* 2001;97:3390–3400.

66. Sandmaier BM, Maloney DG, Hegenbart U, et al. Nonmyeloablative conditioning for HLA-identical related allografts for hematologic malignancies. *Blood* 2000;96:479a.

67. Kobbe g, Aivado M, Huenerlituerkoglu A, et al. High incidence of acute GVHD after allogeneic blood stem cell transplantation following minimal intensive conditioning. *Blood* 2000;96:784a.

68. Bornhauser M, Schuler U, Porksen G, et al. Mycophenolate mofetil and cyclosporine as graft-versus-host disease prophylaxis after allogeneic blood stem cell transplantation. *Transplantation* 1999;67:499–504.

69. Kiehl MG, Armstrong V, Basara N, et al. Intravenous mycophenoate mofetil plus prednisolone and cyclospirne in the prophylaxis of GVHD after stem cell transplantation. *Blood* 1999;94(Suppl 1):153a.

70. Basara N, Blau WI, Kiehl MG, et al. Mycophenolate mofetil for the prophylaxis of acute GVHD in HLA-mismatched bone marrow transplant patients. *Clin Transplant* 2000;14:121–126.

71. Hale G, Jacobs P, Wood L, et al. CD52 antibodies for prevention of graft-versus-host disease and graft rejection following transplantation of allogeneic peripheral blood stem cells. *Bone Marrow Transplant* 2000;26:69–76.

72. Kottaridis PD, Milligan DW, Chopra R, et al. In vivo CAMPATH-2H prevents graft-versus-host disease following nonmyeloabltaive stem cell transplantation. *Blood* 2000;96:2419–2425.

73. Peggs KS, Mahendra P, Milligan DW, et al. Non-myeloablative transplantation using matched unrelated donors – in vivo campath-1H limits graft versus host disease. *Blood* 2000;96:841a.

74. Rizzieri DA, Long GD, Vredenburgh JJ, et al. Chimerism mediated immunotherapy using campath T cell depleted peripheral blood progenitor cells (PBPC) with nonablative therapy provides reliable durable allogeneic engraftment. *Blood* 2000;96:521a.

75. Potter MN, Grace SC, Teehan C, et al. Campath 1 H "in the bag" is an effective method of GVHD prevention in allogeneic stem cell transplantation. *Blood* 2000;96:476a.

76. Durrant S, Mollee P, Morton AJ, Irving I. Combination therapy with tacrolimus and anti-thymocyte globulin for the treatment of steroid-resistant acute graft-versus-host disease developing during cyclosporine prophylaxis. *Br J Haematol* 2001;113:217–223.

77. Furlong T, Storb R, Anasetti C, et al. Clinical outcome after conversion to FK506 (tacrolimus) therapy for acute graft-versus-host disease resistant to cyclosporine or for cyclosporine-assiciated toxicities. *Bone Marrow Transplant* 2000;26:985–991.

78. Koehler MT, Howrie D, Mirro J, et al. FK506 (tacrolimus) in the treatment of steroid-resistant acute graft-versus-host disease in children undergoing bone marrow transplantation. *Bone Marrow Transplant* 1995;15:895–899.

79. Kanamaru A, Takemoto Y, Kakishita E, et al. FK506 treatment of graft-versus-host disease developing or exacerbating during prophylaxis with cyclosporin and/or other immunosuppressants. *Bone Marrow Transplant* 1995;15:885–889.

80. Ihlan O, Celebi H, Arat O, et al. Treatment of acute and chronic graft versus host disease with mycophenolate mofetil. *Blood* 1999;94(Suppl 1):368b.

81. Abhyankar S, Godder K, Christiansen N, et al. Treatment of resistant acute and chronic graft versus host disease with mycophenolate mofetil. *Blood* 1998;92(Suppl 1):340b.

82. Basara N, Kiehl MG, Blau W, et al. Mycophenolate mofetil in the treatment of acute and chronic GVHD in hematopoietic stem cell transplant patients: four years of experience. *Transplant Proc* 2001;33:2121–2123.

83. Ozsahin H, Tuchschmid P, Lauener R, et al. Blockade of acute grade IV skin and eye graft-versus-host disease by anti-interleukin-2 receptor monoclonal antibody in genoidentical bone amrrow transplantation setting. *Turk J Pediatr* 1998;40:231–235.

84. Przepiorka D, Kernan NA Ippoliti C, et al. Daclizumab, a humanized anti-interleukin-2 receptor alpha chain antibody, for treatment of acute graft-versus-host disease. *Blood* 2000;95:83–89.

85. Willenbacher W, Basara N, Blau IW, Fauser AA, Kiehl MG. Treatment of steroid refractory acute and chronic graft-versus-host disease with daclizumab. *Br J Haematol* 2001;112:820–823.

86. Pasquini R, Moreira VA, de Medeiros CR, Bonfim C. Basiliximab (BaMab) – a selective interleukin-2 receptor (IL-2R) antagonist – as therapy for refractory acute graft versus host disease (a-GVHD) following bone marrow transplantation. *Bone Marrow Transplant* 2000;96:177a.

87. Kobbe G, Schneider P, Rohr U, et al. Treatment of severe steroid refractory acute graft-versus-host disease with infliximab, a chimeric human/mouse anti-TNF alpha antibody. *Bone Marrow Transplant* 2001;28:47–49.

88. Andolina M, Rabusin M, Maximova N, Di Leo G. Etanercept in graft-versus-host disease. *Bone Marrow Transplant* 2000;26:929.

89. Lim SH, McWhannell A, Vora AJ, Boughton BJ. Successful treatment with thalidomide of acute graft-versus-host disease after bone-marrow transplantation. *Lancet* 1988;1:117.

90. Ringden O, Aschan J, Westerberg L. Thalidomide for severe acute graft-versus-host disease. *Lancet* 1988;2:568.

91. McCarthy DM, Kanfer E, Taylor J, Barrett AJ. Thalidomide for graft-versus-host disease. *Lancet* 1988;2:1135.

92. Mehta P, Kedar A, Graham-Pole J, Skoda-Smith S, Wingard JR. Thalidomide in children undergoing bone marrow transplantation: series at a single institution and review of the literature. *Pediatrics* 1999;103:e44–e48.

93. Nagler A, Menachem Y, Ilan Y. Amelioration of steroid-resistant chronic graft-versus-host mediated liver disease via tacrolimus treatment. *J Hematother Stem Cell Res* 2001;10:411–417.

94. Redei I, Langston AA, Cherry JK, Allen A, Waller EK. Salvage therapy with mycophenolate mofetil (MMF) for ptients with severe chronic GVHD. *Blood* 1999;94(Suppl 1):159a.

95. Roberts T, Koc Y, Sprague K, et al. Mycophenolate mofetil (MMF) for the treatment of chronic graft versus host disease (cGVHD) of the liver. *Blood* 1999;94(Suppl 1):159a.

96. Pallotta-Filho RS, Barbosa JAL, Macedo MCMA, et al. The use of mycophenolate mofetil in the treatment of refractory chronic graft versus host disease. *Blood* 1998;92(Suppl 1):346b.

97. Busca A, Saroglia EM, Lanino E, et al. Mycophenolate mofetil (MMF) as therapy for refractory chronic GVHD (cGVHD) in children receiving bone marrow transplantation. *Bone Marrow Transplant* 2000;25:1067–1071.

98. Mookerjee B, Altomonte V, Vogelsang G. Salvage therapy for refractory chronic graft-versus-host disease with mycophenolate mofetil and tacrolimus. *Bone Marrow Transplant* 1999;24:517–520.

99. Ratanatharathorn V, Carson E, Reynolds C, et al. Anti-CD20 chimeric monoclonal antibody treatment of refractory immune-mediated thrombocytopenia in a patient with chronic graft-versus-host disease. *Ann Intern Med* 2000;15:275–279.

100. Szabolcs P, Reese M, Yancey K, Hall RP, Kurtzberg J. Combination treatment of bullous skin GVHD and anti-CD20 and anti-CD25 antibodies. *Blood* 2000;96:350b.

101. Arora M, Wagner JE, Davies SM, et al. Randomized clinical trial of thalidomide, cyclosporine and prednisone versus cyclosporine and prednisone as initial therapy for chronic graft-versus-host disease. *Biol Blood Marrow Transplant* 2001;7:265–273.

102. Vogelsang GB, Farmer ER, Hess AD, et al. Thalidomide for the treatment of chronic graft-versus-host disease. *N Engl J Med* 1992;326:1055–1058.
103. Cole CH, Rogers PC, Pritchard S, Phillips G, Chan KW. Thalidomide in the management of chronic graft-versus-host disease in children following bone marrow transplantation. *Bone Marrow Transplant* 1994;14:937–942.
104. Saurat J-H, Camenzind M, Helg C, Chapuis B. Thalidomide for graft-versus-host disease after bone marrow transplantation. *Lancet* 1988;1:359.
105. Heney D, Lewis IJ, Bailey CC. Thalidomide for chronic graft-versus-host disease in children. *Lancet* 1988;2:1317.
106. Heney D, Norfolk DR, Wheeldon J, Bailey CC, Lewis IJ Barnard DL. Thalidomide treatment for chronic graft-versus-host disease. *Br J Haematol* 1991;78:23-27.
107. Parker PM, Chao N, Nademanee A, et al. Thalidomide as salvage therapy for chronic graft-versus-host disease. *Blood* 1995;86:3604–3609.
108. Rovelli A, Arrigo C, Nesi F, et al. The role of thalidomide in the treatment of refractory chronic graft-versus-host disease following bone marrow transplantation in children. *Bone Marrow Transplant* 1998;21:577–581.
109. Browne PV, Weisdorf DJ, DeFor T, et al. Response to thalidomide therapy in refractory chonic graft-versus-host disease. *Bone Marrow Transplant* 2000:26:865–869.
110. van de Poel MH, Pasman PC, Schouten HC. The use of thalidomide in chronic refractory graft versus host disease. *Neth J Med* 2001;59:45–49.
111. Gilman AL, Chan KW, Mogul A, et al. Hydroxychloroquine for the treatment of chronic graft-versus-host disease. *Biol Blood Marrow Transplant* 2000:6:327–334.
112. Hiraoka AF for the Japanese FK506 BMT Study Group. Results of a phase III study on prophylactic use of FK506 for acute GVHD compared with cyclosporine in allogeneic bone marrow transplantation. *Blood* 1997;90:561a.
113. Ratanatharathorn V, Nash RA, Przepiorka D, et al. Phase III study comparing methotrexate and tacrolimus (Prograf, FK506) with methotrexate and cyclosporine for graft-versus-host disease prophylaxis after HLA-identical sibling bone marrow transplantation. *Blood* 1998;92:2303–2314.
114. Nash RA, Antin JH, Karanes C, et al. A phase III study comparing methotrexate and tacrolimus with methotrexate and cyclosporine for prophylaxis of acute graft-versus-host disease after marrow transplantation from unrelated donors. *Blood* 2000;96:2062–2068.
115. Przepiorka D. Prevention of acute graft-versus-host disease. In: Ball ED, Lister J, Law P, eds. *Hematopoietic Stem Cell Therapy*. Churchill Livingstone, Philadelphia, PA, 2000, pp. 452–469.
116. Przepiorka D, Devine SM, Fay JW, Uberti JP, Wingard JR. Practical considerations in the use of tacrolimus for allogeneic marrow transplantation. *Bone Marrow Transplant* 1999;24:1053–1056.
117. Narwani RR, Reddy V, Wingard JR, et al. Topical tacrolimus may be useful for skin manifestations of acute and chronic graft-versus-host disease (GVHD) after bone marrow transplantation (BMT). *Blood* 1999;94(Suppl 1):370b.
118. Carnevale-Schianca F, Martin P, Sullivan K, et al. Changing from cyclosporine to tacrolimus as salvage therapy for chronic graft-versus-host disease. *Biol Blood Marrow Transplant* 2000;6:613–620.
119. Yu C, Seidel K, Nash RA, et al. Synergism between mycophenolate mofetil and cyclosporine in preventing greaft-versus-host disease among lethally irradiated dogs given DLA-nonidentical unrelated marrow grafts. *Blood* 1998;91:2581–2587.
120. Jenke A, Renner U, Richte M, et al. Pharmacokinetics of intravenous mycophenolate mofetil after allogeneic blood stem cell transplantation. *Clin Transplant* 2001;15:176–184.
121. Kiehl MG, Shipkova M, Basara N, et al. Mycophenolate mofetil in stem cell transplant patients in relation to plasma level of active metabolite. *Clin Biochem* 2000;33:203–208.
122. Anasetti C, Hansen JA, Waldmann TA, et al. Treatment of acute graft-versus-host disease with humanized anti-Tac: an antibody that binds to the interleukin-2 receptor. *Blood* 1994;84:1320–1327.
123. Anasetti C, Lin A, Nademanee A, et al. A Phase II/III randomized, double-blind, placebo-controlled multicenter trial of humanized anti-Tac for prevention of acute graft-versus-host disease (GVHD) in recipients of marrow transplants from unrelated donors. *Blood* 1995;86(Suppl 1):621a.
124. Gilleece MH, Dexter TM. Effect of Campath-1H antibody on human hematopoietic progenitors in vitro. *Blood* 1993;82:807–812.
125. Chakrabarti S, Kottaridis P, Ogormon P, et al. High incidence of early and late CMV infection and delayed immune reconstitution after allogeneic transplants with nonmyeloablative conditioning using Campath (anti-CD52 antibody). *Blood* 2000;96:586a.
126. Raefsky EL, Gascon P, Gratwohl A, et al. Biological and immunological characterization of ATG and ALG. *Blood* 1986;68:712-719.
127. Bourdage JS, Hamlin DM. Comparative polyclonal antithymocyte globulin and antilymphocyte/antilymphoblast globulin anti-CD antigen analysis by flow cytometry. *Transplantation* 1995;59:1194–1200.

128. Ourahma S, Talon D, Barrou B, et al. A prospective study on efficacy and tolerance of antithymocyte globulin Fresenius versus thymoglobuline Merieux after renal transplantation. *Transplant Proc* 1997;29:2427.

129. Norrby J, Olausson M. A randomized clinical trial using ATG Fresenius or ATG Merieux as induction therapy in kidney transplantation. *Transplant Proc* 1997;29:3135–3136.

130. Gaber AO, First MR, Tesi RJ, et al. Results of the double-blind, randomized, multicenter, Phase III clinical trial of thymoglobulin versus Atgam in the treatment of acute graft rejection episodes after renal transplantation. *Transplantation* 1998;66:29–37.

131. Baurmann H, Revillard JP, Bonnefoy-Berard N, Schwerdtfeger R. Potent effects of ATG used as part of the conditioning in matched unrealted donor (MUD) transplantation. *Blood* 1998;92(Suppl 1):290a.

132. Eiermann TH, Freitag S, Cortes-Dericks L, Sahm H, Zander AR. Jurkat cell-reactive anti-thymocyte globulin assessed ex vivo by flow cytomtery persists three weeks in ciruclation. *J Hematother Stem Cell Res* 2001;10:395–390.

133. Toren A, Ilan Y, Or R, Kapelushnik J, Nagler A. Impaired liver function tests in patients treated with antithymocyte globulin: implication for liver transplantation. *Med Oncol* 1997;14:125–129.

134. Remberger M, Svahn B-M, Hentschke P, Lôfgren C, Ringden O. Effect on cytokine release and graft-versus-host disease of different anti-T cell antibodies during conditioning for unrelated haematopoietic stem cell transplantation. *Bone Marrow Transplant* 1999;24:823–830.

135. Storb R, Etzioni R, Anasetti C, et al. Cyclophophamide combined with antithymocyte globulin in preparation for allogeneic marrow transplants in patients with aplastic anemia. *Blood* 1994;84:941–949.

136. Holler E, Ledderose G, Knabe H, et al. ATG serotherapy during pretransplant conditioning in unrelated donor BMT: dose dependent modulation of GVHD. *Bone Marrow Transplant* 1998;21(Suppl 1):S30.

137. Kanda Y, Mineishi S, Nakai K, Saito T, Tanosaki R, Takue Y. Frequent detection of rising cytomegalovirus antigenemia after allogeneic stem cell transplantation following a regimen containing antithymocyte globulin. *Blood* 2001;97:3676,3677.

138. Kroger N, Zabelina T, Kruger W, et al. Patient cytomegalovirus seropositivity with or without reactivation is the most important prognostic factor for survival and treatment-related mortality in stem cell transplantation from unrelated donors using pretransplant in vivo T-cell depletion with anti-thymocyte globulin. *Br J Haematol* 2001;113:1060–1071.

139. Hsu B, May R, Carrum G, Krance R, Przepiorka D. Use of antithymocyte globulin for treatment of acute graft-versus-host disease: an international practice survey. *Bone Marrow Transplant* 2001;10:945–950.

140. Boughton BJ, Sheehan TM, Wood J, et al. High-performance liquid chromatography assay of plasma thalidomide: stabilization of specimens and determination of a tentative therapeutic range for chronic graft-versus-host disease. *Ann Clin Biochem* 1995;32:79–83.

141. Schlossberg H, Klumpp T, Sabol P, Herman J, Mangan K. Severe cutaneous ulceration following treatment with thalidomide for GVHD. *Bone Marrow Transplant* 2001;27:229,230.

142. Chao NJ, Parker PM, Niland JC, et al. Paradoxical effect of thalidomide prophylaxis on chronic graft-vs-host disease. *Biol Blood Marrow Transplant* 1996;2:86–92.

17 Posttransplant EBV-Associated Disease

Thomas G. Gross, MD, PhD and Brett J. Loechelt, MD

CONTENTS

EBV AND PTLD
PTLD CLASSIFICATION
RISK FACTORS
TREATMENT
SUMMARY
REFERENCES

1. EBV AND PTLD

Epstein-Barr virus (EBV) is a ubiquitous virus in humans and is carried as a latent asymptomatic infection for the lifetime of infected individuals. Figure 1, illustrates the delicate balance between the host T cell immune response and control of B cell proliferation of latently infected B cells. In a healthy individual, while only 10^{-5}–10^{-6} B-cells are latently infected with EBV, approx 1–5% of all circulating CD8$^+$ T cells are capable of reacting against EBV, illustrating the importance of a qualitatively and quantitatively appropriate T cell response in maintaining homeostasis and preventing B cell proliferation (1–4). Following blood and bone marrow transplant (BMT), EBV transmission is usually from the stem cell graft. It has been shown that the cytoreductive preparative regimen can eliminate the host EBV latent infection, and, in the vast majority of cases of posttransplant lymphoproliferative disease (PTLD) following BMT, the B cells and virus are of donor origin (5–8). Therefore, the development of PTLD is not surprising following BMT, with the intensive immunosuppressive–immunoablative preparative therapy and infusion of EBV infected B cells.

2. PTLD CLASSIFICATION

Complications of EBV infection following BMT cover a spectrum of clinical and morphological lymphoid proliferations (Table 1) (5–7,9–12). Frequently, the definition of PTLD is limited to lymphomatous masses, which are usually multifocal and extranodal. But EBV infection can also present as an infectious mononucleosis-like disease, hepatitis, meningoencephalitis, and lymphocytic interstitial pneumonitis. EBV disease post-BMT may also present as a systemic disease that is often misdiagnosed as sepsis or severe graft-vs-host disease (GVHD) and found only postmortem (7,9,10). Infiltration of organs by polyclonal B cells and T cells, frequently with histiocytes and hemophagocytosis, is observed. This presentation

From: *Current Clinical Oncology: Allogeneic Stem Cell Transplantation*
Edited by: Mary S. Laughlin and Hillard M. Lazarus © Humana Press Inc., Totowa, NJ

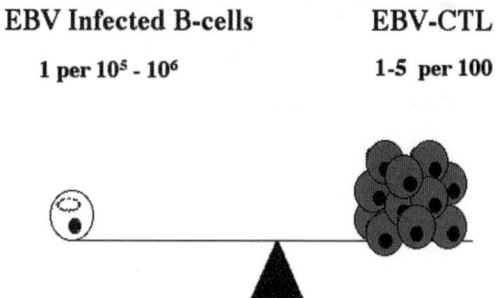

Fig. 1. T cell response required to maintain control of EBV-driven B cell proliferation in an immuno-competent host.

Table 1
Manifestation of EBV Disease Post-BMT

• Asymptomatic infection
• Infectious mononucleosis
    Typical
    Fulminant, severe
• EBV hepatitis
• Lymphocytic interstitial pneumonitis
• Meningoencephalitis
• PTLD

resembles fulminant infectious mononucleosis and is usually rapidly progressive and fatal *(9,13,14)*.

Almost all PTLD is CD20+ and EBV early RNAs (EBER) positive by *in situ* hybridization, whereas immunohistochemistry staining for the LMP-1 protein can be negative in up to 25% of cases *(6,9,15)*. There have been several histologic classifications for PTLD over the years, but the World Health Organization (WHO) has now proposed a classification which includes: (i) polymorphic hyperplasia; (ii) polymorphic PTLD; and (iii) monomorphic PTLD *(16)*.

Polymorphic hyperplasia consists of a mixture of B-cells and infiltrating T cells; whereas, monomorphic PTLD resembles intermediate-to-high grade non-Hodgkin's lymphoma (NHL) *(16)*. Distinguishing polymorphic from monomorphic PTLD can be difficult, and both may be seen in the same patient or even the same lesion. Polymorphic and monomorphic disease can be either polyclonal or monoclonal *(16)*. Determining clonality can be difficult without receptor gene analysis, because up to 50% of PTLD do not express surface immunoglobulin *(6,9)*. Though debated heavily, it has been difficult to demonstrate the prognostic value of morphology and clonality in PTLD, especially following BMT *(6,9,17)*.

3. RISK FACTORS

The risk factors for developing PTLD are well known and are shown in Table 2. Factors that either stimulate B-cell proliferation and/or decrease or delay T-cell immunity will increase the risk of PTLD. PTLD rarely occurs within 30 d of BMT, and the peak incidence is in the third month *(10,18)*. This may represent the time it takes to develop a "critical mass" of proliferating EBV-infected B cells, before development of EBV T cell immunity. Immunity against EBV is one of the first signs of T cell reconstitution. It is common to see cytolytic T lymphocyte (CTL) activity against an EBV lymphoblastoid cell line before a proliferative response to mitogenic stimulation post-BMT (personal observation).

Table 2
Risk Factors for Developing PTLD Following BMT

Risk factor	Relative risk of PTLD (2,8)
Donor sources	
• Allogeneic	
• ≤1 HLA-Ag mismatched related donor	1.0
• >2 HLA-Ag mismatched related	1.5–3.7
• Unrelated marrow donor	3.5
• Unrelated cord blood	1.0 (21)
• Recipient age	1.0
• Donor age	1.04[a]
Preparative regimen	
• TBI, vs no TBI	2.9
Graft manipulation	
• TCD vs no TCD	5.4–9.1
TCD methods	
• CAMPATH-1	2.0
• Elutriation	2.6
• Lectins	4.1
• Anti-T cell MoAb	12.3
• SRBC rosetting	15.6
Immunosuppression	
• ATG/ALG for GVHD prophylaxis or treatment	5.5
• Anti-CD3 MoAb for treatment of GVHD	35.9
Effect of multiple risk factors	
• HLA-mismatched and TCD marrow	15.7
Factors	
• T cell-specific TCD (anti-T cell MoAb or SRBC rosetting)	
• HLA-mismatched (≥2 Ag)	
• Use of ATG/ALG	
• Use of anti-T cell MoAb	
• 2 Factors	8.0
• 3 to 4 Factors 22.3	

Ag, antigen; TBI, total body irradiation; MoAb, monoclonal antibodies; SRBC, sheep red blood cell; ATG, anti-T cell globulin; ALG, antilymphocyte globulin; GVHD, graft-vs-host disease.
[a]Continuous variable.

3.1. Donor Sources

PTLD is rare following autologous BMT, probably because recipients have adequate EBV-CTL recovery by 3 mo (10,19). However, with the advent of more immunosuppressive preparative regimens, especially in autologous BMT for autoimmune disease, PTLD may become more common (20). The incidence of PTLD is low (approx 1%) following BMT with matched related donors (MRD) (10,18). It is not known if the use of cytokine-mobilized peripheral blood stem cell (PBSC) grafts affects the risk of PTLD, but detection of EBV-CTL activity has been detected as early as 30 d posttransplant using PBSC (21). The incidence of PTLD is higher in unrelated donor BMT (10,18). Human leukocyte antigen (HLA) disparity between donor and recipient has repeatedly been shown to be a risk factor for PTLD and may account for the increase incidence of PTLD in unrelated donor BMT. It has been hypothesized that HLA mismatching provides a chronic B cell proliferative stimulus, though delayed EBV-CTL recovery may also play a role (5,21).

Since cord blood does not contain EBV-infected B cells, it was felt PTLD would not occur. However, recent reports show that PTLD does occur following cord blood transplant (CBT), and the incidence is similar to matched related marrow transplant without T cell depletion (TCD) *(22,23)*. If the host latent EBV infection is eradicated by the cytoreductive preparative regimens, then the likely transmission of EBV following CBT is via the natural (oral) route, though blood transfusion cannot be ruled out *(24)*. One may expect the outcome of PTLD in the setting of an EBV naïve donor to be worse, since generation of EBV-CTL is less effective, as opposed to expansion of memory EBV-CTL acquired from an EBV seropositive donor *(21)*. However, there are no data to evaluate the effect of receiving a graft from an EBV naïve donor on the risk or outcome of PTLD. Interestingly, it has been demonstrated that the risk of PTLD increases with donor age, and it has been speculated this is due to fewer or less effective memory EBV-CTL with increasing age *(10)*.

3.2. Immunosuppression

TCD has long been known to significantly increase the risk of PTLD *(5,10,18,25)*. This risk is compounded by HLA mismatching *(10,18)*. It has been demonstrated that TCD methods that specifically remove T cells, e.g., sheep red blood cell (SRBC) rosetting and use of anti-T cell monoclonal antibodies, confer a higher risk of PTLD, than methods that "pan-lymphocyte" deplete the stem cell graft, e.g., CAMPATH-1 monoclonal antibodies or elutriation *(18)*. Since pan-lymphocyte depletion methods decrease the number of EBV-infected B cells as well as T cells, this may delay B cell proliferation from achieving a critical mass until EBV-CTL function recovers *(18,26)*. Though there are no reported data, one would predict that with CD34 positive selection, the incidence of PTLD to be similar to other pan-lymphocyte depletion methods.

Several analyses have shown that anti-T cell antibodies, especially monoclonal antibodies, used to treat GVHD greatly increases the risk of PTLD *(10,18,27,28)*. The increased risk of PTLD using anti-T cell monoclonal antibodies vs polyclonal preparations, i.e., antithymocyte globulin (ATG) or antilymphocyte globulin (ALG), is felt to be due to the increased efficacy in depleting EBV-CTL as well as alloreactive T cells. Data from the solid organ transplant experience suggest that anti-T cell antibodies are the most potent suppressants of EBV-CTL activity, followed by T cell activation inhibitors, i.e., cyclosporin and tacrolimus, while corticosteroids and chemotherapeutic agents, i.e. azathioprine, mycophenolate mofetil, methotrexate, or cyclophosphamide, are much less potent *(29)*. Unfortunately, the latter group has marrow-suppressive effects.

Differences in preparative regimens may increase the risk for PTLD. Total body irradiation (TBI) increases the risk of secondary malignancies and perhaps PTLD *(18,27,28)*. PTLD has been reported with nonmyeloablative preparative regimens *(30)*. Many of these nonmyeloablative regimens are very immunosuppressive and delayed EBV-CTL immunity would be expected. Of interest, PTLD reported following nonmyeloablative regimens appears to develop quite early, i.e., 20–30 d after transplant, raising the question of origin of B cells in these PTLD. It is conceivable that these nonmyeloablative regimens may ablate recipient EBV-CTL, but not recipient EBV-infected B cells.

3.3. Underlying Disease

Finally, several reports have found BMT for immunodeficiency to be a risk factor for PTLD *(10,27)*. Since haploidentical TCD grafts are commonly used for these patients, it is difficult to assess the risk of the underlying disease. These patients are at high risk for developing EBV-associated B cell lymphoproliferative disease without BMT due to their underlying disorder, and a number of patients have developed PTLD following failure to achieve donor engraftment *(10)*.

4. TREATMENT

The mortality of PTLD post-BMT historically has been dismal (> 90%) *(10,31)*. Successful treatment of PTLD necessitates controlling the B cell proliferation and facilitating the development of an appropriate memory cytotoxic T cell (EBV-CTL) response to maintain homeostasis. Additional factors that contribute to the difficulty of treating these patients include increased toxicity from therapy and/or secondary infections and enhancement of alloreactive T cell immunity, thus placing the patient at risk for developing GVHD. Treatment options for PTLD after BMT are shown in Table 3.

4.1. Reduction of Immunosuppression

The first step in treating PTLD is usually reducing immunosuppression. In instances that this can be done, it should be attempted, though this is rarely successful. As opposed to PTLD following solid organ transplantation where lack of EBV-CTL function is usually qualitative, with PTLD following BMT the defect in EBV-CTL function is quantitative. In patients with concurrent GVHD, or when PTLD develops following intensive immunosuppression to treat GVHD, this approach is especially problematic.

4.2. Antiviral Therapy

There is little evidence to demonstrate efficacy of specific antiviral agents, such as acyclovir or ganciclovir, in preventing PTLD since the majority of patients develop PTLD while receiving these agents *(10,17)*. Though antiviral therapy has been reported to be successful in treating some cases of infectious mononucleosis-like disease or meningoencephalitis, the efficacy is controversial, since it is used in conjunction with other potential effective treatments, i.e., reduction of immunosuppression, interferon (IFN)-α, etc. *(10–12,17)*. Because there is little risk of toxicity, antiviral therapy is usually included as part of the treatment. Theoretically, if viral replication, which is lytic to the infected B cells, is inhibited, B cell proliferation could be enhanced and/or recovery of EBV-CTL immunity hindered.

4.3. Local Therapy

Surgical resection and/or radiotherapy can be very effective for localized PTLD, but this is rarely observed following BMT *(5,6,10)*.

4.4. IFN-α

There are numerous anecdotal reports using IFN to treat PTLD. The only published series demonstrated that four out of seven patients had a response to IFN *(10)*. The beneficial effect of IFN in treating PTLD has not been delineated. IFN may have antiviral activity, anti-B cell proliferative activity, and/or T cell-enhancing effects. It has been shown that patients with PTLD demonstrate an imbalance of cytokines in their serum: increased levels of interleukin (IL)-4 (B cell proliferative stimulus) and relatively decreased, or undetectable levels of IFN, compared to healthy EBV seropositive controls *(32)*. Thus, IFN might restore cytokine balance, modifying the milieu that favors proliferation of EBV-transformed B cells. There is a theoretical risk of increasing GVHD with IFN, though this has not been demonstrated. IFN can also be marrow-suppressive, thereby increasing the risk of secondary infection.

4.5. Monoclonal Antibodies

Anti-B cell antibodies have been used successfully to treat PTLD *(33–36)*. Obviously, this approach is directed at decreasing B cell proliferation, and though EBV-CTL development is not directly enhanced, it is not inhibited. The first report used anti-CD21 and anti-CD24 and

Table 3
Treatment for PTLD Post-BMT

Prophylactic therapies
  • Adoptive cellular therapy
    • DLI: mixed results
    • EBV-specific CTL: very effective, costly, and impractical for most centers
  • B cell depletion of stem cell graft: partially effective
Preemptive therapies
  • Monoclonal antibodies (anit-CD20): early results promising
  • GM-CSF: early results promising
Treatment therapies
  • Reduction of immunosuppression: rarely effective
  • Surgical resection/radiation: rarely applicable
  • IFN-α: occasionally effective, potential toxicities
  • Adoptive cellular therapy
    • DLI: mixed results
    • EBV-specific CTL: very effective, costly, and impractical for most centers
  • Monoclonal antibodies (anti-CD20): often effective, relapses occur
  • Chemotherapy: effective, but toxic

showed this to be well tolerated with 35% of the patients achieving long-term disease-free survival: 1 out of 11 patients with monoclonal PTLD and 7 out of 16 patients with polyclonal disease *(33)*. More recently, anti-CD20 or rituximab has been used. Early reports suggest that approx 50% of patients can achieve a complete remission (CR) *(34,35)*. But relapses and severe pulmonary toxicity have been observed *(35)*. Immunoglobulin production may be suppressed for months following rituximab, potentially requiring intravenous immunoglobulin (IVIG) to prevent other infections. Therefore, more experience is required to determine the role of rituximab in treating PTLD following BMT. IL-6 is often elevated in patients with PTLD and is a B cell proliferative stimulus. A recent report in organ transplant patients demonstrated that anti-IL-6 monoclonal antibody therapy was well-tolerated and 8 out of 12 patients responded *(37)*.

4.6. Adoptive Cellular Therapy

Infusion of donor leukocytes (DLI) has been successful in the treatment of PTLD post-BMT *(38,39)*. However, severe GVHD and death due to a "shock-like syndrome" have been reported as complications, and progressive disease may also occur. One study reported that of seven patients treated with DLI, four patients died of progressive PTLD and 1 died of GVHD following CR *(39)*. To circumvent the GVHD problem, investigators have inserted a suicide gene, i.e., herpesvirus thymidine kinase, into donor lymphocytes, so that if GVHD occurs, it could be treated with ganciclovir *(40,41)*. Initial studies demonstrated success with this approach *(40)*. However, in a recent study, 12 patients received DLI containing suicide genes, such as PTLD prophylaxis, but three patients developed PTLD *(41)*. Ex vivo EBV-specific CTLs have been shown to be very effective as prophylaxis and treatment for PTLD without excessive GVHD *(42)*. However, one patient died of PTLD in spite of EBV-CTL therapy, because the in vivo strain of virus was not sensitive to the ex vivo-generated EBV-CTL *(43)*. These studies have provided proof of principle that if adequate EBV-CTL activity can be achieved, PTLD can be prevented and/or cured. However, adoptive cellular therapy with ex vivo-generated EBV-CTL is not cost-effective if used as prophylaxis, since 80–90% of patients will never develop PTLD. Since it requires 4–6 wk to generate EBV-CTL, this must be done in advance or therapy to control the PTLD would be needed until EBV-CTL could be available. Therefore, this approach is not feasible for most centers, due to the cost and regulatory oversight necessary to generate and administer the ex vivo-generated EBV-CTL.

4.7. Cytotoxic Chemotherapy

Chemotherapy has been used to treat resistant PTLD following solid organ transplant *(44,45)*. The attraction of chemotherapy is that it is immunosuppressive enough to control allograft rejection or GVHD, as well as treat PTLD. However, standard dose chemotherapy for treating NHL is too toxic for most posttransplant patients, especially BMT patients within 6 mo posttransplant, and may theoretically inhibit EBV-CTL development. We have had good results using low dose chemotherapy, i.e. cyclophosphamide (20 mg/kg) in solid organ transplant patients with PTLD *(46)*. Of interest, patients receiving the low dose chemotherapy developed normal EBV-CTL numbers (data not shown). Three patients with PTLD post-BMT have been treated with this approach, both patients were >6 mo post-BMT. One patient had no response, two patients achieved a CR, one patient remains alive and in CR, and the other patient died after several months of relapsed leukemia. A low dose chemotherapy approach may be useful in situations where PTLD occurs with GVHD, in patients that are longer post-BMT, or where donor stem cells are available should graft failure occur.

4.8. Prophylactic–Preemptive Therapy

Prevention–prophylaxis against infection and/or early detection of viral infection before clinical disease develops, i.e., preemptive therapy, has been very successful at reducing morbidity and mortality due to CMV posttransplant. As mentioned previously, the role of antiviral prophylaxis with acyclovir or ganciclovir is controversial *(10)*. Using methods that pan-lymphocyte deplete, may help reduce the risk of PTLD by reducing number of EBV-infected B cells infused with the stem cell graft *(10,26)*. Prophylaxis with EBV-CTL infusion is very effective, but not cost effective or feasible for most centers. Therefore, prevention/prophylaxis for PTLD remains problematic.

For preemptive therapy to be successful, one must have a method of reliably identifying patients who are at high risk before they develop disease. Since EBV cannot be cultured, polymerase chain reaction (PCR) of the blood is used to detect infection and/or reactivation and to quantitate EBV DNA in peripheral blood or serum, i.e., viral load. There are many reports that correlate increased viral load with PTLD *(39,41,42)*. However, there are no blinded prospective studies to determine the predictive value of quantitative EBV DNA PCR for the development of PTLD. One must be cautious in interpreting EBV viral load, since there is great variability between different methods and/or laboratories, thus necessitating the use of one laboratory in monitoring a particular patient. It is our experience that very high viral loads, i.e., >1000 copies of EBV DNA/μg DNA, correlate with PTLD in symptomatic patients, i.e., fever, fatigue, and/or adenopathy. In an asymptomatic patient, a single elevated level of EBV DNA appears to correlate poorly with development of PTLD, but persistently positive EBV PCR and especially persistent increases in viral load appear to be predictive for PTLD. Unfortunately, some patients develop PTLD without any detectable EBV DNA in the peripheral blood, or develop PTLD so rapidly that weekly screening has failed to identify patients early.

Investigators are now using anti-CD20 antibody (rituximab) as preemptive therapy *(34,36)*. The rationale is to reduce B cell proliferation until EBV-CTL activity recovers. This approach may also provide the time necessary to generate EBV-CTL in vitro. Early results are very promising, but the numbers are small and the follow-up is very short.

Another approach is to enhance EBV-CTL activity. Currently, EBV vaccination is impractical, since EBV-CTL responses are very HLA restricted, and vaccines would need to be individualized based on HLA typing. Others have used peptide-pulsed dendritic cells to gen-

Table 4
Effect of GM-CSF as Preemptive Therapy for PTLD

Days post-BMT	EBV copies	% EBV-CTL[a]	Symptoms
+50	0	0	—
+97[b]	12,200	0	+
+117	0	8	—
+180	0	10	—

[a]Normal percentage of EBV-CTL, 1–5%.
[b]GM-CSF was initiated.

erate EBV-CTL response posttransplant *(47)*. Again, early results look promising, but this is currently impractical for most centers due to cost, technology needs and the ability to deal with regulatory oversight issues.

In an attempt to stimulate EBV-CTL recovery in vivo, we have used granulocyte-macrophage colony-stimulating factor (GM-CSF) as preemptive therapy *(48)*. GM-CSF can augment a primary immune CTL response to a neoantigen and has been used as a vaccine adjuvant to enhance T cell responses against viruses and cancer, presumably by enhancing antigen presentation *(49)*. A phase I trial of using GM-CSF in 14 BMT patients demonstrated that GM-CSF was well-tolerated with no increase in GVHD *(50)*. Subsequently, five patients, all TCD, matched unrelated donor marrow recipients, were treated with GM-CSF (250 µg/m^2 subcutaneously 3×/wk) when they became EBV PCR positive and had symptoms of EBV infection—i.e., fever, fatigue, nausea and/or vomiting—with no other identifiable etiology. The median time following GM-CSF to resolution of all symptoms was 15 d (7–20 d), and to EBV PCR negativity 20 d (7–32 d). Four patients remain free of symptoms or PTLD. One patient, after GM-CSF was discontinued, developed grade IV GVHD requiring increased immunosuppression including ATG, and subsequently developed PTLD. One patient (*see* Table 4) had EBV-CTL quantitated using multiparametric flow cytometry *(51)*. This patient developed symptoms on d 96 and was treated with GM-CSF. In 3 wk, the patient had resolved all clinical symptoms, the viral load was zero and normal numbers of EBV-CTL were detected. These preliminary results are encouraging and suggest that GM-CSF may be an effective preemptive therapy for post-BMT EBV disease.

5. SUMMARY

EBV-associated disease continues to be problematic following BMT. EBV is such a potent stimulus for B cell proliferation that an immunocompetent host has 3–4 logs more EBV-CTL than latently infected B-cells to maintain homeostasis. Therefore, factors associated with BMT that perturb this balance place patients at risk for developing EBV associated PTLD. The incidence of PTLD is expected to increase with the uses of more alternative donor transplants and more immunosuppressive preparative regimens. The outcome of PTLD has been dismal in the past. Therefore, novel approaches to prevent and treat PTLD are needed. Success depends on the development of nontoxic therapies that reduce B cell proliferation and enhance EBV-CTL recovery post-BMT. Such therapies would ideally be not only effective but affordable and available to all patients. A problem in the treatment of PTLD is the relative rarity of the disorder, so only phase I or phase II pilot studies have been performed. To truly evaluate efficacy of therapies, larger multicenter prospective phase II or phase III studies would be of great benefit.

REFERENCES

1. Tan LC, Gudgeon N, Annels NE, et al. A re-evaluation of the frequency of CD8+ T cells specific for EBV in healthy carriers. *J Immunol* 1999;162:1827–1835.

2. Yang J, Lemas VM, Flinn IW, Krone C, Ambinder RF. Application of the ELISPOT assay to the characterization of CD8⁺ responses to Epstein-Barr virus antigens. *Blood* 2000;95:241–248.

3. Kuzushima K, Hoshino Y, Fujii K, et al. Rapid determination of Epstein-Barr virus-specific CD8⁺ T-cell frequencies by flow cytometry. *Blood* 1999;94:3094–3100.

4. Yang J, Tao Q, Flinn IW, et al. Characterization of Epstein-Barr virus-infected B cells in patients with posttransplantation lymphoproliferative disease: disappearance after rituximab therapy does not predict clinical response. *Blood* 2000;96:4055–4063.

5. Shapiro RS, McClain K, Frizzera G, et al. Epstein-Barr virus associated B cell lymphoproliferative disorders following bone marrow transplantation. *Blood* 1988;71:1234–1243.

6. Swerdlow SH. Post-transplant lymphoproliferative disorders: a morphologic, phenotypic and genotypic spectrum of disease. *Histopathology* 1992;20:373–385.

7. Lones MA, Lopez-Terrada D, Shintaku P, et al. Posttransplant lymphoproliferative disorder in pediatric bone marrow transplant recipients: disseminated disease of donor origin demonstrated by in situ hybridization. *Arch Pathol Lab Med* 1998; 22:708–714.

8. Gratama JW, Oosterveer MA, Zwaan FE, et al. Eradication of Epstein-Barr virus by allogeneic bone marrow transplantation: implication for sites of viral latency. *Proc Natl Acad Sci USA* 1988:85:8693–8696.

9. Greiner TC, Gross TG. Atypical immune lymphoproliferations. In: Hoffman (eds). *Hematology: Basic Principles and Practice*, 3ʳᵈ ed., WB Saunders, Philadelphia, PA, 2000.

10. Gross TG, Steinbuch M, DeFor T, et al. B cell lymphoproliferative disorder following hematopoietic stem cell transplantation: risk factors, treatment and outcome. *Bone Marrow Transplant* 1999;23:251–258.

11. Dellemijn PLI, Brandenburg A, Niesters HGM, et al. Successful treatment with ganciclovir of presumed Epstein-Barr meningo-encephalitis following bone marrow transplant. *Bone Marrow Transplant* 1995;16:311.312.

12. Davis KR, Hinrichs SH, Fidler JL, et al. Post-transplant Epstein-Barr virus associated meningoencephalitis and lymphoid interstitial pneumonitis. *Bone Marrow Transplant* 1999;24:443,444.

13. Okano M, Gross TG. Epstein-Barr virus-associated hemophagocytic syndrome and fatal infectious mononucleosis. *Am J Hematol* 1996;53:111–115.

14. Quintanilla-Martinez L, Kumar S, Fend F, Ret al. Fulminant EBV⁺ T-cell lymphoproliferative disorder following acute/chronic EBV infection: a distinct clinicopathologic syndrome. *Blood* 2000;96:443–451.

15. Dhir RK, Nalesnik MA, Demetris AJ, Randhawa PS. Latent membrane protein expression in posttransplant lymphoproliferative disease. *Appl Immunohistochem* 1995;3:123.

16. Harris NL, Jaffe ES, Diebold J, et al. World Health Organization classification of neoplastic diseases of the hematopoietic and lymphoid tissues: report of the clinical advisory committee meeting-Airlie House, Virginia, November 1997. *J Clin Oncol* 1999;17:3835–3849.

17. Cohen JI : Epstein-Barr virus lymphoproliferative disease associated with acquired immune deficiency. *Medicine* 1991;70:137–160.

18. Curtis RE, Travis LB, Rowlings PA, et al. Risk of lymphoproliferative disorders after bone marrow transplantation: a multi-institutional study. *Blood* 1999;94:2208–2216.

19. Hauke RJ, Greiner TC, Smir BN, et al. Epstein-Barr virus-associated lymphoproliferative disorder after autologous bone marrow transplantation; report of two cases. *Bone Marrow Transplant* 1998;21:1271–1274.

20. Nash RA, Dansey R, Storek J, et al. Epstein-Barr virus lymphoproliferative disorder (PTLD) after high-dose immunosuppressive therapy (HDIT) and autologous CD-34 selected stem cell transplantation (SCT) for severe autoimmune diseases. *Blood* 2000;96:406a.

21. Marshall NA, Howe JG, Formica R, et al. Rapid reconstitution of Epstein-Barr virus-specific T lymphocytes following allogeneic stem cell transplantation. *Blood* 2000;96:2814–2821.

22. Snowden JA, Nivison-Smith I, Atkinson K, et al. First report of Epstein-Barr virus lymphoproliferative disease after cord blood transplantation. *Bone Marrow Transplant* 2000;25:120,121.

23. Barker JN, Martin PL, Defor T, et al. Low incidence of Epstein-Barr virus-associated post-transplant lymphoproliferative disorders (EBV-PTLD) in 263 unrelated donor cord blood transplant recipients. *Blood* 2000;96:206a.

24. Alfieri C, Tanner J, Carpentier L, et al. Epstein-Barr virus transmission from a blood donor to an organ transplant recipient with recovery of the same virus strain from the recipient's blood and oropharynx. *Blood* 1996;87:812–817.

25. Lucas KG, Small TN, Heller G, et al. The development of cellular immunity to Epstein-Barr virus after allogeneic bone marrow transplantation. *Blood* 1996;87:2594–2603.

26. Gross TG, Hinrichs SH, Davis JR, et al. Effect of counterflow elutriation (CE) on Epstein-Barr virus (EBV) infected cells in donor bone marrow. *Exp Hematol* 1998;26:395–399.

27. Bhatia S, Ramsay NKC, Steinbuch M, et al. Malignant neoplasms following bone marrow transplantation. *Blood* 1996;87:3633–3639.

28. Witherspoon RP, Fisher LD, Schoch G, et al. Secondary cancers after bone marrow transplantation for leukemia or aplastic anemia. *N Engl J Med* 1989;784–789.

29. Penn I. The role of immunosuppression in lymphoma formation. *Springer Semin Immunopathol* 1998;20:343–355.
30. Milpied N, Coste-Burel M, Accard F, et al. Epstein-Barr virus-associated B call lymphoproliferative disease after non-myeloablative allogeneic stem cell transplantation. *Bone Marrow Transplant* 1999;23:629,630.
31. Zutter MM, Martin PJ, Sale GE, et al. Epstein-Barr virus lymphoproliferation after bone marrow transplantation. *Blood* 1988;72:520–529.
32. Mathur A, Kamat DM, Filipovich AH, et al. Immunoregulatory abnormalities in patients with Epstein-Barr virus-associated B cell lymphoproliferative disorders. *Transplantation* 1994;57:1042–1045.
33. Benkerrou M, Jais J-P, Leblond V, et al. Anti-B-cell monoclonal antibody treatment of severe post-transplant B-lymphocyte disorder: prognostic factors and long-term outcome. *Blood* 1998;92:3137–3147.
34. Milpied N, Vasseur B, Parquet N, et al. Humanized anti-CD20 monoclonal antibody (Rituximab) in post transplant B-lymphoproliferative disorder: a retrospective analysis on 32 patients. *Ann Oncol* 2000;11:113–116.
35. George D, Small TN, Boulad F, et al. Rituximab for the treatment of Epstein-Barr virus associated lymphoproliferative disorders. *Blood* 2000;96:405a.
36. Kuehnle I, Huls MH, Liu Z, et al. CD20 monoclonal antibody (rituximab) for therapy of Epstein-Barr virus lymphoma after hemopoietic stem-cell transplantation. *Blood* 2000;95:1502–1505.
37. Haddad E, Paczesny S, Leblond V, et al. Treatment of B-lymphoproliferative disorder with a monoclonal anti-interleukin-6 antibody in 12 patients: a multicenter phase 1-2 trial. *Blood* 2001;97:1590–1597.
38. Papadopoulos EB, Ladanyi M, Emanuel D, et al. Infusions of donor leukocytes to treat Epstein-Barr virus-associated lymphoproliferative disorders after allogeneic bone marrow transplantation. *N Engl J Med* 1994;330:1185–1191.
39. Lucas KG, Burton RL, Zimmerman SE, et al. Semiquantitative Epstein-Barr virus (EBV) polymerase chain reaction for determination of patients at risk for EBV-induced lymphoproliferative disease after stem cell transplantation. *Blood* 1998;91:3654–3661.
40. Bonini, C Ferrari G, Verzeletti S,et al. HSV-TK gene transfer into donor lymphocytes for control of allogeneic graft-versus-leukemia. *Science* 1997;276:1719–1724.
41. Tiberghien P, Ferrand C, Lioure B, et al. Administration of herpes simplex-thymidine kinase-expressing donor T-cells with a T-cell-depleted allogeneic marrow graft. *Blood* 2001;97:63–72.
42. Rooney CM, Smith CA, Ng CYC, et al. Infusion of cytotoxic T cells for the prevention and treatment of Epstein-Barr virus-induced lymphoma in allogeneic transplant recipients. *Blood* 1998;92:1549–1555.
43. Gottschalk S, Ng CYC, Perez M, et al. An Epstein-Barr virus deletion mutant associated with fatal lymphoproliferative disease unresponsive to therapy with virus-specific CTLs. *Blood* 2001;97:835–843.
44. Swinnen LJ, Mullen GM, Carr TJ, et al. Aggressive treatment for postcardiac lymphoproliferation. *Blood* 1995;86:3333–3340.
45. Gross TG, Hinrichs SH, Winner J, et al. Treatment of post-transplant lymphoproliferative disease (PTLD) following solid organ transplantation with low dose chemotherapy. *Ann Oncol* 1998;9:339,340.
46. Rooney CM, Loftin S, Holladay MS, et al. Early identification of Epstein-Barr virus-associated post-transplantation lymphoproliferative disease. *Br J Haematol* 1995;89:98–103.
47. Herr W, Ranieri E, Olson W, et al. Mature dendritic cells pulsed with freeze-thaw cell lysates define an effective in vitro vaccine to elicit EBV-specific CD4+ and CD8+ T lymphocyte response. *Blood* 2000;96:1857–1864.
48. Loechelt BJ, Witte DP, Vergamini S, et al. GM-CSF as pre-emptive therapy for post-transplant EBV disease. *Biol Blood Marrow Transplant* 2001;7:80.
49. Armitage JO. Emerging applications of recombinant human granulocyte-macrophage colony-stimulating factor. *Blood* 1998;92:4491–4508.
50. Grimley MS, Lee S, Villaneuva J, et al. Phase I trial of late GM-CSF to promote reconstitution of cell-mediated immunity in pediatric recipients of alternative donor (AD) stem cell transplant (SCT). *Blood* 1999;94:386b.
51. Kuzushima K, Hoshino Y, Yokoyama N, et al. Rapid determination of Epstein-Barr virus-specific CD8+ T-cell frequencies by flow cytometry. *Blood* 1999;94:3094–3100.

V

PREVENTION AND MANAGEMENT OF RELAPSE AFTER ALLOGENEIC TRANSPLANTATION

18 Allogeneic Antitumor Vaccine Strategies

Ginna G. Laport and Carl H. June

CONTENTS

1. INTRODUCTION

The tumor immunosurveillance theory, proposed over 30 yr ago as a cellular immune process to protect against the development of cancer (1), was largely abandoned because most cancers develop in the setting of a normal immune system. However, recently the concept was resurrected when it was demonstrated that lymphocytes and interferon γ collaborate to protect against development of carcinogen-induced sarcomas and spontaneous epithelial carcinomas (2). In addition, it was demonstrated that the immune system selects for cancers with reduced immunogenicity. Therefore, the immune system may function as a tumor-suppressor, and paradoxically, selects for tumors that are more capable of surviving in an immunocompetent host.

Studies during the last decade of the past century documented that the failure of the human immune system to reject tumors was not related to the absence of tumor-associated antigens. Therefore, the realization that human cancers can be responsive to the manipulation of the immune system has only recently been documented. The immune approaches to the treatment of malignancy can be broadly classified into either active or passive immunotherapies. Active or vaccine immunotherapy relies on the stimulation of the host immune system to react against tumors following the administration of biological response-modifying agents and tumor vaccines. Passive immunotherapy involves the delivery of antibodies or lymphocytes with established tumor-immune reactivity, which can directly or indirectly mediate antitumor effects and does not necessarily depend on an intact host immune system. Donor leukocyte infusions are an example of passive immunotherapy currently used in the setting of allogeneic transplantation.

From: *Current Clinical Oncology: Allogeneic Stem Cell Transplantation*
Edited by: Mary S. Laughlin and Hillard M. Lazarus © Humana Press Inc., Totowa, NJ

The history of tumor vaccine therapy extends for about a century *(3)*. William Coley, a surgeon at Memorial Hospital in New York City from 1892 to 1936, carried out the first systematic testing of therapeutic tumor vaccines. He observed tumor regression following nonspecific activation of the immune system in response to potentially fatal bacterial infections/toxins *(4)*. He later devised a vaccine consisting of heat-inactivated cultures of erysipelas and bacillus prodigiousus to deliver what would currently be interpreted as "danger" signals that promote tumor antigen processing and dendritic cell (DC) maturation. In the 1960s, Nadler and Moore combined active and passive immunotherapy with a novel cross vaccination strategy using primed lymphocytes *(5)*. Pairs of cancer patients with incurable tumors were sensitized to each other's tumor by subcutaneous implantation of viable tumor tissue from patient A to patient B and vice versa. Patients were leukapheresed 10–14 d later, and the allogeneic leukocytes were then transferred into the patient that had previously served as a source for cross immunization. Transplantation of tumor did not cause new growth of tumor and toxicity was limited only to erythema and induration at the injection site. Of the 26 patients who were deemed evaluable, seven patients showed tumor regression, including two patients with complete remissions; six of seven responses were observed in patients with malignant melanoma. Their studies were novel, but were poorly documented when compared to today's standards, and efficacy was limited by their inability to achieve sustained engraftment of the primed allogeneic human lymphocytes.

Today, cellular therapy of malignancy has become more feasible with increased understanding of the interactions between immune cells and tumors. Advances in ex vivo bioengineering and recombinant DNA technology have enabled large-scale production of cytotoxic effector lymphocytes, antigen-presenting DCs, and hematopoietic stem and progenitor cells. The general area of cancer vaccines has been reviewed in detail *(6,7)*. This article is a brief review of the current challenges regarding the incorporation of the principles of tumor vaccination into the setting of allogeneic stem cell therapy. The reader is referred to a recent monograph for a comprehensive general review of allogeneic immunotherapy *(8)*. As will become apparent, the selective engineering of the cellular and humoral immune responses to manipulate graft-vs-host disease (GVHD) and graft-vs-tumor (GVT) effects in order to develop effective antitumor vaccination strategies in the setting of allogeneic stem cell transplantation (SCT) holds great promise and challenges.

2. OBSTACLES TO THE INDUCTION OF TUMOR IMMUNITY

It has long been recognized that the host response to the primary tumor is often different from host response to the metastatic tumor. The observation in mice that primary tumors may continue to grow while metastatic tumors regress following vaccination is referred to as "concomitant immunity." Recent studies showed that tumor cells were capable of inducing a protective immune response only if injected as a single-cell suspension *(9)*. In contrast, if they were transplanted as small pieces of intact tumor, the tumors readily grew. The lack of protective tumor immunity to peripheral solid tumors correlates with the failure of tumor cells, and therefore tumor antigens, to reach the draining lymph nodes, and with the absence of primed cytotoxic T cells. These studies reveal the mechanism for a form of immunologic ignorance. Thus, one obstacle to overcome in the induction of tumor immunity is to mediate the efficient delivery of the tumor in an immunogenic form to lymph nodes.

Tumor vaccine strategies require the presence of an intact immune system. Although cancer itself is immunosuppressive, chemotherapy and radiotherapy are the principal contributors to the immunodeficiency state of most cancer patients. Thus, eliciting an adequate immune response to active specific immunotherapy with cancer vaccines is a formidable undertaking.

T cell depletion is the most clinically significant consequence of cytotoxic antineoplastic therapy and allogeneic SCT *(10,11)*. Absolute lymphocyte counts normally recover to baseline values within 3 mo of therapy, with natural killer (NK) populations recovering the fastest. B cell populations normalize in 1–3 mo *(12)*. However, the T cell receptor diversity of patients before and early after allogeneic SCT is reduced, as the patients have markedly skewed repertoires consisting of absent, monoclonal, or oligoclonal profiles for the majority of T cell receptor Vβ subfamilies *(13)*.

In the 1980s, North demonstrated the existence of a T cell-mediated mechanism of immunosuppression that inhibited the capacity of passively transferred tumor-sensitized T cells from mediating regression of tumors in recipient mice *(14)*. This suppressor notion was largely abandoned in the 1990s, but has now resurfaced in mouse models and in human studies. $CD4^+CD25^+$ regulatory T cells (Treg) have recently been shown to inhibit autoimmune diabetes, prevent inflammatory bowel disease, mediate transplantation tolerance, impede antitumor immunity, and prevent the expansion of other T cells in vivo *(15,16)*. In humans, a naturally occurring subpopulation of Treg cells constitutively expressing CD25 (the interleukin [IL]-2 receptor-α chain) comprises approx 15–30% of peripheral blood $CD4^+$ T cells *(17)*. Woo et al. have provided evidence for the contribution of Treg to immune dysfunction in cancer patients *(18)*, as most patients with non-small cell lung cancer and ovarian cancer were found to harbor regulatory T cells with potent immunosuppressive functions at the tumor site *(19)*. Thus, a large body of studies now indicates the existence of naturally occurring tolerogenic T cells in vivo that are responsible for control of self-tolerance and preventing autoimmune disease. Therefore, inhibiting the function of these Treg cells provides a promising new basis for antitumor immunotherapy in order to restore immune function in vivo. Recent studies indicate that the combination of CTLA-4 blockade and depletion of $CD25^+$ Treg cells was synergistic in the induction of potent antitumor immunity in rodents *(20)*.

It is clear that the design of cancer vaccines must include specific measures to overcome tumor-induced immunosuppression as well as postchemotherapy-induced immune deficiency. A considerable advantage of allogeneic vaccine strategies is that in some cases, the donor may be primed, and the T cells later transferred to the host following allogeneic SCT. In principle, this can overcome obstacles of T cell depletion and cellular immunodeficiency that are usually encountered in the setting of autologous SCT.

3. HARNESSING THE ALLOGENEIC IMMUNE RESPONSE

GVHD, an alloimmune attack on host tissues mounted by donor T cells, is the most important toxicity of allogeneic bone marrow transplantation. GVT immune responses are related to GVHD and are a desired and beneficial consequence of allogeneic bone marrow transplantation. Tolerance to human tumors is mediated by two primary mechanisms: either the tumor is ignored by the host immune system or peripheral T cell tolerance is induced. Given the later situation, and the fact that tumor antigens are self-antigens, it is likely that tolerance to the tumor is often induced by the same mechanisms used to avoid autoimmunity. It therefore follows that an extremely attractive means to circumvent this issue is the exploitation of the allogeneic T cell repertoire. This solution is based on the observation that T cell tolerance is self-major histocompatibility complex (MHC) restricted. In addition, allogeneic T cells have the advantage of not having undergone self-MHC-restricted negative selection in the thymus. Studies in rodents indicate that allogeneic T cell cultures can be enriched for T cells that recognize the desired self-MHC/peptide complex and that the resulting cytotoxic T lymphocytes (CTL) exhibit potent antitumor reactivity in vitro and in vivo *(21,22)*.

The allogeneic immune response is the most potent known immune response. For example, in the absence of pharmacological immunosuppression, T cells will destroy an allogeneic solid organ graft within a week of transplantation. The basis for this vigorous and rapid immune response is that unprimed T cells from one individual are strongly stimulated by MHC antigens from other members of the same species. Whereas the precursor T cell frequencies for normal environmental and "self" antigens are of the order of 1 in 1×10^5 to 1×10^6, approx 1–10% of an individual's T cells will respond to the foreign MHC antigens of another individual *(23,24)*. Transplantation of T cells or tumors provides the unique setting in which T cells can be stimulated through two different sets of antigen-presenting cells: donor type and recipient type. Transplantation immunologists have defined "direct" responses as stimulation of recipient alloreactive T cells by donor type antigen-presenting cells and "indirect" responses as stimulation by allopeptides presented in the context of self MHC by recipient type antigen-presenting cells *(25)*. Studies conducted in the 1970s and 1980s established that recipient CD4 and CD8 T cells can recognize intact allogeneic MHC class I and class II molecules on donor antigen-presenting cells. Indirect allorecognition of antigen by CD4 T cells was also demonstrated to occur as a self-restricted presentation of donor allopeptides in the context of self-MHC class II molecules on recipient antigen presenting cells by recipient CD4 T cells. Recent studies have demonstrated that CD8 T cells could recognize exogenous antigen presented in the context of self-MHC class I molecules, a process commonly referred to as "cross presentation" *(26)*. The impressive strength and vigor of the T lymphocyte response to solid organ allografts is thought to result primarily from direct pathway stimulation. Thus, lessons from transplantation immunology provide insight into the development of and rationale for tumor vaccines because of similar issues concerning the nature of the antigen-presenting cell. This is because the use of allogeneic immune systems, as well as the use of allogeneic tumor, is contemplated in some tumor vaccine strategies. In mice, studies indicate that 'immunogenic' tumors that elicit a strong natural immune response do so by accessing lymphoid regions, intermingling with T cells, and allowing direct antigen presentation to T cells to induce anti-tumor immunity *(27)*.

Tumors often express tumor-specific antigens capable of being presented to CD8 T cells by MHC class I molecules. Antigen presentation models predict that the tumor cells expressing MHC class I should present these antigens to T cells. However, self-antigens expressed by solid tumors do not efficiently stimulate naive or activated T cells *(28)*. When conditions for the priming of tumor-specific responses against a B cell lymphoma were examined in mice, no detectable presentation of MHC class I-restricted tumor antigens by the tumor itself was found *(29)*. Rather, host bone marrow-derived cells exclusively presented tumor antigens. Thus, MHC class I-restricted antigens are transferred in vivo to bone marrow-derived antigen-presenting cells, which suggests that human leukocyte antigen (HLA) matching may be less critical in the application of tumor vaccines than was previously thought. However, this issue is controversial, as there are other tumors where cross presentation of MHC class I tumor antigens is not efficient *(27)*.

Recent studies have addressed the nature of antigen presentation cell during the induction of GVHD. In a murine allogeneic bone marrow transplantation model, it was found that, despite the presence of numerous donor antigen-presenting cells, only host-derived antigen-presenting cells initiated GVHD *(30)*. Thus, strategies for augmenting GVT effects should be developed that are based on enhancing the function of host antigen-presenting cells.

4. CURRENT VACCINE APPROACHES IN ALLOGENEIC SCT

Until recently, it was thought that only a few tumors were immunogenic and, therefore, were attractive targets for vaccines. These tumors were hematologic malignancies, such as lympho-

Table 1
Questions in Allogeneic Tumor Vaccine Development

- Optimal tumor antigen.
- Optimal tumor dose and schedule.
- Source of tumor antigen: allogeneic vs autologous.
- Optimal source of donor T cells: peripheral blood, bone marrow, lymph node.
- Optimal formulation of tumor antigen: whole tumor cells, extracts, nucleic acid, etc.

mas, where the waxing and waning clinical course suggested spontaneous natural immune responses, and solid tumors, such as melanoma and renal cell carcinoma, that can have spontaneous regression. Recent vaccine experience indicates that the spectrum of immunogenic tumors is much broader than was realized initially, as the induction of antitumor immunity as well as clinical responses and tumor marker responses have been noted in diverse tumors including melanoma, renal cell carcinoma, prostate, colon, brain, pancreatic, and lung cancer *(31)*.

In a syngeneic mouse myeloablative SCT model, active immunization of donors with tumor antigens has been shown to permit transfer of tumor immunity by adoptive transfer of donor T cells in the posttransplant setting *(32)*. In principle, this general approach could have enhanced efficacy in the allogeneic setting. However, there are several important questions to consider in harnessing the allogeneic immune response to generate antitumor immune responses (Table 1).

First, what is the optimal tumor antigen? Numerous tumor vaccine strategies are under investigation, including vaccination with tumor-associated peptides, tumor cell lysates, nucleic acids, and whole tumor cell-based vaccines, either mixed with adjuvants loaded onto professional antigen-presenting cells or with genetically modified tumor cells *(33,34)*.

Second, what is the optimal dose and schedule for vaccination? The recent ability to precisely measure the appearance of antigen specific T cells following vaccination with antigen-loaded DCs or peptide and adjuvant have shown the kinetics of the human T cell response following priming to a protein antigen *(35,36)*. The nature and dose of the adjuvant is important. For example, incorporation of IL-2 into cancer vaccines can augment the response, but high doses can actually result in immunosuppression *(37)*. Under some circumstances, repetitive vaccination in mice may encourage the appearance of regulatory CD4$^+$ T cells with immunosuppressive effects *(38)*. Preliminary studies in humans indicate that vaccination with immature dendritic cells can induce antigen-specific inhibition of preexisting effector T cells in vivo *(39)*.

The schedule of vaccination with DCs is particularly important and may reflect differences in the requirements for the optimal priming and maintenance of a response to self antigens and to foreign antigens. For example, weekly administration of peptide-pulsed DCs led to diminishing CTL activity after 6 wk of treatment while animals injected with DCs every 3 wk for six treatments, or animals initially given DCs weekly and then injected weekly with antigen-bearing cells, had sustained CTLs *(40)*. Finally, the dose response to vaccines may differ in immunocompromised individuals *(41)*.

Third, should autologous or allogeneic tumors serve as the choice of antigen? Autologous tumors might serve as the ideal choice for therapeutic tumor vaccine because they provide a peptide library of all potential antigens *(42)*. However, practical concerns regarding tumor procurement and processing make this a difficult logistic and labor-intensive process. On the other hand, allogeneic tumor vaccines can be grown in bulk, easing manufacturing processes. The rationale for choosing allogeneic vaccines has been strengthened by the demonstration that antigen presentation with cell-based vaccines can occur through the process of cross-priming on host bone marrow derived antigen-presenting cells, so that HLA matching between the tumor vaccine and the host is unnecessary *(29)*. Kayaga and coworkers found that the allogeneic K1735-M2 (H-2k) melanoma cell vaccine induces a specific protective antitumor response against the syngeneic B16-F10 (H-2b) melanoma tumor in C57BL/6J mice (43). Finally, it has now been demonstrated that many tumor rejection antigens are shared antigens and are present either as tissue-specific targets or as tumor specific targets that can serve as cross-reactive antigens found in many tumors of similar histology (44). There is some concern that the dominant immune response may be allogeneic and will, therefore, deviate the immune response away from the desired tumor- or tissue-specific responses. However, alloantigen stimulation also may prove beneficial in providing immunologic help to maintain CTL responses to weak antigens (45,46).

Fourth, what is the optimal source of donor cells for vaccines in cellular transfer approaches? For many years, passenger T cells have accompanied progenitor cells during allogeneic SCT procedures. Most studies have focused largely on peripheral blood of patients or normal donors as a source of T lymphocytes with potential antitumor reactivity for cellular immunotherapy. However, the T cell subsets in various lymphoid compartments differ, and naïve T cells predominantly reside in lymph nodes. Recent studies show that in short-term culture with autologous DCs prepulsed with tumor lysates from patients with breast cancer, memory T cells from bone marrow, but not peripheral blood, could be specifically reactivated to interferon-γ-producing and cytotoxic effector cells (47). Therefore, at least in the case of breast cancer, vaccine strategies using patients' bone marrow-derived memory T cells rather than peripheral blood should be considered.

Fifth, what is the optimal source of antigen? The reader is referred elsewhere for detailed considerations of tumor vaccine preparation (6,7,31). Our bias is that whole modified tumor cells are optimal sources of antigen for therapeutic vaccination because the entire library of potentially antigenic peptides will be represented. However, experimental head-to-head comparisons of different vaccination strategies are limited. Klein and coworkers compared vaccination of tumor-bearing mice with genetically modified dendritic cells to vaccination with genetically modified tumor cells (48). In a melanoma tumor model, granulocyte-macrophage colony-stimulating factor (GM-CSF)-transduced tumor cells were compared to vaccination with bone marrow-derived DCs engineered to express MAGE-1. Superior results were obtained with vaccination with genetically modified DCs.

Yang has shown that CD80-modified melanoma cells are able to induce primary CTL activity from autologous, HLA class I-matched allogeneic peripheral blood lymphocytes (PBLs) and purified CD8+ T cells in the absence of exogenous cytokines. CTLs generated by CD80 are tumor-specific and HLA class I-restricted, and CD8+ T cells are primarily responsible for this specific cytotoxicity. Furthermore, CTLs generated from HLA class I-matched PBLs by CD80 are cytolytic to tumor cells autologous to the stimulated PBLs. These data suggest that CD80-modified tumor cells can be used as a potential tumor vaccine for both autologous and HLA class I-matched allogeneic patients (49). In mouse models, GM-CSF modification of tumor cells is superior to CD80 modification (34). This may be due to activation of inhibitory CTLA4 signals that are provoked by CD80, and therefore, approaches introducing CD28-specific ligands into tumors may be more attractive.

5. VACCINATION IN THE SETTING OF MYELOABLATIVE AND NONMYELOABLATIVE ALLOGENEIC SCT

Myeloablative conditioning that is given before SCT impairs immune function, and dampens the responsiveness to vaccination. The transfer of memory antibody responses from donor to host occurs following myeloablative SCT (11). Requirements for the transfer of responses to a recently primed response were also evaluated following myeloablative SCT. Donors were immunized with keyhole limpet hemocyanin (KLH) 1 and 3 wk prior to marrow harvest, followed by a T cell-depleted donor marrow infusion *(50)*. Half of the recipients were immunized with KLH pretransplant. IgG antibody levels were only present in recipients that had been preimmunized with KLH and only when the donors had been primed 3 wk before marrow harvest. Thus, in the setting of myeloablative SCT, it is likely that antitumor immunity involving serologic responses will require therapeutic vaccination of donor and host. The use of nonmyeloablative SCT may diminish the host immunosuppression and facilitate tumor vaccination.

During the course of a normal MHC-matched SCT, antigen-naive donor T cells are transferred to the tumor-bearing recipient, and development of GVHD represents a primary immune response to minor histocompatibility antigens (mHAgs). Target organs of GVHD all contain substantial numbers of professional antigen-presenting cells, which may efficiently stimulate primary immune responses to tissue-specific antigens.

It is conceivable that activating and expanding donor T cell populations capable of recognizing only tumor cells could increase the relative potency of GVT activity. An attractive approach is immunization of donors with a recipient-derived tumor cell vaccine before donor cell harvest and transplantation. In a mouse model, Anderson and coworkers immunized normal immunocompetent MHC-matched donors with a recipient-derived tumor cell vaccine to determine if this would substantially increase GVT activity and extend survival of SCT recipients with preexisting micrometastatic tumor *(51)*. They found that pretransplant immunization of allogeneic SCT donors with a recipient-derived whole tumor cell vaccine substantially increased GVT activity but also substantially exacerbated GVHD. In contrast, tumor vaccination of recipients post-SCT against either a fibrosarcoma or a myeloid leukemia produced a substantial increase in GVT activity, which was capable of complete protection against tumor growth and of preventing the growth of preexisting micrometastatic cancer cells. Furthermore, SCT recipients did not develop signs of acute GVHD after tumor cell vaccination, demonstrating that GVT activity could be augmented independently of GVHD *(52)*. In contrast to the toxicity associated with the pretransplant immunization of immunocompetent donors with whole tumor vaccines, studies in mice and humans indicate safety and efficacy of donor immunization with defined antigens. In mice, C3H.SW donors were immunized against a tumor antigen prior to SCT, and CTL were transferred along with bone marrow into irradiated MHC-matched mHAg-mismatched C57BL/6 recipients with established micrometastatic tumors. Donor immunization led to a significant increase in GVT activity, as measured by reduction in tumor growth and enhanced survival *(53)*.

A general impression based on numerous studies was that vaccination of the allogeneic host in the immediate posttransplant period would fail due to the severe immunosuppression of the cellular immune system. A recent study examined the ability of immunization with irradiated GM-CSF-secreting B16 murine melanoma cells to generate specific antitumor immunity after allogeneic SCT *(54)*. They found that this vaccination scheme elicited potent antitumor effects without the induction of GVHD after T cell-depleted allogeneic bone marrow transplant (BMT). In contrast, if animals were vaccinated after a T cell replete BMT, they did not generate tumor immunity, consistent with the immunosuppressive effects of GVHD. It is possible that the mixed hematopoietic chimerism that occurs in the immediate posttransplant setting following T cell-depleted SCT facilitates tumor vaccination, due to the persistence of host antigen presenting cells that may facilitate cross priming to tumor antigens.

6. IMMUNOSUPPRESSION TO ENHANCE ALLOGENEIC VACCINATION

Cytotoxic chemotherapy has diverse effects on the immune system. Cyclophosphamide can be either immunosuppressive or immunopotentiating, depending upon dose and schedule of administration *(55)*. The mechanisms for these paradoxical effects are undoubtedly complex and involve differential depletion of T cell subsets, as well as distinct effects on antigen-presenting cells. Many preclinical studies have shown that cyclophosphamide can augment the acquisition of immunity to new antigens, as well as break immunologic tolerance, perhaps through depletion of regulatory T cells. Cyclophosphamide, doxorubicin, and paclitaxel have been found to have schedule-dependent effects that enhance the antitumor immune response of GM-CSF-secreting whole cell vaccines *(56)*. These agents mediate their effects by enhancing the efficacy of the vaccine rather than via a direct cytolytic effect on cancer cells.

In the autologous SCT setting, the homeostatic mechanisms that regulate T cell mass are different than in steady state lymphopoiesis, permitting augmented clonal expansion of antigen-specific lymphocytes upon priming with tumor antigens, and resulting in enhanced responses to vaccination *(57)*. Borrello and colleagues have shown that vaccination with GM-CSF-modified syngeneic tumor cells in the post-SCT period actually results in a greater degree of antitumor immunity than is achieved following vaccination in the steady state nontransplant setting *(58)*. They employed a mouse B cell lymphoma model to develop strategies that seek to integrate GM-CSF-based tumor cell vaccines in the post-autologous BMT setting. Tumor-specific T cells were shown to undergo a massive clonal expansion and activation in the early posttransplant period, at a time when the recipient was maximally immunosuppressed. Together, these studies suggest that a GVT effect occurs in the autologous BMT setting, but that it is not sustained. Repeated immunizations during immune reconstitution may serve to maintain the antitumor effect.

7. NK CELLS: FRIEND OR FOE?

NK cells and T cells with NK cell receptors (NKT cells) have been described in both human and murine tissues. Unlike T cells, NK cells have limited long-term clonal proliferative capacity but are able to mediate potent MHC-unrestricted cytotoxicity. NK cell killing occurs through specific receptors, which bind to polymorphic determinants of major histocompatibility complex class I molecules and other ligands on cells. One family of receptors on NK cells is a class of inhibitory receptors, a family of immunoglobulin (Ig)-like molecules known as killer cell inhibitory receptors (KIR). KIR genes, each expressed by some of the individual's NK cells, vary considerably among individuals. Because KIRs are specific for MHC class I allotypes, a person's NK cells will not recognize and will, therefore, kill cells from individuals lacking their own KIR ligands. During development, each NK cell precursor makes a random choice of which KIR genes it will express, and therefore, the different combinations of HLA class I molecules select a repertoire of NK cells that express receptors for self HLA class I. Consequently, the NK cells from any given individual will be alloreactive toward cells from others which lack their KIR ligands and, conversely, will be tolerant of cells from another individual who has the same or additional KIR ligands.

The recent identification of ligands for receptors that activate NK cells, and the finding that some of these ligands are restricted in expression to tumor cells has profound implications on the design of tumor vaccine strategies *(59)*. Stimulatory lectin like receptors on NK cells such as NKG2D have recently been shown to bind to MICA, which is an MHC class I homologue whose expression is not readily detected on normal tissue but is expressed on tumor cells of epithelial origin *(60)*. Given the ability of NK cells to kill MHC unrestricted targets, it is likely that successful tumor vaccination strategies in the future will employ combinations of T cells and NK cells, with the NK cells serving to prevent tumor escape from T cells through MHC down-regulation.

Animal models indicate that NK cells can be both helpful and harmful to the host following allogeneic SCT *(61)*. When given early after transplantation, NK cells can prevent GVHD, an effect that is mediated at least in part by transforming growth factor β (TGF-β). In contrast, when NK cells are given late after transplantation, they can exacerbate GVHD.

8. TUMOR VACCINES IN THE CLINIC

Therapeutic vaccines show promise in a variety of cancers; however, to date, efficacy has not been demonstrated with previous vaccine approaches (6). It is possible that current approaches may circumvent the limitations and disappointment of previous approaches. For example, therapeutic vaccination of lymphoma patients with minimal residual disease with idiotype protein and GM-CSF has been shown to induce the clearance of residual tumor cells from blood and is associated with long-term disease-free survival (62). Autologous idiotype-pulsed DCs induced regression in patients with B cell lymphomas (63). In a pilot study to evaluate autologous DCs pulsed with tumor lysate or peptides in patients with metastatic melanoma, objective responses were evident in 5 out of 16 evaluable patients (64).

Response rates in the treatment of metastatic renal cell cancer with chemotherapeutic or hormonal agents are usually less than 10%. Nonmyeloablative allogeneic SCT and donor leukocyte infusions induce a potent antitumor effect in patients with renal cell cancer (65). Preclinical studies indicate that GM-CSF-based tumor cell vaccines have promise for breast cancer in a nonmyeloablative allogeneic SCT in mice (66). Kugler and coworkers described remarkable regressions in patients with metastatic renal cancer using a vaccine therapy based on fusions of allogeneic DCs and tumor cells (67). In this study, allogeneic stimulation of autologous T cells could have contributed to induction of the immune response to the tumor. Phase II or III randomized trials of autologous therapeutic vaccination are presently underway for many cancers, including myeloma, prostate, breast, ovary, colon cancer, and lymphoma (Table 2). It is likely that allogeneic approaches will eventually complement the autologous vaccine approaches that are presently at a more advanced stage of clinical evaluation.

9. CLINICAL CONSIDERATIONS IN THE TESTING OF ALLOGENEIC TUMOR VACCINES

It is currently estimated that more than 10,000 patients with leukemia are now alive following allogeneic SCT (68). Many of these are alive undoubtedly because of alloimmune effects rather than allogeneic stem cell rescue from high dose chemotherapy. The major toxicity faced by these patients is GVHD. It is of interest that in mouse models of GVHD, infusions of activated NK cells following allogeneic stem cell transplantation could suppress GVHD while GVT effects were amplified (61,69). GVHD is also significantly diminished when donor T cells are polarized toward type 2 cytokines (70), and Fowler and colleagues have shown that Th2 cells can prevent GVHD while retaining the GVT activity of donor T cells (71,72).

Autoimmune syndromes may occur spontaneously in patients as a consequence of a natural immune response provoked by the tumor, or following therapeutic vaccination. Antibody and CTL responses have been linked to the occurrence of vitiligo in melanoma patients responding to immunotherapy (73,74). The occurrence of vitiligo is associated with cancer regression in patients with melanoma undergoing immunotherapy. Uveitis has been observed in patients following tumor vaccines (75,76) and in human immunodeficiency virus (HIV)-infected patients who recover immune function on antiviral therapy. Some paraneoplastic disorders represent a convergence of the fields of tumor immunity and autoimmunity. The most striking example is in patients with small cell lung carcinoma and breast and ovarian carcinoma that develop paraneoplastic cerebellar degeneration. These patients often have antibody and CTL response against the cdr2 molecule, which is a protein normally expressed in brain and in some

Table 2
Examples of Ongoing Phase II or III Cancer Vaccine Trials

- A phase III randomized double-blind trial of immunotherapy with a polyvalent melanoma vaccine, CancerVax®, plus BCG vs placebo pluc BCG as a postsurgical treatmen for stage III melanoma: Dr. Donald Morton, John Wayne Cancer Institute.
- Phase III randomized study of high dose IL-2 with or without gp1000 antigen in patients with metastatic cutaneous melanoma: Dr. Douglas Schwartzentruber, National Cancer Institute.
- A phase II study of vaccination with irradiated autologous lung tumor cells mixed with a GM-CSF-secreting bystander cell line (GVAX) in advanced stage nonsmall cell lung cancer: Dr. Kristen Hege, Cell Genesys.
- Phase II pilot study of cyclophosphamide and active imtralymphatic immunotherapy with a vaccine containing IFN-α- or IFN-γ-treated tumor cells followed by sargramostim (GM-CSF) in patients with advanced cancers: Dr. Charles L. Wiseman, St. Vincent Medical Center, Los Angeles, CA.
- Phase I/II stude of Ad2/MART-1v2 and Ad2/gp100v2 melanoma antigen vaccines in patients with stage II, III, or IV melanoma: Genzyme: Frank Haluska, Massachusetts General Hospital.
- Phase I/II study of active immunotherapy with carcinoembryonic antigen (CEA) RNA pulsed autologous DCs in patients with metastic breast cancer who achieve a complete response after high dose chemotherapy and stem cell support: Dr. H. Kimn Lyerly, Duke Comprehensive Cancer Center.
- Phase I/II study of immunization with autologous in vitro-treated tumor cells and DCs in combination with sargramostim (GM-CSF) in patients with stage IV or recurrent melanoma: Dr. Robert O. Dillman, Hoag Memorial Hospital.
- Phase II randomized study of immunization with and HLA-A2 multiepitope peptide vaccine comprised of MART-1:27-35, gp100:209-217 (210M), and tyrosinaseL368-376 (379D) peptides alone or in combination with sargramostim (GM-CSF) and/or IFNα-2b in HlA-A2 positive patients with metastic melanoma: Dr. John Kirkwood, NCI ECOG.

Abbreviations: BCG, bacille Calmette-Guerin.

tumors *(77)*. This naturally occurring immune response occurs in unvaccinated patients and may provide some clinically beneficial antitumor effects as well as toxicity in the form of central nervous system (CNS) autoimmunity.

Most investigators believe that T cells and NK cells mediate protective tumor immunity; however, antibodies may also play a major role in immune protection. Tumor vaccines often elicit cellular and humoral responses, and there is substantial evidence documenting the autoimmune consequences of antibodies induced by growing malignancies, or by passively administered and actively induced antibodies in cancer patients against antigens shared by normal and malignant tissues *(78)*. Antibodies against cell surface or intracellular antigens in the CNS or on epithelial surfaces of normal tissues do not generally result in autoimmunity, but the same types and titers of antibodies against cell surface antigens in the subepidermal skin, peripheral nerves, blood, or vascular sites, such as the spleen and bone marrow, readily induce autoimmunity. Vaccine-induced antibodies against a variety of cancer cell surface antigens have been associated with prevention of tumor recurrence in preclinical models and in vaccinated cancer patients, in the absence of demonstrable autoimmunity. This forms the basis for a series of ongoing phase III trials with single or polyvalent antigen cancer vaccines designed for optimal antibody induction. It was initially thought that antibodies were a form of passive immunity and that they could function in immunosuppressed hosts. However, recent studies show that antibodies require Fc receptors on antigen-presenting cells in order to mediate tumor protective effects *(79)*. It is likely that successful allogeneic vaccines will elicit cellular and humoral responses and that the principles of inducing antibody responses in allogeneic SCT patients will be exploited *(50)*.

The clinical testing of therapeutic cancer vaccines requires different clinical trial designs than used for conventional chemotherapeutic drugs *(80)*. Traditional phase I designs based on escalation from a very low starting dose in cancer patients are not always necessary in cancer vaccine development. The phase I concept of dose escalation to find a maximum-tolerated dose does not apply to most vaccines. This is because most vaccines are incapable of causing immediate serious or life-threatening toxicities at doses feasible to manufacture. In addition, neither toxicity nor efficacy can be assessed in patients with advanced malignant disease associated with a blunted immune response, because both toxicity and efficacy depend on an intact immune response. Consequently, issues of patient selection and end point definition require reconsideration for the early phases of clinical vaccine development. Finally, vaccination strategies often combine multiple agents, each of which needs to be optimized, such as adjuvants, cytokines, or co-stimulatory molecules. Although some of these combination regimens can be optimized in preclinical models, defining the optimal regimen requires clinical testing.

Much of our understanding of the immunobiology of bone marrow transplantation has come from studies in young adult mice reconstituted with T cell-depleted bone marrow after lethal irradiation. Recent evidence indicates, however, that the applicability of conclusions drawn from this model to human BMT may be limited, due to major differences between human and murine immune systems in the mechanisms of T cell homeostasis *(81)*.

10. CONCLUSIONS AND SUMMARY

By priming with the appropriate set of tumor antigens, vaccine therapy can now be directed against virtually any antigen within the human T cell repertoire. Vaccines can be given in either prophylactic or therapeutic settings. Therapeutic vaccines will need to incorporate approaches to overcome inhibition by CTLA4 and regulatory T cells. Genetic screening will increasingly be able to identify people at risk for the development of cancer or patients with early stage premalignant lesions. Gene array technology will likely provide opportunities for the development of prophylactic cancer vaccines using defined antigens. Despite this, tumors will still continue to present at advanced stages, and therapeutic cancer vaccines in the allogeneic setting will be increasingly used. The major remaining question is which antigens are the most suitable targets for tumor vaccination in clinical trials in the allogeneic transplant setting. It is likely that cellular and cytokine therapy, as well as gene therapy, will be required to fully exploit the allogeneic immune responses to tumors.

REFERENCES

1. Burnet FM. The concept of immunological surveillance. *Prog Exp Tumor Res* 1970;13:1–27.
2. Shankaran V, Ikeda H, Bruce AT, White JM, Swanson PE, Old LJ, et al. IFNgamma and lymphocytes prevent primary tumour development and shape tumour immunogenicity. *Nature* 2001;410(6832):1107–1111.
3. Old LJ. Tumor immunology: the first century. *Curr Opin Immunol* 1992;4(5):603–607.
4. Coley WB. The treatment of malignant tumors by repeated inoculations of erysipelas: With a report of ten original cases. *Am J Med Sci* 1893;105(5):487–511.
5. Nadler SH, Moore GE. Clinical immunologic study of malignant disease: response to tumor transplants and transfer of leukocytes. *Ann Surg* 1966;164(3):482–490.
6. Akporiaye E, Hersh EM. Cancer Vaccines: Clinical Applications. In: Devita VT, Hellman S., Rosenberg SA, eds. *Biologic Therapy of Cancer*. Lippincott, Philadelphia, PA, 1999, pp. 635–647.
7. Pardoll DM. Therapeutic vaccination for cancer. *Clin Immunol* 2000;95(1 Pt 2):S44–S62.
8. Barrett J. *Allogeneic Immunotherapy for Malignant Diseases*. Marcel Dekker, New York, 2000.
9. Ochsenbein AF, Klenerman P, Karrer U, Ludewig B, Pericin M, Hengartner H, et al. Immune surveillance against a solid tumor fails because of immunological ignorance. *Proc Natl Acad Sci USA* 1999;96(5):2233–2238.
10. Mackall CL, Fleisher TA, Brown MR, Magrath IT, Shad AT, Horowitz ME, et al. Lymphocyte depletion during treatment with intensive chemotherapy for cancer. *Blood* 1994 84(7):2221–2228.
11. Lum LG. The kinetics of immune reconstitution after human marrow transplantation. *Blood* 1987;69(2):369–380.

12. Small TN, Keever CA, Weiner-Fedus S, Heller G, O'Reilly RJ, Flomenberg N. B-cell differentiation following autologous, conventional, or T-cell depleted bone marrow transplantation: a recapitulation of normal B-cell ontogeny. *Blood* 1990;76(8):1647–1656.

13. Claret EJ, Alyea EP, Orsini E, Pickett CC, Collins H, Wang Y, et al. Characterization of T cell repertoire in patients with graft-versus- leukemia after donor lymphocyte infusion. *J Clin Invest* 1997;100(4):855–866.

14. Dye ES, North RJ. T cell-mediated immunosuppression as an obstacle to adoptive immunotherapy of the P815 mastocytoma and its metastases. *J Exp Med* 1981;154(4):1033–1042.

15. Shimizu J, Yamazaki S, Sakaguchi S. Induction of tumor immunity by removing CD25+CD4+ T cells: a common basis between tumor immunity and autoimmunity. *J Immunol* 1999;163(10):5211–5218.

16. Shevach EM. Regulatory T Cells in Autoimmmunity. *Annu Rev Immunol* 2000;18:423–449.

17. Ng WF, Duggan PJ, Ponchel F, Matarese G, Lombardi G, Edwards AD, et al. Human CD4(+)CD25(+) cells: a naturally occurring population of regulatory T cells. *Blood* 2001;98(9):2736–2744.

18. Woo EY, Chu CS, Goletz TJ, Schlienger K, Coukos G, Rubin SC, et al. Regulatory CD4+CD25+ T cells in tumors from patients with early-stage non small cell lung cancer and late-stage ovarian cancer. *Cancer Res* 2001;61:4766–4772.

19. Woo EY, Yeh H, Chu CS, Schlienger K, Riley JL, Kaiser LR, et al. Cutting edge: regulatory t cells from cancer patients directly inhibit autologous t cell proliferation. *J Immunol* 2002;9:4272–4276.

20. Sutmuller RP, van Duivenvoorde LM, van Elsas A, Schumacher TN, Wildenberg ME, Allison JP, et al. Synergism of cytotoxic T lymphocyte-associated antigen 4 blockade and depletion of CD25(+) regulatory T cells in antitumor therapy reveals alternative pathways for suppression of autoreactive cytotoxic T lymphocyte responses. *J Exp Med* 2001;194(6):823–832.

21. Sadovnikova E, Stauss HJ. Peptide-specific cytotoxic T lymphocytes restricted by nonself major histocompatibility complex class I molecules: reagents for tumor immunotherapy. *Proc Natl Acad Sci USA* 1996;93(23): 13,114–13,118.

22. Sadovnikova E, Jopling LA, Soo KS, Stauss HJ. Generation of human tumor-reactive cytotoxic T cells against peptides presented by non-self HLA class I molecules. *Eur J Immunol* 1998;28(1):193–200.

23. Nisbet NW, Simonsen M, Zaleski M. The frequency of antigen-sensitive cells in tissue transplantation. A commentary on clonal selection. *J Exp Med* 1969;129(3):459–467.

24. Suchin EJ, Langmuir PB, Palmer E, Sayegh MH, Wells AD, Turka LA. Quantifying the frequency of alloreactive T cells in vivo: new answers to an old question. *J Immunol* 2001;166(2):973–981.

25. Shoskes DA, Wood KJ. Indirect pesentation of MHC antigens in transplantation. *Immunol Today* 1994;15:32–38.

26. Heath WR, Kurts C, Miller JFAP, Carbone F. Cross-tolerance: a pathway for inducing tolerance to peripheral tissue antigens. *J Exp Med* 1998;187:1549–1553.

27. Ochsenbein AF, Sierro S, Odermatt B, Pericin M, Karrer U, Hermans J, et al. Roles of tumour localization, second signals and cross priming in cytotoxic T-cell induction. *Nature* 2001;411(6841):1058–1064.

28. Speiser DE, Miranda R, Zakarian A, Bachmann MF, McKall-Faienza K, Odermatt B, et al. Self antigens expressed by solid tumors do not efficiently stimulate naive or activated t cells: implications for immunotherapy. *J Exp Med* 1997;186(5):645–653.

29. Huang AY, Golumbek P, Ahmadzadeh M, Jaffee E, Pardoll D, Levitsky H. Role of bone marrow-derived cells in presenting MHC class I-restricted tumor antigens. *Science* 1994;264(5161):961–965.

30. Shlomchik WD, Couzens MS, Tang CB, McNiff J, Robert ME, Liu J, et al. Prevention of graft versus host disease by inactivation of host antigen-presenting cells. *Science* 1999;285(5426):412–415.

31. Greten TF, Jaffee EM. Cancer vaccines. *J Clin Oncol* 1999;17(3):1047–1060.

32. Hornung RL, Longo DL, Bowersox OC, Kwak LW. Tumor antigen-specific immunization of bone marrow transplantation donors as adoptive therapy against established tumor. *J Natl Cancer Inst* 1995;87(17):1289–1296.

33. Pardoll DM. Cancer vaccines. *Nat Med* 1998;4(Suppl 5):525–531.

34. Mach N, Dranoff G. Cytokine-secreting tumor cell vaccines. *Curr Opin Immunol* 2000;12(5):571–575.

35. Dhodapkar MV, Steinman RM, Sapp M, Desai H, Fossella C, Krasovsky J, et al. Rapid generation of broad T-cell immunity in humans after a single injection of mature dendritic cells. *J Clin Invest* 1999;104(2):173–180.

36. Pittet MJ, Speiser DE, Lienard D, Valmori D, Guillaume P, Dutoit V, et al. Expansion and functional maturation of human tumor antigen-specific CD8+ T cells after vaccination with antigenic peptide. *Clin Cancer Res* 2001;7(Suppl 3):796s–803s.

37. Schmidt W, Schweighoffer T, Herbst E, Maass G, Berger M, Schilcher F, et al. Cancer vaccines: the interleukin 2 dosage effect. *Proc Natl Acad Sci USA* 1995;92(10):4711–4714.

38. Chakraborty NG, Li L, Sporn JR, Kurtzman SH, Ergin MT, Mukherji B. Emergence of regulatory CD4+ T cell response to repetitive stimulation with antigen-presenting cells in vitro: implications in designing antigen-presenting cell-based tumor vaccines. *J Immunol* 1999;162(9):5576–5583.

39. Dhodapkar MV, Steinman RM, Krasovsky J, Munz C, Bhardwaj N. Antigen-specific inhibition of effector T cell function in humans after injection of immature dendritic cells. *J Exp Med* 2001;193(2):233–238.

40. Serody JS, Collins EJ, Tisch RM, Kuhns JJ, Frelinger JA. T cell activity after dendritic cell vaccination is dependent on both the type of antigen and the mode of delivery. *J Immunol* 2000;164(9):4961–4967.

41. Korver K, Boeschoten EW, Krediet RT, van SG, Schellekens PT. Dose-response effects in immunizations with keyhole limpet haemocyanin and rabies vaccine: shift in some immunodeficiency states. *Clin Exp Immunol* 1987;70(2):328–335.

42. Mastrangelo MJ, Lattime EC, Maguire Jr. H, Berd D. Whole Cell Vaccines. In: Devita VT, Hellman S., Rosenberg SA, editors. B*iologic Therapy of Cancer*. Lippincott, Philadelphia, PA, 1999, pp. 648–659.

43. Kayaga J, Souberbielle BE, Sheikh N, Morrow WJ, Scott-Taylor T, Vile R, et al. Anti-tumour activity against B16-F10 melanoma with a GM-CSF secreting allogeneic tumour cell vaccine. *Gene Ther* 1999;6(8):1475–1481.

44. Toes RE, Blom RJ, van d, V, Offringa R, Melief CJ, Kast WM. Protective antitumor immunity induced by immunization with completely allogeneic tumor cells. *Cancer Res* 1996;56(16):3782–3787.

45. Clerici M, Stocks NI, Zajac RA, Boswell RN, Via CS, Shearer GM. Circumvention of defective CD4 T helper cell function in HIV-infected individuals by stimulation with HLA alloantigens. *J Immunol* 1990;144(9):3266–3271.

46. Fabre JW. The allogeneic response and tumor immunity. *Nat Med* 2001;7(6):649–652.

47. Feuerer M, Beckhove P, Bai L, Solomayer EF, Bastert G, Diel IJ, et al. Therapy of human tumors in NOD/SCID mice with patient-derived reactivated memory T cells from bone marrow. *Nat Med* 2001;7(4):452–458.

48. Klein C, Bueler H, Mulligan RC. Comparative analysis of genetically modified dendritic cells and tumor cells as therapeutic cancer vaccines. *J Exp Med* 2000;191(10):1699–1708.

49. Yang S, Darrow TL, Seigler HF. Generation of primary tumor-specific cytotoxic T lymphocytes from autologous and human lymphocyte antigen class I-matched allogeneic peripheral blood lymphocytes by B7 gene-modified melanoma cells. *Cancer Res* 1997;57(8):1561–1568.

50. Wimperis JZ, Gottlieb D, Duncombe AS, Heslop HE, Prentice HG, Brenner MK. Requirements for the adoptive transfer of antibody responses to a priming antigen in man. *J Immunol* 1990;144(2):541–547.

51. Anderson LD, Jr., Petropoulos D, Everse LA, Mullen CA. Enhancement of graft-versus-tumor activity and graft-versus-host disease by pretransplant immunization of allogeneic bone marrow donors with a recipient-derived tumor cell vaccine. *Cancer Res* 1999;59(7):1525–1530.

52. Anderson LD, Jr., Savary CA, Mullen CA. Immunization of allogeneic bone marrow transplant recipients with tumor cell vaccines enhances graft-versus-tumor activity without exacerbating graft-versus-host disease. *Blood* 2000;95(7):2426–2433.

53. Anderson LD, Jr., Mori S, Mann S, Savary CA, Mullen CA. Pretransplant tumor antigen-specific immunization of allogeneic bone marrow transplant donors enhances graft-versus-tumor activity without exacerbation of graft-versus-host disease. *Cancer Res* 2000;60(20):5797–5802.

54. Teshima T, Mach N, Hill GR, Pan L, Gillessen S, Dranoff G, et al. Tumor cell vaccine elicits potent antitumor immunity after allogeneic T-cell-depleted bone marrow transplantation. *Cancer Res* 2001;61(1):162–171.

55. Mastrangelo MJ, Berd D, Maguire H, Jr. The immunoaugmenting effects of cancer chemotherapeutic agents. *Semin Oncol* 1986;13(2):186–194.

56. Machiels JP, Reilly RT, Emens LA, Ercolini AM, Lei RY, Weintraub D, et al. Cyclophosphamide, doxorubicin, and paclitaxel enhance the antitumor immune response of granulocyte/macrophage-colony stimulating factor-secreting whole-cell vaccines in HER-2/neu tolerized mice. *Cancer Res* 2001;61(9):3689–3697.

57. Mackall CL, Bare CV, Granger LA, Sharrow SO, Titus JA, Gress RE. Thymic-independent T cell regeneration occurs via antigen-driven expansion of peripheral T cells resulting in a repertoire that is limited in diversity and prone to skewing. *J Immunol* 1996;156(12):4609–4616.

58. Borrello I, Sotomayor EM, Rattis FM, Cooke SK, Gu L, Levitsky HI. Sustaining the graft-versus-tumor effect through posttransplant immunization with granulocyte-macrophage colony-stimulating factor (GM-CSF)-producing tumor vaccines. *Blood* 2000;95(10):3011–3019.

59. Soloski MJ. Recognition of tumor cells by the innate immune system. *Curr Opin Immunol* 2001;13(2):154–162.

60. Diefenbach A, Jensen ER, Jamieson AM, Raulet DH. Rae1 and H60 ligands of the NKG2D receptor stimulate tumour immunity. *Nature* 2001;413(6852):165–171.

61. Murphy WJ, Longo DL. The potential role of NK cells in the separation of graft-versus-tumor effects from graft-versus-host disease after allogeneic bone marrow transplantation. *Immunol Rev* 1997;157:167–176.

62. Bendandi M, Gocke CD, Kobrin CB, Benko FA, Sternas LA, Pennington R, et al. Complete molecular remissions induced by patient-specific vaccination plus granulocyte-monocyte colony-stimulating factor against lymphoma. *Nat Med* 1999;5(10):1171–1177.

63. Hsu FJ, Benike C, Fagnoni F, Liles TM, Czerwinski D, Taidi B, et al. Vaccination of patients with B-cell lymphoma using autologous antigen-pulsed dendritic cells. *Nature Med* 1996;2(1):52–58.

64. Nestle FO, Alijagic S, Gilliet M, Sun Y, Grabbe S, Dummer R, et al. Vaccination of melanoma patients with peptide- or tumor lysate-pulsed dendritic cells. *Nat Med* 1998;4(3):328–332.

65. Childs RW, Clave E, Tisdale J, Plante M, Hensel N, Barrett J. Successful treatment of metastatic renal cell carcinoma with a nonmyeloablative allogeneic peripheral-blood progenitor-cell transplant: evidence for a graft-versus-tumor effect. *J Clin Oncol* 1999;17(7):2044.

66. Luznik L, Slansky JE, Borrello I, Levitsky HI, Pardoll DM, Fuchs EJ. Successful therapy of metastatic cancer with GM -CSF based tumor cell vaccines after non-myeloablative allogeneic stem cell transplantation. Submitted for publication.

67. Kugler A, Stuhler G, Walden P, Zoller G, Zobywalski A, Brossart P, et al. Regression of human metastatic renal cell carcinoma after vaccination with tumor cell-dendritic cell hybrids. *Nat Med* 2000;6(3):332–336.

68. Horowitz MM, Rowlings PA. An update from the International Bone Marrow Transplant Registry and the Autologous Blood and Marrow Transplant Registry on current activity in hematopoietic stem cell transplantation. *Curr Opin Hematol* 1997;4(6):395–400.

69. Asai O, Longo DL, Tian ZG, Hornung RL, Taub DD, Ruscetti FW, et al. Suppression of graft-versus-host disease and amplification of graft-versus-tumor effects by activated natural killer cells after allogeneic bone marrow transplantation. *J Clin Invest* 1998;101(9):1835–1842.

70. Krenger W, Snyder KM, Byon JC, Falzarano G, Ferrara JL. Polarized type 2 alloreactive CD4+ and CD8+ donor T cells fail to induce experimental acute graft-versus-host disease. *J Immunol* 1995;155(2):585–593.

71. Fowler DH, Breglio J, Nagel G, Eckhaus MA, Gress RE. Allospecific CD8+ Tc1 and Tc2 populations in graft-versus-leukemia effect and graft-versus-host disease. *J Immunol* 1996;157(11):4811–4821.

72. Fowler DH, Gress RE. Th2 and Tc2 cells in the regulation of GVHD, GVL, and graft rejection: considerations for the allogeneic transplantation therapy of leukemia and lymphoma. *Leuk Lymph* 2000;38(3–4):221–234.

73. Rosenberg SA, White DE. Vitiligo in patients with melanoma: normal tissue antigens can be targets for cancer immunotherapy. *J Immunother Emphasis Tumor Immunol* 1996;19(1):81–84.

74. Okamoto T, Irie RF, Fujii S, Huang SK, Nizze AJ, Morton DL, et al. Anti-tyrosinase-related protein-2 immune response in vitiligo patients and melanoma patients receiving active-specific immunotherapy. *J Invest Dermatol* 1998;111(6):1034–1039.

75. Donaldson RC, Canaan SA, Jr., McLean RB, Ackerman LV. Uveitis and vitiligo associated with BCG treatment for malignant melanoma. *Surgery* 1974;76(5):771–778.

76. Allison AC, Byars NE. Immunological adjuvants: desirable properties and side-effects. *Mol Immunol* 1991;28(3):279–284.

77. Albert ML, Darnell JC, Bender A, Francisco LM, Bhardwaj N, Darnell RB. Tumor-specific killer cells in paraneoplastic cerebellar degeneration. *Nat Med* 1998;4(11):1321–1324.

78. Livingston PO, Ragupathi G, Musselli C. Autoimmune and antitumor consequences of antibodies against antigens shared by normal and malignant tissues. *J Clin Immunol* 2000;20(2):85–93.

79. Ravetch JV, Bolland S. IgG Fc receptors. *Annu Rev Immunol* 2001;19:275–290.

80. Simon RM, Steinberg SM, Hamilton M, Hildesheim A, Khleif S, Kwak LW, et al. Clinical trial designs for the early clinical development of therapeutic cancer vaccines. *J Clin Oncol* 2001;19(6):1848–1854.

81. Mackall CL, Gress RE. Pathways of T-cell regeneration in mice and humans: implications for bone marrow transplantation and immunotherapy. *Immunol Rev* 1997;157:61–72.

19 Donor Leukocyte Infusions

Robert H. Collins, Jr, MD

1. INTRODUCTION

Donor leukocyte infusion (DLI) involves infusing leukocytes obtained from a normal donor with the aim of enhancing a particular immunologic effect. In general, the particular effect is graft-vs-leukemia (GVL) or, more broadly, graft-vs-malignancy (GVM) reactivity, although DLI can have other effects, including antiviral activity and enhancement of engraftment. This therapy has great efficacy in certain situations, and the observation that it is possible to harness GVM purposefully has led to development of a new transplant strategy, nonmyeloablative stem cell transplantation. However, it is important to realize that DLI is associated with major drawbacks, including severe graft-vs-host disease (GVHD) and minimal efficacy in many situations. Significant advances in this field will require a better understanding of the basic mechanisms involved in the evolution of GVH and GVL effects.

2. BACKGROUND

Barnes and Loutit first showed an anti-tumor effect of allogeneic immune cells in classic experiments carried out in the 1950s (*1*). In these studies, leukemic mice were treated with total body irradiation followed by either allogeneic or syngeneic bone marrow transplantation (BMT); animals receiving allogeneic marrow were much less likely to relapse than those

From: *Current Clinical Oncology: Allogeneic Stem Cell Transplantation*
Edited by: Mary S. Laughlin and Hillard M. Lazarus © Humana Press Inc., Totowa, NJ

receiving syngeneic marrow. Subsequent animal studies over the ensuing decades have expanded on these findings, clearly demonstrating a GVL effect of allogeneic BMT and, in many instances, shedding light on mechanisms of the effect *(2)* (*see* Chapter 24). Clinical observations in the 1970s and 1980s suggested a GVL effect of human BMT: (i) relapse rates were higher in recipients of syngeneic compared to allogeneic transplants *(3)*; (ii) among recipients of allogeneic transplants, the relapse rates were much lower in patients who developed GVHD *(4,5)*; and (iii) T cell depletion, while decreasing the incidence of GVHD, also significantly increased the incidence of leukemia relapse *(6)*. Horowitz et al. confirmed these findings in a large analysis of International Bone Marrow Transplant Registry (IBMTR) data *(7)*.

Based on an appreciation of the power of the GVL effect, several investigators began attempts to harness it *(8,9)*. These investigators treated patients with recurrent or persistent malignancy after allogeneic BMT with infusions of additional lymphocytes obtained from the original donor, without the cover of immunosuppressive agents. It was anticipated that donor lymphocytes would be effective in this setting because they were not inhibited by immunosuppressive agents and because they had not been inhibited by the tumor escape mechanisms that may have led to the relapse. Complete responses in a significant percentage of patients led to broad application of this approach *(10–22)* (*see* Tables 1 and 2).

3. DISEASE ACTIVITY

3.1. Chronic Myelogenous Leukemia

3.1.1. RESPONSES

Kolb et al. reported on the first three patients with chronic myelogenous leukemia (CML) treated by DLI *(8)*. All three received interferon (IFN)-α as well and achieved long lasting remissions, two in association with GVHD. Numerous additional single-center reports *(10–15,23,24)* and two large registry analyses have confirmed the pronounced sensitivity of CML to DLI (*see* Table 3) *(16,17)*. The overall response rate is roughly 60–80%, with the likelihood of response varying by the extent of disease at the time of DLI. Response rates in hematologic relapse are approx 75%, whereas responses in more advanced disease range from 12.5 to 29%. Responses are better in cytogenetic relapse (82–100%) and molecular relapse (8 of 8 patients in one study) *(25)*, although the number of DLI patients in these categories is relatively low. In the majority of patients with complete remission defined by cytogenetics, there is no evidence of BCR-ABL transcript by polymerase chain reaction (PCR) analysis *(16,17,25)*. The time to complete remission can be quite long, with a median time of 3–4 mo and a range of 1–11 mo or more. Molecular remissions follow cytogenetic remissions by several weeks. Close monitoring with sensitive techniques can define a "critical switch period" of 4–5 wk, during which recipient cell numbers suddenly decrease in association with a sharp decrease in bcr-abl transcripts *(26)*. Other patients manifest a slower, more gradual decline in BCR-ABL transcripts *(27)*.

The most important pre-DLI predictor of response is disease status at the time of DLI *(16,17,25)*. It is unclear whether advanced disease is more resistant because of rapid growth, excessive tumor cell numbers for the number of T cells infused, or intrinsic resistance of tumor cells to GVL mechanisms. Other potential predictive factors have not been consistent from study to study, including prior GVHD and time from BMT to DLI. T cell depletion of the initial BMT was not an important factor in several separate multivariate analyses *(16,17)*. As discussed below, GVHD after DLI is associated with response.

3.1.2. INTERFERON

IFN-α conceivably might increase GVL activity by increasing expression of cell surface molecules necessary for effector and target cell interaction *(28,29)*. Therefore, many patients

Table 1
Indications for DLI

Enhance immune-mediated antitumor activity
    Hematologic malignancies
        CML
        AML
        ALL
        MDS
        Myeloma
        NHL
        Hodgkin's disease
        Others
    Non-hematologic malignances
        Renal cell cancer
        Breast cancer
        Ohters
Enhance immune reconstitution for anti-infection activity
    EBV
    CMV
    Adenovirus
    Others
Enhance donor cell engraftment
    Graft rejection

Table 2
Settings for DLI

Disease status
    Active (DLI used therapeutically).
    High risk (DLI used prophylactically).
Prior therapy
    Standard stem cell transplant.
    Nonmyeloablative stem cell transplant.
    No prior transplant therapy.

Table 3
DLI for CML

	European (16)	North American (17)
Number of patients	84	56
Mononuclear cell dose $\times 10^8$/kg median (range)	3.0 (0.25–12.3)	4.59 (0.79–11.39)
IFN-α	60 (76%)	31 (55%)
Complete remission[a]		
Cytogenetic relapse	14 out of 17 (82%)	3 out of 3 (100%)
Hematologic relapse	39 out of 50 (78%)	25 out of 34 (73.5%)
Transformed relapse	1 out of 8 (12.5%)	5 out of 18 (28%)

[a]Of assessable patients.

have received IFN-α along with DLI. However, multivariate analyses of large numbers of CML patients have not indicated that the response rate is altered by IFN-α *(16,17)*. In addition, high response rates from a large center that does not utilize IFN-α suggests that the drug is not generally necessary *(25)*. However, only a randomized controlled trial would answer this question definitively. Lastly, it is worth noting that occasional patients have seemed to respond only after the addition of IFN *(21)*, suggesting that interferon is required for response in a small percentage of patients.

3.1.3. DURATION OF REMISSION

Remissions appear to be durable in most complete responders who had early-phase relapse at the time of DLI. In one study with a median follow-up time of 39 mo, only 2 of 32 (6%) complete responders treated for early phase disease relapsed compared to 3 of 7 (43%) with advanced phase relapse *(30)*. Another study with median follow-up of 29 mo reported relapse in only 4 of 44 (9%) patients who attained molecular remissions *(25)*. Many patients are now more than 5 yr out from DLI and remain in remission *(18,30)*, and one group has reported 30 patients whose remission duration after DLI exceeds the remission duration after the initial transplant *(25)*. It is unknown whether ongoing molecular remissions are due to the tumor being completely eradicated or to immune surveillance; surveillance by infused T cells can occur in some settings, as shown by the proliferation of gene-marked Epstein-Barr virus (EBV)-specific T cells in response to a flare of EBV, months after initially controlling the disease *(31)*.

3.1.4. LONG-TERM SURVIVAL

Kolb et al. have reported long-term survival data after DLI for CML *(18)*. With median follow-up of approx 2 yr, 80% of patients treated in cytogenetic relapse were alive compared to approx 55% of patients treated in stable phase relapse, and approx 20% of patients treated in transformed phase. Porter et al. reported long-term follow-up for 39 CML patients who had attained a complete remission after DLI *(30)*. The event-free survival at 3 yr was 73%. Seven of 32 patients treated for early phase disease had died, two patiens died of disease, two patients died of GVHD, and three patients died from other causes. Six of seven advanced phase disease patients had died: two patients died of disease, two patients died of GVHD, and two patients died of other causes.

3.2. Acute Myelogenous Leukemia

Acute myelogenous leukemia (AML) is less responsive to DLI than CML. The European registry analysis reported complete remissions in five of 17 AML patients treated with DLI as sole therapy *(16)*, and the North American registry analysis reported complete remissions in six of 39 patients treated in this manner *(17)*. The median time to remission was 34 d *(17)*. It seems likely that earlier relapses, such as molecular or cytogenetic relapses, are more responsive than hematologic relapses to DLI alone, but there are very few data specifically addressing this issue. Ongoing remissions are uncommon in patients with hematologic relapse treated with DLI alone *(18)*; one of 34 such patients remained in remission at 6 mo posttreatment in an unpublished analysis of our database. Thus, DLI as sole therapy in AML patients has very limited efficacy.

Analysis of CML patients has shown that GVL effects typically require several weeks to months to evolve *(16,17,25)*. Thus, diseases such as AML in hematologic relapse may grow too fast for GVL effects to develop. If so, then debulking tumors with chemotherapy before DLI might be advantageous. We have recently completed a study prospectively evaluating this approach *(32)*. Sixty-five patients in hematologic relapse of myeloid malignancy following human leukocyte antigen (HLA)-matched sibling BMT were treated with cytarabine-based chemotherapy followed by granulocyte colony-stimulating factor (G-CSF) primed DLI; prophylactic immunosuppression was not given. Twenty-seven of 57 evaluable patients had a complete response. The complete responders had 1- and 2-yr survival rates of 51 and 41%, respectively, compared to a 1-yr survival rate for nonresponders of only 5%. However, treatment-related mortality was 23%, and 2-yr survival for the entire cohort was only 19%. The most important predictive factor in this study was relapse within 6 mo of BMT, with very few such patients surviving at 1 yr. Post-DLI GVHD was not associated with improved event-free survival. Although these results appear to be superior to those seen with DLI alone, they remain far from satisfactory. Long-term follow-up data from the European registry, which includes patients receiving DLI with or without chemotherapy, confirm the poor results in AML, with 3-yr survival rates of only approx 20% *(18)*.

3.3. Acute Lymphoblastic Leukemia

The large IBMTR registry analysis of GVL by Horowitz et al. showed a GVL effect in acute lymphoblastic leukemia (ALL) that was associated largely with GVHD *(7)*. Thus, one might suspect that it could be possible to harness GVL in ALL through DLI. Anecdotal reports have shown clear responses to DLI in ALL patients *(9,33,34)*; in fact, the first successful DLI was in a patient with ALL *(9)*. However, analyses of larger patient groups have shown that the efficacy of DLI in ALL is quite limited *(16,17,35)*. The European registry includes 43 patients with ALL, with survival at 2 yr close to 0% *(16)*. We have analyzed DLI in 44 ALL patients *(35)*. Of 15 patients who received no pre-DLI chemotherapy, two patients achieved complete remissions, lasting 2+ and 3 yr. Of 29 patients who received DLI either as consolidation of remission or in the nadir period after chemotherapy, only one had ongoing remission. The overall survival at 3 yr was 13%.

3.4. Myelodysplasia

Data are limited regarding DLI in myelodysplasia (MDS) *(16,17,36)*. From published reports, it is often difficult to separate MDS from AML patients, and the two groups are often grouped together for analysis. In the European registry, one of four evaluable patients classified as having MDS responded to DLI *(16)*. In the North American registry, two of five patients responded *(17)*.

3.5. Myeloma

There is clearly a graft-vs-myeloma effect that can be harnessed with DLI. It is unclear, however, where DLI fits into the overall treatment strategy in this disease. Several case reports and small series have shown disease response in myeloma patients receiving DLI *(15,37–42)*; in almost all cases, the response was associated with significant GVHD. Two larger series, of 27 and 25 patients, respectively, have recently appeared in the literature *(43,44)*. In the first series 25 of 27 patients had received a partially T cell-depleted graft from an HLA-matched sibling *(43)*. DLIs were given a median of 30 mo after BMT, with the T cell dose varying between 1×10^6/kg and 5×10^8/kg; doses were escalated if patients did not respond to the earlier dose within 12 wk. Thirteen patients received chemotherapy before the DLI; most responded, but none had a complete response. Outcomes are shown in Table 4. Fourteen (52%) patients responded, with 22% having complete responses. Eight of the 14 responders had ongoing remissions with a median response duration of approx 15 mo. Factors associated with response to DLI were a T cell dose greater than 1×10^8/kg and remission before the initial transplant. GVHD was not associated with response in this study. However, this study did include 13 patients with data updated from an earlier report; in this earlier report, GVHD was associated with response, with 87 and 85% of the responders developing acute and chronic GVHD, respectively *(39)*.

In the second recent series, 23 of the 25 transplants were from HLA-matched related donors; only four patients had had T cell-depleted transplants *(44)*. The median T cell dose of the first

Table 4
DLI for MM

	Lokhorst et al. (43)	Salama et al. (44)
Number of patients	27	25
Responses		
CR to DLI	6 (22%)	4 (18%)[a]
CR to DLI + chemotherapy	—	3 (100%)[b]
PR to DLI	8 (30%)	3 (14%)[a]
Overall	14 (52%)	10 (40%)[c]
Required >1 DLI to respond	6 out of 14 (43%)	5 out of 10 (50%)
Outcome of responders		
Relapse	4 out of 14 (29%)	4 out of 10 (40%)
Died, toxicity	2 out of 14 (14%)	1 out of 10 (10%)
Ongoing CR or PR	8 out of 14 (57%)	5 out of 10 (50%)
No GVHD/responses	6 out of 14 (43%)	0 out of 10 (0%)
Median duration of remission	approx 15 mo	approx 6 mo

[a]Of 22 assessable patients.
[b]Of three assessable patients.
[c]Of the total 25 patients.
CR, complete remission; PR, partial response.

DLI was 1.0×10^8/kg. Nine patients received subsequent DLIs, with a median T cell dose of 3.3×10^8/kg. Three patients received chemotherapy shortly before the DLI; all three completely responded to the combination. Overall, 10 (40%) patients responded to therapy, with seven patients having complete responses. However, because of concomitant chemotherapy the contribution of DLI to response cannot be assessed in three of these patients; thus, four of 22 (18%) patients evaluable for response to DLI alone responded. As in the above study, responses were associated with a higher dose of T cells. Five patients had ongoing remissions with a median duration of response of 6 mo, shorter than that in the other large series discussed above. Also in contrast, all responders in this study had GVHD.

Thus, both of these studies concur in demonstrating a significant GVM effect of DLI, but in a limited number of patients. In the first study, five patients had ongoing remissions more than 30 mo after DLI. In the second study, one patient had an ongoing complete remission at 3 yr,. and another, although relapsing 10 wk after his DLI, had only a very low-level M protein fluctuating between undetectable and 0.5 g/dL for 7.5 yr before succumbing to infection associated with chronic GVHD. Also, both studies concur in suggesting that a high T cell dose is required in myeloma. However, it is also clear that the complete response rate to DLI in myeloma (18–22%) is not as pronounced as in CML. Moreover, the durability of remission is of concern, with the current studies suggesting relapse rates of 29–40%. Lastly, several studies have suggested that few responders escape significant GVHD as a complication; the second series shows a strong correlation between GVHD and GVM (44), as did the initial series of Lokhorst et al. (39). Several smaller series and case reports have also reported a high incidence of GVHD in myeloma patients responding to DLI (41).

3.6. Lymphoma and Chronic Lymphocytic Leukemia

The possibility of a graft-vs-lymphoma effect has been suggested by the lower relapse rate of lymphoma patients treated with allogeneic compared to autologous transplants. Several reports in the early 1990s studied non-Hodgkin's lymphoma (NHL) patients (generally intermediate grade lymphomas) treated with allogeneic BMT if the patient had a matched sibling, and with autologous BMT if not *(45–47)*. These studies concurred in showing significantly reduced relapse rates in recipients of allografts. Large analyses of follicular lymphoma allograft recipients have also suggested a graft-vs-lymphoma effect by showing an apparently flat disease-free survival curve *(48)*. Although follow-up is relatively short, and although it is conceivable that the increased relapse rate in the autograft recipients is explained by marrow tumor contamination, these studies have led to the perception that graft-vs-lymphoma may be a powerful effect. There have now been several reports documenting lymphoid neoplasms responding to DLI, thus confirming the existence of the effect *(49–55)*. However, the data regarding DLI in lymphoma is still rather limited, with most observations limited to case reports and small series. Thus, the likelihood of a given lymphoid neoplasm responding to DLI is difficult to assess. Investigators have reported responses to DLI in follicular lymphoma, chronic lymphocytic leukemia (CLL), diffuse large B cell lymphoma, mantle cell lymphoma, and lymphoblastic lymphoma. There is a perception that graft-vs-lymphoma may be particularly effective in low-grade B cell neoplasms, but an estimate of the likelihood of response in these lymphomas, as well as others, must await larger series.

3.7. Solid Tumors

Data regarding DLI in solid tumors are very preliminary. Early results in renal cell cancer are promising. As part of a nonmyeloablative transplant strategy, Childs and colleagues have treated renal cell cancer patients with DLI and observed clear responses *(56)*. Additional studies in renal cell cancer patients are ongoing. Conversely, nonmyeloablative transplants with planned DLI have not been successful in melanoma (R. Childs, personal communication). Limited observations suggest the possibility of a graft-vs-breast cancer effect *(57,58)*. Studies are ongoing, in particular at the U.S. National Institutes of Health, to assess the possibility of an antitumor effect of donor leukocytes in a variety of solid tumors.

4. DLI FOR INDICATIONS OTHER THAN MALIGNANCY

DLI is usually used for malignant diseases. However, the infusion of immunocompetent cells can be of use in other clinical situations, including infections and graft failure.

4.1. EBV-Associated Lymphoproliferative Disorder

EBV-infected B cells are normally kept under surveillance by EBV-specific T cells. These T cells are present at high frequencies, ranging from 1 in 400 to 1 in 3000 *(59)*. Under conditions of intensive immunosuppression, such as after bone marrow or solid organ transplantation, these T cells are reduced to the point where EBV-infected B cells can proliferate. This can lead to a lymphoma-like illness caused by polyclonal or monoclonal B cells *(60,61)*. In the post-BMT setting, EBV-lymphoproliferative disorder (LPD) occurs in the context of severe T cell depletion (generally in recipients of T cell depleted transplants) and results in a rapidly progressive and uniformly fatal course. The disorder almost always involves donor-derived B cells. On the assumption that increased T cell numbers might restore anti-EBV immunity, Papadopoulos et al. gave donor leukocytes to five patients with EBV-LPD *(62,63)*. All patients had had T cell-depleted transplants and anti-thymocyte globulin in the peritransplant period. The patients were treated with infusions of 1×10^6 T cells/kg. This dose was chosen because the threshold T cell dose for inducing GVHD in HLA-matched siblings is 1×10^5 T cells/kg at the time of transplantation, and animal studies suggest that a dose 10–50× greater than that required to induce GVHD can be tolerated without causing GVHD if given 3 or more weeks after transplantation. All five patients had complete remissions to DLI which were ongoing in three patients at several months. All three of these patients developed chronic GVHD as well.

Two patients who had begun to have respiratory failure, presumably due to pulmonary involvement with EBV-LPD, worsened after DLI and died. Neither patient had any evidence of EBV-LPD at autopsy; the cause of the respiratory failure could not be ascertained. Thus, these results show that anti-EBV immunity can be reconstituted and can rapidly eliminate EBV-infected B cells causing EBV-LPD; the adverse outcome, however, in two patients suggests that caution is required when utilizing this therapy. Other groups have studied DLI for this indication as well. One group observed no responses in three patients (64). Another group gave donor-derived EBV-specific cytotoxic T lymphocyte lines to 10 allograft recipients (65). Three patients with evidence of EBV reactivation responded within 3 wk of therapy, including a patient with overt EBV-LPD. This group has shown that EBV-specific T cells (genetically marked with the neomycin resistance gene) can persist for as long as 38 mo after infusion (31,66). A recent report of a larger number of patients confirmed the earlier encouraging findings, showing that such cell lines could prevent EBV-LPD and could successfully treat established disease (66). Others have reported success with irradiated donor lymphocytes and rituximab in the management of EBV-LPD after haploidentical BMT (67). Experience with DLI for solid organ transplant-associated EBV-LPD is limited, but successfully treated cases have been reported (68). EBV-LPD in the solid organ transplant setting is usually of recipient origin. Thus, donor cells must be chosen from a donor who is EBV seropositive, and who shares with the recipient HLA antigens that present EBV-derived peptides. DLI in this setting carries not only the risk of GVHD but of organ graft rejection as well.

4.2. Other Infections

Infusions of small numbers of donor leukocytes can be associated with rapid restoration of CD3+, CD4+, and CD8+ T cell numbers, and an increase in antigen-specific T cell responses. Some (69,70) (but not all [71]) patients have a broadening of the immune repertoire after DLI. Thus, it seems reasonable that DLI might be used to reconstitute immunity and treat infectious diseases after BMT. A variety of infections have been treated with DLI, including cytomegalovirus (CMV) (69,72) and adenovirus (73,74); however, data are relatively limited. The main risk, of course, for any such intervention, is the development of GVHD. Walter and colleagues have reported infusion of CD8+ CMV-specific cytotoxic T-cell clones in 14 patients at risk for CMV reactivation and disease after allogeneic BMT (72). The transfused clones persisted for at least 12 wk and were associated with an increase in cytotoxic activity against CMV. Neither CMV viremia nor CMV disease developed in any of the 14 patients. However, cytotoxic T cell activity declined in patients deficient in CMV-specific CD4+ T helper cells; this observation has led to ongoing studies involving both CD4+ and CD8+ CMV-specific clones (75).

4.3. Graft Failure

Stem cell transplant rejection is mediated by persistent host cells that prevent establishment of donor hemoatopoiesis. Infusions of unmanipulated DLI, without additional chemotherapy or immunosuppressive therapy, can reverse rejection and result in complete hematopoietic recovery (76).

5. COMPLICATIONS (TABLE 5)

5.1. GVHD

GVHD is the most significant complication of DLI. In the European registry analysis, 59% of the patients developed acute GVHD, with 41% requiring treatment (16); chronic GVHD was not detailed in this study. In the North American registry analysis, 60% of the patients developed acute GVHD (17). The median time post-DLI to the development of acute GVHD was

Table 5
Complications of DLI *(16,17)*

GVHD	
Acute, grade II–IV	41–46%
Acute, grade III–IV	22%
Chronic, extensive	32%
Chronic, limited	29%
Pancytopenia	20%
Nonrelapse mortality, 1-yr	14–18%

32 d *(17)*. The incidence of grade II–IV acute GVHD was 46%, and the incidence of grade III–IV acute GVHD was 22%. The incidence of chronic GVHD in this study was 61%, with 47% of the chronic GVHD patients having limited disease, and 53% having extensive disease. Factors predictive of GVHD in the European study were IFN treatment and T cell depletion of the initial BMT. Interferon was also predictive of GVHD in the North American study, as was post-BMT chronic GVHD; however, T cell depletion of the initial BMT was not predictive of GVHD in this study. Several modifications of DLI have been attempted to reduce GVHD and are discussed in more detail below.

5.2. Pancytopenia

Pancytopenia occurs in approx 20% of patients *(16,17)*. The likelihood of pancytopenia depends on the status of the disease. It occurs in as many as 50% of CML patients in hematologic relapse, but is very infrequent in patients with cytogenetic or molecular relapse *(14,25)*. Pancytopenia correlates with a low degree of donor-derived hematopoiesis at the time of DLI *(77)*. This supports the hypothesis that pancytopenia results when donor lymphocytes ablate recipient cells, but donor stem cells are inadequate to allow recovery of hematopoiesis. Patients may recover with observation-alone, with a course of G-CSF, or with infusion of bone marrow or peripheral blood stem cells. One might suspect that infusion of stem cells along with DLI would prevent pancytopenia, but one study suggests that this strategy is inadequate (discussed in Section 10.1.6.) *(78)*. Probably the best way to avoid pancytopenia is to treat the patient early in the course of relapse.

5.3. Treatment-Related Mortality

In the European registry study, 17 of the 135 patients died in remission *(16)*. Six died with myelosuppression, four patients died with GVHD, four patients died with the combination of GVHD and myelosuppression, and three patients died with other causes. The actuarial probability of death in remission at 1 yr for CML patients was 18%. In the North American study, 17 of the 140 patients died from causes other than progressive disease *(17)*. Eight patients died from GVHD, six patients died from infection, and patients died from other causes. The probability of death not related to malignancy was 14% at 1 yr and 18% at 2 yr.

6. ASSOCIATION OF GVHD WITH RESPONSE

GVHD is closely correlated with response. In the North American registry study, 42 of 45 assessable complete responders developed acute GVHD, and 36 of 41 assessable complete responders developed chronic GVHD *(17)*. The correlation of acute and chronic GVHD with complete remission was highly statistically significant ($p < 0.00001$). In this study, of the 23 patients who did not develop either acute or chronic GVHD, only three patients attained complete remission. However, it is important to point out that many responders have been reported in the literature who did not develop clinically detectable GVHD. For example, although the European registry analysis reported a high response rate in CML patients who developed GVHD or myelosuppression (91%), they also reported that 45% of patients without any GVHD or myelosuppression had responses (however, it should be noted that this group did not report data regarding chronic GVHD) *(16)*. Almost all reports of DLI have included at least a small number of patients who responded without GVHD, and in some studies, this number has been fairly high *(23,24,79)*. Thus, while GVHD is usually associated with response in patients receiving standard DLI, the observation of apparent GVL without GVHD in some patients is encouraging and has led to a variety of approaches aimed at separating the two phenomena.

7. ASSOCIATION OF CELL DOSE WITH GVHD

Animal and human BMT studies suggest that a given T cell dose is more or less likely to cause GVHD depending on how soon it is given after the transplant preparative regimen. The milieu of excessive inflammatory cytokines characteristic of the early period posttransplant is especially likely to activate potentially alloreactive cells *(80)*. Animal studies show that 10–50× more T cells than the usual number required to induce GVHD can be tolerated without causing GVHD if given 3 or more weeks after transplantation *(81)*. In human BMT, the threshold T cell dose for inducing GVHD in HLA-matched siblings is 1×10^5/kg at the time of transplantation *(82)*. Mackinnon et al. showed that up to 1×10^7 T cells/kg could be given without causing GVHD when infused 9 mo to several years after the initial transplant *(23)*. Additional human DLI studies suggest that such a cell dose is more likely to cause GVHD if given closer to transplant. For example, in one study, 100% of patients developed GVHD when given prophylactic DLI—1×10^7 T cells/kg—at d 30 posttransplant despite concomitant prophylactic immunosuppression *(83)*. Although it is apparent that T cells are more likely to cause GVHD the closer they are given to transplantation, it is difficult to translate this into a specific recommendation regarding the safe T cell dose at a given interval posttransplant. The safe dose probably depends on several other factors in addition to timing, including preparative regimen (e.g., myeloablative vs nonmyeloablative), the patient's clinical status (e.g., actively infected vs not), and the particular minor histocompatibility differences in a given donor–recipient pair.

8. LONG-TERM FOLLOW-UP

As noted above, long-term follow-up of CML patients has suggested that the majority of remissions are durable in patients with molecular, cytogenetic, or hematologic relapse *(18,25,30)*. However, overall survival is limited to some degree by mortality from nonrelapse causes, and in patients with more advanced disease, by relapse (Fig. 1). An interesting pattern of relapse has been reported in AML and myeloma patients, with some patients recurring in extramedullary sites, while the bone marrow remains free of disease *(84–86)*. This suggests that appropriate homing is likely a critical component of successful DLI, with lymphocytes homing to certain areas (and not to others) based on the expression of certain cell surface molecules *(87)*.

9. DLI FROM PATIENTS OTHER THAN MATCHED SIBLINGS

One recent report has looked specifically at the outcomes of DLIs from unrelated donors *(88)*. This report included 25 CML patients, 23 AML patients, seven ALL patients, and three patients with other diseases. The complete response rates for evaluable patients were 46% for CML, 42% for AML, and 50% (2 out of 4) for ALL. Disease-free survival at 1 yr after complete

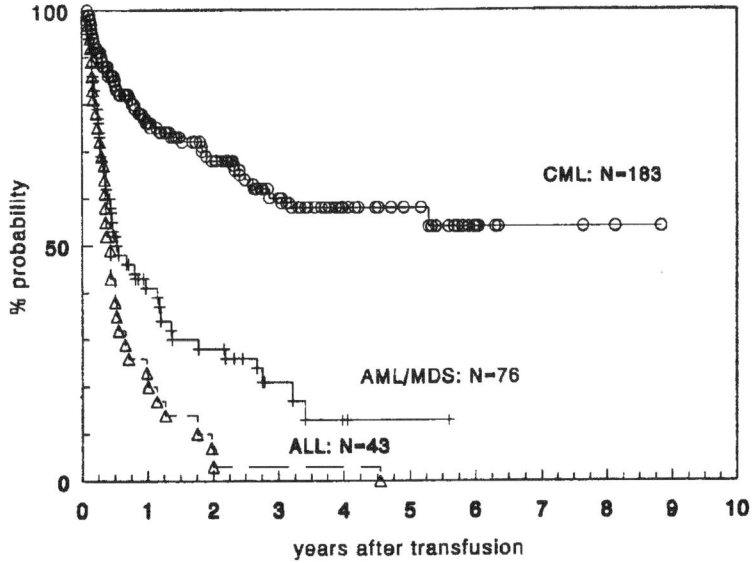

Fig. 1. Long-term survival data from the European survey by Kolb et al. *(18).*

remission was 65% for CML, 23% for AML, and 30% for ALL. Interestingly, the incidence and severity of acute and chronic GVHD did not appear to be worse than that seen in DLI from matched siblings. A possible explanation for this finding is that patients who relapse after unrelated BMT may be a selected group with a lower risk of GVHD; the most susceptible patients to severe GVHD may have died of GVHD after the initial transplant or have had severe enough GVHD after transplant that they were deemed to be poor candidates for DLI. Another interesting finding of this study was that cell dose did not correlate with response, survival, or GVHD. Because there was no association between cell dose and GVHD, the authors of this study recommended $0.1–1.0 \times 10^8$ mononuclear cells (MNC)/kg as a reasonable dose in unrelated DLI. The only factors predictive of improved survival and disease-free survival were the intervals from BMT to relapse and BMT to DLI, respectively; patients treated within 1 year of BMT had an increased incidence of disease-related death, probably because patients relapsing and requiring treatment earlier have more aggressive disease.

There are very few data regarding DLI from HLA-mismatched family members. The few cases reported suggest that the treatment may have the potential for disease activity but carries a high risk of GVHD *(89).*

10. MODIFICATIONS OF DLI

10.1. Attempts to Lessen Toxicity (Table 6)

10.1.1. ESCALATING DOSES

As noted above, most early DLIs have involved large cell doses, generally on the order of 1×10^8 T cells/kg; GVHD is commonly observed after infusion of these doses. Several groups have studied lower doses to determine if there might be a dose at which GVL occurs but GVHD does not *(9,23,24).* Mackinnon et al. studied 22 patients with relapsed CML: eight patients in cytogenetic or molecular relapse, 10 patients in chronic phase, and four patients in accelerated phase *(23).* Patients received escalating doses of T cells at intervals of 4- to 33-wk, with eight dose levels between 1×10^5 and 5×10^8/kg. Nineteen of 22 patients achieved remission, with remissions achieved at the following doses: 1×10^7 $(n = 8)$, 5×10^7 $(n = 4)$, 1×10^8 $(n = 3)$, and 5×10^8 $(n = 4)$. GVHD correlated with the T cell dose given, with only 1 of the 8 patients who

Table 6
Attempts to Lessen Toxicity of DLI

Escalating doses
CD8+ depletion
T cell lines and clones
Suicide gene-transduced T cells
Irradiated DLI
G-CSF mobilization

attained remission at 1×10^7/kg developing GVHD, while eight of the 11 responders who received doses of $\geq 5 \times 10^7$/kg developed GVHD. It should be noted that in patients treated with escalating doses, it is difficult to tell which dose an individual responds to. Since response to DLI can take many weeks to occur, it is always possible that a response to an escalated dose is actually a response to an earlier, lower dose. In addition, it should be noted that most of the responses to lower cell doses in this study occurred in patients with molecular or cytogenetic relapses. Regardless, the observation of GVL without clinical GVHD is important. Whether this represents a true leukemia-specific response is unclear (discussed below).

Others have also reported patients treated with escalating doses of T cells. Dazzi et al. reported that patients treated with an escalating dose regimen were as likely to respond as patients treated with a single bulk dose *(24)*; however, the incidence of GVHD was much lower in the group receiving escalating doses (10 vs 44%). A very interesting analysis of this study concerned only a subset of patients treated by bulk dose vs escalating doses, in which the final cell doses infused were comparable; the incidence and severity of acute and chronic GVHD were significantly lower for the group of patients treated with escalating doses. This finding suggests that the incidence of GVHD associated with escalating doses is low not because the final cell dose is small, but because lymphocytes were given over a prolonged period. The mechanisms underlying this observation are unknown. The authors propose two possibilities. First, that the escalating dose regimen may be associated with less GVHD because the full cell dose is infused later after the BMT than it is in patients receiving bulk doses (this explanation could be compatible with animal studies suggesting that delayed infusion is associated with less GVHD). The second possibility is that the initial infused cells may be anergized and play a regulatory role by inhibiting alloresponses of subsequent T cell infusions. It should be noted, however, that this particular subset analysis involved relatively small numbers of patients (e.g., only 12 patients were in the escalating dose group); additional studies are needed to confirm the observation.

10.1.2. CD8+-DEPLETED DLI

Animal and clinical studies have suggested that depletion of CD8+ T cells from the bone marrow inoculum may reduce the incidence of GVHD *(90,91)*. Based on these observations, two groups have investigated DLI-depleted of CD8+ cells *(79,92)*. In the first study, 10 CML patients received a mean cell dose of 4.65×10^7 CD4+ and 0.6×10^6 CD8+ T cells/kg *(79)*. Six patients achieved remissions, with GVHD developing in three patients (acute, 2; chronic, 1). In the second study, 40 patients with hematologic malignancies (CML, 25; multiple myeloma [MM], 7; others, 8) received targeted doses of CD4+ T-cells *(92)*. Cohorts received 0.3, 1.0, or 1.5×10^8 CD4+ cells/kg. Six of 27 patients (22%) who received 0.3×10^8 CD4+ cells/kg developed GVHD, compared with 6 of 11 (55%) who received $\geq 1.0 \times 10^8$ CD4+ cells/kg. All patients in this trial who developed GVHD also had a response; however, 48% of responding patients did not develop GVHD. Thus, these studies suggest that CD8+ depletion may result in less GVHD, but larger studies are required to allow firm conclusions.

10.1.3. CELL LINES AND CLONES

Antigen-specific T cell lines and clones represent the most rational way to deliver specific immunity while avoiding GVHD. However, relatively few groups have applied to the clinic the difficult technology involved in growing large numbers of these cells. This approach is most feasible when viruses are the targets of immunotherapy and, as discussed above, two groups have reported fairly large groups of patients treated with CMV-specific T cell clones or EBV-specific cytotoxic T cell lines *(65,66,72)*. The study of leukemia-reactive cytotoxic T cell lines has been more limited. Falkenburg et al. reported a patient with CML in accelerated phase after allogeneic BMT *(93,94)*. This patient had a suboptimal response to an unmanipulated DLI. Cytotoxic T cell lines were then generated from her HLA identical donor using a modification of a limiting dilution assay. The cells were selected based on their ability to inhibit the growth of CML progenitor cells in vitro and then expanded in vitro to generate cytotoxic T cell lines. Three lines lysed patient leukemic cells as well as inhibiting the growth of leukemic progenitor cells; the cells did not react with lymphocytes from the recipient. Shortly after infusion of a cumulative cell dose of 3.2×10^9 cytotoxic T cells, the patient had a complete molecular response. Additional investigators are exploring the use of cytotoxic T cell lines directed against hematopoietic tissue-restricted minor histocompatibility antigens, but clinical results have not been reported *(95)*.

10.1.4. SUICIDE GENE-TRANSDUCED DONOR T CELLS

Cycling T cells transduced with the HSV1 thymidine kinase (HSV-TK) gene are susceptible to killing by ganciclovir *(96–101)*. Thus, conceivably, GVH reactions initiated by HSV-TK-transduced T cells might be ameliorated by administration of ganciclovir *(98)*. (Other potential suicide genes exist, but to date, clinical studies have involved HSV-TK.) Bonini et al. reported eight patients with relapsed malignancy post-BMT who received escalating doses of HSV-TK transduced lymphocytes from their original HLA-matched sibling donor *(97)*. Patients received a range of $0.5–38.6 \times 10^6$ transduced T cells/kg. Gene modified cells were detected repeatedly in blood, marrow, and tissue biopsies in all but one patient. The percentage of transduced cells among circulating lymphocytes ranged from 1 in 104 to 13.4% and could be detected for more than 12 mo after the last infusion. Five patients had disease responses, and three patients developed GVHD. Two patients with acute GVHD had complete resolution of all signs of GVHD after treatment with ganciclovir; a third patient with chronic GVHD had a partial response to ganciclovir, but despite prolonged treatment with ganciclovir, all gene-modified cells were not eliminated. The two patients with complete disease responses who received ganciclovir for GVHD remained in complete remission. Tiberghien et al. have treated 12 patients with HSV-TK-transduced T cells given concomitantly with a T cell-depleted BMT *(100)*. Cohorts of patients received gene-modified T cells at one of three dose levels, 2×10^5, 6×10^5, or 20×10^5 cells/kg. These cells circulated for a prolonged time and induced GVHD in four patients. Two of three patients who developed acute GVHD responded to treatment with ganciclovir, as did the one patient who developed chronic GVHD.

Thus, this area of research has promise. However, potential obstacles should be appreciated. First, the technical challenges of vector design, and optimal cell transduction, expansion, and selection are formidable. In addition, even if technical issues are completely solved, potential theoretical challenges remain: even if all transduced T cells are eliminated, it is conceivable that a downstream cascade of secondary effectors involved in GVHD will have been initiated that cannot be stopped; if GVHD is completely abrogated, it is conceivable that GVL will be abrogated as well; as the suicide gene is a foreign protein, it may induce an immune response, resulting in elimination of transduced cells *(102)*.

10.1.5. Irradiated DLI

Irradiated T cells retain cytotoxic activity against tumor cells. Because these cells are not able to proliferate, their ability to cause GVHD should be limited. Waller et al. have demonstrated in an animal model that irradiated donor T cells facilitate engraftment and mediate GVL (103,104). Early clinical trials assessing this approach are under way. Success of this approach will be limited if significant proliferation of T cells is required for optimal GVL.

10.1.6. Mobilizing DLI with G-CSF to Avoid Pancytopenia

As discussed above, it is considered likely that pancytopenia results after DLI when donor lymphocytes eliminate recipient hematopoiesis and inadequate donor cells are present to reconstitute hematopoiesis (77). If so, then infusing hematopoietic stem cells along with lymphocytes (most easily accomplished by collecting the DLI after mobilization with G-CSF) might lessen the likelihood of pancytopenia. However, one study suggests that this approach does not prevent aplasia (78). In a nonrandomized comparison of two groups receiving DLI—one with G-CSF-mobilized cells and one without—G-CSF mobilization did not result in any difference in incidence, time to onset, or duration of cytopenia. This suggests that some patients may have failure of hematopoiesis from other, as yet undefined, mechanisms. Lastly, some studies suggest that G-CSF administration alters the cytokine profiles of dendritic cells and T cells (105–107); the clinical significance of these effects in terms of disease response is unknown.

10.2. Attempts to Improve Disease Activity (Table 7)

10.2.1. Pre-DLI Chemotherapy

GVL effects can take several weeks to evolve in DLI recipients; therefore, it is conceivable that the reason why some patients with extensive or fast-growing disease do poorly with DLI is that GVL effects do not have sufficient time to evolve. If so, then debulking disease with pre-DLI chemotherapy may be a necessary intervention. The study discussed in Section 3.2., involving this approach in AML, suggests that pre-DLI chemotherapy may somewhat improve the outcome of patients with advanced disease treated with DLI, but it must be noted that the overall outcome is still fairly poor, with overall disease-free survival of less than 20% (32). This suggests that poor results in these patients are due to more than just fast growth rate. Given the excellent activity of imatinib (STI-571, Gleevec) in CML (108,109), some have suggested that this agent might be used to debulk CML before DLI. Because complete response rates are so high with this agent, lower cell doses would likely be sufficient, with a lower risk of GVHD. If, however, CML cells presenting antigen are required for GVL, then debulking CML below a certain level with imatinib might prevent GVL effects from developing.

10.2.2. Administration of DLI in the Minimal Residual Disease State

Almost all patients with cytogenetic or molecular relapses of CML have complete responses to DLI. Moreover, these responses can often be obtained without GVHD by using lower T cell doses or the escalating dose regimen of Dazzi et al. discussed above (23,24). Thus, one could argue that CML patients should be followed closely with PCR, preferably quantitative PCR, and treated at the earliest sign of relapse. However, it should be noted that some investigators have raised questions about the reliability of the PCR in predicting full-blown relapse.

Some investigators have argued that DLI's success in salvaging early relapse of CML after allogeneic BMT suggests an alteration of the general transplant strategy for this disease (110,111). These investigators have suggested that patients first receive a T cell-depleted transplant; patients curable with high-dose therapy alone will be cured and will incur much less risk of GVHD. Those patients who require GVL effects for cure would be detected by close monitoring after BMT and early intervention with DLI; DLI for early relapse could be given

Table 7
Attempts to Improve Disease Activity of DLI

Pre-DLI chemotherapy
Administration in the Minimal Residual Disease State
DLI and IL-2
T cell lines and clones
Immunization of the donor

at a lower dose with less risk of GVHD. One study of this approach reports a 4% treatment-related mortality and an 80% 5-yr survival rate *(110)*.

Patients with certain diseases and disease statuses are at very high risk of relapse after allogeneic BMT. Some investigators have studied the potential role of prophylactic DLI in this setting. The Seattle group reported a randomized trial several years ago, in which the study group received additional buffy coat cells in the peritransplant period *(112)*. This was associated with a very high rate of severe GVHD, which likely cancelled out any possible antitumor benefit. Since then, animal studies have suggested that GVHD may be minimized by infusing lymphocytes later after the transplant *(113,114)*. Thus, more recent studies of prophylactic DLI have given the cells several weeks after the transplant *(83,115–117)*. It is too early to assess the benefit of this strategy, although the incidence of GVHD still appears to be fairly high. One study suggests that delaying the infusion past d 45 may result in an acceptable incidence of GVHD *(83)*.

10.2.3. DLI PLUS INTERLEUKIN-2

Several patients have received interleukin (IL)-2 with DLI *(9,118)*. Slavin et al. have reported a strategy of allogeneic cell therapy involving, first, escalating doses of unmanipulated DLI, followed in nonresponders by DLI plus IL-2, followed by, in patients who still do not respond, donor leukocytes activated in vitro with IL-2 and given along with IL-2 *(9)*. Ten of 17 patients with acute and chronic leukemia in relapse achieved complete remission. Four patients with cytogenetic relapses responded to DLI alone, whereas five of six patients with overt hematologic relapse responded only after additional activation of cells with IL-2. Since responses to DLI can take several weeks to occur, it is possible that responses to DLI plus IL-2 were actually responses to previous DLI.

10.2.4. IMMUNIZATION OF THE DONOR WITH TUMOR-SPECIFIC PROTEIN BEFORE DLI

The immunoglobulin idiotype serves as a tumor-specific protein in myeloma and B cell lymphomas and might be used to vaccinate the donor before DLI. Clinical experience with this approach is limited, but encouraging findings have included the detection of idiotype-specific T cell responses in vivo after BMT, and a complete and prolonged remission after DLI in one patient *(119,120)*.

11. NONMYELOABLATIVE STEM CELL TRANSPLANTS

The successes of DLI have led many groups to explore new ways of carrying our transplants that emphasize the GVM effects of donor leukocytes and minimize reliance on toxic doses of chemotherapy and radiotherapy. Investigators of nonmyeloablative stem cell transplantation (NST) have developed preparative regimens that are less toxic than standard transplant regimens, but are nevertheless immunosuppressive enough to allow donor cell engraftment; engrafted donor immune cells, it is hoped, will then mediate antitumor effects (*see* Chapter 13) *(121–123)*. Responses have been observed in several malignancies, sometimes only after additional DLIs have been given to boost antitumor activity; GVHD and treatment-related mortality may be less frequent than seen after standard transplant, but these problems can continue to be quite substantial. Additional studies along these lines will investigate increasingly reliable and well-tolerated preparative regimens. However, experience with DLI has taught that many diseases are unresponsive to graft-vs-tumor mechanisms and that cellular therapy can frequently be associated with serious toxicity. Thus, major strides in this area will require an improved understanding of basic mechanisms involved in GVHD, GVM, and engraftment.

12. MECHANISMS OF DLI

Our current understanding of the mechanisms of human GVL is relatively limited (*see* Chapters 24 and 25 for more thorough discussion of GVL mechanisms). It is likely that the mechanisms of GVL vary among different diseases and even among different individuals with the same disease. Possible target antigens include antigens expressed only by leukemic cells (true GVL targets), antigens expressed by both leukemic cells and normal nonhematopoietic cells (GVH targets), and antigens which are expressed by both normal and malignant hematopoietic tissue *(124)*. Additional possible target antigens are antigens shared between donor and host, in effect autoantigens. T cells with high affinity for self antigens are deleted in the thymus and the periphery, but T cells with low affinity for self antigens can persist and become pathogenic under certain circumstances. Potential effectors in GVL reactions include T cells with αβT cell receptors, T cells with γδ receptors, and natural killer (NK) cells. In addition, it is possible that various cytokines released in a dysregulated fashion as part of an exuberant immune reaction could affect leukemia cells nonspecifically *(80)*. Recent findings suggest that hematopoietic tissue-restricted antigens can be the targets of GVL reactions *(125–127)*. One might expect such reactions to occur without GVHD. However, clinical observations have shown that disparity for a single hematopoietic tissue-restricted minor histocompatibility antigen, HA-1, is associated with a high risk of GVHD *(128)*. A possible explanation for this is that activation of the T cells specific for HA-1 might lead to production of cytokines that stimulate other, more broadly alloreactive T cell clones *(126)*.

Clinical observations of DLI patients suggest that the mechanism of response to DLI may involve alloreactive T cells. GVHD and GVL are often closely correlated, as discussed above *(17)*. In addition, resolution of CML in one study was associated with the conversion of mixed T cell chimerism to full donor T cell chimerism, even in patients who did not develop GVHD, suggesting that the target antigen was shared between leukemic and normal cells (T cells usually are not involved in the CML clone) *(23)*. However, these observations do not rule out the possibility that GVHD and GVL were mediated by separate GVH- and GVL-specific clones that expanded simultaneously.

Most supposition about GVL mechanisms derives from extrapolation from animal models or from after-the-fact inferences about clinical events. However, DLI represents a unique opportunity to study GVL mechanisms by allowing careful study of patients during the evolution of actual tumor responses. A few groups have taken this approach. In particular, the group led by J. Ritz has studied the T-cell repertoire of several CML and myeloma patients during response to DLI *(42,70,129,130)*. In each responding patient, these investigators were able to identify the expansion of at least one Vβ gene subfamily that occurred simultaneously with cytogenetic response *(70,129)*. In one patient, further study showed that the Vβ gene subfamily expansion was associated with the appearance of clonal T cells. This clone was further characterized by direct sequencing of the CDR3 region. Further characterization of T cell clones associated with GVL is ongoing. An additional study by this group has used SEREX technology to show that antibodies specific for certain proteins are temporally associated with the response to DLI, suggesting a role for B cell immunity in GVL *(130)*. Others have attempted to study GVL mechanisms by studying cells collected from the patient at the time of disease response. Bunjes et al. documented increased patient-reactive helper T lymphocyte precursor frequencies in association with the development of acute GVHD and bone marrow aplasia in DLI patients *(131)*, and Jiang et al. showed modest increases in the cytotoxic lymphocyte precursor frequency against leukemic cells and an increase in NK cell activity in CML patients responding to DLI *(132)*. Smit et al. developed additional assays to look specifically at antihost progenitor cell activity and showed that the GVL effect in responding CML patients was associated with T cells recognizing leukemic CD34+ progenitor cells *(133)*. Thus, these early studies suggest the promise of studying cell populations during actual GVL. More sophisticated assays of antigen-specific T cells, using, for example, tetramer analysis or intracellular cytokine expression will likely shed further light on the nature and specificity of immune cells mediating GVL *(134–136)*.

A relatively little-studied aspect of DLI involves sensitivity of tumor tissue to potential GVL effectors. An effective immune response requires not only appropriate effector cells, but also proper antigen processing, presentation of antigen in the presence of co-stimulatory molecules by tumor cells or professional antigen-presenting cells, expression of adhesion molecules by tumor cells, and intact pathways allowing the target cell to undergo apoptosis. Deficiency in any one of these components would impair GVL reactivity *(137)*. Conceivably, study of patients relapsing from previous DLI-induced responses might lead to insights into mechanisms of resistance. Along these lines, Dermine et al. studied patients relapsing after transplant and showed that many critical cell surface molecules involved in immune responses had been downregulated in leukemia cells at the time of relapse compared to pretransplant cells; this was associated with a decrease in responsiveness to lysis by cytotoxic T cells and NK cells *(138)*.

13. ALTERNATIVES TO DLI (TABLE 8)

A variety of other treatments have been used in patients with relapsed malignancy after allogeneic BMT. Second transplants have been applied successfully in relapsed patients but the approach is associated with significant morbidity and mortality *(139–142)* *(see* Chapter XX for discussion). IFN-α has been used to treat CML in relapse *(143–145)*. This treatment induces durable complete remission in approx 25% of patients treated in hematologic relapse. Results appear to be better in patients with cytogenetic relapse. Higano et al. reported complete remissions in 12 of 14 patients with cytogenetic relapse treated with IFN-α at doses starting at 1–3 million $U/m^2/d$ and adjusted as needed to maintain modest cytopenia *(144)*. The treatment was generally well-tolerated, with only one patient stopping therapy because of toxicity. Complete remission occurred at a median of 7.5 mo, and eight patients (57%) remained in remission with follow-up ranging from 10+ to 54+ mo. Discontinuation of immunosuppression can result in remission in CML as well as other malignancies *(146–149)*. Most patients reported have had CML, with remissions reported in all phases of relapse, although responses are more likely in patients with cytogenetic relapses. In one study, 10 of 20 patients with CML had complete remissions after immunosuppression withdrawal *(148)*. Responses were associated with GVHD. Given the frequency of remission to this maneuver, it is likely that many cases reported as responses to DLI were actually responses to the discontinuation of immunosuppression that preceded DLI. Lastly, G-CSF has been reported to result in remission in patients with CML, AML, and ALL *(150,151)*. The mechanism of this effect is unknown; some (but not all) of these patients had discontinuation of immunosuppression before G-CSF administration, suggesting that some of the patients may have developed GVL on this basis. The new agent imatinib (STI-571) has pronounced activity in CML and minimal toxicity *(108,109)*; its use in

Table 8
Alternatives to DLI

Second tranplant
IFN-α
Discontinuation of immunosuppression
G-CSF
Imatinib (STI-571)

the posttransplant relapse setting is under study. Thus, there are many alternatives to DLI in the management of relapsed disease, but comparative trials are needed. Comparative trials in CML should ensure that groups of treated patients are comparable; a recently published risk assessment tool incorporating five prognostic factors will be useful in this regard (152).

14. DLI IN PERSPECTIVE

The use of DLI to induce remission of relapsed disease after BMT has generated a great deal of enthusiasm. This enthusiasm is justified in certain instances, CML in particular. Many would argue that the current treatment of choice in relapsed CML is DLI, given in as early a relapse as possible, and using a dose escalating scheme. However, the risk assessment system mentioned above would suggest that some patients with relapsed CML have a long expected survival regardless (152). Lastly, given the activity and minimal toxicity of imatinib (STI-571), one has to wonder if it will supplant DLI in managing relapsed disease.

However, the enthusiasm for DLI is not justified in several other areas. There is very minimal activity in ALL with minimal chance of long-term survival. Likewise, AML patients usually do not benefit from the treatment; this is especially so for patients who require treatment within 6 mo of BMT. One could argue that ALL and AML patients should not be treated with DLI except in the context of well-designed clinical trials investigating novel approaches. The usefulness of DLI remains unclear in myeloma, as current studies are somewhat conflicting. Certainly the likelihood of remission in this disease is much less than in CML, although durable remissions are sometimes seen. Although there seems to be a great deal of excitement about DLI in low-grade NHL and CLL, it should be noted that there are currently few data concerning DLI in these diseases. The role of DLI in solid tumors requires a great deal more investigation at this point. It must be kept in mind that DLI remains a toxic and risky procedure with a significant risk of debilitating GVHD or death; although some new approaches show promise in being able to ameliorate GVHD, data regarding their use are relatively limited.

The successes of DLI have led to a general embracing of NST as a new treatment modality, which aims to emphasize GVL in the clinic (121–123). However, based on the experience with DLI, it is likely that NST will have many of the same problems, including low response rates in certain diseases and significant morbidity and mortality due to GVHD and infection.

DLI has done a great deal to show us that GVL can be purposefully harnessed, and it has led to completely new ways of thinking about allogeneic transplantation. Certain avenues of clinical and translational research have great promise in this field, in particular antigen-specific T cell clones and lines. However, at this point, meaningful advances in this area will likely require a much better understanding of the basic mechanisms underlying GVL.

REFERENCES

1. Barnes D, Loutit J, Neal F. Treatment of murine leukemia with x-rays and homologous bone marrow. *Bri Med J* 1956;2:626–630.
2. Truitt RL, Johnson B. Principles of graft-vs.-leukemia reactivity. *Biol Blood Marrow Transplant* 1995;1:61–68.

3. Gale RP, Champlin RE. How does bone-marrow transplantation cure leukaemia? *Lancet* 1984;2:28–30.
4. Weiden PL, Flournoy N, Thomas ED, et al. Antileukemic effect of graft-versus-host disease in human recipients of allogeneic-marrow grafts. *N Engl J Med* 1979;300:1068–1073.
5. Weiden PL, Sullivan KM, Flournoy N, Storb R, Thomas ED. The Seattle Marrow Transplant Team: antileukemic effect of chronic graft-versus-host disease. Contribution to improved survival after allogeneic marrow transplantation. *N Engl J Med* 1981;304:1529.
6. Mitsuyasu RT, Champlin RE, Gale RP, et al. Treatment of donor bone marrow with monoclonal anti-T-cell antibody and complement for the prevention of graft-versus-host disease. A prospective, randomized, double-blind trial. *Ann Intern Med* 1986;105:20–26.
7. Horowitz MM, Gale RP, Sondel PM, et al. Graft-versus-leukemia reactions following bone marrow transplantation in humans. *Blood* 1990;75:555–562.
8. Kolb HJ, Mittermuller J, Clemm C, et al. Donor leukocyte transfusions for treatment of recurrent chronic myelogenous leukemia in marrow transplant patients. *Blood* 1990;76:2462–2465.
9. Slavin S, Naparstek E, Nagler A, Ackerstein A, Samuel S, Kapelushnik J. Allogeneic cell therapy with donor peripheral blood cells and recombinant human interleukin-2 to treat leukemia relapse after allogeneic bone marrow transplantation. *Blood* 1996;87:2195–2204.
10. Bar BM, Schattenberg A, Mensink EJ, et al. Donor leukocyte infusions for chronic myeloid leukemia relapsed after allogeneic bone marrow transplantation. *J Clin Oncol* 1993;11:513–519.
11. Drobyski WR, Keever CA, Roth MS, et al. Salvage immunotherapy using donor leukocyte infusions as treatment for relapsed chronic myelogenous leukemia after allogeneic bone marrow transplantation: efficacy and toxicity of a defined T-cell dose. *Blood* 1993;82:2310–2318.
12. Hertenstein B, Wiesneth M, Novotny J, et al. Interferon-a and donor buffy coat transfusions for treatment of relapsed chronic myeloid leukemia after allogeneic bone marrow transplantation. *Transplantation* 1993;56:1114–1118.
13. Porter DL, Roth MS, McGarigle C, Ferrara JL, Antin JH. Induction of graft-versus-host disease as immunotherapy for relapsed chronic myeloid leukemia. *N Engl J Med* 1994;330:100–106.
14. van Rhee F, Lin f, Cullis JO, et al. Relapse of chronic myeloid leukemia after allogeneic bone marrow transplant: the case for giving donor leukocyte transfusions before the onset of hematologic relapse. *Blood* 1994;83:3377–3383.
15. Collins Jr. RH, Pineiro LA, Nemunaitis JJ, et al. Transfusion of donor buffy coat cells in the treatment of persistent or recurrent malignancy after allogeneic bone marrow transplantation. *Transfusion* 1995;35:891–898.
16. Kolb HJ, Schattenberg A, Goldman JM, et al. Graft-versus-leukemia effect of donor lymphocyte transfusions in marrow grafted patients. European Group for Blood and Marrow Transplantation Working Party Chronic Leukemia. *Blood* 1995;86:2041–2050.
17. Collins RH, Jr., Shpilberg O, Drobyski WR, et al. Donor leukocyte infusions in 140 patients with relapsed malignancy after allogeneic bone marrow transplantation. *J Clin Oncol* 1997;15:433–444.
18. Kolb HJ. Donor leukocyte transfusions for treatment of leukemic relapse after bone marrow transplantation. EBMT Immunology and Chronic Leukemia Working Parties. *Vox Sang* 1998;74:321–329.
19. Porter DL, Antin JH. The graft-versus-leukemia effects of allogeneic cell therapy. *Annu Rev Med* 1999;50:369–386.
20. Dazzi F, Szydlo RM, Goldman JM. Donor lymphocyte infusions for relapse of chronic myeloid leukemia after allogeneic stem cell transplant: where we now stand. *Exp Hematol* 1999;27:1477–1486.
21. Mackinnon S. Who may benefit from donor leucocyte infusions after allogeneic stem cell transplantation? *Br J Haematol* 2000;110:12–17.
22. Alyea E. Adoptive immunotherapy: insights from donor lymphocyte infusions. *Transfusion* 2000;40:393–395.
23. Mackinnon S, Papadopoulos EB, Carabasi MH, et al. Adoptive immunotherapy evaluating escalating doses of donor leukocytes for relapse of chronic myeloid leukemia after bone marrow transplantation: separation of graft-versus-leukemia responses from graft-versus-host disease. *Blood* 1995;86:1261–1268.
24. Dazzi F, Szydlo RM, Craddock C, et al. Comparison of single-dose and escalating-dose regimens of donor lymphocyte infusion for relapse after allografting for chronic myeloid leukemia. *Blood* 2000;95:67–71.
25. Dazzi F, Szydlo RM, Cross NCP, et al. Durability of responses following donor lymphocyte infusions for patients who relapse after allogeneic stem cell transplantation for chronic myeloid leukemia. *Blood* 2000;96:2712–2716.
26. Baurmann H, Nagel S, Binder T, Neubauer A, Siegert W, Huhn D. Kinetics of the graft-versus-leukemia response after donor leukocyte infusins for relapsed chronic myeloid leukemia after allogeneic bone marrow transplantation. *Blood* 1998;92:3582–3590.
27. Raanani P, Dazzi F, Sohal J, et al. The rate and kinetics of molecular response to donor leucocyte transfusions in chronic myeloid leukaemia patients treated for relapse after allogeneic bone marrow transplantation. *Br J Haematol* 1997;99:945–950.
28. Balkwill FR. Interferons. *Lancet* 1989;1:1060–1063.

29. Upadhyaya G, Guba SC, Sih SA, et al. Interferon-alpha restores the deficient expression of the cytoadhesion molecule lymphocyte function antigen-3 by chronic myelogenous leukemia progenitor cells. *J Clin Invest* 1991;88:2131–2136.

30. Porter DL, Collins Jr. RH, Shpilberg O, et al. Long-term follow-up of patients who acheived complete remission after donor leukocyte infusions. *Biol Blood Marrow Transplant* 1999;5:253–261.

31. Heslop HE, Ng CYC, Smith CA, et al. Long-term restoration of immunity against Epstein-Barr virus infection by adoptive transfer of gene-modified virus-specific T lymphocytes. *Nat Med* 1996;2:551–555.

32. Levine JE, Braun T, Penza SL, et al. A Prospective Trial of Chemotherapy and Donor Leukocyte Infusions for Relapse of Advanced Myeloid Malignancies following Allogeneic Stem Cell Transplantation. *J Clin Oncol* 2002;2:405–412.

33. Yazaki M, Andoh M, Ito T, Ohno T, Wada Y. Successful prevention of hematological relapse for a patient with Philadelphia chromosome-positive acute lymphoblastic leukemia after allogeneic bone marrow transplantation by donor leukocyte infusion. *Bone Marrow Transplant* 1997;19:393,394.

34. Atra A, Millar B, Shepherd V, et al. Donor lymphocyte infusion for childhood acute lymphoblastic leukaemia relapsing after bone marrow transplantation. *Br J Haematol* 1997;97:165–168.

35. Collins Jr. RH, Goldstein S, Giralt S, et al. Donor leukocyte infusions in acute lymphocytic leukemia. *Bone Marrow Transplant* 2000;26:511–516.

36. Porter DL, Roth MS, Lee SJ, McGarigle C, Ferrara JLM, Antin JH. Adoptive immunotherapy with donor mononuclear cell infusions to treat relapse of acute leukemia or myelodysplasia after allogeneic bone marrow transplantation. *Bone Marrow Transplant* 1996;18:975–980.

37. Verdonck LF, Lokhorst HM, Dekker AW, Nieuwenhuis HK, Petersen EJ. Graft-versus-myeloma effect in two cases. *Lancet* 1996;347:800,801.

38. Tricot G, Vesole DH, Jagannath S, Hilton J, Munshi N, Barlogie B. Graft-versus-myeloma effect: proof of principle. *Blood* 1996;87:1196–1198.

39. Lokhorst HM, Schattenberg A, Cornelissen JJ, Thomas LLM, Verdonck LF. Donor leukocyte infusions are effective in relapsed multiple myeloma after allogeneic bone marrow transplantation. *Blood* 1997;90:4206–4211.

40. van der Griend R, Verdonck LF, Petersen EJ, Veenhuizen P, Bloem AC, Lokhorst HM. Donor leukocyte infusions inducing remissions repeatedly in a patient with recurrent multiple myeloma after allogeneic bone marrow transplantation. *Bone Marrow Transplant* 1999;23:195–197.

41. Mehta J, Singhal S. Graft-versus-myeloma. *Bone Marrow Transplant* 1998;22:835–843.

42. Orsini E, Alyea EP, Schlossman R, et al. Changes in T cell receptor repertoire associated with graft-versus-tumor effect and graft-versus-host disease in patients with relapsed multiple myeloma after donor lymphocyte infusion. *Bone Marrow Transplant* 2000;25:623–632.

43. Lokhorst HM, Schattenberg A, Cornelissen JJ, et al. Donor lymphocyte infusions for relapsed multiple myeloma after allogeneic stem-cell transplantation: predictive factors for response and long-term outcome. *J Clin Oncol* 2000;18:3031–3037.

44. Salama M, Nevill T, Marcellus D, et al. Donor leukocyte infusions for multiple myeloma. *Bone Marrow Transplant* 2000;26:1179–1184.

45. Jones RJ, Ambinder RF, Piantadosi S, Santos GW. Evidence of a graft-versus-lymphoma effect associated with allogeneic bone marrow transplantation. *Blood* 1991;77:649–653.

46. Ratanatharathorn V, Uberti J, Karanes C, et al. Prospective comparative trial of autologous versus allogeneic bone marrow transplantation in patients with non-Hodgkin's lymphoma. *Blood* 1994;84:1050–1055.

47. Chopra R, Goldstone AH, Pearce R, et al. Autologous versus allogeneic bone marrow transplantation for non-Hodgkin's lymphoma: a case-controlled analysis of the European Bone Marrow Transplant Group Registry data. *J Clin Oncol* 1992;10:1690–1695.

48. van Besien K, Sobocinski KA, Rowlings PA, et al. Allogeneic bone marrow transplantation for low-grade lymphoma. *Blood* 1998;92:1832–1836.

49. Rondon G, Giralt S, Huh Y, et al. Graft-versus-leukemia effect after allogeneic bone marrow transplantation for chronic lymphocytic leukemia. *Bone Marrow Transplant* 1996;18:669–672.

50. van Besien KW, de Lima M, Giralt SA, et al. Management of lymphoma recurrence after allogeneic transplantation: the relevance of graft-versus-lymphoma effect. *Bone Marrow Transplant* 1997;19:977–982.

51. Mandigers CM, Meijerink JP, Raemaekers JM, Schattenberg AV, Mensink EJ. Graft-versus-lymphoma effect of donor leucocyte infusion shown by real-time quantitative PCR analysis of t(14;18). *Lancet* 1998;352:1522,1523.

52. Khouri IF, Keating M, Korbling M, et al. Transplant-lite: induction of graft-versus-malignancy using fludarabine- based nonablative chemotherapy and allogeneic blood progenitor-cell transplantation as treatment for lymphoid malignancies. *J Clin Oncol* 1998;16:2817–2824.

53. Sykes M, Preffer F, McAfee S, et al. Mixed lymphohaemopoietic chimerism and graft-versus-lymphoma effects after non-myeloablative therapy and HLA-mismatched bone-marrow transplantation. *Lancet* 1999;353(9166):1755–1759.

54. Khouri IF, Lee MS, Romaguera J, et al. Allogeneic hematopoietic transplantation for mantle-cell lymphoma: molecular remissions and evidence of graft-versus-malignancy. *Ann Oncol* 1999;10:1293–1299.

55. Sohn SK, Baek JH, Kim DH, et al. Successful allogeneic stem-cell transplantation with prophylactic stepwise G-CSF primed-DLIs for relapse after autologous transplantation in mantle cell lymphoma: a case report and literature review on the evidence of GVL effects in MCL. *Am J Hematol* 2000;65:75–80.

56. Childs R, Chernoff A, Contentin N, et al. Regression of metastatic renal-cell carcinoma after nonmyeloablative allogeneic peripheral-blood stem-cell transplantation. *N Engl J Med* 2000;343:750–758.

57. Eibl B, Schwaighofer H, Nachbaur D, et al. Evidence for a graft-versus-tumor effect in a patient treated with marrow ablative chemotherapy and allogeneic bone marrow transplantation for breast cancer. *Blood* 1996;88:1501–1508.

58. Ueno NT, Rondon G, Mirza NQ, et al. Allogeneic peripheral-blood progenitor-cell transplantation for poor-risk patients with metastatic breast cancer. *J Clin Oncol* 1998;16:986–993.

59. Bourgault I, Gomez A, Gomard E, Levy JP. Limiting-dilution analysis of the HLA restriction of anti-Epstein-Barr virus-specific cytolytic T lymphocytes. *Clin Exp Immunol* 1991;84:501–507.

60. Harris NL, Ferry JA, Swerdlow SH. Posttransplant lymphoproliferative disorders: summary of Society for Hematopathology Workshop. *Semin Diagn Pathol* 1997;14:8–14.

61. Paya CV, Fung JJ, Nalesnik MA, et al. Epstein-Barr virus-induced posttransplant lymphoproliferative disorders. ASTS/ASTP EBV-PTLD Task Force and The Mayo Clinic Organized International Consensus Development Meeting. *Transplantation* 1999;68:1517–1525.

62. Papadopoulos EB, Ladanyi M, Emanuel D, et al. Infusions of donor leukocytes to treat Epstein-Barr virus-associated lymphoproliferative disorders after allogeneic bone marrow transplantation. *N Engl J Med* 1994;330:1185–1191.

63. O'Reilly RJ, Small TN, Papadopoulos E, Lucas K, Lacerda J, Koulova L. Biology and adoptive cell therapy of Epstein-Barr virus-associated lymphoproliferative disorders in recipients of marrow allografts. *Immunol Rev* 1997;157:195–216.

64. Gross TG, Steinbuch M, DeFor T, et al. B cell lymphoproliferative disorders following hematopoietic stem cell transplantation: risk factors, treatment and outcome. *Bone Marrow Transplant* 1999;23:251–258.

65. Rooney CM, Smith CA, Y C Ng C, et al. Use of gene-modified virus-specific T lymphocytes to control Epstein-Barr-virus-related lymphoproliferation. *Lancet* 1995;345:9–13.

66. Rooney CM, Smith CA, Ng CYC, et al. Infusion of cytotoxic T cells for the prevention and treatment of Epstein-Barr virus-induced lymphoma in allogeneic tranplant recipients. *Blood* 1998;92:1549–1555.

67. McGuirk P, Seropian S, Howe G, Smith B, Stoddart L, Cooper DL. Use of rituximab and irradiated donor-derived lymphocytes to control Epstein-Barr virus-associated lymphoproliferation in patients undergoing related haplo-identical stem cell transplantation. *Bone Marrow Transplant* 1999;24:1253–1258.

68. Emanuel DJ, Lucas KG, Mallory GB, Jr., et al. Treatment of posttransplant lymphoproliferative disease in the central nervous system of a lung transplant recipient using allogeneic leukocytes. *Transplantation* 1997;63:1691–1694.

69. Small TN, Papadopoulos EB, Bouland F, et al. Comparison of immune reconstitution after unrelated and related T-cell-depleted bone marrow transplantation: effect of patient age and donor leukocyte infusions. *Blood* 1999;93:467–480.

70. Orsini E, Alyea EP, Chillemi A, et al. Conversion to full donor chimerism following donor lymphocyte infusion is associated with disease response in patients with multiple myeloma. *Biol Blood Marrow Transplant* 2000;6:375–386.

71. Verfuerth S, Peggs K, Vyas P, Barnett L, O'Reilly RJ, Mackinnon S. Longitudinal monitoring of immune reconstitution of CDR3 size spectratyping after T-cell-depleted allogeneic bone marrow transplant and the effect of donor lymphocyte infusions on T-cell repertoire. *Blood* 2000;95:3990–3995.

72. Walter EA, Greenberg PD, Gilbert MJ, et al. Reconstitution of cellular immunity against cytomegalovirus in recipients of allogeneic bone marrow by transfer of T-cell clones from the donor. *N Engl J Med* 1995;333:1038–1044.

73. Bordigoni P, Carret AS, Venard V, Witz F, Le Faou A. Treatment of adenovirus infections in patients undergoing allogeneic hematopoietic stem cell transplantation. *Clin Infect Dis* 2001;32:1290–1297.

74. Smith FO, Thomson B. T-cell recovery following marrow transplant: experience with delayed lymphocyte infusions to accelerate immune recovery or treat infectious problems. *Pediatr Transplant* 1999;3 (Suppl 1):59–64.

75. Riddell SR, Greenberg PD. T-cell therapy of cytomegalovirus and human immunodeficiency virus infection. *J Antimicrob Chemother* 2000;45(Suppl T3):35–43.

76. Godder KT, Abhyankar SH, Lamb LS, et al. Donor leukocyte infusion for treatment of graft rejection post partially mismatched related donor bone marrow transplant. *Bone Marrow Transplant* 1998;22:111–113.

77. Keil F, Haas OA, Fritsch G, Kalhs P, Lechner K, Mannhalter C. Donor leukocyte infusion for leukemia relapse after allogeneic marrow transplantation: lack of residual donor hematopoiesis predicts aplasia. *Blood* 1997;89:3113–3117.

78. Flowers ME, Leisenring W, Beach K, et al. Granulocyte colony-stimulating factor given to donors before apheresis does not prevent aplasia in patients treated with donor leukocyte infusion for recurrent chronic myeloid leukemia after bone marrow transplantation. *Biol Blood Marrow Transplant* 2000;6:321–326.

79. Giralt S, Hester J, Huh Y, et al. CD8-depleted donor lymphocyte infusion as treatment for relapsed chronic myelogenous leukemia after allogeneic bone marrow transplantation. *Blood* 1995;86:4337–4343.

80. Ferrara JL, Levy R, Chao NJ. Pathophysiologic mechanisms of acute graft-vs.-host disease. *Biol Blood Marrow Transplant* 1999;5:347–356.

81. Johnson BD, Brobyski WR, Truitt RL. Delayed infusion of normal donor cells after MHC-matched bone marrow transplantation provides an antileukemia reaction without graft-versus-host disease. B*one Marrow Transplant* 1993;11:329–336.

82. Kernan NA, Collins NH, Juliano L, et al. Clonable T lymphocytes in T-cell depleted bone marrow transplants correlates with development of graft versus host diseases. *Blood* 1986;68:770–773.

83. Barrett AJ, Mavroudis D, Tisdale J, et al. T cell-depleted bone marrow transplantation and delayed T cell add-back to control acute GVHD and conserve a graft-versus-leukemia effect. *Bone Marrow Transplant* 1998;21:543–551.

84. Berthou C, Leglise MC, Herry A, et al. Extramedullary relapse after favorable molecular response to donor leukocyte infusions for recurring acute leukemia. *Leukemia* 1998;12:1676–1681.

85. Zomas A, Stefanoudaki K, Fisfis M, Papadaki T, Mehta J. Graft-versus-myeloma after donor leukocyte infusion: maintenance of marrow remission but extramedullary relapse with plasmacytomas. *Bone Marrow Transplant* 1998;21:1163–1165.

86. Grigg AP. Multiply recurrent extramedullary plasmacytomas without marrow relapse in the context of extensive chronic GVHD in a patient with myeloma. *Leuk Lymphom*a 1999;34:635,636.

87. Butcher EC, Picker LJ. Lymphocyte homing and homeostasis. *Science* 1996;272:60–66.

88. Porter DL, Collins Jr. RH, Hardy C, et al. Treatment of relapsed leukemia after unrelated donor marrow transplantation with unrelated donor leukocyte infusions. *Blood* 2000;95:1214–1221.

89. Pati AR, Godder K, Lamb L, Gee A, Henslee-Downey PJ. Immunotherapy with donor leukocyte infusions for patients with ralapsed acute myeloid leukemia following partially mismatched related donor bone marrow transplantation. *Bone Marrow Transplant* 1995;15:979–981.

90. Sprent J, Korngold R. T cell subsets controlling graft-v-host disease in mice. *Transplant Proc* 1987;19:41–47.

91. Nimer SD, Giorgi J, Gajewski JL, et al. Selective depletion of CD8+ cells for prevention of graft-versus-host disease after bone marrow transplantation. A randomized controlled trial. *Transplantation* 1994;57:82–87.

92. Alyea EP, Soiffer RJ, Canning C, et al. Toxicity and efficacy of defined doses of CD4(+) donor lymphocytes for treatment of relapse after allogeneic bone marrow transplant. *Blood* 1998;91:3671–680.

93. Falkenburg JH, Wafelman AR, Joosten P, et al. Complete remission of accelerated phase chronic myeloid leukemia by treatment with leukemia-reactive cytotoxic T lymphocytes. *Blood* 1999;94:1201–1208.

94. Smit WM, Rijnbeek M, van Bergen CA, Willemze R, Falkenburg JH. Generation of leukemia-reactive cytotoxic T lymphocytes from HLA- identical donors of patients with chronic myeloid leukemia using modifications of a limiting dilution assay. *Bone Marrow Transplant* 1998;21:553–560.

95. Mutis T, Verdijk R, Schrama E, Esendam B, Brand A, Goulmy E. Feasibility of immunotherapy of relapsed leukemia with ex vivo-generated cytotoxic T lymphocytes specific for hematopoietic system-restricted minor histocompatibility antigens. *Blood* 1999;93:2336–2341.

96. Bonini C. Transfer of the HSV-TK gene into donor peripheral blood lymphocytes for in vivo immuno-modulation of donor anti-tumor immunity after allo-BMT. *Blood* 1994;84:110.

97. Bonini C, Ferrari G, Verzeletti S, Servida P, Zappone E, Ruggieri L. HSV-TK gene transfer into donor lymphocytes for control of allogeneic graft-versus-leukemia. *Science* 1997;276:1719–1724.

98. Bonini C, Ciceri F, Marktel S, Bordignon C. Suicide-gene-transduced T-cells for the regulation of the graft-versus- leukemia effect. *Vox Sang* 1998;74:341–343.

99. Tiberghien P, Reynolds CW, Keller J, et al. Ganciclovir treatment of herpes simplex thymidine kinase-transduced primary T lymphocytes: an approach for specific in vivo donor T-cell depletion after bone marrow transplantation? *Blood* 1994;84:1333–1341.

100. Tiberghien P, Ferrand C, Lioure B, et al. Administration of herpes simplex-thymidine kinase-expressing donor T cells with a T-cell-depleted allogeneic marrow graft. *Blood* 2001;97:63–72.

101. Kuhlcke K, Ayuk FA, Li Z, et al. Retroviral transduction of T lymphocytes for suicide gene therapy in allogeneic stem cell transplantation. *Bone Marrow Transplant* 2000;25(Suppl 2):S96–98.

102. Riddell SR, Elliott M, Lewinsohn DA, et al. T-cell mediated rejection of gene-modified HIV-specific cytotoxic T lymphocytes in HIV-infected patients. *Nat Med* 1996;2:216–223.

103. Waller EK, Ship AM, Mittelstaedt S, et al. Irradiated donor leukocytes promote engraftment of allogeneic bone marrow in major histocompatibility complex mismatched recipients without causing graft-versus-host disease. *Blood* 1999;94:3222–3233.

104. Waller EK, Boyer M. New strategies in allogeneic stem cell transplantation: immunotherapy using irradiated allogeneic T cells. *Bone Marrow Transplant* 2000;25(Suppl 2):S20–24.

105. Pan L, Teshima T, Hill GR, et al. Granulocyte colony-stimulating factor-mobilized allogeneic stem cell transplantation maintains graft-versus-leukemia effects through a perforin-dependent pathway while preventing graft-versus-host disease. *Blood* 1999;93:4071–4078.

106. Arpinati M, Green CL, Heimfeld S, Heuser JE, Anasetti C. Granulocyte-colony stimulating factor mobilizes T helper 2-inducing dendritic cells. *Blood* 2000;95:2484–2490.

107. Rutella S, Rumi C, Lucia MB, Sica S, Cauda R, Leone G. Serum of healthy donors receiving granulocyte colony-stimulating factor induces T cell unresponsiveness. *Exp Hematol* 1998;26:1024–1033.

108. Druker BJ, Lydon NB. Lessons learned from the development of an abl tyrosine kinase inhibitor for chronic myelogenous leukemia. *J Clin Invest* 2000;105:3–7.

109. Druker BJ, Talpaz M, Resta DJ, et al. Efficacy and safety of a specific inhibitor of the BCR-ABL tyrosine kinase in chronic myeloid leukemia. *N Engl J Med* 2001;344:1031–1037.

110. Drobyski WR, Hessner MJ, Klein JP, et al. T-cell depletion plus salvage immunotherapy with donor leukocyte infusions as a strategy to treat chronic-phase chronic myelogenous leukemia patients undergoing HLA-identical sibling marrow transplantation. *Blood* 1999;94:434–441.

111. Alyea E, Weller E, Schlossman R, et al. T-cell-depleted allogeneic bone marrow transplantation followed by donor lymphocyte infusion in patients with multiple myeloma: induction of graft-versus-myeloma effect. *Blood* 2001;98:934–939.

112. Sullivan KM, Storb R, Buckner CD, et al. Graft-versus-host disease as adoptive immunotherapy in patients with advanced hematologic neoplasms. *N Engl J Med* 1989;320:828–834.

113. Johnson BD, Truitt RL. Delayed infusion of immunocompetent donor cells after bone marrow transplantation breaks graft-host tolerance allows for persistent antileukemic reactivity without severe graft-versus-host disease. *Blood* 1995;85:3302–3312.

114. Johnson BD, Becker EE, Truitt RL. Graft-vs.-host and graft-vs.-leukemia reactions after delayed infusions of donor T-subsets. *Biol Blood Marrow Transplant* 1999;5:123–132.

115. Schaap N, Schattenberg A, Bar B, Preijers F, van de Wiel van Kemenade E, de Witte T. Induction of graft-versus-leukemia to prevent relapse after partially lymphocyte-depleted allogeneic bone marrow transplantation by pre- emptive donor leukocyte infusions. *Leukemia* 2001;15:1339–1346.

116. Lee CK, Gingrich RD, deMagalhaes-Silverman M, et al. Prophylactic reinfusion of T cells for T cell-depleted allogeneic bone marrow transplantation. *Biol Blood Marrow Transplant* 1999;5:15–27.

117. de Lima M, Bonamino M, Vasconcelos Z, et al. Prophylactic donor lymphocyte infusions after moderately ablative chemotherapy and stem cell transplantation for hematological malignancies: high remission rate among poor prognosis patients at the expense of graft-versus-host disease. *Bone Marrow Transplant* 2001;27:73–78.

118. Mehta J, Powles R, Singhal S, et al. Cytokine-mediated immunotherapy with or without donor leukocytes for poor-risk acute myeloid leukemia relapsing after allogeneic bone marrow transplantation. *Bone Marrow Transplant* 1995;16:133–137.

119. Kwak LW, Taub DD, Duffey PL, et al. Transfer of myeloid idiotype-specific immunity from an actively immunised marrow donor. *Lancet* 1995;345:1016–1020.

120. Cabrera R, Diaz-Espada F, Barrios Y, et al. Infusion of lymphocytes obtained from a donor immunised with the paraprotein idiotype as a treatment in a relapsed myeloma. *Bone Marrow Transplant* 2000;25:1105–1108.

121. Little MT, Storb R. The future of allogeneic hematopoietic stem cell transplantation: minimizing pain, maximizing gain. *J Clin Invest* 2000;105:1679–1681.

122. Carella AM, Champlin R, Slavin S, et al. Mini-allografts: ongoing trials in humans. *Bone Marrow Transplant* 2000;25:345–350.

123. Slavin S, Nagler A, Naparstek E, et al. Nonmyeloablative stem cell transplantation with lethal cytoreduction for the treatment of malignant and nonmalignant hematologic diseases. *Blood* 1998;91:756–763.

124. Barrett AJ, Malkovska V. Graft-versus-leukaemia: understanding and using the alloimmune response to treat haematological malignancies. *Br J Haematol* 1996;93:754–761.

125. Fontaine P, Roy-Proulx G, Knafo L, Baron C, Roy DC, Perreault C. Adoptive transfer of minor histocompatibility antigen-specific T lymphocytes eradicates leukemia cells without causing graft-versus-host disease. *Nat Med* 2001;7:789–794.

126. Dazzi F, Simpson E, Goldman JM. Minor antigen solves major problem. *Nat Med* 2001;7:769,770.

127. Molldrem JJ, Lee PP, Wang C, et al. Evidence that specific T lymphocytes may participate in the elimination of chronic myelogenous leukemia. *Nat Med* 2000;6:1018–1023.

128. Goulmy E, Schipper R, Pool J, et al. Mismatches of minor histocompatibility antigens between HLA-identical donors and recipients and the development of graft-versus-host disease after bone marrow transplantation. *N Engl J Med* 1996;334:281–285.

129. Claret EJ, Alyea EP, Orsini E, et al. Characterization of T cell repertoire in patients with graft-versus-leukemia after donor lymphocyte infusion. *J Clin Invest* 1997;100:855–866.

130. Wu CJ, Yang XF, McLaughlin S, et al. Detection of a potent humoral response associated with immune-induced remission of chronic myelogenous leukemia. *J Clin Invest* 2000;106:705–714.

131. Bunjes D, Theobald M, Hertenstein B, et al. Successful therapy with donor buffy coat transfusions in patients with relapsed chronic myeloid leukemia after bone marrow transplantation is associated with high frequencies of host-reactive interleukin 2- secreting T helper cells. *Bone Marrow Transplant* 1995;15:713–719.

132. Jiang YZ, Cullis JO, Kanfer EJ, Goldman JM, Barrett AJ. T cell and NK cell mediated graft-versus-leukaemia reactivity following donor buffy coat transfusion to treat relapse after marrow transplantation for chronic myeloid leukaemia. *Bone Marrow Transplant* 1993;11:133–138.

133. Smit WM, Rijnbeek M, van Bergen CA, Fibbe WE, Willemze R, Falkenburg JH. T cells recognizing leukemic CD34(+) progenitor cells mediate the antileukemic effect of donor lymphocyte infusions for relapsed chronic myeloid leukemia after allogeneic stem cell transplantation. *Proc Natl Acad Sci USA* 1998;95:10,152–10,157.

134. Mutis T, Gillespie G, Schrama E, Falkenburg JH, Moss P, Goulmy E. Tetrameric HLA class I-minor histocompatibility antigen peptide complexes demonstrate minor histocompatibility antigen-specific cytotoxic T lymphocytes in patients with graft-versus-host disease. *Nat Med* 1999;5:839–842.

135. Maino VC, Picker LJ. Identification of functional subsets by flow cytometry: intracellular detection of cytokine expression. *Cytometry* 1998;34:207–215.

136. Picker LJ. Proving HIV-1 immunity: new tools offer new opportunities. *J Clin Invest* 2000;105:1333,1334.

137. Guinan EC, Gribben JG, Boussiotis VA, Freeman GJ, Nadler LM. Pivotal role of the B7:CD28 pathway in transplantation tolerance and tumor immunity. *Blood* 1994;84:3261–3282.

138. Dermime S, Mavroudis D, Jiang YZ, Hensel N, Molldrem J, Barrett AJ. Immune escape from a graft-versus-leukemia effect may play a role in the relapse of myeloid leukemias following allogeneic bone marrow transplantation. *Bone Marrow Transplant* 1997;19:989–999.

139. Radich JP, Sanders JE, Buckner CD, et al. Second allogeneic marrow transplantation for patients with recurrent leukemia after initial transplant with total-body irradiation- containing regimens. *J Clin Oncol* 1993;11:304–313.

140. Mrsic M, Horowitz MM, Atkinson K, et al. Second HLA-identical sibling transplants for leukemia recurrence. *Bone Marrow Transplant* 1992;9:269–275.

141. Blau IW, Basara N, Bischoff M, et al. Second allogeneic hematopoietic stem cell transplantation as treatment for leukemia relapsing following a first transplant. *Bone Marrow Transplant* 2000;25:41–45.

142. Mehta J, Powles R, Treleaven J, et al. Outcome of acute leukemia relapsing after bone marrow transplantation: utility of second transplants and adoptive immunotherapy. *Bone Marrow Transplant* 1997;19:709–719.

143. Higano CS, Chielens D, Bryant EM. Alfa-2A-interferon produces durable complete cytogenetic responses in patients with cytogenetic relapse of chronic myelogenous leukemia after marrow transplantaiton. *Blood* 1995;86:566.

144. Higano CS, Chielens D, Raskind W, et al. Use of α-2a-interferon to treat cytogenetic relapse of chronic myeloid leukemia after marrow transplantation. *Blood* 1997;90:2549–2554.

145. Pigneux A, Devergie A, Pochitaloff M, et al. Recombinant alpha-interferon as treatment for chronic myelogenous leukemia in relapse after allogeneic bone marrow transplantation: a report from the Societe Francaise de Greffe de Moelle. *Bone Marrow Transplant* 1995;15:819–824.

146. Collins Jr. RH, Rogers ZR, Bennett M, Kumar V, Nikein A, Fay JW. Hematologic relapse of chronic myelogenous leukemia following allogeneic bone marrow transplantation: apparent graft-versus-leukemia effect following abrupt discontinuation of immunosuppression. *Bone Marrow Transplant* 1992;10:391–395.

147. Higano CS, Brixey M, Bryant EM, et al. Durable complete remission of acute nonlymphocytic leukemia associated with discontinuation of immunosuppression following relapse after allogeneic bone marrow transplantation. A case report of a probable graft-versus-leukemia effect. *Transplantation* 1990;50:175–177.

148. Elmaagacli AH, Beelen DW, Schaefer UW. A retrospective single centre study of the outcome of five different therapy approaches in 48 patients with relapse of chronic myelogenous leukemia after allogeneic bone marrow transplantation. *Bone Marrow Transplant* 1997;20:1045–1055.

149. Brandenburg U, Gottlieb D, Bradstock K. Antileukemic effects of rapid cyclosporin withdrawal in patients with relapsed chronic myeloid leukemia after allogeneic bone marrow transplantation. *Leuk Lymphoma* 1998;31:545–550.

150. Giralt S, Escudier S, Kantarjian H, et al. Preliminary results of treatment with filgrastim for relapse of leukemia and myelodysplasia after allogeneic bone marrow transplantation. *N Engl J Med* 1993;329:757–761.

151. Bishop MR, Tarantolo SR, Pavletic ZS, et al. Filgrastim as an alternative to donor leukocyte infusion for relapse after allogeneic stem-cell transplantation. *J Clin Oncol* 2000;18:2269–2272.

152. Guglielmi C, Arcese W, Hermans J, et al. Risk assessment in patients with Ph+ chronic myelogenous leukemia at first relapse after allogeneic stem cell transplant: an EBMT retrospective analysis. *Blood* 2000;95:3328–3334.

20

Second Hematopoietic Stem Cell Transplantation for the Treatment of Graft Failure, Graft Rejection, or Relapse

Steven N. Wolff, MD

CONTENTS

1. INTRODUCTION

Two circumstances have required a second hematopoietic stem cell (HSC) transplant: (i) graft failure or rejection (dysfunction), and (ii) disease relapse without graft dysfunction. Each warrant specific consideration based on frequency, pathogenesis, and treatment. This review will focus on the transplantation of substantial numbers of HSC given to augment graft function after a first transplant or the performance of a complete second transplant with cytotoxic therapy for disease relapse. Recently, donor lymphocytes infusions (DLI) without HSC mobilization have been increasingly used to treat relapse of malignant disease. DLI will, however, be discussed in another chapter.

2. DEFINITIONS

Engraftment can be defined by the absolute presence or by a specified number of donor cells in the recipient, further characterized as hematopoietic or lymphoid. Compounding this definition, and making historical comparisons difficult, is the increasing sophistication of technology able to identify and distinguish exceedingly small cell populations (1). Engraftment, on a functional basis, may be defined as the first day of achieving a peripheral blood neutrophil count of donor origin greater than 500/μL for 3 consecutive days. Graft failure is the inability to demonstrate any donor cells using polymerase chain reaction (PCR) methodology at 4 wk after transplantation. Rejection is the substantial diminution of donor cells after successful engraftment beyond 4 wk after transplantation, characterized as early (before 60 d) or late (after

From: *Current Clinical Oncology: Allogeneic Stem Cell Transplantation*
Edited by: Mary S. Laughlin and Hillard M. Lazarus © Humana Press Inc., Totowa, NJ

Table 1
Parameters Associated with Marrow Dysfunction

Quantitative HSC issues:
    Inadequate number of transfused stem cell.
    Splenomegaly.
Qualitative marrow issues:
    Perturbed marrow microenvironment.
Immunologic issues:
    Blood or cellular component transfusion.
    T cell depletion.
    Donor and recipient HLA disparity.
    Donor and recipient ABO disparity.
    Diseases of marrow failure states.
    Diseases of perturbed erythropoiesis.
    Reduced cytotoxic conditioning ("nonablative").
    Constrained GVHD prophylaxis.
Environmental issues:
    CMV infection.
    HV-6 and HHV-8 infection.
    Parvovirus infection.

60 d) rejection. However, many reports do not distinguish between failure to engraft or graft rejection, have vague times for the occurrence of graft failure, and report only the interval between initial transplantation and the maneuver used to overcome graft dysfunction.

3. INTRODUCTION TO GRAFT DYSFUNCTION

Successful allogeneic donor engraftment is achieved when HSC are transplanted within a recipient milieu of adequate immunosuppression. Failure to engraft after marrow ablative therapy is life-threatening, but fortunately occurs at an overall frequency of less than 5% (2–4).

Graft failure may be due to an inadequate number of transplanted HSC or by the failure of adequate numbers of cells to survive. The barriers to engraftment include immunologic destruction, infectious agents, drug toxicity or a poor marrow microenvironment (5). Each of these components individually and together has been demonstrated to result in graft failure (Table 1).

3.1. Factors Influencing Graft Dysfunction

Pioneering work led to the recognition that the dose of HSC is crucial to engraftment (6). In patients with severe aplastic anemia (sAA) prepared with cyclophosphamide, a dose of $>3 \times 10^8$/kg nucleated cells increased the likelihood of engraftment. In multivariate analysis, other parameters that hindered engraftment included previous blood transfusions and reactivity in a mixed lymphocyte reaction. These observations demonstrate the interaction of the transfused donor HSC and the sensitized immune state of the recipient. In this early series, optimal immunosuppression was not achieved, since most patients received only methotrexate for graft-vs-host disease (GVHD) prophylaxis, and additional donor lymphocytes (buffy coat) infusions facilitated sustained engraftment, albeit with an increase in chronic GVHD.

An update of the Seattle experience reviewed 333 patients with sAA transplanted between 1970 and 1996 (7). Reflecting the changing process of transplantation practices, the rate of rejection decreased from 35% in the period of 1970–1976, to 12% in the period of 1977–1981 ($p < 0.001$) and ultimately to 9% in the period of 1982–1996. Additionally, the onset of graft dysfunction was delayed in the latter period with a median onset of 180 d (range 22–583).

Twelve patients in the period of 1982–1996 received a second transplant prepared with the addition of antithymocyte globulin (ATG) to cyclophosphamide conditioning and cyclosporine to methotrexate for GVHD prophylaxis. These patients demonstrated a reduced rejection rate of 25% compared to the first transplant. A subsequent third transplant was performed in three patients, and all subsequently engrafted. Overall, patients conditioned for a second transplant with cyclophosphamide and ATG, and given cyclosporine with methotrexate had a probability of 83% of long-term survival. The improved outcome was related to having more untransfused patients, γ-irradiating blood transfusions and increasing the dose of infused HSC, along with better GVHD prophylaxis and improved supportive care, especially the prevention and treatment of severe infections. Other series of sAA patients using more profound cytotoxic therapy (e.g., total body irradiation [TBI]) and GVHD prophylaxis (cyclosporine) have demonstrated significant reduction of graft dysfunction with an estimated frequency of approx 10% (8,9).

However, sAA should not be used as a standard measure for graft failure, since the primary disease itself is frequently immune-mediated. In other diseases, the incidence of graft failure is substantially less frequent. Supporting this observation is the reduced rejection rate (4.0%) observed after transplantation for hepatitis-induced sAA, which is a disorder felt not to be immunologically based (8). In addition to sAA, graft dysfunction is more problematic in diseases such as sickle cell anemia and thalassemia, since all patients have been extensively transfused without chronic immunologic suppression caused by previous cytotoxic therapy.

Graft dysfunction is more common with disparate donor (e.g., haploidentical related, unrelated marrow and umbilical cord) transplants, after T cell-depleted marrow transplants, or with reduced intensity preparative regimens (10–23). In unrelated marrow transplants, disparity in class I, especially human leukocyte antigen (HLA)-C, was associated with graft dysfunction (24,25). A case report and similar observations demonstrate that as little as one amino acid difference between HLA-B alleles was able to elicit a host cytotoxic T cell (CTL) response leading to donor HSC graft rejection (26,27). Other reports suggest that residual recipient natural killer (NK) cells can mediate graft dysfunction (28–30).

Aside from disease or immunologic mechanisms of graft dysfunction, the compromised marrow microenvironment of heavily pretreated recipients or the occurrence of viral infections, such as cytomegalovirus (CMV) or human herpes virus (HHV) infections have been implicated to cause graft failure (31–34).

Although graft rejection usually occurs within the first 6 mo after transplantation, very late graft rejection has been reported in sAA, even with intense conditioning (35). Rejection may be heralded by incomplete and decreasing donor chimerism, allowing the reexpression of host T cell function (36–38). One case report demonstrated graft rejection 8 yr after transplantation precipitated by an undefined viral infection (39).

Graft dysfunction is an ominous circumstance and may herald relapse of neoplasm with restoration of host hematopoiesis. In sAA, restoration of autolgous hematopoiesis after nonmarrow ablative cytotoxic therapy conditioning can occur as a result of the transplant immunosuppression abrogating host autoimmunity. This observation led to the use of immunosuppression as an effective treatment for sAA (40,41). Autologous recovery after graft dysfunction has occurred, even after regimens (e.g., TBI) thought to be marrow ablative. An interesting report of graft rejection after HLA-identical HSC transplantation for sickle cell anemia demonstrated perturbed autologous hematopoietic recovery, producing high levels of hemoglobin F, thus leading to a salutary clinical outcome (10).

3.2. Management of Graft Dysfunction

Whatever the etiology, the occurrence of graft failure or rejection should be identified early and recognized as a serious and life-threatening process requiring intervention. Management has consisted of augmentation of hematopoiesis by hematopoietic growth factors without additional HSC infusions, infusions of HSC without additional cytotoxic therapy (boost), or the performance of a complete second transplant with preinfusion conditioning.

3.2.1. USE OF AUTOLOGOUS BACK-UP HSC INFUSION

Patients able to store autologous HSC have been reinfused after graft dysfunction following allogeneic HSC transplantation *(42)*. An occasional patient has even been noted to subsequently experience long-term disease-free survival (DFS). The rather infrequent occurrence of graft dysfunction and the inherent difficulty of collecting uncontaminated HSC in patients with hematologic neoplasms make a routine decision to collect autologous HSC problematic. Specific consideration could be given to patients undergoing transplantation processes at high risk for graft dysfunction. However, even in this situation, preference would be for an allogeneic source of additional HSC.

3.2.2. USE OF GROWTH FACTORS TO ENHANCE HEMATOPOIESIS AFTER GRAFT DYSFUNCTION

Some patients, especially those with HLA disparate or ABO-mismatched transplants, may manifest slow engraftment and transient periods of dysfunction commonly associated with GVHD *(43)*. One of the earliest large reports of cytokine support for graft dysfunction used granulocyte-macrophage colony-stimulating factor (GM-CSF) between 21 and 171 d after allogeneic transplantation *(44)*. Nine of 15 patients increased absolute neutrophil counts from <100/μL to >500/μL within 14 d of beginning GM-CSF. Eight of the responders maintained counts after discontinuation of GM-CSF, and none had exacerbation of GVHD. Greater responses were seen in those patients having at least partial donor hematopoietic chimerism.

Another study using GM-CSF reported that two out of seven patients with graft failure concomitantly given infusions of additional HSC, and 10 out of 11 patients with graft rejection (without additional HSC) achieved a granulocyte response to >500/μL *(45)*. Sustained neutrophil recovery was generally noted only in those patients receiving additional stem cells, and some responders had autologous recovery. Despite cytokine and HSC treatment, the actuarial probability of survival at more than 1 yr after treatment was only 16%.

The combination of GM-CSF followed by granulocyte colony-stimulating factor (G-CSF) was compared to GM-CSF alone in patients with graft failure or rejection predominantly after related or unrelated allogeneic transplantation *(46)*. More than 85% of patients responded within a median of 9 d with an increase of neutrophils to >500/μL. As anticipated by the lineage specificity of these cytokines, salutary effect on red blood cell and platelet recovery was not noted. In this series, the 100-d survival after cytokine therapy was substantial (>70%) and statistically improved in those patients receiving only GM-CSF.

Nonetheless, it is still not clear what is the role for the commercially available growth factors to abrogate graft dysfunction after allogeneic transplantation. Certainly, hematopoietic growth factors should be considered an adjunct in the management of graft dysfunction, especially with partial donor chimerism. A primary role for hematopoietic growth factors has not been established.

3.2.3. THE EFFECT OF HSC DOSE ON GRAFT DYSFUNCTION

Augmentation of HSC dose has been assumed to reduce the likelihood of graft dysfunction, since "inadequate" dose is related to the occurrence of graft dysfunction. Supporting this hypothesis is "megadose" HSC infusion as a successful measure to avoid rejection in T cell-depleted haploidentical peripheral blood stem cell transplantation *(47)*. In this study, 41 out of 43 patients initially engrafted after receiving large doses of peripheral blood HSC, and those with graft dysfunction underwent successful second HSC transplants from a different donor.

What is the ideal HSC dose to help prevent dysfunction has not been established, although this study administered a mean of $>10 \times 10^6$/kg of CD34$^+$ cells.

3.2.4. SECOND HSC TRANSPLANTATION FOR GRAFT DYSFUNCTION

There are many reports of second HSC transplants for graft dysfunction. Unfortunately, clinical and treatment heterogeneity issues, such as additional conditioning and immunosuppression, the source of HSC, or the use of a different donor remain unanswered. Nonetheless, the performance of a second HSC infusion offers survival potential as demonstrated in patients with sAA after graft dysfunction, of who few survive without additional HSC. As noted previously, the utility of second HSC transplants for sAA was associated with long-term survival of 83% *(7)*.

A retrospective multicenter review from the Société Française de Greffe de Moelle (SFGM) analyzed 82 second early allogeneic HSC transplants for graft dysfunction in patients treated between 1985 and 1997 for acute leukemia, chronic myeloid leukemia, or sAA *(48)*. Approximately one-third of the patients had graft failure with the remainder graft rejection. The median time from first to second transplant was 62 d (range 32–307); 46 d (range 32–116) for graft failure, and 84 d (range 34–307) for graft rejection. Primary transplant T cell depletion was more common early in the study period, but used only for alternative donors transplants in the later time frame. Conditioning for the second transplant consisted of cytotoxic therapy in most patients, although 13 received only anti-T cell serotherapy. The same donor was used in 68% of second transplants, and 20 patients received additional hematopoietic growth factors. Overall, neutrophil recovery was 73%, with peripheral blood as the HSC source associated with a more rapid recovery. The probability of grade II–IV and III–IV GVHD was 41 and 17% respectively. Estimates of the 3-yr overall survival and d 100 transplant-related mortality were 30 and 53%, respectively. Recipient age <34 yr, an intertransplant time of approx 80 d, the use of cyclosporine alone for GVHD prophylaxis and positive recipient CMV serology were predictors of a better outcome. Twelve percent of successfully engrafted patients developed second graft dysfunction and one of five patients receiving a third transplant survived more than 3 yr. Issues not resolved in this retrospective review were the best source of HSC (blood vs peripheral mobilized) and, if available, the use of a new donor. Similar to previous reports, survival after graft failure was inferior to that after graft rejection, suggested by the improved results of second transplants when performed approx 80 d after the first transplant.

Second infusions of marrow HSC were reviewed at one institution from 1974 to 1992 *(4)*. Previous transplants included related or unrelated donor for the treatment of malignant disorders or marrow failure states. Variation of the second conditioning regimen and GVHD prophylaxis occurred. After primary graft failure, 57% (12 of 21) of reinfused patients engrafted with estimated survival at 1 year of 24% (95% cumulative incidence [CI]: 6–42%). After secondary graft failure (rejection), 12 patients received an additional HSC transplant with 33% (4 of 12) engrafting with survival of 25% (95% CI: 0–50%) at 1 yr. GVHD occurred in 52% of evaluable patients. Long-term survival was approx 20% without significant effect noted of primary or secondary graft failure.

The evidence for the avoidance of additional cytotoxic therapy was raised in a report of 20 patients (4% of all allogeneic patients) who received a second HSC infusion for failure to establish stable engraftment (leucocytes or platelets), graft rejection, or the persistence of donor immune cells causing hemolysis *(49)*. No additional chemotherapy or radiation conditioning was administered, although four received ATG. HSC sources included marrow and peripheral blood-mobilized cells. GVHD prophylaxis generally included cyclosporine continuing from the first transplant. Except for one patient, GVHD after the second HSC infusion was not substantial. Fifteen patients showed an improvement of neutrophil count to >500/μL or became platelet transfusion-independent. Overall survival after HSC boost was 43% at 3 yr with better outcome after graft rejection and after related marrow transplantation. The heterogeneity of this patient population make firm conclusions difficult but suggest that boost HSC can be effective after graft rejection.

The contribution of a conditioning regimen was, however, suggested in a report of a patient with Fanconi's anemia who rejected a graft from a matched sibling after preparation with low-dose cyclophosphamide (40 mg/kg), anti-T cell serotherapy, and cyclosporine for GVHD prophylaxis (50). The second transplant decreased the dose of cyclophosphamide (20 mg/kg) and continued anti-T cell serotherapy, but added total lymphoid irradiation (600 cGy) which resulted in engraftment with full donor chimerism.

Second marrow HSC transplants from unrelated donors were described in 12 patients with graft dysfunction (51). For primary transplantation, patients received T cell-depleted marrow (median cell dose of 5.6×10^8/kg) matched at the molecular level (HLA-A, -B, -DR, and -DQ) for two-thirds of patients, with the remainder one allelic mismatched (three class I and one class II). Anti-T cell serotherapy was given to all patients followed by aggressive cytotoxic conditioning and cyclosporine GVHD prophylaxis. The median time from the first HSC infusion to the second was 5 mo (range 1–13) with five from the original donor and seven were from another donor. The degree of disparity was not improved for patients receiving a second infusion from a different donor (median cell dose 5.7×10^8/kg). The additional cytotoxic conditioning was generally less intense compared to the primary transplant; no second infusion was T cell depleted, although most patients received anti-T cell serotherapy. Nine of ten evaluable patients engrafted at a median time of 17 d (range 12–39); one patient failed to engraft and one rejected the second infusion. GVHD occurred in a total of nine patients and was severe in three. Five patients survived 21–66 mo after the second infusion, although not all remain free of primary disease.

Although all patients in the above unrelated donor series received conditioning prior to the second infusion, a report described one patient who underwent a second unrelated donor infusion without cytotoxic conditioning (52). The first infusion was HLA-A, -B, -DRβ1, -DRQ1 matched and conditioned with TBI, cyclophosphamide and anti-T cell serotherapy with GVHD prophylaxis consisting of cyclosporine, methotrexate, and prednisolone. Due to technical issues with the marrow harvest, a modest cell dose (0.7×10^6/kg CD34$^+$ and 1.4×10^8/kg nucleated cells) was administered, which required the use of G-CSF (G-CSC) after infusion. Functional engraftment did not occur, but donor cells were identified by DNA studies of the peripheral blood. After 2 d of high-dose prednisolone, an infusion from a similarly matched but different unrelated donor was administered 25 days after the first HSC infusion. An increased cell dose (2.5×10^6/kg CD34$^+$ cells) from the second donor was followed by cyclosporine and Prednisolone GVHD prophylaxis. At 38 d after post-first BMT, chimerism studies revealed cells from both donors, but predominantly from the first donor; at 60 d chimerism revealed equality from both donors; at 73 d chimerism was predominantly from the second donor; at 86 d only the second donor cells were detected. Unfortunately, the patient died 104 d after the first infusion with tri-lineage engraftment of the second donor without GVHD.

3.2.5. The Source of HSC for Second Transplants

The best HSC source remains unclear, although higher cell doses are generally achieved with the use of cytokine mobilized HSC resulting in a trend for this source for the treatment of graft dysfunction. Two children with sAA and sickle cell anemia after graft rejection were successfully treated with additional cytotoxic therapy, cyclosporine GVHD prophylaxis, and G-CSF-mobilized HSC (53). Two adults with acute myeloid leukemia (AML) who experienced graft failure were successfully engrafted after unsuccessful G-CSF treatment using a second HSC transplant with ATG conditioning *(54)*. HSC were obtained from a different donor in one patient and the same donor in the other patient by apheresis of G-CSF-mobilized peripheral HSC. A patient with β-thalassemia undergoing T cell-depleted HLA-related phenotypic-matched HSC transplant prepared with busulfan, cyclophosphamide, and total lymphoid irradiation manifested only minimal donor chimerism (4–7%). Due to low transfusion requirements, a second transplant was delayed until 5 yr later. After preparation with hydroxyurea and cyclophosphamide and no other immunosuppression. G-CSF-mobilized peripheral HSC from the same donor, established 100% donor reconstitution. Another report used G-CSF mobilized peripheral stem cells with lymphocytes for persistence of substantial recipient isohemagglutinins 6 mo after first marrow HSC infusion *(55)*. The HSC-enhanced DLI suppressed residual recipient cells and reduced host immunologic reactivity against donor cells, resulting in improved erythropoiesis.

4. SECOND HSC TRANSPLANTATION FOR RELAPSE

Disease relapse is an ominous occurrence after allogeneic HSC transplantation. Results are poor with cytotoxic therapy alone, and second HSC transplants have been associated with substantial regimen-related toxicity (RRT) *(56–69)*. Nonetheless, considering the alternatives, second HSC should be entertained with consideration for the selection of donor, the extent of cytotoxic therapy, and the intensity of immunosuppression. Summaries have been published from many large cooperative groups demonstrating reasonable long-term survival even with substantial risk of treatment-related mortality (TRM). The value of DLI (without HSC or conditioning therapy) for neoplastic disease relapse will be the subject of another chapter, although case reports demonstrate DLI failure with subsequent salvage by another full transplant *(70)*.

4.1. General Outcome for Relapse

The International Blood and Marrow Transplant Registry (IBMTR) reported 145 second HSC transplants from 1978 to 1989; 114 HLA-matched siblings and the remainder from a variety of donors *(71)*. This retrospective review was heterogenous, but all patients received cytotoxic conditioning prior to the second infusion. After the second infusion, GVHD, hepatic venoocclusive disease (VOD), and pulmonary interstitial pneumonia increased with a 2-yr probability of TRM of 41%. The risk of TRM was 3.9× greater in patients receiving a second HSC within 6 mo of the first HSC infusion. The 2-yr probability of relapse after the second transplant was 65% and more frequent in patients not having achieved remission from the first transplant. The 2-yr probability of leukemia-free survival (LFS) was 21% and correlated best with a diagnosis of chronic myeloid leukemia (CML), acute leukemia in remission, initial remission greater than 6 mo, and better performance status.

The Gruppo Italiano Trapianto di Midolo Osseo (GITMO) reported their experience with second HSC transplants from 1987 to 1994 (72). Thirty-eight patients (median age 19 yr with range 2–46) had acute lymphoblastic leukemia (ALL) or AML in relapse or remission induced by additional cytotoxic treatment. The second HSC transplant was performed at a median time of 13 mo (range 4–88) after the first HSC transplant. All received second transplants from a genotypic HLA identical sibling (four not being the original donor) with intensive conditioning determined by the prior administration of TBI. GVHD prophylaxis was given to most patients. Prompt hematopoietic recovery occurred in all evaluable patients resulting in a 3-yr probability of event-free survival (EFS) of 42% improved for AML compared to ALL, but not improved in remission compared to relapse. Early TRM was 18.4% with a 3-yr probability of 28%. Acute GVHD increased after the second HSC transplant and was noted in 15 of 25 patients who apparently did not develop GVHD after the first transplant.

The SFGM reviewed 6709 allogeneic HSC transplant patients from 1984 to 1996 and noted 150 who underwent second HSC for relapse of acute or chronic leukemia *(73)*. Their median age was 25 yr (range 1.5–46) with 107 adults and 43 children. Diagnoses consisted of AML ($n = 61$), ALL ($n = 47$), or CML ($n = 42$); most patients were in complete remission or for CML, in chronic phase at the time of the initial transplant. At the time of the second transplant, a variety of treatments were undertaken with all patients receiving cytotoxic conditioning, 83% having the same donor, 20% receiving no GVHD prophylaxis, 7% receiving mobilized peripheral blood HSC, 2% receiving T cell-depleted HCS, and two syngeneic patients receiving a second allogeneic HSC infusion. Engraftment occurred in 93% of patients, 57% developed GVHD grade II–IV, 23% had severe grade III–IV GVHD, and 38% developed chronic GVHD. With a median follow-up of 30 mo, 24% of patients relapsed and 68% of patients died of TRM, resulting in an overall 5-yr DFS of 30%. In multivariate analysis, five factors correlated with improved survival (overall and disease free): age <16 yr, relapse >1 yr after the first transplant, absence of acute GVHD, occurrence of chronic GVHD, and the use of a female donor. Statistical limitations prevented analysis of the impact of the state of disease prior to second transplantation.

The Seattle group reported their results of second HSC transplantation for recurrent leukemia (CML, AML, and ALL) after initial transplantation with a TBI containing regimen (74). Despite treatment at a single institution, second treatment varied reflecting the current clinical practice at the time of second HSC transplant. The median time from first to second transplant was 28 mo (range 3–187), all patients used the same donor, had evidence of prior lymphoid engraftment and received cytotoxic chemotherapy conditioning regimens. GVHD prophylaxis had varying combinations of T cell depletion, immunosuppressive agents, and anti-T cell serotherapy. Sustained engraftment occurred in all evaluable patients. Severe RRT occurred in 39%, reflecting a greater than fourfold increase compared to the initial transplant; 62% of all patients developed VOD. At 1 yr after second transplantation, nonrelapse-related mortality was 45%, and relapse was 70%, resulting in an overall DFS probability of 14%, which was slightly improved for CML patients (28%). Severe VOD, age >10 yr, and GVHD <grade II adversely affected DFS.

4.1.1. COMPARISON OF AUTOLOGOUS VS ALLOGENEIC SECOND HCS TRANSPLANT

The decision to perform a second transplant using autologous or allogeneic HSC was discussed by the European Cooperative Group for Blood and Marrow Transplantation (EBMT) with a review of 2752 patients from 1981 through 1997, who relapsed after undergoing primary autologous HSC for AML in remission *(75)*. Ninety-four and 74 patients, respectively, underwent allogeneic or autologous second HSC transplant. TRM at 2 yr was 51% in recipients of matched allografts and 26% following an autograft ($p \leq 0.05$). Two-year DFS was 27% and 35% in the two groups, respectively ($p = $ NS). TRM was increased in patients who were in second or later remission at the time of the initial autograft ($p \leq 0.05$) and recipients of a second allograft ($p \leq 0.05$). Relapse was more common in patients with ALL ($p \leq 0.001$), patients >25 yr of age ($p \leq 0.02$), first autografts performed later than 1991 ($p \leq 0.05$), and with second autografts ($p \leq 0.05$). LFS was decreased in patients > 25 yr of age ($P \leq 0.01$) if the interval from first autograft to relapse was 8 mo or less ($p \leq 0.01$) and if TBI was used at first autograft ($p \leq 0.05$). Reviews like this indicate that second HSC should be considered without defining whether the outcome will be affected by the choice of an allogeneic or autolgous source of cells.

4.1.2. THE SOURCE OF HSC FOR SECOND HSC TRANSPLANT

The outcome using mobilized peripheral blood allogeneic HSC for second transplant was described in 10 patients after receiving an initial marrow HSC transplant *(76)*. Substantial heterogeneity of the small group was noted although hematopoietic recovery was more rapid

Table 2

Evaluations for Graft Dysfunction

- Were adequate initial HSC cells (e.g., CD34+) infused?
- Was the recipient heavily transfused or previously exposed to donor cells?
- Did the first transplant have an augmented risk of immunologic graft dysfunction such as T cell depletion, HLA disparity, or reduced intensity conditioning?
- Is there a hindrance to engraftment such as massive splenomegaly?
- Did the stem cells initially engraft?
- Was adequate GVHD prophylaxis administered?
- Did rejection occur after engraftment?
- Was an infection such as CMV, HHV-6, HHV-8, or parvovirus noted?
- Is there evidence of residual host immunity (CTL or NK) directed against donor cells?

by approx 1 wk in the second HSC transplant with survival of four out of six patients having an inter-transplant time greater than 1 yr. Other small studies confirm that G-CSF-mobilized stem cells result in rapid engraftment similar to primary transplantation *(77)*. However, considering the benefit of GVHD, the use of G-CSF mobilized peripheral cells as a source for second transplantation needs to be evaluated, since G-CSF-mobilization can perturb lymphocyte function, perhaps constraining a graft-vs-leukemia effect *(78)*. The overall benefit of peripheral compared to marrow cells has not been established although, the former will invariably result in a larger cell dose, more rapid engraftment, and perhaps reduced early morbidity *(79,80)*.

4.2. Cost-Effectiveness for Second HSC Transplant

Cost analysis of a second HSC transplant compared to conventional (nontransplant) options was performed in a retrospective study *(81)*. Data was derived from patients with acute leukemia who failed a first allogeneic HSC transplant. Patients from five second HSC transplant series ($n = 167$) and two nontransplant series ($n = 299$) were analyzed with outcome derived using survival extrapolation. Improved long-term ($p < 0.001$) and median survival ($p < 0.001$) of 20% and 10 mo compared to 0% and 3 mo was noted for the HSC transplant group and conventional therapy group, respectively. The estimated cost was $150,000 for HSC transplantation (range $90,000–$200,000) and $60,000 for conventional treatment. The analysis noted a cost benefit for HSC transplantation of $52,215 per life year gained extrapolated from a survival gain of 19.6 discounted months for the transplant group. Although substantial, this magnitude of cost was judged reasonable and justifiable in comparison with other oncologic interventions, especially with the observation of long-term EFS.

4.3. Decision Analysis for a Second HSC Transplant

The occurrence of severe graft dysfunction or malignant disease relapse is an indication for consideration of a second HSC transplant. However, some patients, especially those undergoing HLA disparate or ABO incompatible transplants, may experience sluggish engraftment and transient periods of lowered counts, especially with acute or chronic GVHD. In any case, hematopoietic growth factors should be utilized, especially with evidence of partial donor chimerism. The persistence of partial host chimerism, even without graft dysfunction, is a harbinger of disease relapse and warrants similar consideration, although DLI (without HSC infusion) may be an alternative since prospective comparison with full transplants have not been performed.

An evaluation for the cause of graft dysfunction should be instituted to determine whether the patient received an ample HSC infusion together with sufficient immunosuppression to blunt the likelihood of residual host immunity (Table 2). If a cause of graft dysfunction is noted,

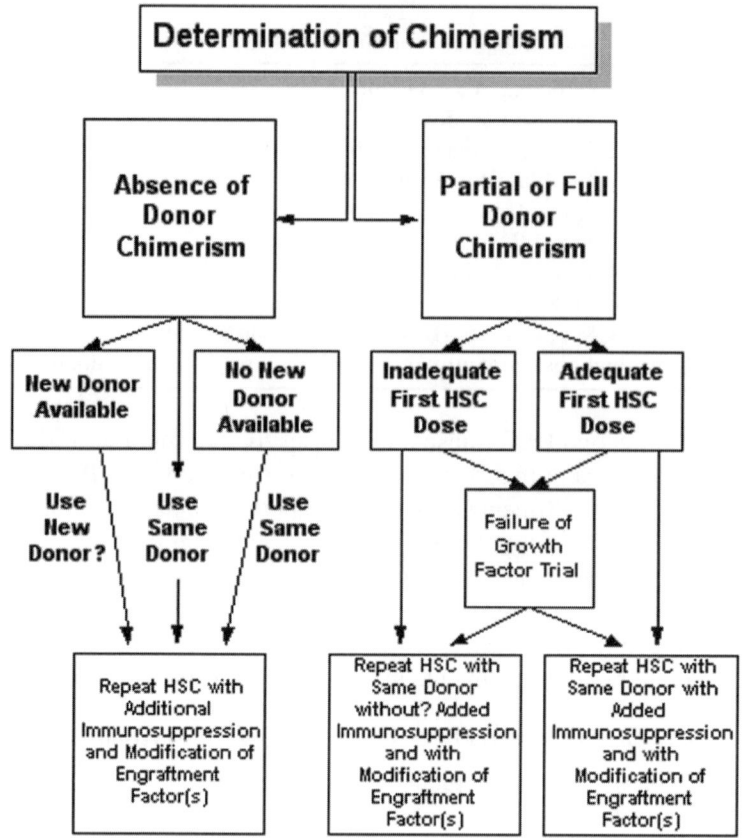

Fig. 1. Algorithm for a second HSC infusion for a graft dysfunction.

then specific modifications for the second HSC transplant should be undertaken. If no known cause is determined, then an immunologic mechanism must be considered and the second transplant should be undertaken with augmented immunosuppressive measures (82). Despite the lack of prospective randomized trials, there are basic tenets for a second HSC transplant. A generalized summary of the decision algorithm for a second HSC transplant for graft dysfunction is shown in Fig. 1. Nonetheless, there are still many unanswered questions that make absolute recommendations difficult.

4.3.1. ASSUMED TENETS FOR A SECOND HSC TRANSPLANT

1. Graft failure (absence of donor chimerism) without specific cause, especially with an adequate number of infused HSC, suggests a potent host immunologic mechanism of graft dysfunction. In this case, the second HSC transplant should be performed with enhanced immunosuppression including additional cytotoxic therapy, a large dose of HSC, and minimization of features associated with graft dysfunction. This would include avoiding or reducing T cell depletion and averting reduced intensity conditioning regimens (83). If available, consideration should be undertaken for the use of a different donor, especially if HLA disparity is not increased.
2. Infections associated with graft dysfunction should be treated and controlled prior to a second HSC transplant.
3. Graft dysfunction with substantial donor chimerism can be treated with growth factors (myeloid and erythroid) until it is determined that transfusion independence is not likely to be obtained.

A second HSC infusion (boost) using the same donor can be performed without cytotoxic conditioning by augmenting the dose of HSC with peripheral blood-mobilized HSC collections. However, unless immunologic mechanisms of graft dysfunction can be dismissed, the second infusion could be accompanied by additional immunosuppression to alleviate residual host immune mechanisms for marrow dysfunction. This can be accomplished by anti-T cell serotherapy with the consideration of additional cytotoxic immunosuppressive therapy *(84)*.

4.4. Remaining Questions for Second HSC

1. When should graft dysfunction with substantial donor chimerism be treated with growth factors and sustained observation prior to a second HCT?
2. When should a different donor be used?
3. Should HSC infusion without additional cytotoxic therapy (boost) ever be used, or should all second HSC infusions be performed with a minimum of additional immunosuppressive treatment?
4. With partial donor chimerism, is anti-T cell serotherapy followed by HSC infusion adequate for graft dysfunction or should additional cytotoxic immunosuppression be added?
5. What role does DLI have in ameliorating residual partial host chimerism to improve graft function?
6. What is the role of DLI compared to a second HSC transplant for the treatment of disease relapse?

5. SUMMARY

With fastidious management of the patient having graft dysfunction, this once formidable complication can be overcome with a second HSC infusion. However, graft dysfunction is still an adverse event reducing overall survival. The prognosis for long-term survival is improved with graft dysfunction occurring well after initial infusion and with evidence of partial donor chimerism. Second HSC transplantation for graft dysfunction should be considered a standard of practice. The relapse of malignant disease can also be overcome with a complete second HSC transplant, although results are still unsatisfactory compared to first transplants and alternatives should be investigated.

REFERENCES

1. Blau IW, Basara N, Serr A, et al. A second unrelated bone marrow transplant: successful quantitative monitoring of mixed chimerism using a highly discriminative PCR-STR system. *Clin Lab Haematol* 1999;21(2):133–138.
2. Thomas E, Storb R, Clift RA, et al. Bone-marrow transplantation (first of two parts). *N Engl J Med* 1975;292(16):832–843.
3. Thomas ED, Storb R, Clift RA, et al. Bone-marrow transplantation (second of two parts). *N Engl J Med* 1975; 292(17):895–902.
4. Davies SM, Weisdorf DJ, Haake RJ, et al. Second infusion of bone marrow for treatment of graft failure after allogeneic bone marrow transplantation. *Bone Marrow Transplant* 1994;14(1):73–7.
5. Donohue J, Homge M, Kernan NA. Characterization of cells emerging at the time of graft failure after bone marrow transplantation from an unrelated marrow donor. *Blood* 1993;82(3):1023–1029.
6. Storb R, Prentice RL, Thomas ED, et al. Factors associated with graft rejection after HLA-identical marrow transplantation for aplastic anaemia. *Br J Haematol* 1983;55(4):573–585.
7. Stucki A, Leisenring W, Sandmaier BM, et al. Decreased rejection and improved survival of first and second marrow transplants for severe aplastic anemia (a 26-year retrospective analysis). *Blood* 1998;92(8):2742–2749.
8. McCann SR, Bacigalupo A, Gluckman E, et al. Graft rejection and second bone marrow transplants for acquired aplastic anaemia: a report from the Aplastic Anaemia Working Party of the European Bone Marrow Transplant Group. *Bone Marrow Transplant* 1994;13(3):233–237.
9. Champlin RE, Horowitz MM, van Bekkum DW, et al. Graft failure following bone marrow transplantation for severe aplastic anemia: risk factors and treatment results. *Blood* 1989;73(2):606–613.
10. Ferster A, Corazza F, Vertongen F, et al. Transplanted sickle-cell disease patients with autologous bone marrow recovery after graft failure develop increased levels of fetal haemoglobin which corrects disease severity. *Br J Haematol* 1995;90(4):804–808.
11. Martin PJ, Akatsuka Y, Hahne M, et al. Involvement of donor T-cell cytotoxic effector mechanisms in preventing allogeneic marrow graft rejection. *Blood* 1998;92(6):2177–2181.

12. Beatty PG, Clift RA, Mickelson EM, et al. Marrow transplantation from related donors other than HLA-identical siblings. *N Engl J Med* 1985;313(13):765–771.

13. Anasetti C, Amos D, Beatty PG, et al. Effect of HLA compatibility on engraftment of bone marrow transplants in patients with leukemia or lymphoma. *N Engl J Med* 1989;320(4):197–204.

14. Beatty PG, Hansen JA, Longton GM, et al. Marrow transplantation from HLA-matched unrelated donors for treatment of hematologic malignancies. *Transplantation* 1991;51(2):443–447.

15. Kernan NA, Bartsch G, Ash RC, et al. Analysis of 462 transplantations from unrelated donors facilitated by the National Marrow Donor Program. *N Engl J Med* 1993;328(9):593–602.

16. McGlave P, Bartsch G, Anasetti C, et al. Unrelated donor marrow transplantation therapy for chronic myelogenous leukemia: initial experience of the National Marrow Donor Program. *Blood* 1993;81(2):543–550.

17. Bosserman LD, Murray C, Takvorian T, et al. Mechanism of graft failure in HLA-matched and HLA-mismatched bone marrow transplant recipients. *Bone Marrow Transplant* 1989;4(3):239–245.

18. Bunjes D, Wiesneth M, Hertenstein B, et al. Graft failure after T cell- depleted bone marrow transplantation: clinical and immunological characteristics and response to immunosuppressive therapy. *Bone Marrow Transplant* 1990;6(5):309–314.

19. Lamb LS, Szafer F, Henslee-Downey PJ, et al. Characterization of acute bone marrow graft rejection in T cell-depleted, partially mismatched related donor bone marrow transplantation. *Exp Hematol* 1995;23(14):1595–1600.

20. Lienert-Weidenbach K, Valiante NM, Brown C, et al. Mismatches for two major and one minor histocompatibility antigen correlate with a patient's rejection of a bone marrow graft from a serologically HLA-identical sibling. *Biol Blood Marrow Transplant* 1997;3(5):255–260.

21. Carella AM, Champlin R, Slavin S, et al. Mini-allografts: ongoing trials in humans. *Bone Marrow Transplant* 2000;25(4):345–350.

22. Bacigalupo A. Hematopoietic stem cell transplants after reduced intensity conditioning regimen (RI-HSCT): report of a workshop of the European group for Blood and Marrow Transplantation (EBMT). *Bone Marrow Transplant* 2000;25(8):803–805.

23. Bierer BE, Emerson SG, Antin J, et al. Regulation of cytotoxic T lymphocyte-mediated graft rejection following bone marrow transplantation. *Transplantation* 1988;46(6):835–839.

24. Petersdorf EW, Longton GM, Anasetti C, et al. Association of HLA-C disparity with graft failure after marrow transplantation from unrelated donors. *Blood* 1997;89(5):1818–1823.

25. Bishara A, Amar A, Brautbar C, et al. The putative role of HLA-C recognition in graft versus host disease (GVHD) and graft rejection after unrelated bone marrow transplantation (BMT). *Exp Hematol* 1995;23(14):1667–1675.

26. Fleischhauer K, Kernan NA, O'Reilly RJ, et al. Bone marrow- allograft rejection by T lymphocytes recognizing a single amino acid difference in HLA-B44. *N Engl J Med* 1990;323(26):1818–1822.

27. Marijt WA, Kernan NA, Diaz-Barrientos T, et al. Multiple minor histocompatibility antigen-specific cytotoxic T lymphocyte clones can be generated during graft rejection after HLA-identical bone marrow transplantation. *Bone Marrow Transplant* 1995;16(1):125–132.

28. Goss GD, Wittwer MA, Bezwoda WR, et al. Effect of natural killer cells on syngeneic bone marrow: in vitro and in vivo studies demonstrating graft failure due to NK cells in an identical twin treated by bone marrow transplantation. *Blood* 1985;66(5):1043–1046.

29. Dennert G, Anderson CG, Warner J. T killer cells play a role in allogeneic bone marrow graft rejection but not in hybrid resistance. *J Immunol* 1985;135(6):3729–3734.

30. Grigoriadou K, Menard C, Perarnau B, et al. MHC class Ia molecules alone control NK-mediated bone marrow graft rejection. *Eur J Immunol* 1999;29(11):3683–3690.

31. Quinones RR. Hematopoietic engraftment and graft failure after bone marrow transplantation. *Am J Pediatr Hematol Oncol* 1993;15(1):3–17.

32. Rosenfeld CS, Rybka WB, Weinbaum D, et al. Late graft failure due to dual bone marrow infection with variants A and B of human herpesvirus-6. *Exp Hematol* 1995;23(7):626–629.

33. Steffens HP, Podlech J, Kurz S, et al. Cytomegalovirus inhibits the engraftment of donor bone marrow cells by downregulation of hemopoietin gene expression in recipient stroma. *J Virol* 1998;72(6):5006-5015.

34. Johnston RE, Geretti AM, Prentice HG, et al. HHV-6-related secondary graft failure following allogeneic bone marrow transplantation. *Br J Haematol* 1999;105(4):1041–1043.

35. Eapen M, Davies SM, Ramsay NK. Late graft rejection and second infusion of bone marrow in children with aplastic anaemia. Br J Haematol, 1999. 104(1):186-8.

36. Bader P, Holle W, Klingebiel T, et al. Mixed hematopoietic chimerism after allogeneic bone marrow transplantation: the impact of quantitative PCR analysis for prediction of relapse and graft rejection in children. *Bone Marrow Transplant* 1997;19(7):697–702.

37. Cimino G, Rapanotti MC, Elia L, et al. A prospective molecular study of chimaerism in patients with haematological malignancies receiving unrelated cord blood or bone marrow transplants: detection of mixed chimaerism predicts graft failure with or without early autologous reconstitution in cord blood recipients. *Br J Haematol* 1999;104(4):770–777.

38. Gyger M, Baron C, Forest L, et al. Quantitative assessment of hematopoietic chimerism after allogeneic bone marrow transplantation has predictive value for the occurrence of irreversible graft failure and graft-vs.-host disease. *Exp Hematol* 1998;26(5):426–434.

39. Dufour C, Dallorso S, Casarino L, et al. Late graft failure 8 years after first bone marrow transplantation for severe acquired aplastic anemia. *Bone Marrow Transplant* 1999;23(7):743–745.

40. Bacigalupo A, Bruno B, Saracco P, et al. Antilymphocyte globulin, cyclosporine, prednisolone, and granulocyte colony-stimulating factor for severe aplastic anemia: an update of the GITMO/EBMT study on 100 patients. European Group for Blood and Marrow Transplantation (EBMT) Working Party on Severe Aplastic Anemia and the Gruppo Italiano Trapianti di Midolio Osseo (GITMO). *Blood* 2000;95(6):1931–1934.

41. Marsh J, Schrezenmeier H, Marin P, et al. Prospective randomized multicenter study comparing cyclosporin alone versus the combination of antithymocyte globulin and cyclosporin for treatment of patients with nonsevere aplastic anemia: a report from the European Blood and Marrow Transplant (EBMT) Severe Aplastic Anaemia Working Party. *Blood* 1999;93(7):2191–2195.

42. Shing MM, Vowels M. Role of second bone marrow transplants. *Bone Marrow Transplant* 1993;12(1):21–25.

43. Beguin Y, Collignon J, Laurent C, et al. Spontaneous complete remission and recovery of donor haemopoiesis without GVHD after relapse and apparent marrow graft rejection in poor-prognosis myelodysplastic syndrome. *Br J Haematol* 1996;94(3):507–509.

44. Nemunaitis J, Singer JW, Buckner CD, et al. Use of recombinant human granulocyte-macrophage colony-stimulating factor in graft failure after bone marrow transplantation. *Blood* 1990;76(1):245–253.

45. Sierra J, Terol MJ, Urbano-Ispizua A, et al. Different response to recombinant human granulocyte-macrophage colony-stimulating factor in primary and secondary graft failure after bone marrow transplantation. *Exp Hematol* 1994;22(7):566–572.

46. Weisdorf DJ, Verfaillie CM, Davies SM, et al. Hematopoietic growth factors for graft failure after bone marrow transplantation: a randomized trial of granulocyte-macrophage colony-stimulating factor (GM-CSF) versus sequential GM-CSF plus granulocyte-CSF. *Blood* 1995;85(12):3452–3456.

47. Aversa F, Tabilio A, Velardi A, et al. Treatment of high-risk acute leukemia with T-cell-depleted stem cells from related donors with one fully mismatched HLA haplotype. *N Engl J Med* 1998;339(17):1186–1193.

48. Guardiola P, Kuentz M, Garban F, et al. Second early allogeneic stem cell transplantations for graft failure in acute leukaemia, chronic myeloid leukaemia and aplastic anaemia. French Society of Bone Marrow Transplantation. *Br J Haematol* 2000;111(1):292–302.

49. Remberger M, Ringden O, Ljungman P, et al. Booster marrow or blood cells for graft failure after allogeneic bone marrow transplantation. *Bone Marrow Transplant* 1998;22(1):73–78.

50. O'Donnell J, Roberts I, De la Fuente J, et al. Successful second bone marrow transplant for Fanconi's anaemia following escalation of conditioning. *Br J Haematol* 1997;98(3):772–774.

51. Grandage VL, Cornish JM, Pamphilon DH, et al. Second allogeneic bone marrow transplants from unrelated donors for graft failure following initial unrelated donor bone marrow transplantation. *Bone Marrow Transplant* 1998;21(7):687–690.

52. Wolff D, Becker C, Kubel M, et al. Second unrelated bone marrow transplantation without additional conditioning therapy after engraftment failure. *Bone Marrow Transplant* 1998;21(3):315–317.

53. Zecca M, Perotti C, Marradi P, et al. Recombinant human G-CSF- mobilized peripheral blood stem cells for second allogeneic transplant after bone marrow graft rejection in children. *Br J Haematol* 1996;92(2):432–434.

54. Molina L, Chabannon C, Viret F, et al. Granulocyte colony-stimulating factor-mobilized allogeneic peripheral blood stem cells for rescue graft failure after allogeneic bone marrow transplantation in two patients with acute myeloblastic leukemia in first complete remission. *Blood* 1995;85(6):1678,1679.

55. Selleri C, Raiola A, De Rosa G, et al. CD34+-enriched donor lymphocyte infusions in a case of pure red cell aplasia and late graft failure after major ABO-incompatible bone marrow transplantation. *Bone Marrow Transplant* 1998;22(6):605–607.

56. Barrett AJ, Locatelli F, Treleaven JG, et al. Second transplants for leukaemic relapse after bone marrow transplantation: high early mortality but favourable effect of chronic GVHD on continued remission. A report by the EBMT Leukaemia Working Party. *Br J Haematol* 1991;79(4):567–574.

57. Miniero R, Busca A, Vai S, et al. Second bone marrow transplant for children who relapsed or rejected their first graft: experience of the Italian Pediatric Hematology and Oncology Group (AIEOP). *Bone Marrow Transplant* 1996;18(Suppl 2):135–138.

58. Wagner JE, Santos GW, Burns WH, et al. Second bone marrow transplantation after leukemia relapse in 11 patients. *Bone Marrow Transplant* 1989;4(1):115–118.

59. Kishi K, Takahashi S, Gondo H, et al. Second allogeneic bone marrow transplantation for post-transplant leukemia relapse: results of a survey of 66 cases in 24 Japanese institutes. *Bone Marrow Transplant* 1997;19(5):461–466.

60. Tsai T, Goodman S, Saez R, et al. Allogeneic bone marrow transplantation in patients who relapse after autologous transplantation. *Bone Marrow Transplant* 1997;20(10):859–863.

61. Aschan J, Remberger M, Carlens S, et al. Unrelated donor stem cell transplantation after autologous transplantation: experience of a single center. *Bone Marrow Transplant* 1999;24(3):279–282.

62. Spinolo JA, Yau JC, Dicke KA, et al. Second bone marrow transplants for relapsed leukemia. *Cancer* 1992;69(2):405–409.

63. Chiang KY, Weisdorf DJ, Davies SM, et al. Outcome of second bone marrow transplantation following a uniform conditioning regimen as therapy for malignant relapse. *Bone Marrow Transplant* 1996;17(1):39–42.

64. Lipton JH, Messner H. The role of second bone marrow transplant using a different donor for relapsed leukemia or graft failure. *Eur J Haematol* 1997;58(2):133–136.

65. Aoki Y, Takahashi S, Okamoto S, et al. Graft-versus-leukemia after second allogeneic bone marrow transplantation. *Blood* 1994;84(11):3983.

66. Mattot M, Ninane J, Vermylen C, et al. Second bone marrow transplantation in eight children. *Pediatr Hematol Oncol* 1992;9(4):353–357.

67. Mahon FX, Marit G, Viard F, et al. Second bone marrow transplantation for leukemic relapse without graft-vs.-host disease prophylaxis. *Am J Hematol* 1993;43(4):324,325.

68. Martino R, Badell I, Brunet S, et al. Second bone marrow transplantation for leukemia in untreated relapse. *Bone Marrow Transplant* 1994;14(4):589–593.

69. Mehta J, Powles R, Treleaven J, et al. Outcome of acute leukemia relapsing after bone marrow transplantation: utility of second transplants and adoptive immunotherapy. *Bone Marrow Transplant* 1997;19(7):709–719.

70. Ashida T, Kawanishi K, Ariyama T, et al. Successful graft-versus- leukemia effect of second bone marrow transplantation on relapsed leukemia cutis that was refractory to intensive chemotherapy and donor lymphocyte transfusions in a patient with acute monocytic leukemia. *Int J Hematol* 2000;71(4):385–388.

71. Mrsic M, Horowitz MM, Atkinson K, et al. Second HLA-identical sibling transplants for leukemia recurrence. *Bone Marrow Transplant* 1992;9(4):269–275.

72. Bosi A, Bacci S, Miniero R, et al. Second allogeneic bone marrow transplantation in acute leukemia: a multicenter study from the Gruppo Italiano Trapianto Di Midollo Osseo (GITMO). *Leukemia* 1997;11(3):420–424.

73. Michallet M, Tanguy ML, Socie G, et al. Second allogeneic haematopoietic stem cell transplantation in relapsed acute and chronic leukaemias for patients who underwent a first allogeneic bone marrow transplantation: a survey of the Societe Francaise de Greffe de moelle (SFGM). *Br J Haematol* 2000;108(2):400–407.

74. Radich JP, Sanders JE, Buckner CD, et al. Second allogeneic marrow transplantation for patients with recurrent leukemia after initial transplant with total-body irradiation-containing regimens. *J Clin Oncol* 1993;11(2):304–313.

75. Ringden O, Labopin M, Frassoni F, et al. Allogeneic bone marrow transplant or second autograft in patients with acute leukemia who relapse after an autograft. Acute Leukaemia Working Party of the European Group for Blood and Marrow Transplantation (EBMT). *Bone Marrow Transplant* 1999;24(4):389–396.

76. Russell JA, Bowen T, Brown C, et al. Second allogeneic transplants for leukemia using blood instead of bone marrow as a source of hemopoietic cells. *Bone Marrow Transplant* 1996;18(3):501–505.

77. Bensinger WI, Martin PJ, Storer B, et al. Transplantation of Bone Marrow as Compared with Peripheral-Blood Cells from HLA-Identical Relatives in Patients with Hematologic Cancers. *N Engl J Med* 2001;344(3):175–181.

78. Gyger M, Stuart RK, Perreault, C. Immunobiology of allogeneic peripheral blood mononuclear cells mobilized with granulocyte-colony stimulating factor. *Bone Marrow Transplant* 2000;26(1):1–16.

79. Arslan O, Seferoglu A, Gurman G, et al. Resistant graft failure overcome with allogenic peripheral blood plus bone marrow stem cells. *Haematologia* 1998;29(1):47–50.

80. Cobos E, Keung YK, Morgan D, et al. Successful engraftment using allogeneic peripheral blood progenitor cells in a patient with primary bone marrow graft failure. *J Hematother* 1995;4(1):37–40.

81. Messori A, Costantini M, Bonistalli L, et al. Second bone marrow transplantation in non-Hodgkin's lymphoma. *J Clin Oncol* 1998;16(2):804–806.

82. Or R, Mehta J, Kapelushnik J, et al. Total lymphoid irradiation, anti- lymphocyte globulin and Campath 1-G for immunosuppression prior to bone marrow transplantation for aplastic anemia after repeated graft rejection. *Bone Marrow Transplant* 1994;13(1):97–99.

83. Herve P, Cahn JY, Flesch M, et al. Successful graft-versus-host disease prevention without graft failure in 32 HLA-identical allogeneic bone marrow transplantations with marrow depleted of T cells by monoclonal antibodies and complement. *Blood* 1987;69(2):388–393.

84. Byrne JL, Stainer C, Cull G, et al. The effect of the serotherapy regimen used and the marrow cell dose received on rejection, graft-versus-host disease and outcome following unrelated donor bone marrow transplantation for leukaemia. *Bone Marrow Transplant* 2000;25(4):411–417.

VI PRECLINICAL STUDIES IN ALLOGENEIC TRANSPLANTATION

The Role of T Cell Depletion
in Bone Marrow Transplantation

Yair Reisner, PHD and Massimo F. Martelli, MD, PHD

1. INTRODUCTION

New advances in the understanding of the complex mechanisms underlying acute and chronic graft-vs-host disease (GVHD) revealed the role of key cytokines and chemokines involved in the outbreak of the "cytokine storm," which follows the initial allostimulation in vivo *(1–4)*. However, to date, none of the attempts to translate these new insights into clinical interventions have led to a major improvement in the control of GVHD. Clearly, containing such a multifactorial outbreak by a single or even a double agent is enormously difficult, if not impossible.

In contrast, numerous murine and clinical studies during the past three decades have demonstrated that effective T cell depletion of bone marrow preparations can completely prevent the development of both acute and chronic GVHD in the absence of any posttransplant prophlyaxis *(5–16)*. However, the benefit of this simple modality of GVHD prevention was found to enhance the risk of graft failure and leukemia relapse *(17)*.

These obstacles, which are largely caused by the absence of GVHD, were addressed during the past decade either by modifications introduced to the conditioning protocols or by manipulating the composition of the graft. In the present chapter, the outcome of these "fine tuning" attempts to enable successful use of T cell depletion, primarily in the treatment of leukemia, is reviewed.

2. HAPLOIDENTICAL TRANSPLANTS IN SEVERE COMBINED IMMUNE DEFICIENCY: PROOF OF PRINCIPLE

Early studies in murine models of marrow transplantation demonstrated that GVHD is initiated by thymus-derived T lymphocytes of donor origin. Transplantation of allogeneic

From: *Current Clinical Oncology: Allogeneic Stem Cell Transplantation*
Edited by: Mary S. Laughlin and Hillard M. Lazarus © Humana Press Inc., Totowa, NJ

hematopoietic tissues deficient in T lymphocytes, such as early fetal liver *(5)*, adult spleen, or marrow cells from mice thymectomized in the neonatal period *(13)*, or marrow or spleen cells pretreated with a cytotoxic antiserum specific for T lymphocytes *(12)*, resulted in stable chimeras without GVHD. Such transplants have regularly produced immunologically vigorous long-lived chimeras when donor and recipient are haploidentical (e.g., parent—F1). Production of long-lived chimeras was less consistent when fully allogeneic transplants were performed, due in part to a reduced incidence of engraftment and also, possibly, to genetic restrictions on cooperation between donor lymphoid cells and host elements in the generation of effective immune responses *(18)*.

Based on the insight that GVHD is triggered by T cells, several techniques were developed during the 1970s that are effective in depleting alloreactive T lymphocytes from mouse marrow or spleen cells. These included: (i) physical separation of the stem cells either by discontinuous gradient of bovine serum albumin or by velocity sedimentation *(7)*; (ii) in vitro "suicide" techniques *(11)*; (iii) pre-treatment with antibodies specific for the Th1 antigen present on thymic and circulating T lymphocytes *(12)*; and (iv) selective fractionation of hematopoietic precursors with plant lectins *(8)*.

The first successful clinical application of T cell-depleted 3-loci-mismatched parental bone marrow transplant was achieved in the early 1980s in the treatment of patients with severe combined immune deficiency (SCID) *(14)*. The problem of GVHD, which is almost uniformly lethal in such transplants, was completely prevented by 3 log T cell depletion using soybean lectin and E-rosetting *(9,10,14)*.

In this initial study, in two of three transplanted patients, engraftment and development of parental lymphoid cells was associated with normalization of T cell numbers, full reconstitution of in-vitro transformation responses to mitogens and antigens, development of the capacity to generate cytokines in vitro, and in vivo delayed type hypersensitive responses to dinitrochloroenzene (DNCB). The engrafted parental lymphocytes were also capable of allospecific response, as indicated by their strong reactivity to third party cells in mixed leukocyte culture (MLC) *(14)*. Reactivity of engrafted parental T cells against host cells in vitro was markedly reduced, thus demonstrating that tolerance towards host antigens had been established, as previously documented in animal models (Table 1).

Since this initial study, more than 300 transplants from haploidentical donors have been carried out worldwide with a high rate of long-term partial or complete immune reconstitution, confirming that GVHD can be completely prevented in SCID patients by 3 log T cell depletion *(19–22)*.

Interestingly, these patients frequently develop a unique state of split lymphoid chimerism having T cells of donor origin and non-T cells, which are predominantly or exclusively of host origin. Rosenkrantz *(23)* studied the immunologic recognition of donor, host, or third party alloantigens.

When compared with freshly isolated donor lymphocytes, the engrafted donor cells exhibited markedly reduced to absent responses toward host antigen (Ag) in primary or secondary MLC and cell-mediated lympholysis assays. However, under limiting dilution conditions, cytotoxic responses to host Ag could be demonstrated, indicating that small numbers of host-reactive cells were present, although down-regulated at high responder cell doses *(23)*. These results are consistent with prior observations in limiting dilution cultures that indicate that cells with the potential to lyse autologous target cells exist in the peripheral blood of all normal individuals. The number of host reactive cells present in these patients is significantly less than that present in cells isolated directly from the marrow donors, and is also less than the number of autocytotoxic cells normally seen in peripheral blood. Together, these observations indicate that two mechanisms contribute to donor host tolerance in these patients. The majority of host-reactive cells appear to have undergone clonal deletion or inactivation, whereas the small residual host-reactive population appears to be under ongoing immunoregulatory control.

Table 1
MLC Posttransplantation of Patient UPN 75 (In Vitro Incorporation of 14C-Thymidine [net cpm])[a]

	Stimulators			
	Patient's[b] non-T lymphocytes	Father's non-T lymphocytes	Mother's non-T lymphocytes	Unrelated pool
Responders				
Paternal lymphocytes	5.843	685	9.038	7.773
Engrafted paternal T lymphocytes	350	80	8950	3242

[a]Reprinted from ref. *(14)*.
[b]Non-T lymphocytes express HLA phenotype of the patient.

3. T CELL DEPLETION IN THE TREATMENT OF LEUKEMIA

3.1. HLA Identical Related Donors

Following the encouraging results in SCID patients, it was reasonable to assume that in leukemia patients pretreated by supralthal radiochemotherapy, the remaining immunity at the day of the transplant is dramatically reduced as in SCID patients and, therefore, graft rejection should not represent a major problem. However, early results suggested that this was not the case, and a high rate (>50%) of graft rejection was documented *(17,24,25)*. Similar to findings in the mouse *(26)* and primate *(27)* models, Kernan et al. *(28)* and Butturini et al. *(29)* found evidence that rejection of human leukocyte antigen (HLA)-nonidentical marrow grafts was associated with the emergence of host-derived specific anti-donor cytotoxic T lymphocytes (CTLs) directed against major HLA class 1 determinants.

Significant rates (10–20%) of graft rejection were also documented upon the initial attempts to employ T cell-depleted HLA identical transplants in leukemia patients *(25,30–36)*. This problem was contained to some extent in the mid 1980s by adding antithymocyte globulin (ATG) and steroids to the conditioning protocol, as well as to the immediate posttransplant period. However, the slight improvement in engraftment was offset by an increased rate of Epstein-Barr virus (EBV) lymphoproliferative disease *(37)*. Thus, ATG inclusion in the preparative regimen was limited to the pretransplant period.

Further improvement of engraftment without adverse effects was achieved in the early 1990s by the addition of thiotepa to the conditioning protocol. This modality, based on a preclinincal study in the mouse model *(38)*. was initially used in the treatment of leukemia patients by Aversa et al. *(39)*, and subsequently adopted by the Sloan-Kettering group *(40)*, with both teams employing identical conditioning and both making use of bone marrow depleted of T cells by soybean agglutination and E-rosetting technique. In the former study, this approach was tested in 54 consecutive patients with acute leukemia (median age 30 yr) who received transplants from HLA-identical sibling donors or, in two cases, from family donors mismatched at D-DR. No posttransplant immunosuppressive treatment was given as GVHD prophylaxis. Neither graft rejection nor GVHD occurred. Transplant-related deaths occurred in six (16.6%) of 36 patients in remission and in seven (38.8%) of 18 patients in relapse at the time of transplantation. The probability of relapse was 0.12 for patients with acute myeloid leukemia (AML) and 0.28 for patients with acute lymphoblastic leukemia (ALL) who received transplants at the first or second remission. At a median follow-up of 6.9 yr (minimum follow-up, 4.9 yr), disease-free survival (DFS) for patients who received transplants while in remission was 0.74 for AML patients and 0.59 for ALL patients. (Fig. 1). All surviving patients had 100% performance status.

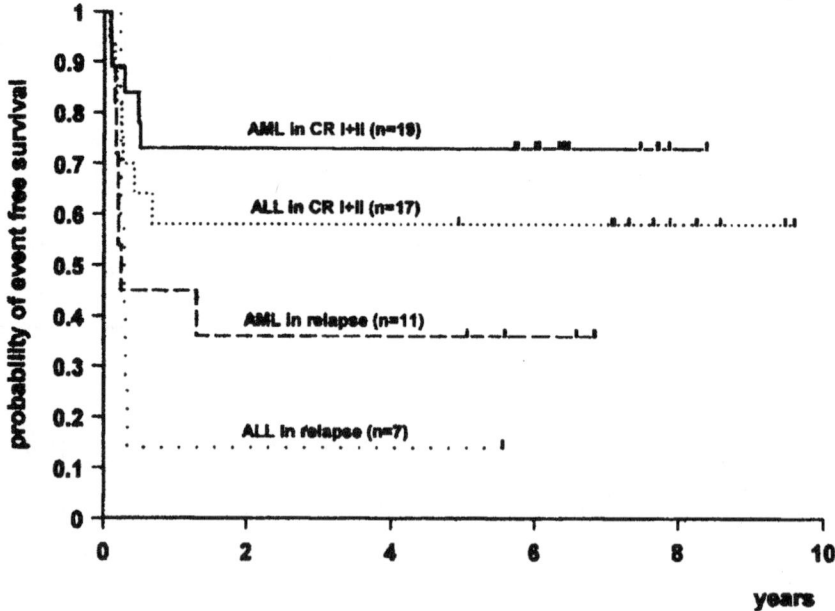

Fig. 1. Probability of event-free survival for patients with acute leukemia who underwent BMT while in first or second remission (upper curves) or while in relapse (lower curves). The tick marks represent patients alive and disease-free at the time of analysis. Reprinted with permission from ref. *(39)*.

The second study reported the results of 31 consecutive patients with AML in first remission (median age 36.7) and 8 in second remission (median age 32.9) who have achieved a median follow-up duration of approx 4.8 and 4 yr, respectively. DFS probabilities were 77 and 50%, respectively (Fig. 2). Probabilities for relapse were 3.2 or 12.5%, respectively, and 19.4 or 37.5%, respectively, for nonleukemic mortality. There were no cases of immune-mediated graft rejection and no cases of grade II to IV acute GVHD. All but two survivors enjoy performance scores of 100%.

Altogether, these similar studies strongly suggest that engraftment without GVHD can now be attained in recipients of T cell-depleted HLA identical transplants without an adverse effect on relapse rate.

An essentially similar outcome was also documented recently in AML patients in first remission, pretreated with anti-CD52 (CAMPATH-1G) to overcome graft rejection and receiving HLA identical bone marrow depleted of T cells with CD52 (CAMPATH-1M) *(41)*. No posttransplant immunosuppression was given. Results were compared with two control groups: (i) 50 patients who received bone marrow depleted with CAMPATH-1M, but no CAMPATH-1G in vivo; and (ii) 459 patients reported to the International Bone Marrow Transplant Registry (IBMTR) who received nondepleted grafts and conventional GVHD prophylaxis with cyclosporin A (CyA) and methotrexate (MTX). The incidence of acute GVHD was 4% in the treatment group compared with 35% in the CyA/MTX group ($p < 0.001$). Chronic GVHD was also relatively low in the treatment group (3 vs 36%; $p < 0.001$). The problem of graft rejection, which had been frequent in the historic CAMPATH-1M group (31%), was largely overcome in the treatment group (6%). Thus, transplant-related mortality of the treatment group (15% at 5 yr) was lower than for the CyA/MTX group (26%; $p = 0.04$). There was little difference in the risk of leukemia relapse between the treatment group (30% at 5 yr) and the CyA/MTX group (29%). Survival of the treatment group at 6 mo was better than the CyA/MTX group (92 vs 78%), although at 5 yr the difference was not significant (62 vs 58%) and neither was the difference in leukemia-free survival (60 vs 52%).

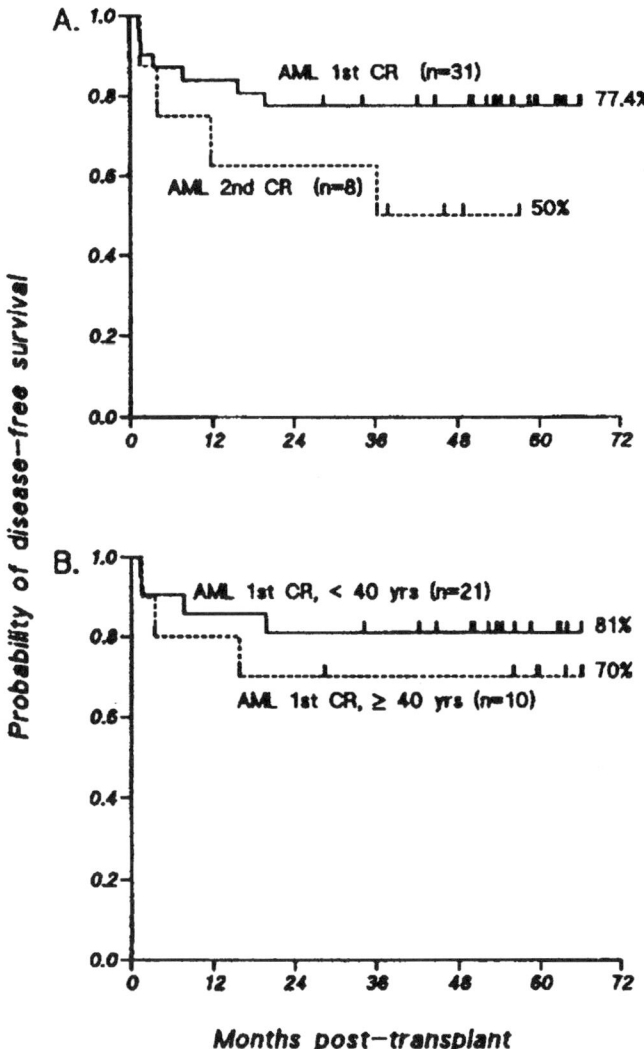

Fig. 2. Kaplan-Meier estimates of probability of DFS for patients transplanted with T cell-depleted allografts for AML. **(A)** Patients with AML transplaned in first CR compared with those transplanted in second CR. **(B)** Patients with AML transplanted in first CR, analyzed according to age at time of BMT; *p* value was not significant. Reprinted with permission from ref. *(40)*.

Very recently, similar preliminary results were obtained at six centers when the same approach was studied in 187 consecutive patients who received granulocyte colony-stimulating factor (G-CSF)-mobilized peripheral blood cell transplants from HLA-matched siblings between 1997 and 1999 *(42)*.

In contrast to results obtained with T cell depletion in acute leukemia, the outcome of such transplants in chronic myeloid leukemia (CML) patients was clearly associated with a markedly enhanced relapse rate and, therefore, for almost 10 yr beginning in the mid 1980s, when this problem was initially recognised *(17)*, T cell-depleted transplants were not used in the treatment of CML. However, with the advent of donor lymphocyte infusion (DLI) *(22,43–48)*, the road was opened to a "comeback" of T cell depletion in CML.

In 1995, Mackinnon et al. *(49)* investigated whether a DLI dose capable of inducing remission without GVHD could be found. They demonstrated that while only one of the eight patients who achieved remission at a T cell dose of 1×10^7/kg developed GVHD, this complication developed in 8 of the 11 responders who received a T cell dose of less than or equal to 5×10^7/kg. Thus, they concluded that in many patients this potent graft-vs-leukemia (GVL) effect can occur in the absence of clinical GVHD. Alternatively, Naparstek et al. (50), advocated the treatment of hematological malignancies with T cell-depleted transplants followed by DLI prophylaxis in every patient. However, the role of DLI in acute leukemia is still controversial and the GVHD rate associated with this form of DLI may not result in an improved DFS.

One remaining difficulty associated with T cell depletion in adult and to a lesser degree in childhood leukemia, is the slow immune recovery. Roosnek, Rous, and coworkers studied the repopulation of the T cell compartment in 27 patients transplanted with bone marrow from an HLA identical sibling (51). Significant differences were found between recipients of unmanipulated and T cell-depleted grafts. Analysis of the T cells by a method based on amplification of minisatellite DNA regions showed that without depletion, >99.9% of the clones responding to a mitogenic stimulus after transplantation were of donor origin. In contrast, when the graft had been depleted with CAMPATH-1M plus complement, a significant part of the T cells clones during the first weeks after transplantation comprised recipient T cells that had survived the preconditioning. Analysis of the T cell receptor repertoire showed that in recipients of a T cell-depleted graft, the recipient as well as the donor T cells that repopulated the peripheral T cell pool during the first month were the progeny of a limited number of precursors. Clearly, without depletion, larger numbers of donor T cells are being cotransfused with the marrow and, consequently, the repertoire is much more diverse. These data show that immediately after transplantation, the peripheral pool is repopulated primarily through expansion of circulating T cells.

More recently, the same group studied the reconstitution of the T cell compartment after bone marrow transplantation (BMT) in five patients who received a GVHD prophylaxis consisting of MTX, Cy, and 10 daily injections (d 24–15) of CAMPATH-1G (52). This treatment eliminated virtually all T cells and enabled the analysis of the thymus-dependent and -independent pathways of T cell regeneration. Based on the levels of $CD4^+$ $CD45RA^+$ RO^- and $CD4^+$ $CD45RA^+$ RO^- T cells in the peripheral blood and on T cell repertoire analyzed by T cell receptor (TCR) spectra typing, the authors concluded that after BMT, the thymus is essential for the restoration of the T cell repertoire. Because the thymic activity is restored in adults with a lag time of approx 6 mo, this might explain why, particularly in recipients of a T cell-depleted graft, immune recovery is delayed.

Similar studies were conducted by the Sloan Kettering group investigating immune reconstitution in patients transplanted with lectin-separated HLA identical marrow, from sibling (37) or from unrelated donors (53). However, while in agreement that the immune deficit is associated with recipient age, the authors did not find a major difference between adult recipients of T cell-depleted and -nondepleted marrow from matched sibling donors. In addition, these studies suggested that a CD4 cell count above 200/mm^2 might be useful in predicting which patients are at increased risk of developing opportunistic infections following successful engraftment.

3.2. HLA Identical Unrelated Donors

Altogether, the modifications introduced in the late 1980s into the conditioning of leukemic recipients of T cell-depleted HLA identical marrow from sibling donors have now been evaluated in a large number of patients with a long follow-up period. The encouraging DFS rate attained with an extremely low incidence of GVHD and in the absence of posttransplant prophylaxis prompted further investigation of the role of T cell depletion in matched unrelated transplants. Recent results in children suggest comparable efficacy to that found in matched sibling transplants *(53–55)*, but in adult recipients there seems to be a more profound deficit in immune recovery following transplantation of matched unrelated T cell-depleted transplants *(53)*. Small et al. suggest that several factors could be hypothesized to account for the more profound and prolonged immunological deficiencies observed among recipients of transplants from unrelated donors *(54)*. First, major or microvariant HLA disparities between donor and host might, on the one hand, alter the capacity of the donor's lymphoid progenitors to migrate to or mature within the host thymus or, on the other hand, stimulate clinical or subclinical GVHD, thereby further potentiating thymic injury. In this context, it is possible that mild clinical or even subclinical forms of GVHD could contribute to the extended immunodeficiency observed after unrelated BMT.

A second factor that most likely contributes to the delayed and incomplete immune reconstitution of T cells observed in adults is the involution of the thymus, which normally occurs in adulthood, beginning late in the second decade of life (reviewed in ref. *56*). Interestingly, the authors showed that the immune deficit in these patients can be partially corrected by adoptive cell therapy with small numbers of donor T cells. As in the treatment of CML relapse, GVHD associated with DLI was more likely to be prevented if DLI was administered at time points greater than 4 mo posttransplant.

Very recently Champlin et al. reviewed data of 870 patients with leukemia who received T cell-depleted transplants from unrelated or HLA-mismatched related donors from 1982 to 1994 *(57)*. Outcomes were compared with those of 998 non-T cell-depleted transplants. Five categories of T cell-depletion techniques were compared: (i) narrow-specificity antibodies, (ii) broad-specificity antibodies, (iii) CAMPATH antibodies, (iv) elutriation, and (v) lectins. Strategies resulting in similar DFS were pooled to compare T cell depleted with non-T cell-depleted transplants. Recipients of transplants T cell depleted by narrow-specificity antibodies had lower treatment failure risk (higher DFS) than recipients of transplants T cell depleted by other techniques. Compared with non-T cell-depleted transplants (5-yr probability of DFS, 31%), 5-yr DFS was 29% (P = NS) after transplants T cell depleted by narrow-specificity antibodies and 16% (p < 0.0001) after transplants T cell depleted by other techniques.

While this retrospective study is important in establishing relevant factors underlying the outcome of T cell-depleted unrelated transplants, this study ignores the advances in T cell depletion made in the late 1980s in the treatment of acute leukemia patients or in the mid 1990s in the treatment of CML (see above). Thus, by including CML patients treated before DLI was introduced or AML and ALL treated between 1984 and 1990 (before thiotepa was added to the conditioning of acute leukemia recipients of lectin-separated grafts and before CAMPATH-1G was introduced to the conditioning of recipients of CAMPATH-1M treated grafts), the results were biased against T depletion techniques, such as lectin or CAMPATH-1M, which afford effective T cell depletion.

Further analysis of the same data basis, taking into account the importance of the modifications specifically aimed at compensating for the withdrawal of the alloreactive effects associated with GVHD, is warranted.

3.3. HLA Haploidentical Donors

3.3.1. T Cell Depletion Ex Vivo Combined with Posttransplant GVHD Prophylaxis

While the mild adverse effects of T cell depletion in HLA identical leukemic recipients, namely graft rejection and relapse, were monitored and dealt with as described above by slight modifications to the treatment protocols, the high rate of graft rejection in 3 loci haploidentical recipients precluded for almost a decade the use of T cell depletion in the latter group of patients.

This resistance to engraftment was shown to be mediated primarily by host-derived CTLs, and therefore subsequent research with animal models was focused on the host immunity remaining after lethal total body irradiation (TBI) *(26–29)*, as well as on new approaches to overcome this barrier to bone marrow allografting. These murine models have shown that incompatible T cell-depleted transplants can be successfully performed by manipulating the preparative regimen and/or the graft composition. Immunologic response of the remaining recipient immune system against the graft can be overcome by increasing the dose of TBI *(26,58,59)* or by adding selective anti-T measures with low extrahematological toxicity, such as splenic irradiation *(60)* or in vivo treatment with anti-T monoclonal antibodies *(61,62)*. Engraftment is also improved by increasing the myeloablative effect of the conditioning regimen, through the use of dimethyl-myleran, busulfan *(63)*, or thiotepa *(38)*, given with TBI. The use of intensified conditioning protocol, combined with less extensive T cell depletion ex vivo and GVHD prophylaxis in vivo, was carried out primarily in pediatric patients by Henslee-Downey *(64)*. Sixty-seven patients, 43 with ALL and 24 with AML, were transplanted with bone marrow from related donors. Two to three loci HLA disparity was detected in two-thirds of the donor–recipient pairs. Conditioning therapy, including TBI and chemotherapy followed by GVHD (GvHD) prophylaxis with partial T cell depletion of the graft using T10B9 or OKT3, was combined with posttransplantation immunosuppression.

Estimated probability (EP) of engraftment was 0.96 and was not affected by donor–antigen mismatch. EP of grades II–IV acute GVHD was 0.24, and EP of DFS was 0.26 at 3 yr ,but improved to 0.45 when donors were younger than 30 yr ($P < 0.001$). EP of relapse at 3 yr was 0.41 and was reduced with younger donors' age. For patients who were in relapse at the time of transplantation, absence of blasts was associated with a lower relapse rate (0.46 vs 0.84; $p = 0.083$), similar to that of patients in remission.

While acute and chronic GVHD were not prevented successfully in these partially matched transplants (only 40% of the donor–host pairs were 3 loci mismatched) compared to other T cell-depletion methods making use of CD34 selection, lectin agglutination, or treatment with CAMPATH, the authors argue that DFS was not inferior. However, preliminary data from studies using megadose CD34 transplants in childhood leukemia, preventing completely GVHD or graft rejection in children, seem to induce superior immune reconstitution and are associated with lower infection-related mortality (*see* Section 3.3.2.). Clearly, further evaluation and better controlled trials are required.

3.3.2. The Megadose Approach

An alternative approach to overcome rejection of T cell-depleted bone marrow in the mouse model, is by using cell dose escalation *(63,65,66)*. Thus, full donor-type engraftment was demonstrated even under the most difficult experimental conditions, for instance in mice presensitized with donor lymphocytes or partially reconstituted before the transplant by adding back graduated numbers of recipient mature thymocytes *(63)*. Likewise, escalation of T cell-depleted bone marrow doses leads to full donor type chimerism in mice pretreated with sublethal doses (5.5–7.5 Gy) of TBI, which spare a substantial number of recipient T lymphocytes *(67)*.

In 1993 it first became possible to test the concept of stem cell dose escalation in humans by supplementing bone marrow with peripheral blood progenitor cells (PBPCs) collected after administration of G-CSF to the donor *(68)*. ATG and thiotepa were added to TBI and cyclophosphamide (CY) to boost both myeloablation and immunosuppression. This first pilot study (performed in Perugia between 1993–1995) included 36 high-risk acute leukemia patients with a median age of 23. All patients received a full haplotype-mismatched transplant, consisting of bone marrow and PBPCs, each depleted of T lymphocytes by soybean agglutination and E-rosetting. The final inoculum contained a mean of 10×10^6 CD34$^+$ cells/kg bosy weight (bw) and 2×10^5 CD3$^+$ cells/kg bw. Eighty percent of patients achieved primary sustained engraftment. Although no posttransplant immunosuppressive therapy was used as prophylaxis, the incidence of GVHD was only approx 20%. It should be noted that in an earlier phase of the study, with a group of patients who received the same conditioning protocol and standard doses of T cell-depleted mismatched bone marrow cells, rejection was observed in all.

The 1993–1995 study showed for the first time that in humans as in mice, cell dose escalation facilitated engraftment of T cell-depleted mismatched transplants. The fundamental role of CD34$^+$ cell dose escalation in promoting engraftment across the HLA-barriers was further confirmed in a second study in which megadose-purified CD34$^+$ cells were used instead of T cell-depleted transplants (69). To eliminate GVHD, the number of T lymphocytes in the inoculum was reduced to a mean of 2×10^4/kg bw, 1 log less than in the previous series. This level was reached by processing peripheral blood mononuclear cells by one-round E-rosetting followed by a positive immunoselection of the CD34$^+$ cells with a Ceprate column.

To reduce extra hematological toxicity, the conditioning regimen was modified by substituting fludarabine for Cy. This new strategy was used in 43 acute leukemia patients, with a median age of 22 yr. The great majority of these patients were at high risk for both transplant-related mortality and leukemia relapse. A full donor-type engraftment was achieved in all patients, including two who required second transplants. No case of GVHD occurred, although no postgrafting immunosuppressive treatment was employed as GVHD prophylaxis. The extrahematological toxicity of the conditioning protocol was minimal in these heavily pre-treated patients.

Similar results were achieved lately when the CD34$^+$ cell selection was carried out by a one-step procedure using the Myltenni Clinimax devise .

Other recent reports have shown that the same excellent engraftment rates can be obtained following conditioning protocols based on chemotherapy alone. By using busulphan, thiotepa, and Cy in combination with either ATG or OKT3, Handgretinger et al. (70) obtained a high engraftment rate in children with acute leukemia.

Remarkably, the growing experience over the past 8 yr indicates that leukemia relapse rate was relatively low in patients with acute leukemia in first or second remmision. Ruggeri et al. suggested recently that donor natural killer (NK) alloreactivity, a biological phenomenon unique to mismatched transplants, could play a role in a GVL effect (71). They found that newly formed incompatible donor type NK cells are not blocked by host cells which fail to express killer cell inhibitory receptor (KIR) inhibitory class I allele(s), and therefore, the low relapse rate observed in haploidentical transplants in remission might be attributed in part to the robust NK recovery during the early posttransplant period.

While the beneficial effect of alloreactive NK cells in haploidentical transplants might be translated to a relatively lower relapse rate, compared to the HLA identical setting in which NK donor cells are blocked by the KIR, in haploidentical transplants the ability to use DLI once relapse occurs is markedly hampered by the severity of GVHD. Thus, treatment of CML patients in chronic phase with haploidentical transplants is currently not encouraged due the expected high risk for relapse. Further attempts to explore the potential of alloreactive NK cells in the treatment of CML relapse might enable the use of this modality as a substitute for DLI in the haploidentical setting. Alternatively, the use of specific antitumor or antiminor histocompatability antigens, expressed exclusively on host hematopoietic or leukemic cells, emerges as a promising selective approach avoiding the lethal risk of GVHD (72–74).

One major problem, at least in adults that appears to be common to all T cell-depleted transplants is the slow recovery of the antimicrobial and antiviral responses. Thus, while Handgretinger et al. showed that in children the immune reconstitution is attained promptly (70), Aversa et al. showed that 40% of the mortality in haploidentical transplants was caused

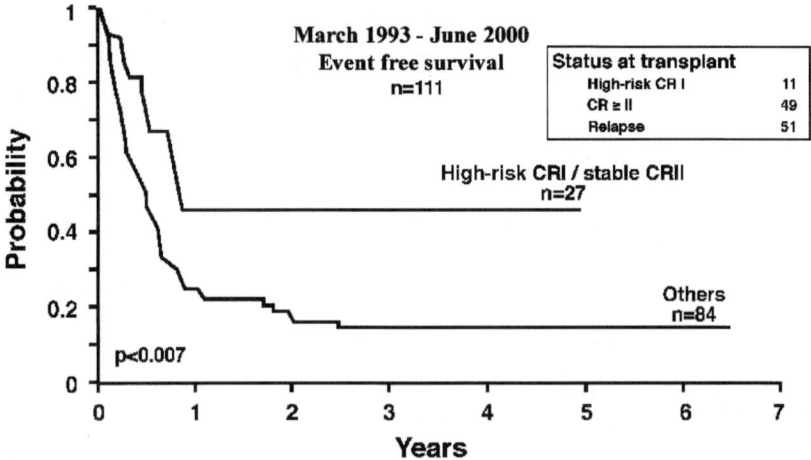

Fig. 3. Full haplotype mismatched transplantation for acute leukemia. With permission from the Hematopoetic Stem Cell Transplantation Program, University of Perugia.

by infections. As in recipients of HLA indentical transplants, the slow immune recovery in recipients of full-haplotype-mismatched transplants is attributable to the low number of T cells that can be infused safely with the graft (i.e., without causing GVHD) and to the decreased thymic function in adult recipients. Considering that these limitations are fixed variables, new insights into the forces that drive the T cells in the graft to undergo homeostatic expansion in the lymphopenic host might unravel new ways to improve survival.

Velardi et al. *(76)* have recently shown that antigen presentation plays a pivotal role in the recovery of the postgrafting immune system and have identified measures which, by improving antigen-presenting cell (APC) function, impact dramatically on the postgrafting immune recovery. Specifically, they demonstrated that G-CSF administration posttransplant blocks interleukin (IL)-12 production in APCs and, thereby, may exert strong immune suppressive effects. This observation prompted the elimination of the G-CSF administration to the recipients. While no unwanted effects were noted on the engraftment rate, IL-12 as detected by mRNA expression in monocytes and dendritic cells was restored by the second month posttransplant, and recovery of CD4+ cells was much faster than previously observed *(75)*.

Very recently, Aversa et al. analysed 111 consecutive patients with acute leukemia who were transplanted since March 1993 in Perugia (Fig. 3). This analysis shows that only 27 patients were in first or second stable complete remission (CR). None of these patients were included in the first 36 patients treated between 1993 and 1995. Altogether, for this group of patients, the probability of relapse and for DFS at 5 yr was approx 10 and 45%, respectively, compared with 69 and 14% in the other 84 patients. These results strongly suggest that mismatched transplants can compare favorably with conventionally matched unrelated transplants, if applied for the treatment of poor prognostic acute leukemia patients in first or second CR (at least 2 mo of therapy) or patients in early relapse before the risk of infection has accelerated. Haploidentical transplants in ALL in refractory relapse are not recommended.

Furthermore, we also analyzed the impact of the new protocol employed in Perugia since January 1999, using one-step positive selection CD34 cells with Clinimax and avoiding G-CSF in the posttransplant period. Thus, out of 32 patients with acute leukemia, 10 AML patients and one ALL patient could be classified as "good CR patients," that is in either first hematological and cytogenetical CR or second CR lasting at least 2 mo of therapy with good performance status and without major lung infection prior to transplantation.

Although the follow-up is short, the results show that transplant mortality was extremely low with only one patient dying from toxicity of the conditioning, and the probability of event-free survival at 1 yr was approx 70%. Clearly, if this promising trend continues, the outcome of haploidentical megadose transplants will be comparable to the results described above for matched related transplants.

These suggestions of Aversa et al. were presented recently at two special meetings dedicated to haploidentical transplantation, which took place in Perugia and in Chicago, with the purpose of defining a consensus for a controlled trial in Europe and in the U.S. Clearly, further evaluation of the megadose approach could be carried out in a well-defined population for which the intent to treat will be decided. Such a population will be referred to as HLA identical matched related, unrelated, or haploidentical donors, depending upon availability within the first 2 mo after initiation of the search.

A very intriguing basic question raised by the CD34 megadose transplants is how do these cells overcome the barrier presented by host CTL-precursor (CTL-p)? Very recently, this question was answered in part by the finding that cells within the CD34 fraction are endowed with potent veto activity *(76)*. The term veto related to the ability of cells to neutralize CTL-p directed against their antigens *(77–79)*. Thus, when purified CD34 cells were added to bluk mixed leukocyte reaction (MLR), they suppressed CTLs against match stimulators, but not against stimulators from a third party *(76)*. The effective CD34$^+$ cell number required for the veto effect was found to be at a veto/effector ratio of about 0.5–1.0.

After 5 d of primary MLR culture in the presence of CD34$^+$ cells, fluorescence-activated cell sorter (FACS) analysis showed the CD34$^+$ cells are not killed by the alloreactive T cells, although CD34$^+$ cells are lysed if used as target cells at the end of MLR, which did not contain CD34$^+$ cells from the begining. The addition of CD34$^+$ cells to MLR cultures was effective only during the first 48 h of culture. Thereafter, it seems that the veto effect of these cells is directed at CTL-ps, but does not affect differentiated antidonor CTLs. IL-2 and γ-interferon (IFN) production, as measured by intracellular staining or by Elispot analysis, are specifically reduced in CD8+ T cells from the cultures inhibited by CD34$^+$ cells. It could be agrued that the unique phenotype of cells within the CD34$^+$ compartment, lacking B7, might have induced anergy in the responder cells due to inappropriate antigen presentation. However, removal of the CD34$^+$ cells after 5 d of culture prior to the secondary challenge with the stimulator cells, in the presence of exogenous IL-2, could not reverse the inhibition of antidonor CTLs. Moreover, addition of anti-CD28 antibody to the primary MLR did not block the inhibition, thus further ruling out an anergy-based mechanism *(80)*. Very recently, Bachar-Lustig, Gur, and coworkers found that in mice, early hematopoietic Sca-1$^+$Lin$^-$ bone marrow cells, similarly to human CD34$^+$ cells, are endowed with veto activity *(81)*. In the future, the mechanisms mediating this intriguing activity of cells within the progenitor cell compartment might be identified by taking advantage of different mutants or knock-out strains of mice, which are impaired in crucial regulatory molecules. Furthermore, if the veto cells within the hematopoietic progenitors are showm to be distinct from the pluripotential hematopoietic stem cells, then it might be more feasible to expand the veto cells ex vivo and use them together with a small number of pluripotential stem cells, for transplantation.

4. CONCLUDING REMARKS

The concerns raised in the early 1980s—that T cell-depleted transplants are associated with marked leukemia relapse and graft rejection rates—were adequately addressed toward the end of the past decade by compensating for the absence of GVHD with a slightly intensified conditioning, adding either thiotepa or CAMPATH-1G. In addition, T cell-depleted transplants were limited to patients with acute leukemia, avoiding transplantation in CML patients who were at the highest risk for relapse. However, with the advent of DLI in the mid-1990s, the road was opened for the use of T cell depletion even in this difficult setting, and several groups are currently evaluating the potential of this modality to completely prevent the risk for lethal GVHD in CML, while dealing with the risk for relapse by using graduated numbers of donor T cells. It is hoped that further progress in the treatment of CML will be afforded by the new availability of specific CTLs directed against tumor-specific or minor hiscompatability hematopoietic peptides. Delayed immune reconstitution remains a problem in allogeneic BMT. As described here, several studies have shown that this barrier is not unique to T cell-depleted transplants, but rather is typical of adult recipients of allogeneic BMT. Thymic involution is clearly a major factor, but it is also aggravated by the supralethal preparatory protocols, as well as by clinical or even subclinical alloreactivity against the thymic stroma.

Extensive work is currently dedicated to addressing the problem of immune reconstitution in adult leukemic recipients of allogeneic transplants. In particular, it is hoped that donor T lymphocytes directed against specific sources of infection will prove useful. In addition, basic studies in animal models might lead to the development of new means to improve the thymic function and the ability of the thymic precursors to develop within the rudimentary thymus epithelium, which is most likely severely affected by the supralethal chemoradiotherapy. In this context, exciting possibilities have been indicated by two major findings showing that keratinocyte growth factor (KGF) can induce protection from thymic epithelial injury if given prior to BMT (82) and that IL-7 can facilitate thymic and extrathymic T cell differentiation and expansion (83).

Alternatively, promising nomyeloablative protocols with lowered extra medullary toxicity are currently being investigated in elderly patients. Conventional unseparated bone marrow or peripheral blood stem cell transplants following a nonmyeloablative conditioning are currently employed extensively in HLA identical leukemic recipients. These are associated with marked alloreactivity due to the large number of T cells in the transplant innoculum, which in most instances eradicates recipient hematopoiesis. Clearly, this alloreactivity is also associated with a significant incidence of lethal GVHD. The major challenge, therefore, for future years is to achieve engraftment of allogeneic hematopoietic cells following nonmyeloablative conditioning in the absence of alloreactive T cells.

In humans, nonalloreactive T cells can be generated by removal of $CD25^+$ (84) or $CD69^+$ (85) activated cells following stimulation against host cells, or by anergy induction making use of co-stimulation blockade with CTLA4 (86,87). However, these approaches, which make use of T cell stimulation with the very antigens against which tolerance is desired, might involve some risk for generating committed CTLs, if any of the CTL-p escape deletion or anergy induction. Once such anti-host CTLs are generated, it is very difficult to suppress their alloreactivity in vivo.

An alternative approach is based on earlier studies, which showed that $CD8^+$ CTL clones possess extremely high veto activity (78). Thus, we focus our attempts on ex vivo expansion and selection of nonalloreactive clones (88), and we test their capacity to facilitate engraftment of purified Sca-1$^+$Lin$^-$ hematopoietic progenitors in sublethally irradiated mismatched recipients. If successful, these studies could lead to safe mismatched hematopoietic transplants in patients for whom the risk of supralethal radiochemotherapy is not justified, such as patients with thalassemia, sickle cell anemia, and several enzyme deficiencies. Furthermore, induction of substantial durable chimerism could be used to induce tolerance toward subsequent solid organ transplants from the original stem cell donor or as a prelude for adaptive cell therapy in cancer patients.

REFERENCES

1. Ferrera JLM, Deeg HJ, Burakoff SG. *Graft-Versus-Host Disease*. Marcell Decker, New York, 1997.
2. Krenger W, Hill GR, Ferrera JLM. Cytokine cascades in acute graft-versus-host disease. *Transplantation* 1997;64:553.
3. Serody JS, Cook DN, Kirby SL, Reap E, Shea TC, Frelinger JA. Murine T lymphocytes incapable of producing macrophage inhibitory protein-1 are impaired in causing graft versus host disease across a class 1 but not class 11 major histocompatibility complex barrier. *Blood* 1999;93:43.
4. Murphy WJ, Blazar BR. New strategies for preventing graft-versus-host disease. *Curr Opin Immunol* 1999;11:509.
5. Uphoff DE. *J Natl Cancer Inst* 1958;20:625.
6. Muller-Ruchholtz W, Wottge H-U, Muller-Hermelink HK. Bone marrow transplantation in rats across stron histocompatibility barriers by selective elimination of lymphoid cells in donor marrow. *Transplant Proc* 1976;8:537–541.
7. Dicke KA, van Bekkum DW. Allogeneic bone marrow transplantation after elimination of immunocompetent cells by means of density gradient centrifugation. *Transplant Proc* 1971;3:666.
8. Reisner Y, Itzicovitch L, Meshorer A, Sharon N. Hemopoietic stem cell transplantation using mouse bone marrow and spleen cells fractionated by lectins. *Proc Natl Acad Sci USA* 1978;75:2933.
9. Reisner Y, Kapoor N, O'Reilly RJ, Good RA. Allogeneic bone marrow transplantation using stem cells fractionated by sheep red blood cells and soybean agglutinin. *Lancet* 1980;ii:1320.
10. Reisner Y, Kapoor N, Kirkpatrick D, et al. Transplantation for acute leukemia with HLA-A and B non0identical parental marrow cells fractionated with soybean agglutinin and sheep red blood cells. *Lancet* 1981;ii:327.
11. Rich RR, Kirkpatrick CH, Smith TK.Simultaneous suppression of responses to allogeneic tissue in vitro and vivo. *Cell Immunol* 1972;5:190.
12. Von Boehmer H, Sprent J, Nabholz M. Tolerance to histocompatibility determinants in tetraparental bone marrow chimeras. *J Exp Med* 1975;141:322.
13. Yunis EJ, Good RA, Smikth J, Stutman O. Protection of lethally irradiated mice by spleen cells from neonatally thymectomized mice. *Proc Natl Acad Sci USA* 1974;71:2544.
14. Reisner Y, Kapoor N, Kirkpatrick D, et al. Transplantation for severe combined immunodeficiency with HLA-A,B.D.DR incompatible parental marrow cells fractionated by soybean agglutinin and sheep red blood cells. *Blood* 1983;61:341.
15. O'Reilly RJ, Kapoor N, Kirkpatrick D, et al. Transplantation for severe combined immunodeficiency using histoincompatible parental marrow fractionated by soybean agglutinin and sheep red blood cells: experience in six consecutive cases. *Transplant Proc* 1983;15:1431.
16. Friedrich W, Goldmann SF, Vetter U, et al. Immunoreconstitution in severe immunodeficiency following transplantation of HLA-haploidentical, T-cell depleted bone marrow. *Lancet* 1984;i:761.
17. Gale RP, Reisner Y. Graft rejection and graft-versus-host disease: mirror images. *Lancet* 1986;i:1468.
18. Zinkernagel RM, Althage A, Callahan G, Welsh RMJ. On the immunocompetence of H-2 incompatible irradiaation bone marrow chimeras. *J Immunol* 1980;124:2356.
19. Haddad E, Landais P, Friedrich W, et al. Long-term immune reconstitution and outcome after HLA-nonidentical T-cell-depleted bone marrow transplantation for severe combined immunodeficiency: a european retrospective study of 116 patients. *Blood* 1998;91:3646.
20. O'Reilly RJ, Keever CA, Small TN, Brochstein J. The use of HLA-non-identical T-cell depleted marrow transplants for correction of severe combined immunodeficiency disease. *Immunodefic Rev* 1989;1:273.
21. Buckley RH. Bone marrow reconstitution in primary immunodeficiency, In Rich RR (eds): *Clinical Immunology*. Mosby, St. Louis, MO, 1996, p. 1813.
22. Buckley RH, Schiff SE, Schiff RI, et al. Hematopoietic stem-cell transplantation for the treatment of severe combined immunodeficiency. *N Engl J Med* 1999;349:508.
23. Rosenkrantz K, Keever C, Bhimani K, et al. Both ongoing suppression and clonal elimination contribute to graft-host tolerance after transplantation of HLA mismatched T cell-depleted marrow for severe combined immunodeficiency. *J Immunol* 1990;144:1721.
24. O'Reilly RJ, Collins NH, Kernan N. *Transplant Proc* 1985;17:455.
25. O'Reilly RJ, Collins N, Dinsmore R, et al. Transplantation of HLA-mismatched marrow depleted of T-cells by lectin agglutination and E-rosette depletion. *Tokai J Exp Clin Med* 1985;10:99.
26. Schwartz E, Lapidot T, Gozes D, Singer TS, Reisner Y. Abrogation of bone marrow allograft resistance in mice by increased total body irradiation correlaates with eradication of host clonable T cells and alloreactive cytotoxic precursors. *J Immunol* 1987;138:460.
27. Reisner Y, Ben-Bassat I, Douer D, Kaploon A, Schwartz E, Ramot B. Demonstration of clonable alloreactive host T cells in a primate model for bone marrow transplantation. *Proc Natl Acad Sci USA* 1986;83:4012.

28. Kernan NA, Flomenberg N, Dupont B, O'Reilly RJ. Graft rejection in recipients of T-cell-depleted HLA-nonidentical marrow transplants for leukemia. Identificaation of host-derived antidonor allocytotoxic T lymphocytes. *Transplantation* 1987;43:842.

29. Butturini A, Seeger RC, Gale RP. Recipient immune-competent T lymphocytes can survive intensive conditioning for bone marrow transplantation. *Blood* 1986;68:954.

30. Slavin S, Waldmann H, Or R, et al. Prevention of graft-versus-host disease in allogeneic bone marrow transplantation for leukemia by T cell depletion in vitro prior to transplantation. *Transplant Proc* 1985;17:465.

31. Bordignon C, Keever CA, Small TN, et al.. Graft failure after T-Cell-depleted human leukocyte antigen identical marrow transplants for leukemia: II. In vitro analyses of host effector mechanisms. *Blood* 1989;74:2237.

32. Hale G, Cobbold S, Waldmann H. CAMPATH-1 Users: T cell depletion with CAMPATH-1 in allogeneic bone marrow transplantation. *Transplantation* 1988;45:753.

33. Patterson J, Prentice HG, Brenner MK, et al. Graft rejection following HLA matched T-lymphocyte depleted bone marrow transplantation. *Br J Haematol* 1986;63:221.

34. Mitsuyasu RT, Champlin RE, Gale RP, Ho WG, Lenarsky C, Winston D. Treatment of donor bone marrow with monoclonal anti-T cell antibody and complement for the prevention of graft-versus-host disease. *Ann Intern Med* 1986;105:20.

35. Filipovich AH, Vallera DA, Youle RJ, et al. Graft versus host disease prevention in allogeneic bone marrow transplantation from histocompatible siblings. *Transplantation* 1987;44:62.

36. Martin PJ, Hansen JA, Buckner CD, et al. Effects of in vitro depletion of T-cells in HLA-identical allogeneic marrow grafts. *Blood* 1985;66:664.

37. Small TN, Avigan D, Dupont B, et al. Immune reconstitution following T-cell depleted bone marrow transplantation: effect of age and posttransplant graft rejection prophylaxis. *Biol Blood Marrow Transplant* 1997;3:65.

38. Terenzi A, Lubin I, Lapidot T, et al. Enhancement of T-cell depleted bone marrow allografts in mice by thiotepa. *Transplantation* 1990;50:717.

39. Aversa F, Terenzi A, Carotti A, et al. Improved outcome with T-cell-depleted bone marrow transplantation for acute leukemia. *J Clin Oncol* 1999;17:1545.

40. Papadopoulos EB, Carabasi MH, Castro-Malaspina H, et al. T-cell-depleted allogeneic bone marrow transplanation as postremission therapy for acute myelogenous leukemia: freedom from relapse in the absence of graft-versus-host disease. *Blood* 1998;91:1083.

41. Hale G, Zhang M-J, Bunjes D, et al. Improving the outcome of bone marrow transplantation by using CD52 monoclonal antibodies to prevent graft-versus-host disease and graft rejection. *Blood* 1998;92:4581.

42. Hale G, Jacobs P, Wood L, et al. CD52 antibodies for prevention of graft-versus-host disease and graft rejection following transplantaation of allogeneic peripheral blood stem cells. *Bone Marrow Transplant* 2000;26:69.

43. Kolb HJ, Mittermuller J, Clemm CH, et al. Donor leukocyte transfusions for treatment of recurrent chronic myelogenous leukemia in marrow transplant patients. *Blood* 1990;76:2462.

44. Drobyski WR, Keever CA, Roth MS, et al. Salvage immunotherapy using donor leukocyte infusions as treaatment for relaapsed chronic myelogenous leukemia after allogeneic bone marrow transplantation: efficacy and toxicity of a defined T-cell dose. *Blood* 1993;82:2310.

45. Porter DL, Roth MS, McGarigle C, et al. Induction of graft-versus-host disease as immunotherapy for relapsed chronic myeloid leukemia. *N Engl J Med* 1994;330:100.

46. Helg C, Roux E, Beris P, et al. Adoptive immunotherapy for recurrent CML after BMT. *Bone Marrow Transplant* 1993;12:125.

47. van Rhee F, Lin F, Cullis JO, et al. Relapse of chronic myeloid leukemia after allogeneic bone marrow transplant: The case for giving donor leukocyte transfusions before the onset of hematologic relapse. *Blood* 1994;83:3377.

48. Slavin S, Naparstek E, Nagler A, et al. Allogeneic cell therapy for relapsed leukemia after bone marrow transplantation with donor peripheral blood lymphocytes. *Exp Hematol* 1995; 23:1553.

49. Mackinnon S, Papadopoulos EB, Carabasi MH, et al. Adoptive immunotherapy evaluating escalating doses of donor leukocytes for relapse of chronic myeloid leukemia after bone marrow transplantation: separation of graft-versus-leukemia responses from graft-versus-host disease. *Blood* 1995;86:1261.

50. Naparstek E, Nagler A, Or R, et al. Allogeneic cell-mediated immunotherapy using donor lymphocytes for prevention of relapse in patients treaated with allogeneic bone marrow transplantation for hematological malignancies. *Clin Transplant* 1996;281–290.

51. Roux E, Helg C, Dumont-Girard F, et al. Analysis of T-cell repopulation after allogeneic bone marrow transplantation: significant differences between recipients of T-cell depleted and unmanipulated grafts. *Blood* 1996;87:3984.

52. Dumont-Girard F, Roux E, van Lier RA, et al. Reconstitution of the T-cell compartment after bone marrow transplantation: restoration of the repertoire by thymic emigrants. *Blood* 1998;92:4464.

53. Small TN, Papadopoulos EB, Boulad F, et al. Comparison of immune reconstitution after unrelated and related T-cell-depleted bone marrow transplantation: effect of patient age and donor leukocyte infusions. *Blood* 1999;93:467.
54. Oakhill A, Pamphilon DH, Otter MN, et al. Unrelated donor bone marrow transplantation for children with relapsed acute lymphoblastic leukaemia in second complete remission. *Br J Haematol* 1996;94:574.
55. Green A, Clarke E, Hunt L, et al. Children with acute lymphoblastic leukemia who receive T-cell-depleted HLA mismatched marrow allografts from unrelaated donors have an increaased incidence of primary graft failure but a similar overall transplant outcome. *Blood* 1999;94:2236.
56. Sprent J. T lymphocytes and the thymus, In Paul WE (ed). *Fundamental Immunology* 3rd ed., Raven, New York, 1993, p. 75.
57. Champlin RE, Passweg JR, Zhang M-J, et al. T-cell depletion of bone marrow transplants for leukemia from donors other than HLA-identical siblings: advantage of T-cell antibodies with narrow specificities. *Blood* 2000;95:3996.
58. Salomon O, Lapidot T, Terenzi A, et al. Induction of donor-type chimerism in murine recipients of bone marrow allografts by different radiation regimens currently used in treatment of leukemia patients. *Blood* 1990;76:1872.
59. Ferrara JL, Michaelson J, Burakoff SJ, et al. Engraftment following T cell-depleted bone marrow transplantation. III. Differential effects of increased total-body irradiation on semiallogeneic recipients. *Transplantation* 1988;45:948.
60. Lapidot T, Singer TS, Salomon O, et al. Booster irradiation to the spleen following total body irradiation: a new immunosuppressive approach for allogeneic bone marrow transplantation. *J Immunol* 1988;141:2619.
61. Soderling CC, Song CW, Blazer BR, et al. A correlation between conditioning and engraftment in recipients of MHC mismatched T cell-depleted murine bone marrow transplants. *Immunology* 1985;135:941.
62. Cobbold SP, Martin G, Qin S, et al. Monoclonal antibodies to promote marrow engraftment and tissue graft tolerance. *Nature* 1986;323:164.
63. Lapidot T, Terenzi A, Singer TS, et al. Enhancement by dimethyl myleran of donor type chimerism in murine recipients of bone marrow allografts. *Blood* 1989;73:2025.
64. Godder KT, Hazlett LJ, Abhyankar SH, et al. Partially mismatched related-donor bone marrow transplantation for pediatric patients with acute leukemia: younger donors and absence of peripheral blasts improve outcome. *J Clin Oncol* 2000;18:1856.
65. Lapidot T, Terenzi A, Singer TS, et al. Size of bone marrow inoculum versus number of donor-type cells used for presensitization: a murine model for bone marrow allograft rejection in leukemia patients. *Blood* 1987;70:309a.
66. Uharek L, Gassmann W, Glass B, et al. Influence of cell dose and graft-versus-host reactivity on rejection rats after allogeneic bone marrow transplantation. *Blood* 1992;79:1612.
67. Bachar-Lustig E, Rachamim N, Li HW, et al. Megadose of T cell-depleted bone marrow overcomes MHC barriers in sublethally irradiated mice. *Nat Med* 1995;1:1268.
68. Aversa F, Tabilio A, Terenzi A, et al. Successful engraftment of T-cell-depleted haploidentical "three-loci" incompatible transplants in leukemia patients by addition of recombinant human granulocyte colony-stimulating factor-mobilized peripheral blood progenitor cells to bone marrow inoculum. *Blood* 1994;84:3948.
69. Aversa F, Tabilio A, Velardi A, et al. Treatment of high-risk acute leukemia with T-cell-depleted stem cells from related donors with one fully mismatched HLA haplotype. *N Eng J Med* 1998;339:1186.
70. Handgretinger R, Schumm M, Lang P, et al. Transplantation of megadoses of purified haploidentical stem cells. *Ann NY Acad Sci* 1999;872:351.
71. Ruggeri L, Capanni M, Casucci M, et al. Role of natural killer cell alloreactivity in HLA-mismatched hematopoietic stem cell transplantation. *Blood* 1999;94:333.
72. Goulmy E, Schipper R, Pool J, et al. Mismatches of Minor histocompatibility antigens between HLA-identical donors and recipients and the development of graft-versus-host disease after bone marrow transplantation. *N Engl J Med* 1996;334:281.
73. Falkenburg JHF, Wafelman AR, Joosten P, et al. Complete remission of accelerated phase chronic myeloid leukemia by treatment with leukemia-reactive cytotoxic T lymphocytes. *Blood* 1999;94:1201.
74. Molldrem JJ, Lee PP, Wang C, et al. Evidence that specific T lymphocytes may participate in the elimination of chronic myelogenous leukemia. *Nat Med* 2000;6:1018.
75. Volpi I, Perruccio K, Ruggeri L, et al. G-CSF blocks IL-12 production by antigen presenting cells: implications for improved immune reconstitution after haploidentical hematopoietic transplantation. *Blood* 1999;94:640a.
76. Min D, Taylor P, Chung B, et al. Protection from thymic epithelial cell (TEC) injury by pre-BMT keratinocyte growth factor (KGF): a new approach to speed thymic reconstitution after lethal irradiation. 42nd Annual Meeting of the American Society of Hematology, San Francisco, CA, December 1–5. *Blood* 2000;96:474a
77. Bolotin E, Smogorzewska M, Smith S, et al. Enhancement of thymopoiesis after bone marrow transplant by in vivo interleukin-7. *Blood* 1996;88:1887.

78. Cavazzana Calvo M, Stephan JL, Sarnacki S, et al. Attenuation of graft-versus-host disease and graft rejection by ex vivo immunotoxin elimination of alloreactive T cells in an H-2 haplotype disparate mouse combination. *Blood* 1994;83:288.

79. Koh MB, Prentice HG, Lowdell MW. Selective removal of alloreactive cells from haematopoietic stem cell grafts: graft engineering for GVHD prophylaxis. *Bone Marrow Transplant* 1999;23:1071.

80. Boussiotis VA, Gribben JG, Freeman GJ, et al. Blockade of the CD28 co-stimulatory pathway: a means to induce tolerance. *Curr Opin Immunol* 1994;6:797.

81. Gribben JG, Guinan EC, Boussiotis VA, et al. Complete blockade of B7 family-mediated costimulation is necessary to induce human alloantigen-specific anergy: a method to ameliorate graft-versus-host disease and extend the donor pool. *Blood* 1996;87:4887.

82. Sambhara SR, Miller RG.: Programmed cell death of T cells signaled by the T cell receptor and the alpha 3 domain of class I MHC. *Science* 1991;252:1424.

83. Reich-Zeliger S, Zhao Y, Krauthgamer R, et al. Anti-third party CD8+ CTLs as potent veto cells: coexpression of CD8 and FasL is a prerequisite. *Immunity* 2000;13:507.

22 Minimal Residual Disease in Allogeneic Recipients

Jerald P. Radich, MD

1. INTRODUCTION

Relapse after stem cell transplant (SCT) is a major obstacle to cure. Sensitive methods can identify patients that harbor minimal residual disease (MRD) while appearing in morphological remission after myeloablative therapy. Often, the detection of MRD is the harbinger of relapse in these patients. The study of MRD aims to differentiate patients with residual leukemia destined for relapse as opposed to patients with stable or declining residual disease. Once identified, patients with a high risk of relapse could potentially undergo additional preemptive therapy to abort relapse.

2. METHODS OF MRD DETECTION

Several techniques can define residual disease below the threshold of conventional pathological examination. These include "classic" metaphase and molecular cytogenetics, cell "flow"cytometric studies, and the polymerase chain reaction (PCR) detection of specific genetic targets (Table 1). Each method takes advantage of differences in phenotypic and genotypic characteristics of the tumor cell compared to the normal cell, and each has relative advantages, disadvantages, and differences in sensitivity. Conventional metaphase cytogenetics can detect approx one leukemia cell in 10–100 normal cells (denoted as 10^{-1} sensitivity) if 20–50 metaphases are counted *(1,2)*. Cytogenetics is limited by sampling only those few cells that divide in culture. Fluorescence *in situ* hybridization (FISH) uses chromosome-specific or locus-specific probes to identify genetic targets in metaphase or interphase cells and is most useful in detecting simple losses or gains of chromosomes and chromosomal translocations *(3)*.

From: *Current Clinical Oncology: Allogeneic Stem Cell Transplantation*
Edited by: Mary S. Laughlin and Hillard M. Lazarus © Humana Press Inc., Totowa, NJ

Table 1
Methods to Detect Minimal Residual Disease

Detection method	Target	Sensitivity
Pathologic examination	Cellular morphology	5%
Cytogenetics	Chromosome structure	1–5%
FISH	Chromosome structure	1%
Flow cytometry	Surface antigen expression	0.1–1%
PCR	DNA or RNA sequence	0.0001–0.1%

Cell surface antigen expression can distinguish malignant from normal cells. While truly tumor-specific antigens are rare, malignant cells often express cell surface antigens in more subtly different patterns than normal cells *(4,5)*. By using combinations of multiple antibodies, "multiparametric" flow cytometric assays uses aberrant antigen expression patterns to "fingerprint" the malignant clone. If combinations of several antibodies are used to define the aberrant antigen expression, the sensitivity can reach as low as 10^{-2}–10^{-3} in experienced hands.

The most sensitive approach to detect MRD involves nucleic acid amplification using the PCR *(6)*. Unlike conventional cytogenetics or flow cytometry, however, a specific genetic lesion target is the fingerprint of the malignancy in order for PCR-driven analyses to have the desired sensitivity and specificity. Gene translocations, such as the t(9;22) in chronic myeloid leukemia (CML), and the t(15:17), t(8;21), and inversion *(16)* found in acute myeloid leukemia (AML) cases, are the most straightforward leukemia-specific markers for the detection of MRD *(7–13)*. However, there is a rapidly expanding list of disease-specific translocations, and now translocations can be detected and amplified in 40–50% of acute myeloid leukemias (AML) and acute lymphoblastic leukemia (ALL) *(14)*. Another type of leukemia-specific fingerprints takes advantage of the rearrangement of the immunoglobulin heavy chain and T cell receptor genes that occur normally in B and T cell lymphoid development *(15,16)*.

3. MRD DETECTION IN CML

CML has been the paradigm for many facets of leukemia research. It was the first disease associated with a specific chromosomal abnormality *(17)* and among the first translocations successfully amplified by PCR *(18)*. It also may be the strongest example of the power of MRD detection to shape therapy and potentially prevent relapse. The qualitative detection of *bcr-abl* post-SCT is associated with relapse, but the strength of the effect varies according to the type of transplant and the time from transplant *(19–26)*. Quantitative PCR of the *bcr-abl* burden may refine and strengthen the predictive value of residual disease detection. Note that in the following sections, it is implied that the detection of MRD occurs in patients who appear to be in remission by conventional pathological techniques.

3.1. Risk of Relapse and Time from Transplant

The highest risk of relapse associated with *bcr-abl* detection appears to be associated "early" (≤12 mo post-SCT) after transplant *(21,22,25)*. For example, we examined 346 patients post-SCT and found that a single positive assay for *bcr-abl* was associated with an elevated risk of relapse *(25)*. The predictive value of *bcr-abl* detection was strongest at 6–12 mo post-bone marrow transplantation (BMT), where the presence of *bcr-abl* was associated with a 42% risk of relapse at a median of 200 d from the first PCR-positive result, as opposed to a 3% risk of relapse in PCR-negative patients. Tests earlier than 3 mo post-SCT were not strongly associated with relapse. The relative risk of relapse associated with MRD was approx 30-fold even after controlling for clinical variables associated with relapse, such as phase of disease and graft-vs-host disease (GVHD) status.

MRD can be detected for years post-SCT. *Bcr-abl* has been detected in 25–50% of patients ≥3 yr posttransplant, with subsequent relapse rates of approx 10–20% *(25–28)*. Costello et al. found that 66 out of 117 (56%) of CML patients were positive ≥3 yr post-BMT, but only 8% subsequently relapsed *(27)*. Further follow-up of nearly 400 patients have shown that 25% of patients will have at least one *bcr-abl*-positive assay ≥18 mo post-SCT, but that only 16% will relapse, compared to 1% in *bcr-abl*-negative patients *(28)*. Van Rhee et al. reported 19 patients in complete remission for more that 10 yr post-BMT, two patients of whom were still positive for *bcr-abl (29)*. A semiquantitative assay demonstrated that *bcr-abl* transcript levels were very low in these patients. In summary, these data suggest that MRD in CML patients years post-SCT may not be a harbinger of relapse, and these patients may, thus, not be appropriate candidates for intervention trials of treating molecular relapse.

3.2. Risk of Relapse and Donor Status

The immunological effect associated with an allograft may influence the risk of relapse associated with *bcr-abl* detection. Unrelated donor (URD) transplants, which have a lower risk of relapse after SCT compared to allogeneic-related-matched transplants presumably owing to the graft-vs-leukemia (GVL) effect, had a similar prevalence of *bcr-abl* -positivity at 6–12 mo post-SCT compared to related SCT patients (25 vs 30%), but the subsequent relapse rate was much greater in the *bcr-abl*-positive-related donor group compared to the *bcr-abl*-positive URD, recipients (approx 60 vs 10%) *(25)*. This suggests that in the URD the GVL effect may be working to control the leukemic clones that have escaped the conditioning regimen. Curiously, the subsequent study of late *bcr-abl* positivity showed no difference of relapse rate of URD compared to matched-related transplants *(28)*. This may reflect the immune tolerance that occurs in URD patients as time elapses, ameliorating the GVL effect.

More evidence of the power of an immunologic effect in controlling relapse was found by Pichert and colleagues *(26)*, who studied 48 T cell depleted and 44 untreated marrow transplant patients. They found that over 80% of patients receiving T cell-depleted marrow were *bcr-abl* positive 6–24 mo posttransplant, compared to 25% of patients receiving unmanipulated marrow. *Bcr-abl* detection was highly associated with relapse, which occurred predominately in the T cell-depleted patients. Furthermore, Mackinnon et al. studied 36 patients following T cell-depleted marrow graft (30). Thirty of 36 (83%) were positive for *bcr-abl* post-SCT, and 60% of these MRD-positive patients relapsed. Of the 20 patients who became MRD-positive within 6 mo posttransplant, 15 patients (84%) eventually relapsed. Thus, while T cell depletion limits the morbidity of GVHD, the burden of relapse is greater and may necessitate donor T cell infusions in those patients who are MRD-positive posttransplant.

3.3. "Dormancy" in CML Posttransplant

Why don't all CML patients with residual disease relapse? Several possibilities, which are not mutually exclusive, include: (i) Patients who harbor MRD years post-BMT are a select population that exhibit an enduring GVL effect, curbing the outgrowth of malignant clones; (ii) the *bcr-abl*-positive cells might be lymphoid in origin, and not of myeloid lineage that is presumably responsible for relapse. A few patients receiving T cell-depleted transplants have had marrow samples used to establish erythroid, granulocytic, and macrophage colony formation, and 5% of the total colonies across all cell lineages demonstrated *bcr-abl* expression *(31)*; (iii) the persisting *bcr-abl*-expressing cells may need further genetic "hits" to become frankly leukemic, or conversely, have substained additional genetic mutations that decrease their proliferative capacity. Of interest is a recent report that patients bound to relapse also exhibit the "p190" *bcr-abl* variant associated with Philadelphia chromosome (Ph)+ ALL *(32)*. However, since p190 *bcr-abl* can be seen in virtually all CML at diagnosis (due to a splicing variation of p210 *bcr-abl* expression), the above observation may be simply an artifact of the high expression of p210 *bcr-abl* naturally seen with CML relapse, rather than causal *(33,34)*. Another explanation of dormancy is that MRD reflects slow-growing CML cells bound to recapitulate the natural history of CML, with a slow accumulation of disease burden resulting in relapse years later.

Very few patients who are *bcr-abl*-negative post-BMT relapse *(24–28)*. Does this mean that there are no, or very few, residual CML cells in these patients, or could there be a pool of slowly proliferating CML cells that express little or no *bcr-abl* mRNA and thus escape detection? Cases where genomic Bcr-Abl is detected without *bcr-abl* mRNA expression are unusual *(35–39)* and suggest that patients who are PCR-negative for *bcr-abl* mRNA do not commonly have a reservoir of cells that might become positive at a later time. Thus, it is unlikely that there is a large pool of *bcr-abl*-negative patients at risk for relapse.

3.4. Quantitative PCR for bcr-abl in CML

The predictive value of MRD detection in CML may be strengthened by *bcr-abl* quantification (called Q-PCR) *(40–45)*. The use of quantitative PCR (Q-PCR) has been pioneered in the study of MRD in CML. Lin and colleagues studied 69 patients with a competitive Q-PCR and demonstrated that the kinetics of *bcr-abl* level over time described both impending relapse and response to donor leukocyte infusion after relapse *(40)*. Low (or no) residual *bcr-abl* was associated with a very low risk of relapse (1%), compared to 75% relapse rate in patients with increasing or persistently high *bcr-abl* levels. Patients who relapsed had doubling times of the *bcr-abl* transcript level twice that of patients who failed to relapse (15 vs 25 d). Recently, Olavarria et al. studied 138 CML patients early (3–5 mo) posttransplant and showed that the *bcr-abl* level was highly correlated with relapse *(45)*. Patients with no evidence of *bcr-abl* had a 9% risk of subsequent cytogenetic or hematologic relapse, whereas patients defined as having a low burden of disease (<100 *bcr-abl* transcripts/μg RNA) or high level of transcripts (>100 copies/μg) had a cumulative relapse rate of 30 and 74%, respectively. These results are consistent with the high risk of relapse associated with early qualitative *bcr-abl* positivity at 6 mo post-BMT formerly reported *(20,25)*. In addition, we evaluated the qualitative and quantitative assessment of MRD in 379 CML patients "late" (>18 mo) post-SCT *(28)*. Ninety patients (24%) had at least one assay positive for *bcr-abl,* and 13 out of 90 patients (14%) relapsed. Conversely, 3 out of 289 patients who were persistently *bcr-abl*-negative relapsed (hazard ratio of relapse = 19). Quantification of *bcr-abl* level was performed on 344 samples from 85 patients, and a rising *bcr-abl* heralded eventual relapse. Thus, a simple qualitative reverse transcription-PCR (RT-PCR) assay for *bcr-abl* can flag patients who need close follow-up, while quantification can indicate those who might benefit from early therapeutic intervention.

In summary, these qualitative and quantitative MRD data confirm that molecular relapse of *bcr-abl* is common in CML patients following transplantation. While the *bcr-abl* assay must be carefully controlled for issues of false positivity and other technical issues, a qualitative *bcr-abl* result has prognostic importance, and further refinement by quantitative assays target patients who would benefit from early intervention. Of considerable interest are those patients that remain with detectable molecular disease, as their study may further our insight into the mechanisms that dictate remission or relapse.

4. MRD DETECTION IN ACUTE LEUKEMIA

In CML the detection of MRD is simplified by the occurrence of a unique genetic marker (the Ph) in essentially all cases. Unfortunately, such is not the case in the acute leukemias, where multiple genetic abnormalities have been described, so that approx 40% of cases will have some variety of genetic fingerprint *(14)*. Furthermore, the detection of MRD is made more difficult since the acute leukemias grow faster than CML, greatly increasing the likelihood of tumors evading detection if the testing intervals are not frequent enough.

In ALL, clonal immunoglobulin heavy chain (IgH V-D-J) or T cell receptor (TCR) gene rearrangements can be used to follow MRD in many cases. This method takes advantage of the unique gene rearrangements that occur in these genes as cells develop into functional B and T cells. While all individual normal B and T cells should have unique gene rearrangements, a clonal outgrowth of malignant cells should all have identical gene rearrangements, and this fingerprint can later be used to distinguish malignant vs normal cells in remission samples. The detection of MRD in ALL, either by PCR or flow cytometry, has been shown to be highly predictive of relapse in the conventional chemotherapy setting, particularly in the pediatric population *(46–51)*. Following allogeneic transplantation, however, the data is sparse. IgH V-D-J detection was used in 20 allogeneic transplant patients to detect MRD, and it was found that the presence of MRD within the first 100 d after transplant was associated with a 6-fold increase in relapse rate compared to PCR-negative patients *(52)*. Indeed, all patients who were PCR-positive died after transplant; the median time from first PCR-positive assay to relapse was 30 d (median, 6–250 d). A subsequent study of 71 pediatric ALL patients after allogeneic transplant demonstrated that MRD detection at any time after transplant was a poor prognostic sign *(53)*. Of the 32 patients who relapsed, 16 patients were persistently positive for MRD, while 12 patients became positive at a median of 3 mo prior to frank relapse. Of the 36 patients who remained in remission, only eight patients were MRD positive at any time post-SCT. The odds ratio for relapse associated with MRD detection in the first 3 mo following transplantation was ninefold, quite similar to the earlier study cited above. The importance of MRD detection in remission patients prior to transplant also seems important in predicting outcome *(54)*. Using a semi-quantitative assay to catagorize patients of having no, low, or high MRD burden, the level of MRD in remission patients was strongly associated with subsequent outcome after transplant, with the 2-yr event-free survival for no, low, and high MRD disease being 73, 36, and 0%, respectively.

A careful evaluation of mixed chimerism may also identify patients at a high risk of relapse after SCT. In a small study of 12 patients, Zetterquist et al. found that five patients had evidence of mixed chimerism as determined by variable number tandem repeat (VNTR) analysis of B lineage cells *(55)*. Four of the patients with mixed chimerism relapsed. However, to obtain sufficient sensitivity, the authors performed cell cytometry sorting of the CD19 lymphoid lineage cells and performed chimerism analysis on the selected population. This rather labor-intensive analysis would seem no easier than PCR-driven detection of IgH V-D-J markers.

The Ph chromosome can be found in 5–25% of pediatric and adult ALL patients and is the MRD marker of choice in these patients. In Ph+ ALL, however, PCR must be performed for both variants of the *bcr-abl* chimeric mRNA, the "p210" *bcr-abl* variant (found in CML and some ALL), and the "p190" *bcr-abl* (found only rarely in CML but common in ALL). Miyamura et al. *(56)* studied 13 patients after allogeneic (*n* = 8) and autologous (*n* = 5) transplant and found that a positive PCR assay for *bcr-abl* in the first 12 mo following transplant was predictive of relapse. All seven patients who were PCR-positive relapsed, whereas only one out of six MRD-negative patients relapsed. A later study of 37 Ph+ ALL patients *(57)* showed the clinical utility of *bcr-abl* detection and fundamental differences in p190 and p210 Ph+ ALL. The relative risk of relapse of patients with a positive PCR (either p210 or p190) post-BMT compared to PCR-negative patients was approx sixfold. Those patients with p190 *bcr-abl* had an 88% relapse rate in comparison to 12% for patients who expressed the p210 *bcr-abl* transcript.

There are few studies documenting the prevalence and significance of MRD in AML following SCT. This is largely due to the fact that the most common translocations found in AML (the t(15;17), t(8;21), and inversion *[16]* gene rearrangements), while occurring in aggregate in 20–30% of AML cases, are associated with intermediate or good outcomes with conventional chemotherapy and, thus, are underrepresented in the transplant population. What little data that exists suggests that the significance of MRD depends on the specific type of genetic subtype of AML. Thus in t(15;17) AML, the detection of the promyelocyte leukemia/retinoic receptor α (PML/RARα) transcript following SCT is highly correlated with relapse, albeit it warned that the number of patients was small *(58,59)*. This follows the data following conventional chemotherapy, where the molecular detection of PML/RARα is highly correlated with relapse *(60,61)*. In t(8;21), conversely, the detection of AM1/ETO is often found in patients for years following conventional chemotherapy and, thus, is not tightly linked to outcome *(62,63)*. Remarkably, this appears to be the case even after allogeneic transplant, where many patients remain with evidence of MRD, yet do not relapse *(64–66)*. In the largest study of t(8;21) AML, nine of ten patients examined after SCT were positive from 7–83 mo post-BMT, and none relapsed *(64)*. There are few cases of inversion *(16)* detection described, and it is difficult to make a conclusion as to the significance of MRD *(67,68)*. In all of the above cases, however, it seems that the risk of relapse associated with the absence of MRD is quite low.

This persistence of molecular disease seen in t(8;21) AML has been also noted in most patients after years in remission following conventional chemotherapy *(62,63)*. In t(8;21) AML, molecular evidence of the AML1/ETO fusion mRNA can be found in a minority of lymphoid and erthyroid colonies taken from remission samples *(69)*, implying that (i) the disease may be stem cell in origin; and (ii) that MRD detection may sometimes detect non-myeloid cells bearing the translocation. Of additional interest is the observation that pediatric ALL patients who relapsed after >10 yr of remission following conventional chemotherapy relapse with a leukemia possessing the same clonal IgH V-D-J gene rearrangement as initially present at diagnosis *(70)*. The apparent persistency of dormancy in a disease as aggressive as ALL is quite provocative. What could be the mechanism of dormancy in acute leukemia? The mechanisms may or may not be the same following conventional chemotherapy or allogeneic transplantation. One can imagine several, nonmutually exclusive mechanisms including: (i) prolonged immune surveillance, especially in the transplant setting; (ii) the detection of cells whose lineage is not principally involved (for unknown reasons) with the leukemia; (iii) the persistence of "preleukemic" clonal disease without the full complement of genetic lesions required for the development of frank malignancy; or (iv) the presence of a secondary genetic lesion that may render the leukemic progenitor cells relatively quiescent. Regardless, it is likely that a functional "cure" of leukemia is not equivalent to the total eradication of all leukemic or preleukemic cells. The discovery of the mechanisms of dormancy may lead to inroads in defining what it takes to cure leukemia.

Lastly, the use of the tumor suppressor WT1 has been used in a marker of MRD following SCT *(71)*. This gene is found elevated in AML and ALL compared to bone marrow and peripheral blood and, thus, has some potential for a marker of MRD. Elmaagacli et al. studied 38 patients post-SCT, and 14 out of 38 patients were positive for elevated WT1 at least once posttransplant. Of the 14 patients positive for MRD, seven patients relapsed, compared to five patient relapses in the 34 patients without MRD. In 17 of these patients, translocation markers were available, and the authors were able to test the concordance of the leukemia-specific translocation and WT1 expression. These assays were concordant 70% of the time; in the discordant 30%, roughly one-half were positive for the leukemia-specific marker and negative of WT1; the other half visa-versa. Thus, while not absolutely predictive of relapse, the WT1 assay may be a relative universal tool for assessing risk of relapse.

5. MRD IN LYMPHOMA AND MYELOMA

Allogeneic SCT is relatively uncommon for lymphoma or myeloma, so it is not surprising that there is little data concerning the significance of MRD detection in these diseases in the allogeneic setting. IgH V-D-J rearrangements can also be used in multiple myeloma to detect MRD in a similar manner. Two relatively small studies have shown that approx one-half of patients will become MRD-negative, but the relapse rate appears similar in the MRD-positive and -negative group *(72,73)*. Most patients who achieve a complete remission (CR) become MRD-negative after 6 mo posttransplant, but many take less than 2 yr (one remarkable case took 6 yr to achieve MRD-negative). One worries, however, about the influence of selection bias in these studies, as relapses in these cohorts have been surprising infrequent.

The strategy of MRD detection can also be used in chronic lymphocytic leukemia (CLL). Mattson et al. studied six CLL patients posttransplant by both IgH V-D-J rearrangement and chimerism studies of the CD19+ cell population *(74)*. Chimerism of the CD19+ population correlated with IgH V-D-J status in the vast majority of cases. Five of six patients obtained a CR, and many had evidence of MRD despite CR, even up to 2 yr posttransplant. This has also been seen after nonmyeloablative mini-transplants, where some patients became MRD-negative after 6 mo posttransplant of an allogeneic-related immune system *(75)*. These results imply that clearance of disease following transplant may be remarkably slow and facilitated largely by immune mechanisms.

6. THE TREATMENT OF MRD

The underlying premise of MRD detection is the potential use of preemptive therapy to curtail relapse. Is there any evidence that the treatment of lesser disease burden works? The proof-of-principle for treating MRD disease has been demonstrated by van Rhee et al. *(76)*, who treated 14 CML patients who relapsed hematologically, cytogenetically, or molecularly (i.e., *bcr-abl*-positive) with donor leukocyte infusions (DLI). Of the seven patients with hematologic relapse, three patients had a complete cytogenetic response to DLI; however, two of these patients developed aplasia. Three patients with hematologic relapse and two patients with only *bcr-abl* molecular positivity were treated; all had a complete response, and there were no aplastic events. There was no clear difference in the incidence of severe GVHD among the three groups. Thus, patients treated earlier in the course of relapse had improved response and fewer complications. Further studies of DLI administration post-SCT have also suggested the potential increased efficacy of treating a lower disease burden afforded by MRD testing *(77–79)*. Lastly, single patient reports exist showing the resolution of MRD as detected by WT1 or inversion *(16)* detection in AML post-SCT *(80)*. Both reports note the resolution of MRD after DLI given for MRD up to 21 and 16 mo of follow-up, respectively.

In the near future, novel therapeutic approaches may be used to treat MRD in the post-SCT setting. For example, the tyrosine kinase inhibitor STI571 has shown remarkable promise in the treatment of interferon-resistant CML *(81)* and, given it's low toxicity profile, seems a logical choice for the treatment of MRD in CML patients. Antibody therapy, such as Mylotarg *(82)*, which is directed against the CD33 antigens present in most myeloid precursors and AML blasts, may also be considered as a possible choice in the MRD setting, but utmost caution must be taken given the higher toxicity profile of these agents. In all cases, it cannot be emphasized enough that any treatment of MRD post-SCT is investigation, and should take place only in the context of a research trial.

7. CONCLUSION

The primary goal of MRD research is to redefine remission, so that those patients at a high risk of relapse can be detected early and treated with preemptive therapy designed to squash

Table 2
MRD Detection Post-SCT

Disease	Genetic target	Associated with relapse?	Comments
ALL	IgH V-D-J	Yes	Detection before and after SCT is meaningful.
Ph+	bcr-abl	Yes	p190 bcr-abl may be worse than p210.
AML t(15;17)	PML/RARα	Yes	Levels >10^{-3} associated with relapse after conventional therapy.
t(8;21)	AML1-ETO	Maybe	Even "cured" patients are often PCR+; quantfication will likely help.
inversion (16)	CFBF-MYH11	Maybe	Unclear association.
CML	bcr-abl	Yes	Relapse risk higher in T cell depleted. Quantification helps define relapse risk.
Myeloma, CLL	IgH V-D-J	Maybe	Very few studies.
AML, ALL, CML	WT1	Maybe	Variable association with relapse after conventional treatment and SCT.

the leukemia prior to frank relapse. MRD detection after SCT is highly associated with subsequent relapse in CML and ALL; it is likely that the association will hold true in AML and other hematological malignancies as well, but the data in these diseases are slim in comparison (Table 2). The study of MRD has shown that, in many diseases, detectable amounts of disease persist in patients who remain in a long-term remission. This must be telling us something important about the nature of a cure in leukemia, in that cure apparently does not equate with the total absence of all detectable disease. The investigation of the processes that govern dormancy may yield new insights and approaches to curing leukemia.

REFERENCES

1. Arthur CK, Apperley JF, Guo AP, et al. Cytogenetic events after bone marrow transplantation for chronic myeloid leukemias in chronic phase. *Blood* 1988;71:1179–1186.
2. Hook EB. Exclusion of chromosomal mosaicism: tables of 90%, 95%, and 99% confidence limits and comments on use. *Am J Hum Genet* 1977;29:94–99.
3. Tkachuk DC, Westbrook CA, Andreeff M, et al. Detection of BCR-ABL fusion in chronic myelogenous leukemia by two-color fluorescence *in situ* hybridization. *Science* 1990;250:559–562.
4. Compana D, Coustan-Smith E, Janossy G. The immunologic detection of minimal residual disease in acute leukemia. *Blood* 1990;76:163–171.
5. Sievers EL, Lange BJ, Buckley JD, et al. Prediction of relapse of pediatric acute myeloid leukemia by use of multidimensional flow cytometry. *J Nat Cancer Inst* 1996;88:1483–1488.
6. Saiki RK, Gelfand DH, Stofffel S, et al. Primer-directed enzymatic amplification of DNA with a thermostable DNA polymerase. *Science* 1988;239:487–491.
7. Kawasaki ES, Clark SS, Coyne MY, et al. Diagnosis of chronic myeloid and acute lymphocytic leukemias by detection of leukemia-specific mRNA sequences amplified *in vitro*. *Proc Natl Acad Sci USA* 1988;85:5698–5702.
8. Miller WH, Levine K, DeBlasio A, et al. Detection of minimal residual disease in acute promyelocytic leukemia by a reverse transcription polymerase chain reaction assay for the PML/RARα fusion mRNA. *Blood* 1993;82:1689–1694.
9. Kusec R, Laczika K, Knobl P, et al. AML1/ETO fusion mRNA can be detected in remission blood samples of all patients with t(8;21) acute myeloid leukemia after chemotherapy or autologous bone marrow transplantation. *Leukemia* 1994;8:735–739.
10. Maruyama F, Stass SA, Estey EH, et al. Detection of AML1/ETO fusion transcript as a tool for diagnosing t(8;21) positive acute myelogenous leukemia. *Leukemia* 1994;8:40–45.
11. Claxton DF, Liu P, Hsu HB, et al. Detection of fusion transcripts generated by the inversion 16 chromosome in acute myelogenous leukemia. *Blood* 1994;83:1750–1756.
12. Hebert J, Cayuela JM, Daniel MT, et al. Detection of minimal residual disease in acute myelomonocytic leukemia with abnormal marrow eosinophils by nested polymerase chain reaction with allele specific amplification. *Blood* 1994;84:2291–2296.

13. Lee MS, Chang KS, Cabanillas F, et al. Detection of minimal residual cells carrying the t(14;18) by DNA sequence amplification. *Science* 1987;237:175–178.
14. Pallisgaard N, Hokland P, Riishoj DC, et al. Multiplex reverse transcript-polymerase chain reaction for simultaneous screening of 29 translocation and chromosomal aberrations in acute leukemia. *Blood* 1998;93:574–588.
15. Wasserman R, Galili N, Ito Y, et al. Residual disease at the end of induction therapy as a predictor of relapse during therapy in childhood B-lineage acute lymphoblastic leukemia. *J Clin Onc* 1989;10:1879–1884.
16. Yamada M, Wasserman R, Lange B, et al. Minimal residual disease in childhood B-lineage lymphoblastic leukemia. Persistence of leukemia cells during the first 18 months of treatment. *N Engl J Med* 1990;323:448–455.
17. Nowell PC, Hungerford DA: A minute chromosome in human chronic granulocytic leukemias. *Science* 1960;14:97.
18. Lee MS, Chang KS, Freireich EJ, et al. Detection of minimal residual *bcr/abl* transcripts by a modified polymerase chain reaction. *Blood* 1988;72:893–897.
19. Roth MS, Antin JH, Bingham EL, Ginsburg D. Detection of Philadelphia chromosome-positive cells by the polymerase chain reaction following bone marrow transplant for chronic myelogenous leukemia. *Blood* 1989;74:882–885.
20. Sawyers CCL, Timson L, Kawasaki ES, et al. Molecular relapse in chronic myelogenous leukemia patients after bone marrow transplantation detected by polymerase chain reaction. *Proc Natl Acad Sci USA* 1990;87:563–567.
21. Hughes TP, Morgan GJ, Martiat P, Goldman JM. Detection of residual leukemia after bone marrow transplant for chronic myeloid leukemia: role of the polymerase chain reaction in predicting relapse. *Blood* 1991;77:874–878.
22. Roth MS, Antin JH, Ash R, et al. Prognostic significance of Philadelphia chromosome-positive cells detected by the polymerase chain reaction after a allogeneic bone marrow transplant for chronic myelogenous leukemia. *Blood* 1992;79:276–282.
23. Lion T, Henn T, Gaiger A, et al. Early detection of relapse after bone marrow transplantation in patients with chronic myelogenous leukemia. *Lancet* 1993;341:275,276.
24. Miyamura K, Tahara T, Tanimoto M, et al. Long persistent *bcr-abl* positive transcript detected by polymerase chain reaction after marrow transplant for chronic myelogenous leukemia without clinical relapse: A study of 64 patients. *Blood* 1993;81:1089–1094.
25. Radich J, Gehly G, Gooley T, et al. PCR detection of the *bcr-abl* fusion transcript after allogeneic marrow transplantation for chronic myeloid leukemia: results and implications in 346 patients. *Blood* 1995;85:2632–2638.
26. Pichert G, Roy DC, Goin R, et al. Distinct patterns of minimal residual disease associated with graft-versus-host disease after allogeneic bone marrow transplantation for chronic myelogenous leukemia. *J Clin Oncol* 1995;13:1704–1713.
27. Costello RT, Kirk J, Gabert J. Value of PCR analysis for long term survivors after allogeneic bone marrow transplant for chronic myelogenous leukemia: a comparative study. *Leuk Lymphoma* 1996;20:239–243.
28. Radich JP, Gooley T, Bryant E, Chauncey T, et al. The significance of BCR-ABL molecular detection in CML patients "late" (≥18 months) post-transplant. *Blood* 2001;6:1701–1707.
29. van Rhee F, Lin F, Cross NCP, et al. Detection of residual leukaemia more than 10 years after allogeneic bone marrow transplantation for chronic myelogenous leukaemia. *Bone Marrow Transplant* 1994;14:609–612.
30. Mackinnon S, Barnett L, Heller G. Polymerase chain reaction is highly predictive of relapse in patients following T cell-depleted allogeneic bone marrow transplantation of chronic myeloid leukemia. *Bone Marrow Transplant* 1996;17:643–647.
31. Pichert G, Alyea EP, Soiffer RJ, et al. Persistence of myeloid progenitor cells expressing BCR-ABL mRNA after allogeneic bone marrow transplantation for chronic myelognous leukemia. *Blood* 1994;84:2109–2114.
32. Saglio G, Pane F, Gottardi E, et al. Consistent amounts of acute leukemia-associated P190BCR/ABL transcripts are expressed by chronic myelogenous leukemia patients at diagnosis. *Blood* 1996;87:1075–1080.
33. van Rhee F, Hochhaus A, Lin F, et al. p190 BCR-ABL mRNA is expressed at low levels in p210-positive chronic myeloid and acute lymphoblastic leukemias. *Blood* 1996;87:5213–5217.
34. Serrano J, Roman J, Sanchez J, et al. Molecular analysis of lineage-specific chimerism and minimal residual disease by RT-PCR of p210^{BCR-ABL} and p190^{BCR-ABL} after allogeneic bone marrow transplantation for chronic myeloid leukemia: increasing mixed myeloid chimerism and p190^{BCR-ABL} detection precede cytogenetic relapse. *Blood* 2000;95:2659–2665.
35. Zhang JG, Goldman JM, Cross NCP. Characterization of genomic BCR-ABL breakpoints in chronic myeloid leukaemia by PCR. *Br J Haematol* 1995;90:138–146.
36. Zhang JG, Lin F, Chase A, et al. Comparison of genomic DNA and cDNA for detection of residual disease after treatment of chronic myeloid leukemia with allogeneic bone marrow transplantation. *Blood* 1996;87:2588–2593.
37. Chomel J-C, Brizard F, Veinstein A, et al. Persistence of BCR-ABL genomic rearrangement in chronic myeloid leukemia patients in complete and sustained cytogenetic remission after interferon-α therapy or allogeneic bone marrow transplantation. *Blood* 2000;95:404–408.
38. Chase A, Parker S, Kaeda J, et al. Absence of host-derived cells in the blood of patients in remission after allografting for chronic myeloid leukemia. *Blood* 2000;96:777,778.

39. Deininger M, Lehmann T, Krahl R, et al. No evidence for persistence of BCR-ABL-positive cells in patients in molecular remission after conventional allogeneic transplantation for chronic myeloid leukemia. *Blood* 2000;96:778,779.

40. Lin F, van Rhee F, Goldman JM, Cross NCP. Kinetics of increasing BCR-ABL transcript numbers in chronic myeloid leukemia patients who relapse after bone marrow transplantation. *Blood* 1996;87:4473–4478.

41. Lion T, Izraelli S, Henn T, et al. Monitoring of residual disease in chronic myelogenous leukemia by quantitative polymerase chain reaction. *Leukemia* 1992;6:495–499.

42. Mensink E, van de Locht A, Schattenberg A, et al. Quantitation of minimal residual disease in Philadelphia chromosome positive chronic myeloid leukaemia patients using real-time quantitative RT-PCR. *Br J Haematol* 1998;102:768–774.

43. Preudhomme C, Revillion F, Merlat A, et al. Detection of BCR-ABL transcripts in chronic myeloid leukemia (CML) using a "real time" quantitative RT-PCR assay. *Leukemia* 1999;13:957–964.

44. Branford S, Hughes TP, Rudzski Z. Monitoring chronic myeloid leukaemia therapy by real-time quantitative PCR in blood is a reliable alternative to bone marrow cytogenetics. *Br J Haematol* 1999;107:587–599.

45. Olavarria E, Kanfer E, Szydlo et al. Early detection of BCR-ABL transcripts by quantitative reverse transcriptase-polymerase chain reaction predicts outcome after allogeneic stem cell transplantation for chronic myeloid leukemia. *Blood* 2001;97:1560–1565.

46. Yamada M, Hudson S, Tournay O, et al. Detection of minimal disease in hematopoietic malignancies of the B-cell lineage by using third-complementarity-determining region (CDR-III)-specific probes. *Proc Natl Acad Sci USA* 1989;86:5123–5127.

47. Rovera G, Wasserman R, Yamada M. Detection of minimal residual disease in childhood leukemia with the polymerase reaction. *N Engl J Med* 1991;324:774–781.

48. Brisco MJ, Hughes E, Neoh SH, et al. Relationship between minimal residual disease and outcome in adult acute lymphoblastic leukemia. *Blood* 1996;87:5251–5256.

49. Sikes PJ, Snell LE, Brisco MJ, Neoh SH, et al. The use of monoclonal gene rearrangement for detection of minimal residual disease in acute lymphoblastic leukemia of childhood. *Leukemia* 1997;11:153–158.

50. Roberts WM, Estrov Z, Ouspenskaia MV, et al. Measurement of residual leukemia during remission in childhood acute lymphoblastic leukemia. *New Engl J Med* 1997;336:317–323.

51. Cave H, van der Werff ten Bosch J, Suciu S, et al. Clinical significance of minimal residual disease in childhood acute lymphoblastic leukemia. *N Engl J Med* 1998;339:591–598.

52. Radich J, Ladne P, Gooley T. Polymerase chain reaction-based detection of minimal residual disease in acute lymphoblastic leukemia predicts relapse after allogeneic BMT. *Biol Blood Marrow Transplant* 1995;1:24–31.

53. Knechtli CJC, Goulden NJ, Hancock JP, et al. Minimal residual disease status as a predictor of relapse after allogeneic bone marrow transplantation for children with acute lymphoblastic leukaemia. *Br J Haematol* 1998;102:860–871.

54. Knechtli CJC, Goulden NJ, Hancock JP, et al. Minimal residual disease status before allogeneic bone marrow transplantation is an important determinant of successful outcome for children and adolescents with acute lymphoblastic leukemia. *Blood* 1998;92:4072–4079.

55. Zetterquist H, Mattsson J, Uzunel M, et al. Mixed chimerism and minimal residual disease in patients with pre-B acute lymphoblastic leukemia. *Bone Marrow Transplant* 2000;25:843–851.

56. Miyamura K, Tanimoto M, Morishima Y, et al. Detection of Philadelphia chromosome-positive acute lymphoblastic leukemia by polymerase chain reaction: Possible eradication of minimal residual disease by marrow transplantation. *Blood* 1992;79:1366–1371.

57. Radich J, Gehly G, Lee A, et al. Detection of *bcr-abl* transcripts in Philadelphia chromosome-positive acute lymphoblastic leukemia after marrow transplantation. *Blood* 1997;89:2602–2609.

58. Perego RA, Marenco P, Bianchi C, et al. PML/RARa transcripts monitored by polymerase chain reaction in acute promyelocytic leukemia during complete remission, relapse and after bone marrow transplantation. *Leukemia* 1996;10:207–212.

59. Roman J, Martin C, Torres A, et al. Absence of detectable PML-RARa fusion transcripts in long-term remission patients after BMT for acute promyelocytic leukemia. *Bone Marrow Transplant* 1997;9:679–683.

60. Mandelli F, Diverio D, Avvisati G, et al. Molecular remission in PML/RARa-positive acute promyelocytic lelukemia by combined all-*trans* retinoic acid and idarubicin (AIDA) therapy. *Blood* 1997;1014–1021.

61. Diverio D, Rossi V, Avvisati G, et al. Early detection of relapse by prospective reverse transcriptase-polymerase chain reaction analysis of the PML/RARa fusion gene in patients with acute promyelocytic leukemia enrolled in the GIMEMA-AIEOP multicenter "AIDA" trial. *Blood* 1998;92:784–789.

62. Kusec R, Laczika K, Knobl P, et al. AML1/ETO fusion mRNA can be detected in remission blood samples of all patients with t (8;21) acute myeloid leukemia after chemotherapy or autologous bone marrow transplantation. *Leukemia* 1994; 8:735–739.

63. Miyamoto T, Nagafuji K, Harada M, et al. Quantitative analysis of AML1/ETO transcripts in peripheral blood stem cell harvests from patients with t(8;21) acute myelogenous leukemia. *Br J Haematol* 1995;91:132–138.

64. Jurlander J, Caligiuri MA, Ruutu T, et al. Persistence of the AML1/ETO fusion transcript in patients treated with allogeneic bone marrow transplantation for t(8;21) leukemia. *Blood* 1996;88:2183–2191.

65. Sugimoto T, Das H, Imoto S, et al. Quantitation of minimal residual disease in t(8;21)-positive acute myelogenous leukemia patients using real-time quantitative RT-PCR. *Am J Hematol* 2000;64:101–106.

66. Marcucci G, Livak KJ, Bi W, et al. Detection of minimal residual disease in patients with AML1/ETO-associated acute myeloid leukemia using a novel quantitative reverse transcription polymerase chain reaction assay. *Leukemia* 1998;12:1482–1489.

67. Laczika K, Novak M, Hilgarth B, et al. Competitive CBFβ/MYH11 reverse-transcriptase polymerase chain reaction for quantitative assessment of minimal residual disease during postremission therapy in acute myeloid leukemia with inversion(16): a pilot study. *J Clin Oncol* 1998;16:1519–1525.

68. Elmaagacli AH, Beelen DW, Kroll M, et al. Detection of CBFβ/MYH11 fusion transcripts in patients with inv(16) acute myeloid leukemia after allogeneic bone marrow or peripheral blood progenitor cell transplantation. *Bone Marrow Transplant* 1998;21:159–166.

69. Miyamoto T, Kagafuji K, Akashi K, et al. Persistence of multipotent progenitors expressing AML1/ETO transcripts in long-term remission patients with t(8;21) acute myelogenous leukemia. *Blood* 1996;87:4789–4796.

70. Vora A, Frost L, Goodeve A, et al. Late relapsing childhood lymphoblastic leukemia. *Blood* 1998; 92:2334–2337.

71. Elmaagacli AH, Beelen DW, Trenschel R, Schaefer UW. The detection of wt-1 transcripts is not associated with an increased leukemic relapse rate in patients with acute leukemia after allogeneic bone marrow or peripheral blood stem cell transplantation. *Bone Marrow Transplant* 2000;25:91–96.

72. Corradini P, Voena C, Tarella C, et al. Molecular and clinical remission in multiple myeloma: role of autologous and allogeneic transplantation of hematopoetic cells. *J Clin Oncol* 1999;17:208–215.

73. Cavo M, Terrangna C, Martinelli G, et al. Molecular monitoring of minimal residual disease in patients in long-term complete remission after allogeneic stem cell transplantation for multiple myeloma. *Blood* 2000;96:355–357.

74. Mattsson J, Uzunel M, Remberger M, et al. Minimal residual disease is common after allogeneic stem cell transplantation in patients with B cell chronic lymphocytic leukemia and may be controlled by graft-versus-host disease. *Leukemia* 2000;14:247–254.

75. McSweeney PA, Niederwieser D, Shizuru JA, et al. Hematopoietic cell transplantation in older patients with hematologic malignancies: replacing high-dose cytotoxic therapy with graft-versus-tumor effects. *Blood* 2001;11:3390–3400.

76. van Rhee F, Lin F, Cullis JO, et al. Relapse of chronic myeloid leukemia after allogeneic bone marrow transplant: the case for giving donor leukocyte transfusions before the onset of hematologic relapse. *Blood* 1994;83:3377–3383.

77. Au WY, Lie AKW, Lee CCK, et al. Donor lymphocyte infusion induced molecular remission in relapse of acute myeloid leukaemia after allogeneic bone marrow transplantation. *Bone Marrow Transplant* 1999;23:1201–1203.

78. Formankova R, Honzatkova L, Moravcova J, et al. Prediction and reversion of post-transplant relapse in patients with chronic myeloid leukemia using mixed chimersim and residual disease detection and adoptive immunotherapy. *Leuk Res* 2000;24:339–347.

79. Dazzi F, Szydlo RM, Cross NCP et al. Durability of responses following donor lymphocyte infusions for patients who relapse after allogeneic stem cell transplantation for chronic myeloid leukemia. *Blood* 2000;96:2712–2716.

80. Ogawa A, Tsuboi A, Oji Y, et al. Successful donor leukocyte transfusion at molecular relapse for a patient with acute myeloid leukemia who was treated with allogeneic bone marrow transplantation: importance of the monitoring minimal residual disease by WT1 assay. *Bone Marrow Transplant* 1998;21:525–527.

81. Druker BJ, Talpaz M, Resta DJ, et al. Efficacy and safety of a specific inhibitor of the BCR-ABL tyrosine kinase in chronic myeloid leukemia. *N Engl J Med* 2001;344:1031–1037.

82. Sievers EL, Larson RA, Stadtmauer EA, et al. Efficacy and safety of gemtuzumab ozogamicin in patients with CD33-positive acute myeloid leukemia in first relapse. *J Clin Oncol* 2001;19:3244–3254.

23 Nonhuman Primate Models of Hematopoietic Stem Cell Transplantation

Steven M. Devine and Ronald Hoffman

CONTENTS

1. INTRODUCTION

Recent advances in hematopoietic stem cell (HSC) transplantation have occurred in large measure due to the development of reliable animal model systems. Clearly, the most widely used models are rodent, particularly the mouse. The murine system has been uniquely suited for studies defining the genetics and pathogenesis of graft-vs-host disease (GVHD), as well as for determining the requirements for successful engraftment of histoincompatible HSC. Nevertheless, sole reliance on the murine systems to create models, which parallel human hematopoiesis and the effects of HSC transplantation, is less than ideal for a number of important reasons. For instance, mice require approx one-half to one full log less bone marrow cells than do nonhuman primates or humans in order to survive a lethal dose of myelosuppressive conditioning (1–3). This alone is a simple yet important demonstration of the intrinsic differences in the properties of primate and murine HSC. Furthermore, there are marked differences between mice and humans with regard to the patterns of GVHD observed following stem cell transplantation (4). For example, mice initially tolerate the engraftment of fully major histocompatibility complex (MHC)-mismatched bone marrow, whereas the engraftment of fully mismatched or even haploidentical non-T cell-depleted bone marrow in humans or monkeys is associated with acute and often lethal acute GVHD (2,4).

From: *Current Clinical Oncology: Allogeneic Stem Cell Transplantation*
Edited by: Mary S. Laughlin and Hillard M. Lazarus © Humana Press Inc., Totowa, NJ

Due to their phylogenetic proximity to humans, the relatedness of their MHC complex, naturally outbred nature, similar hematopoietic response to total body irradiation (TBI), requirements for roughly equivalent doses of either autologous and allogeneic bone marrow cells for rescue following TBI, and comparable responses to human hematopoietic cytokines, nonhuman primates are theoretically a superior target for the development of HSC transplantation models. Nevertheless, due to the high cost of maintaining transplanted animals, difficulty in handling large species, and the difficulties encountered in accurately defining the MHC compatibility between donor–recipient pairs, there exist only a handful of investigators who have made a long-term investment into the development of nonhuman primate models of HSC transplantation.

In this chapter, we review several areas of investigation in which nonhuman primate models have provided data that has proven either highly translatable to the human setting or has served as the basis for the development of clinical protocols. New avenues for research, in which the nonhuman primate model could be further exploited, will also be presented.

2. ALLOGENEIC HSC TRANSPLANT MODELS

Dogs have been the preferred large animal model with which to study HSC transplantation due to their large litter sizes and relatively fast breeding, resulting in a significant number of available dog leukocyte antigen (DLA)-matched siblings (5–9). In contrast, fully MHC-matched siblings are very difficult to identify in nonhuman primates due to their breeding patterns and longer gestation periods. In addition, posttransplantation care is easier to administer to dogs than to nonhuman primates. However, dogs tolerate radiation less well than rhesus monkeys, baboons, or humans (doses greater than 7Gy are not well-tolerated) (1,2,7,9,10). Also, there are significant differences in the number of T cells transplanted when comparing primate and canine bone marrow (4). Furthermore, canine cells do not cross-react with many of the available human hematopoietic cytokines or many other monoclonal antibodies that are recognized by both human and nonhuman primate cells. Finally, the phylogenetic proximity between humans and nonhuman primates would imply they represent a more reliable model of human transplantation (11).

Early work by groups led by VanBekkum and Dicke suggested that the rhesus macaque could be used effectively to study GVHD reactions (2,4,12–15). In contrast to mice, grafting of MHC identical sibling marrow was almost always associated with lethal acute GVHD in rhesus monkeys not given posttransplant immunoprophylaxis, as is the case clinically (4,12,13). The presenting features and histopathology of acute GVHD in the rhesus monkey bear close resemblance to human acute GVHD (16,17). Studies performed in the late 1960s through mid-1970s demonstrated that the nonhuman primate model could be used to evaluate strategies designed to mitigate or prevent GVHD (12,15). Pretreatment of MHC identical rhesus monkeys with antilymphocyte serum prevented GVHD (15). Furthermore, effective T cell depletion of MHC-incompatible rhesus marrows (3 to 4 log T cell depletion) could in fact lessen or in some cases prevent GVHD (12). These findings proved to be highly translatable to the clinical setting inasmuch as T cell depletion has consistently been demonstrated to effectively prevent or limit acute GVHD in both the MHC-matched and -mismatched settings (18–20). The rhesus monkey was also used to demonstrate that in vivo T cell depletion using antilymphocyte globulin could effectively treat established GVHD (14).

The baboon system has been used to demonstrate the hematopoietic potential of CD34+ bone marrow cells, first in an autologous setting and later in an MHC-matched allogeneic setting (21,22). Five baboons administered bone marrow selected for CD34+ cells by avidin–biotin immunoadsorption promptly reconstituted hematopoiesis following lethal irradiation, whereas two baboons given marrow depleted of CD34+ cells either died without engraftment or remained pancytopenic for more than 100 d, demonstrating that marrow cells containing the CD34 antigen were enriched for cells with long-term repopulating potential *(22)*. Later, the same group demonstrated that allogeneic marrow cells could be enriched for CD34+ cells, which retained the capacity to reconstitute hematopoiesis in MHC compatible recipients *(21)*. Two of these baboons remained full chimeras between 5 and 6 yr following transplantation and had fully reconstituted their immune system, further proof that CD34+ cells were capable of fully reconstituting lymphohematopoiesis *(23)*. These studies served as the basis for clinical trials evaluating CD34+ selection, using either autologous or allogeneic grafts. The results of these human studies have provided evidence that data obtained in the baboon model are predictive of clinical outcomes *(24–27)*.

While clearly demonstrative of the power of the nonhuman primate model, the studies performed by Andrews and colleagues have also demonstrated the pitfalls of this model *(21)*. These investigators evaluated more than 30 potential donor–recipient pairs before they were able to identify mixed lymphocyte culture nonreactive, presumably MHC-compatible siblings. Furthermore, following allogeneic HSC transplantation, baboons are difficult to support without rigorous standards. In the report by Andrews, three out of five MHC-compatible baboons died of infectious complications between 1 and 4 mo following transplantation *(21)*.

Without sophisticated support measures, extensive personnel, and great expense, it is very difficult to identify and support fully MHC-compatible nonhuman primate donor–recipient pairs *(21)*. In the absence of gene sequencing, which is an expensive and cumbersome task, one cannot reliably determine nonhuman primate histocompatibility without knowledge of the animal's pedigree. In practical terms, allogeneic HSC transplantation can only be performed consistently in these models using either fully MHC mismatched or at best haploidentical donor–recipient pairs. With the advent of the National Marrow Donor Program (NMDP) in 1987 and the clinical development of volunteer unrelated donor protocols, emphasis shifted away from MHC-mismatched (haploidentical) related transplants to volunteer unrelated donor transplants. Due to breeding patterns, lack of multiple births, and long duration of gestation (approx 180 d in the baboon), nonhuman primates are impractical as a model of unrelated donor transplantation since the numbers of monkeys maintained at all the primate centers worldwide would be insufficient to provide enough unrelated yet MHC-matched donor–recipient pairs. In contrast, given the large litter size and fast breeding of dogs, the canine model has been exploited for studying unrelated donor transplants. Only recently, given the renewed interest in haploidentical-related transplants spurred by encouraging clinical results, has interest been rekindled in the use of a nonhuman primate model for MHC-mismatched but related HSC transplantation *(28–30)*. Furthermore, interest in the use of hematopoietic cells for the induction of transplantation tolerance has led to the development of nonhuman primate allograft transplantation models, in which fully MHC-mismatched HSC and solid organs can be transplanted serially or simultaneously *(31,32)*. Nevertheless, over the past 15 yr, the nonhuman primate has been used more to evaluate the effects of human hematopoietic cytokines on hematopoiesis and stem cell mobilization in models of ex vivo HSC expansion and, lastly, as a model of gene therapy. Several of the important studies performed in these settings will be described below.

3. HEMATOPOIETIC GROWTH FACTORS

The baboon and macaque (Rhesus, cynomolgus) species have been used to study the in vivo effects of putative human hematopoietic growth factors. Studies have focused on the effects of growth factors during both steady state or following perturbations of hematopoiesis. Despite potential limitations due to the development of neutralizing antibodies, most of these models have yielded data which has facilitated the design of clinical trials. Non-human primate models have been used to study numerous growth factors including granulocyte colony-stimulating factor (G-CSF) *(33,34)*, granulocyte-macrophage colony-stimulating factor (GM-CSF) *(35–39)*, interleukin-3 (IL-3) *(37,39–41)*, IL-6 *(40–42)*, IL-11 *(43)*, stem cell factor (SCF) *(44)*, leukemia inhibitory factor (LIF) *(45)*, thrombopoietin (TPO) *(46)*, megakaryocyte growth and development factor (MGDF) *(47–49)*, daniplestim *(50)*, and myelopoietin *(51)*. A selected group of trials are listed in Table 1. In many instances, these models have provided reliable data regarding the relative safety of and potential toxicities associated with these molecules. Interestingly, the first in vivo demonstration of the effects of SCF on mast cell expansion and degranulation was demonstrated in both baboons and cynomolgus monkeys prior to the demonstration of this effect in humans *(52)*. These nonhuman primate models afford the capacity to study potential synergistic interactions between cytokines and to develop optimized schedules of administration. The effects of human cytokines on hematopoiesis in both baboons and rhesus monkeys have been highly predictive of outcomes observed in clinical trials. Notwithstanding, it is reasonable to apply caution when interpreting the results obtained in these models. For instance, human growth factors must often be given in much higher doses in comparison to humans in order to achieve a biological effect in these xenogeneic systems. At such supraphysiological doses, effects on other endogenous cytokines may be provoked, theoretically making an accurate quantification of the effects of a single cytokine difficult. Additionally, since these animals have not previously been treated with chemotherapy or radiation, it is often difficult to extrapolate data obtained in chemotherapy-naïve animals to describe or predict responses likely to occur in heavily pretreated patients. Nevertheless, it has been quite striking to note how often nonhuman primate models have successfully predicted the effects of many human hematopoietic growth factors on human biological responses. This is most evident when evaluating the effects of hematopoietic growth factors on the mobilization of hematopoietic stem and progenitor cells into the peripheral blood *(53–61)*. The baboon model has been used to assess the capacity of G-CSF, SCF, and Flt3 ligand given singly or in combination to mobilize cells possessing the capacity to rescue animals from otherwise lethal irradiation *(53–55,60)*. The baboon was the first system to demonstrate the synergistic effects of G-CSF with SCF on stem cell mobilization, an effect later realized and exploited clinically *(54,55,62,63)*. The baboon has also been used to demonstrate the importance of adhesive interactions on stem cell mobilization. It was recently demonstrated that an anti-integrin antibody (antiVLA-4) given in combination with G-CSF or SCF enhanced the mobilization of hematopoietic progenitor cells *(56)*. The rhesus monkey has also been exploited to study the safety and efficacy of novel chimeric hematopoietic agonists on progenitor cell mobilization *(58,64)*. Table 2 provides a selected list of studies using the nonhuman primate to assess the capacity of human hematopoietic growth factors to mobilize HSC.

4. GENE THERAPY

Nonhuman primate models have proven to be a powerful preclinical tool for analyzing the in vivo effects of various gene transduction strategies *(3,65,66)*. Such models have demonstrated many of the potential barriers to successful gene therapy in humans. Despite the success predicted by murine models, nonhuman primate systems have clearly established where the murine models fall short. This is particularly true in the case of strategies targeting hematopoietic stem and progenitor cells *(66)*. In early nonhuman primate studies, the efficiency of gene transfer into hematopoietic repopulating cells was consistently lower than that achieved using murine HSC *(3,65)*. Differences in the density of expression of retroviral receptors on primate

Table 1
Selected Hematopoietic Cytokine Studies Performed in Nonhuman Primates

Ref.	Cytokine	Species	Model	Result
34	G-CSF	Cynomolgus	CIM/RIM	Shortened duration of myelosuppression.
35	GM-CSF	Rhesus	RIM/BMT	Reduced duration of neutropenia following radiation and BMT.
36	GM-CSF	Rhesus	RIM	Enhanced granulocyte recovery in animals receiving GM-CSF.
39	IL-3 +/- GM-CSF	Rhesus	SSA	Sequential administration of IL-3 followed by GM-CSF increased thrombopoiesis.
37	IL-3 +/- GM-CSF	Rhesus	RIM	Sequential administration of IL-3 followed by GM-CSF did not improve hematopoietic recovery compared to GM-CSF alone.
41	IL-3 +/- IL-6	Rhesus	CIM	IL-6 was effective in shortening duration of thrombocytopenia.
40	IL-3 +/- IL-6	Rhesus	RIM	IL-6 enhanced platelet recovery following radiation. Sequential IL-3/IL-6 not clearly superior.
42	IL-6	Rhesus	RIM	IL-6 induced accelerated recovery of neutrophils and platelets.
44	SCF	Baboon	SSA	SCF caused rise in BM cellularity and CFU-GM and BFU-E formation.
45	LIF	Rhesus	RIM	LIF decreased duration of thrombocytopenia; no effect on neutrophil recovery.
43	IL-11	Cynomolgus	CIM/RIM	IL-11 improved platelet recovery following chemotherapy or radiation induced myelosuppression.
46	TPO +/- G-CSF	Rhesus	TBI/ BMT	No improvement in platelet recovery observed.
49	MGDF +/- G-CSF	Rhesus	CIM	Improvement in both neutrophil and platelet recovery.
47	MGDF	Baboon	SSA or CIM	MGDF enhanced steady state platelet/megakaryocyte production; modestly improved platelet recovery after 5-FU.
48	MGDF +/- G-CSF	Rhesus	RIM	Pegylated MGDF enhanced multi-lineage recovery when combined with G-CSF.
50	Daniplestim	Rhesus	RIM	Enhanced platelet recovery and raised neutrophil nadir after radiation.
51	Myelopoietin	Rhesus	RIM	Improved neutrophil and platelet recovery observed.

G-CSF, granulocyte colony-stimulating factor; GM-CSF, granulocyte-macrophage colony-stimulating factor; IL-3, interleukin-3; IL-6, interleukin-6; IL-11, interleukin-11; SCF, stem cell factor; LIF, leukemia-inhibitory factor; TPO, thrombopoietin; MGDF, megakaryocyte growth and development factor; CIM, chemotherapy-induced myelosuppression; RIM, radiation-induced myelosuppression; BMT, bone marrow transplantation; SSA, steady state administration; CFU-GM, colony forming unit-granulocyte macrophage; BFU-E, burst forming unit-erythrocyte; 5-FU, 5 flourouracil.

Table 2
Hematopoietic Cytokine Mobilization Studies in Nonhuman Primates

Ref.	Cytokine(s) studied	Species	Result
53	SCF	Baboon	SCF alone mobilized cells capable of rescuing lethally irradiated baboons.
52	SCF	Baboon or Cynomolgus	SCF administration resulted in marked expansion of mast cells in a variety of tissues.
57	IL-3 + GM-CSF	Rhesus	Combining IL-3 with GM-CSF followed by large volume apheresis resulted in collection of increased numbers of hematopoietic progenitors in comparison to untreated controls.
54	G-CSF +/- SCF	Baboon	Demonstrated dose and schedule dependent effects of combination G-CSF and SCF on progenitor cell mobilization.
55	G-CSF +/- SCF	Baboon	Blood cells mobilized by combination G-CSF and SCF engrafted lethally irradiated recipients more rapidly than cells mobilized by G-CSF alone.
60	FL +/- G-CSF	Baboon	Demonstrated synergistic effects of combination FL and G-CSF on mobilization of hematopoietic progenitor cells.
56	G-CSF/FL/SCF	Baboon	Anti-integrin treatment with an anti-VLA-4 antibody resulted in a synergistic hematopoietic progenitor cell mobilization when combined with human hematopoietic cytokines.
58	Myelopoietin/Daniplestim/G-CSF	Rhesus	Myelopoietin administration resulted in mobilization of larger numbers of hematopoietic progenitors in comparison to treatment with Daniplestim or G-CSF alone.

G-CSF, granulocyte colony-stimulating factor; GM-CSF, granulocyte-macrophage colony-stimulating factor; IL-3, interleukin-3; SCF, stem cell factor; FL, Flt-3 ligand.

HSC, or the requirements for growth factors in culture, have been significant and highlight the fundamental problems when extrapolating from murine studies. Intrinsic differences in the properties of primate and murine HSC are also likely important enough to account for many of the difficulties encountered to date. Studies demonstrating fundamental differences between murine and nonhuman primate HSC will be discussed in the section on hematopoiesis.

Xenogeneic assays of human hematopoiesis using the non-obese diabetic/severe combined immunodeficiency (NOD/SCID) mouse and the fetal sheep have been used as in vivo models to study the efficiency of gene transfer into human HSC *(67–70)*. However, the effects of a xenogeneic microenvironment on the behavior and function of human HSC in these models remains unclear at present, calling into question the reliability of these systems for predicting human in vivo hematopoiesis. Secondly, the immunosuppressed milieu inherent in these models does not allow for an accurate prediction of the effects of an otherwise intact human immune system in response to genetically modified human hematopoietic cells. Importantly, an in vivo immunologic response to green fluorescent protein (GFP) transduced human hematopoietic cells has recently been demonstrated in a rhesus model *(71)*. On the other hand, autologous transplantation models using nonhuman primates seem superior for evaluating engraftment, proliferation, and differentiation of transduced HSC and for predicting the effects of an intact immune system. Moreover, such models can be exploited to examine the effects of and requirements for conditioning of a recipient prior to the infusion of gene-modified HSC. Numerous groups have used either the rhesus or baboon models in order to optimize gene transfer conditions, the effects to retroviral vector pseudotyping, the effects of novel retroviruses such as lentiviruses, and to determine the requirements for conditioning necessary to achieve stable gene expression *(61 65,66,72–89)*. Table 3 lists some of the gene therapy strategies that have been used in nonhuman primate models.

5. PRIMATE HEMATOPOIESIS

Within a typical 2-yr lifespan, a mouse makes about the same amount of red blood cells in its entire lifetime as does a man in 1 d *(90)*. This suggests that the demands placed on murine and primate HSC vary. For these reasons, we and others have studied hematopoiesis in nonhuman primates during both steady state and following perturbation. In the rhesus monkey, Kim and colleagues described the tracking of clonal contributions to hematopoiesis of autologous mobilized peripheral blood cells infused following lethal TBI by using retroviral insertion site analysis *(91)*. In two animals studied, 48 clones were identified up to 18 mo following transplantation, and multiple clones were shown to contribute to hematopoiesis at two or more time points. These data contrast sharply with what is known of murine hematopoiesis at steady state and underscore the importance of using nonhuman primates in order to accurately describe human hematopoiesis.

Our group has used continuous bromodeoxyuridine (BrDU) labeling to study stem cell cycling behavior at both steady state or following human growth factor administration in a baboon model *(92)*. We found that in contrast to murine HSC, baboon HSC remained largely quiescent over prolonged periods. Nevertheless, they do eventually cycle, but at far longer time intervals in comparison to mice. At times of stress, as mimicked by the administration of G-CSF, baboon HSC could be rapidly recruited into cycle, presumably in order to meet increased demands. This demonstration of the striking differences in stem cell behavior between nonhuman primate and murine HSC may indeed help explain the difficulties that have been encountered in gene therapy trials targeting human HSC *(93,94)*. They also caution against the over interpretation of murine HSC transplantation models to describe human hematopoiesis following stem cell transplantation. This is particularly true when describing effects of HSC trans-

Table 3
Selected Nonhuman Primate Gene Therapy Models

Ref.	Species	Strategy	Result
72	Rhesus	Transduction of cytokine mobilized hematopoietic progenitors.	Cytokine priming resulted in collection of more primitive cells with improved susceptibility to retroviral transduction.
78	Baboon	Competitive repopulation assay.	GALV pseudotyped vector more efficiently transduced baboon hematopoietic progenitors in comparison to amphotropic vector.
79	Baboon	Fibronectin fragment used to enhance transduction efficiency.	Gene transfer efficiency was improved when cells were transduced in the presence of fibronectin fragment (CH-296).
73	Rhesus	In vivo tracking of nonexpressed transgenes.	AAV vector resulted in higher short-term in vivo marking of T lymphocytes in comparison to retroviral vector.
61	Rhesus	In vivo tracking of gene marked CD34+ cells.	Nonmyeloablative conditioning permitted long-term persistence of gene-marked cells in multiple hematopoietic lineages.
82	Baboon	Use of helper-dependent ("gutless") vectors to evade immune recognition.	A helper-dependent adenoviral vector system resulted in reduced immunogenicity of transduced cells.
80	Rhesus	Injection of human Factor IX via adenoviral vector.	Administration of high doses of adenoviral vector resulted in dose-limiting hepatic toxicity.
71	Rhesus	EGFP marking of hematopoietic cells.	Demonstrated development of immune response to EGFP expressing hematopoietic cells.

AAV, adeno-associated virus; GALV, Gibbon ape leukemia virus; EGFP, enhanced green fluorescent protein.

plantation following in vitro exposure to agents inducing cell cycling in an effort to "expand" stem or progenitor cells.

6. EX VIVO EXPANSION

The possibility of expanding in vitro the numbers of primitive hematopoietic cells capable of long-term bone marrow reconstitution is of great interest, due to the potential for both gene therapeutic and transplantation applications *(95)*. Encouraging data have been obtained using various murine models, including the SCID-Hu and NOD/SCID mouse systems *(96–98)*. Nevertheless, in some studies, stem cell cycling following in vitro exposure to various hematopoietic cytokines has been associated with either loss of repopulating potential or the development of a marrow homing defect *(99–101)*. In addition, early clinical trials evaluating the transplantation of ex vivo-expanded adult bone marrow or umbilical cord blood cells have failed to demonstrate a significant improvement in engraftment kinetics *(95,102,103)*. In order to attempt to explain this and better resolve the controversies surrounding the results of murine studies, several groups have turned to the nonhuman primate system. Tisdale and colleagues retrovirally transduced G-CSF/SCF-mobilized peripheral blood CD34+ cells obtained from rhesus monkeys with the neomycin resistance gene *(104)*. Following transduction, an aliquot of cells were either frozen without further manipulation or further expanded with cytokines for 10–14 d in vitro. Following TBI, both non-expanded and expanded cells were co-infused. Despite five- to 13-fold greater numbers, dose of total cells ,as well as colony forming units (CFU) transfused with the expanded product, the nonexpanded cells made far greater contributions to both short- and long-term hematopoiesis in all animals transplanted. Using adult baboon bone marrow expanded ex vivo in the presence of human hematopoietic cytokines and porcine microvascular endothelial cells (PMVEC), our group demonstrated that hematopoietic reconstitution was delayed in recipients of lethal TBI given a graft containing only ex vivo-expanded cells in comparison to recipients given similar doses of unmanipulated bone marrow cells *(105)*. While the expanded cell population was capable of eventually reconstituting hematopoiesis in this system, the observed delay in engraftment is compatible with the acquisition of an engraftment defect associated with in vitro stem cell cycling. Such data strongly suggest that further strategies designed to improve upon current results using novel in vitro expansion systems should heavily emphasize a demonstration of safety and efficacy obtained first in a nonhuman primate system before moving forward with clinical protocols. This point cannot be overemphasized in light of the recent safety concerns that have arisen in the context of human gene therapy trials *(106)*.

7. TRANSPLANTATION TOLERANCE

Organ transplants in nonhuman primates provide a model that closely simulates the biological conditions encountered in human organ allograft transplantation, due to the similarities in structure and expression between human and nonhuman primate MHC (class I and II) molecules. The establishment of stable unbreakable host–donor transplantation tolerance remains the "Holy Grail" of solid organ transplantation *(31,32,107,108)*. While stable tolerance has been achieved in numerous rodent systems using a multitude of strategies, achievement of tolerance in the nonhuman primate has remained a far more elusive target *(31,109)*. Strategies focusing on the induction of stable mixed donor–host hematopoietic chimerism are now being actively pursued in primate systems since both rodent and swine models have clearly demonstrated that mixed chimerism leads to robust donor–host tolerance and long term acceptance of vascularized organs, and more importantly, skin allografts, which is the most stringent experimental test of tolerance *(31,32,110,111)*. Mixed chimerism has been shown to lead to tolerance, predominantly due to the development of intrathymic clonal deletion of donor reactive cells *(32)*. The potential for this strategy to apply clinically was recently demonstrated in a patient with advanced multiple myeloma, who first underwent a bone marrow transplantation (BMT) followed 10 wk later by a renal allograft from the original bone marrow donor *(112)*. The patient and her renal allograft were surviving more than 22 mo following transplantation, off of all immunosuppression.

Recently, a protocol utilizing an effective T cell depleting antibody–toxin conjugate demonstrated that stable mixed chimerism across MHC barriers could be established in the miniature swine *(110)*. In these studies, high doses of donor peripheral blood progenitor cells were administered to animals following an anti-CD3 immunotoxin and with thymic irradiation. This nonmyeloblative approach led to stable donor lymphoid chimerism, although myleoid chimerism was low. Efforts are ongoing to establish similar systems in nonhuman primates.

In a cynomolgus monkey renal transplantation model, recipients were conditioned with antithymocyte globulin, fractionated TBI (3Gy), local thymic irradiation (7Gy), and splenectomy followed by transplantation of unfractionated bone marrow and a kidney allograft from the same donor *(113)*. Recipients were also administered cyclosporine for 4 wk after BMT, but none thereafter. Multilineage chimerism was detected in the recipients peripheral blood up to 68 d, and long-term renal allograft function was achieved despite loss of donor hematopoietic chimerism. In a separate experiment, treatment of the recipient with a monoclonal antibody to CD154 led to enhanced hematopoietic chimerism and abrogated the requirement for splenectomy *(114)*. To date, however, long-term stable mixed lymphohematopoietic chimerism has yet to be reliably achieved in a nonhuman primate *(31)*.

Since stable mixed chimerism may also be able to reverse the phenotype of patients with hemoglobinopathies, particularly sickle cell disease, we are currently pursuing a strategy in the baboon, which combines conditioning of recipients with low doses of TBI (250–375 cGy) combined with co-stimulatory blockade using the anti-CD154 monoclonal antibody followed by transplantation of high doses of bone marrow or peripheral blood from haploidentical donors. Such studies should determine whether the encouraging results obtained in murine systems using this approach will be effectively translated into the clinic.

8. MESENCHYMAL STEM CELL TRANSPLANTATION

Recently, a process for the isolation, culture, and expansion of a human bone marrow-derived cell capable of multilineage mesenchymal cell differentiation has been described *(115)*. These cells, referred to as mesenchymal stem cells or MSC, offer the potential for the regeneration and repair of numerous mesenchymal tissues. Since MSC gives rise to a number of the cells that comprise the bone marrow stroma and are themselves capable of supporting hematopoiesis in vitro, interest in the HSC transplant community has been focused on the potential capacity for these cells to enhance hematopoietic engraftment, perhaps through the capacity to repair or rejuvenate the host bone marrow microenvironment damaged by prior therapy *(116,117)*. Currently, clinical trials evaluating the safety and efficacy of intravenously infused ex vivo-expanded populations of donor-derived MSC, together with either HLA-matched bone marrow or peripheral blood, or following unrelated umbilical cord blood transplantation, are ongoing. Such attempts imply the capacity for systemically infused MSC to home to and engraft within the host bone marrow microenvironment. However, most of the available clinical data suggest that stromal cells remain of host origin following conventional HSC transplantation *(116,117)*. Although there are a number of potential explanations for this, it is most likely a result of the paucity of stromal cells or MSC contained within a typical allograft. A fundamental question remaining is whether giving a graft containing an expanded

Table 4
Relative Advantages and Disadvantages of Various Animal Model Systems

	Mouse	Fetal sheep	Dog	Nonhuman primate
Advantages	Well-defined genetics.	Well-defined hematopoietic assay.	Fast breeding and large litters.	Phylogenetic proximity to man.
	Availability of disease models.	Provides xenogeneic model.	Relatively easy to handle.	Translatability highest.
	Availability of reagents.	Gestation period well-defined.	Some disease models.	Predictable response to human cytokines.
	Ease of handling.	Model for in utero transplantation.	MHC typing available.	Stem cell behavior similar to humans.
	Affords mechanistic understanding.		Clinically translatable.	Immunologically competent.
	Short gestation/rapid breeding.		Immunologically competent.	
	Less expensive than other systems.			
Disadvantages	Clinical relevance unclear.	Clinical relevance unclear.	Lack of reagents.	Expensive.
	Xenogeneic microenvironment for study of human cells.	Few facilities available.	Expense.	Few facilities available.
	Stem cell behavior differs from humans.	Lack of disease models.	Large facility required for handling.	Lack of disease models.
		Xenogeneic microenvironment for study of human cells.	Response to radiation and chemotherapy differs from primates.	MHC typing difficult.
		Immunologically incompetent.		Difficulty handling.
				Long gestation periods.

dose of MSC would increase the likelihood of detecting donor stromal cell chimerism within the recipient following transplantation.

Our group has used the baboon model system to address this and other fundamental questions related to the transplantation of MSC. We have been able to establish that baboon MSC, collected and expanded under essentially the same conditions as for human MSC, are phenotypically and functionally similar to human MSC (118). Following intravenous administration, baboon MSC safely distribute to multiple nonhematopoietic tissues as well as bone marrow, and can be detected in recipients for up to 21 mo following transplantation. Posttransplant bone marrow biopsies have been repeatedly positive by polymerase chain reaction (PCR) analysis for the presence of transplanted MSC. The actual levels of engraftment are likely low, however. Interestingly, conditioning does not appear to be requisite for long-term MSC engraftment, and fully MHC-incompatible MSC also appear to be accepted by the recipients long-term, without deleterious effects. We are continuing to use the baboon model to answer a number of questions vital to support future clinical trials, such as the relationship between MSC dose and engraftment, the necessity for conditioning and engraftment, as well as the optimal route and schedule of MSC administration.

9. CONCLUSION

Multiple animal model systems, each with its own distinct set of advantages and disadvantages, are currently available for the study of cellular transplantation (Table 4). Despite being resource-intensive, expensive, and time-consuming, the nonhuman primate model systems currently in use complement the other model systems, as they provide invaluable insights into our understanding of HSC biology and the effects of transplantation. In the future, it is difficult to envision a scenario in which significant improvements in the outcomes in gene therapy, ex vivo stem cell expansion, MSC transplantation, or induction of transplantation tolerance are achieved without first evaluating novel strategies in the nonhuman primate. Furthermore, with the emergence of embryonic stem cell research and recent interest generated in adult somatic stem cell plasticity, important observations made in rodent systems will inevitably require additional study in nonhuman primate models before the full clinical potential of this exciting new avenue of research can be realized.

REFERENCES

1. van Bekkum DW. Radiation sensitivity of the hemopoietic stem cell. *Radiat Res* 1991;128(1 Suppl):S4–8.
2. van Bekkum DW. The rhesus monkey as a preclinical model for bone marrow transplantation. *Transplant Proc* 1978;10(1):105–111.
3. Hanazono Y, Terao K, Ozawa K. Gene transfer into nonhuman primate hematopoietic stem cells: implications for gene therapy. *Stem Cells* 2001;19(1):12–23.
4. van Bekkum DW. Biology of acute and chronic graft-versus-host reactions: predictive value of studies in experimental animals. *Bone Marrow Transplant* 1994;14(Suppl 4):S51–55.
5. Ladiges WC, Storb R, Thomas ED. Canine models of bone marrow transplantation. *Lab Anim Sci* 1990;40(1):11–15.
6. Storb R, Rudolph RH, Thomas ED. Marrow grafts between canine siblings matched by serotyping and mixed leukocyte culture. *J Clin Invest* 1971;50(6):1272–1275.
7. Storb R, Rudolph RH, Kolb HJ, Graham TC, Mickelson E, Erickson V, et al. Marrow grafts between DL-A-matched canine littermates. *Transplantation* 1973;15(1):92–100.
8. Storb R, Gluckman E, Thomas ED, Buckner CD, Clift RA, Fefer A, et al. Treatment of established human graft-versus-host disease by antithymocyte globulin. *Blood* 1974;44(1):56–75.
9. Storb R, Weiden PL, Graham TC, Thomas ED. Studies of marrow transplantation in dogs. *Transplant Proc* 1976;8(4):545–549.
10. Wagemaker G, Vriesendorp HM, van Bekkum DW. Successful bone marrow transplantation across major histocompatibility barriers in rhesus monkeys. *Transplant Proc* 1981;13(1 Pt 2):875–880.

11. Prilliman K, Lawlor D, Ellexson M, McElwee N, Confer D, Cooper DK, et al. Characterization of baboon class I major histocompatibility molecules. Implications for baboon-to-human xenotransplantation. *Transplantation* 1996;61(7):989–996.

12. Dicke KA, van Bekkum DW. Allogeneic bone marrow transplantation after elimination of immunocompetent cells by means of density gradient centrifugation. *Transplant Proc* 1971;3(1):666–668.

13. Dicke KA, Tridente G, van Bekkum DW. The selective elimination of immunologically competent cells from bone marrow and lymphocyte cell mixtures. 3. In vitro test for detection of immunocompetent cells in fractionated mouse spleen cell suspensions and primate bone marrow suspensions. *Transplantation* 1969;8(4):422–434.

14. Dicke KA, Spitzer G, Peters L, Stevens EE, Hendriks W, McCredie t. Approaches to graft-versus-host disease following bone marrow transplantation in monkeys and man. *Transplant Proc* 1978;10(1):217–221.

15. van Bekkum DW, Balner H, Dicke KA, van den Berg FG, Prinsen GH, Hollander CF. The effect of pretreatment of allogeneic bone marrow graft recipients with antilymphocytic serum on the acute graft-versus-host reaction in monkeys. *Transplantation* 1972;13(4):400–407.

16. Woodruff JM, Eltringham JR, Casey HW. Early secondary disease in the Rhesus monkey. I. A comparative histopathologic study. *Lab Invest* 1969;20(6):499–511.

17. Woodruff JM, Butcher WI, Hellerstein LJ. Early secondary disease in the rhesus monkey. II. Electron microscopy of changes in mucous membranes and external epithelia as demonstrated in the tongue and lip. *Lab Invest* 1972;27(1):85–98.

18. Goker H, Haznedaroglu IC, Chao NJ. Acute graft-vs-host disease: pathobiology and management. *Exp Hematol* 2001;29(3):259–277.

19. Cornelissen JJ, Lowenberg B. Developments in T-cell depletion of allogeneic stem cell grafts. *Curr Opin Hematol* 2000;7(6):348–352.

20. Champlin RE, Passweg JR, Zhang MJ, Rowlings PA, Pelz CJ, Atkinson KA, et al. T-cell depletion of bone marrow transplants for leukemia from donors other than HLA-identical siblings: advantage of T-cell antibodies with narrow specificities. *Blood* 2000;95(12):3996–4003.

21. Andrews RG, Bryant EM, Bartelmez SH, Muirhead DY, Knitter GH, Bensinger W, et al. CD34+ marrow cells, devoid of T and B lymphocytes, reconstitute stable lymphopoiesis and myelopoiesis in lethally irradiated allogeneic baboons. *Blood* 1992;80(7):1693–701.

22. Berenson RJ, Andrews RG, Bensinger WI, Kalamasz D, Knitter G, Buckner CD, et al. Antigen CD34+ marrow cells engraft lethally irradiated baboons. *J Clin Invest* 1988;81(3):951–955.

23. Andrews RG, Winkler A, Potter J, Bryant E, Knitter GH, Bernstein ID, et al. Normal immunologic response to a neoantigen, bacteriophage phiX-174, in baboons with long-term lymphohematopoietic reconstitution from highly purified CD34+ Lin- allogeneic marrow cells. *Blood* 1997;90(4):1701–1708.

24. Gorin NC, Lopez M, Laporte JP, Quittet P, Lesage S, Lemoine F, et al. Preparation and successful engraftment of purified CD34+ bone marrow progenitor cells in patients with non-Hodgkin's lymphoma. *Blood* 1995;85(6):1647–1654.

25. Bensinger WI, Buckner CD, Shannon-Dorcy K, Rowley S, Appelbaum FR, Benyunes M, et al. Transplantation of allogeneic CD34+ peripheral blood stem cells in patients with advanced hematologic malignancy. *Blood* 1996;88(11):4132–4138.

26. Urbano-Ispizua A, Rozman C, Martinez C, Marin P, Briones J, Rovira M, et al. Rapid engraftment without significant graft-versus-host disease after allogeneic transplantation of CD34+ selected cells from peripheral blood. *Blood* 1997;89(11):3967–3973.

27. Vescio R, Schiller G, Stewart AK, Ballester O, Noga S, Rugo H, et al. Multicenter phase III trial to evaluate CD34(+) selected versus unselected autologous peripheral blood progenitor cell transplantation in multiple myeloma. *Blood* 1999;93(6):1858–1868.

28. Aversa F, Tabilio A, Velardi A, Cunningham I, Terenzi A, Falzetti F, et al. Treatment of high-risk acute leukemia with T-cell-depleted stem cells from related donors with one fully mismatched HLA haplotype. *N Engl J Med* 1998;339(17):1186–1193.

29. Henslee-Downey PJ, Abhyankar SH, Parrish RS, Pati AR, Godder KT, Neglia WJ, et al. Use of partially mismatched related donors extends access to allogeneic marrow transplant. *Blood* 1997;89(10):3864–3872.

30. Sykes M, Preffer F, McAfee S, Saidman SL, Weymouth D, Andrews DM, et al. Mixed lymphohaemopoietic chimerism and graft-versus-lymphoma effects after non-myeloablative therapy and HLA-mismatched bone-marrow transplantation. *Lancet* 1999;353(9166):1755–1759.

31. Wekerle T, Sykes M. Mixed chimerism and transplantation tolerance. *Annu Rev Med* 2001;52:353–370.

32. Sykes M. Mixed chimerism and transplant tolerance. *Immunity* 2001;14(4):417–424.

33. Welte K, Bonilla MA, Gillio AP, Boone TC, Potter GK, Gabrilove JL, et al. Recombinant human granulocyte colony-stimulating factor. Effects on hematopoiesis in normal and cyclophosphamide-treated primates. *J Exp Med* 1987;165(4):941–948.

34. Welte K, Bonilla MA, Gillio AP, Gabrilove JL, O'Reilly RJ, Souza LM. Recombinant human granulocyte-colony stimulating factor: in vivo effects on myelopoiesis in primates. *Behring Inst Mitt* 1988(83):102–106.

35. Monroy RL, Skelly RR, MacVittie TJ, Davis TA, Sauber JJ, Clark SC, et al. The effect of recombinant GM-CSF on the recovery of monkeys transplanted with autologous bone marrow. *Blood* 1987;70(5):1696–1699.

36. Monroy RL, Skelly RR, Taylor P, Dubois A, Donahue RE, MacVittie TJ. Recovery from severe hematopoietic suppression using recombinant human granulocyte-macrophage colony-stimulating factor. *Exp Hematol* 1988;16(5):344–348.

37. Farese AM, Williams DE, Seiler FR, MacVittie TJ. Combination protocols of cytokine therapy with interleukin-3 and granulocyte-macrophage colony-stimulating factor in a primate model of radiation-induced marrow aplasia. *Blood* 1993;82(10):3012–3018.

38. Stahl CP, Winton EF, Monroe MC, Holman RC, Zelasky M, Liehl E, et al. Recombinant human granulocyte-macrophage colony-stimulating factor promotes megakaryocyte maturation in nonhuman primates. *Exp Hematol* 1991;19(8):810–816.

39. Stahl CP, Winton EF, Monroe MC, Haff E, Holman RC, Myers L, et al. Differential effects of sequential, simultaneous, and single agent interleukin-3 and granulocyte-macrophage colony-stimulating factor on megakaryocyte maturation and platelet response in primates. *Blood* 1992;80(10):2479–2485.

40. MacVittie TJ, Farese AM, Patchen ML, Myers LA. Therapeutic efficacy of recombinant interleukin-6 (IL-6) alone and combined with recombinant human IL-3 in a nonhuman primate model of high-dose, sublethal radiation-induced marrow aplasia. *Blood* 1994;84(8):2515–2522.

41. Winton EF, Srinivasiah J, Kim BK, Hillyer CD, Strobert EA, Orkin JL, et al. Effect of recombinant human interleukin-6 (rhIL-6) and rhIL-3 on hematopoietic regeneration as demonstrated in a nonhuman primate chemotherapy model. *Blood* 1994;84(1):65–73.

42. Patchen ML, MacVittie TJ, Williams JL, Schwartz GN, Souza LM. Administration of interleukin-6 stimulates multilineage hematopoiesis and accelerates recovery from radiation-induced hematopoietic depression. *Blood* 1991;77(3):472–480.

43. Goldman SJ. Preclinical biology of interleukin 11: a multifunctional hematopoietic cytokine with potent thrombopoietic activity. *Stem Cells* 1995;13(5):462–471.

44. Andrews RG, Bartelmez SH, Knitter GH, Myerson D, Bernstein ID, Appelbaum FR, et al. A c-kit ligand, recombinant human stem cell factor, mediates reversible expansion of multiple CD34+ colony-forming cell types in blood and marrow of baboons. *Blood* 1992;80(4):920–927.

45. Farese AM, Myers LA, MacVittie TJ. Therapeutic efficacy of recombinant human leukemia inhibitory factor in a primate model of radiation-induced marrow aplasia. *Blood* 1994;84(11):3675–3678.

46. Neelis KJ, Dubbelman YD, Wognum AW, Thomas GR, Eaton DL, Egeland T, et al. Lack of efficacy of thrombopoietin and granulocyte colony-stimulating factor after high dose total-body irradiation and autologous stem cell or bone marrow transplantation in rhesus monkeys. *Exp Hematol* 1997;25(10):1094–1103.

47. Andrews RG, Winkler A, Myerson D, Briddell RA, Knitter GH, McNiece IK, et al. Recombinant human ligand for MPL, megakaryocyte growth and development factor (MGDF), stimulates thrombopoiesis in vivo in normal and myelosuppressed baboons. *Stem Cells* 1996;14(6):661–677.

48. Farese AM, Hunt P, Grab LB, MacVittie TJ. Combined administration of recombinant human megakaryocyte growth and development factor and granulocyte colony-stimulating factor enhances multilineage hematopoietic reconstitution in nonhuman primates after radiation-induced marrow aplasia. *J Clin Invest* 1996;97(9):2145–2151.

49. Harker LA, Marzec UM, Kelly AB, Cheung E, Tomer A, Nichol JL, et al. Prevention of thrombocytopenia and neutropenia in a nonhuman primate model of marrow suppressive chemotherapy by combining pegylated recombinant human megakaryocyte growth and development factor and recombinant human granulocyte colony-stimulating factor. *Blood* 1997;89(1):155–165.

50. Farese AM, Herodin F, McKearn JP, Baum C, Burton E, MacVittie TJ. Acceleration of hematopoietic reconstitution with a synthetic cytokine (SC-55494) after radiation-induced bone marrow aplasia. *Blood* 1996;87(2):581–591.

51. MacVittie TJ, Farese AM, Smith WG, Baum CM, Burton E, McKearn JP. Myelopoietin, an engineered chimeric IL-3 and G-CSF receptor agonist, stimulates multilineage hematopoietic recovery in a nonhuman primate model of radiation-induced myelosuppression. *Blood* 2000;95(3):837–845.

52. Galli SJ, Iemura A, Garlick DS, Gamba-Vitalo C, Zsebo KM, Andrews RG. Reversible expansion of primate mast cell populations in vivo by stem cell factor. *J Clin Invest* 1993;91(1):148–152.

53. Andrews RG, Bensinger WI, Knitter GH, Bartelmez SH, Longin K, Bernstein ID, et al. The ligand for c-kit, stem cell factor, stimulates the circulation of cells that engraft lethally irradiated baboons. *Blood* 1992;80(11):2715–2720.

54. Andrews RG, Briddell RA, Knitter GH, Opie T, Bronsden M, Myerson D, et al. In vivo synergy between recombinant human stem cell factor and recombinant human granulocyte colony-stimulating factor in baboons enhanced circulation of progenitor cells. *Blood* 1994;84(3):800–810.

55. Andrews RG, Briddell RA, Knitter GH, Rowley SD, Appelbaum FR, McNiece IK. Rapid engraftment by peripheral blood progenitor cells mobilized by recombinant human stem cell factor and recombinant human granulocyte colony-stimulating factor in nonhuman primates. *Blood* 1995;85(1):15–20.

56. Craddock CF, Nakamoto B, Andrews RG, Priestley GV, Papayannopoulou T. Antibodies to VLA4 integrin mobilize long-term repopulating cells and augment cytokine-induced mobilization in primates and mice. *Blood* 1997;90(12):4779–4788.

57. Hillyer CD, Swenson RB, Hart KK, Lackey DA, 3rd, Winton EF. Peripheral blood stem cell acquisition by large-volume leukapheresis in growth factor-stimulated and unstimulated rhesus monkeys: development of an animal model. *Exp Hematol* 1993;21(11):1455–1459.

58. MacVittie TJ, Farese AM, Davis TA, Lind LB, McKearn JP. Myelopoietin, a chimeric agonist of human interleukin 3 and granulocyte colony-stimulating factor receptors, mobilizes CD34+ cells that rapidly engraft lethally x-irradiated nonhuman primates. *Exp Hematol* 1999;27(10):1557–1568.

59. McNiece IK, Briddell RA, Hartley CA, Smith KA, Andrews RG. Stem cell factor enhances in vivo effects of granulocyte colony stimulating factor for stimulating mobilization of peripheral blood progenitor cells. *Stem Cells* 1993;11(Suppl 2):36–41.

60. Papayannopoulou T, Nakamoto B, Andrews RG, Lyman SD, Lee MY. In vivo effects of Flt3/Flk2 ligand on mobilization of hematopoietic progenitors in primates and potent synergistic enhancement with granulocyte colony-stimulating factor. *Blood* 1997;90(2):620–629.

61. Rosenzweig M, MacVittie TJ, Harper D, Hempel D, Glickman RL, Johnson RP, et al. Efficient and durable gene marking of hematopoietic progenitor cells in nonhuman primates after nonablative conditioning. *Blood* 1999;94(7):2271–2286.

62. Basser RL, To LB, Begley CG, Maher D, Juttner C, Cebon J, et al. Rapid hematopoietic recovery after multicycle high-dose chemotherapy: enhancement of filgrastim-induced progenitor-cell mobilization by recombinant human stem-cell factor. *J Clin Oncol* 1998;16(5):1899–1908.

63. Shpall EJ, Wheeler CA, Turner SA, Yanovich S, Brown RA, Pecora AL, et al. A randomized phase 3 study of peripheral blood progenitor cell mobilization with stem cell factor and filgrastim in high-risk breast cancer patients. *Blood* 1999;93(8):2491–2501.

64. MacVittie TJ, Farese AM, Herodin F, Grab LB, Baum CM, McKearn JP. Combination therapy for radiation-induced bone marrow aplasia in nonhuman primates using synthokine SC-55494 and recombinant human granulocyte colony-stimulating factor. *Blood* 1996;87(10):4129–4135.

65. Dunbar CE, Tisdale J, Yu JM, Soma T, Zujewski J, Bodine D, et al. Transduction of hematopoietic stem cells in humans and in nonhuman primates. *Stem Cells* 1997;15(Suppl 1):135–139; discussion 139,140.

66. Donahue RE, Dunbar CE. Update on the use of nonhuman primate models for preclinical testing of gene therapy approaches targeting hematopoietic cells. *Hum Gene Ther* 2001;12(6):607–617.

67. Barquinero J, Segovia JC, Ramirez M, Limon A, Guenechea G, Puig T, et al. Efficient transduction of human hematopoietic repopulating cells generating stable engraftment of transgene-expressing cells in NOD/SCID mice. *Blood* 2000;95(10):3085–3093.

68. Schiedlmeier B, Kuhlcke K, Eckert HG, Baum C, Zeller WJ, Fruehauf S. Quantitative assessment of retroviral transfer of the human multidrug resistance 1 gene to human mobilized peripheral blood progenitor cells engrafted in nonobese diabetic/severe combined immunodeficient mice. *Blood* 2000;95(4):1237–1248.

69. Tran ND, Porada CD, Almeida-Porada G, Glimp HA, Anderson WF, Zanjani ED. Induction of stable prenatal tolerance to beta-galactosidase by in utero gene transfer into preimmune sheep fetuses. *Blood* 2001;97(11):3417–3423.

70. Zanjani ED, Anderson WF. Prospects for in utero human gene therapy. *Science* 1999;285(5436):2084–2088.

71. Rosenzweig M, Connole M, Glickman R, Yue SP, Noren B, DeMaria M, et al. Induction of cytotoxic T lymphocyte and antibody responses to enhanced green fluorescent protein following transplantation of transduced CD34(+) hematopoietic cells. *Blood* 2001;97(7):1951–1959.

72. Dunbar CE, Seidel NE, Doren S, Sellers S, Cline AP, Metzger ME, et al. Improved retroviral gene transfer into murine and Rhesus peripheral blood or bone marrow repopulating cells primed in vivo with stem cell factor and granulocyte colony-stimulating factor. *Proc Natl Acad Sci USA* 1996;93(21):11,871–11,876.

73. Hanazono Y, Brown KE, Handa A, Metzger ME, Heim D, Kurtzman GJ, et al. In vivo marking of rhesus monkey lymphocytes by adeno-associated viral vectors: direct comparison with retroviral vectors. *Blood* 1999;94(7):2263–2270.

74. Heim DA, Hanazono Y, Giri N, Wu T, Childs R, Sellers SE, et al. Introduction of a xenogeneic gene via hematopoietic stem cells leads to specific tolerance in a rhesus monkey model. *Mol Ther* 2000;1(6):533–544.

75. Hirata RK, Miller AD, Andrews RG, Russell DW. Transduction of hematopoietic cells by foamy virus vectors. *Blood* 1996;88(9):3654–3661.

76. Huhn RD, Tisdale JF, Agricola B, Metzger ME, Donahue RE, Dunbar CE. Retroviral marking and transplantation of rhesus hematopoietic cells by nonmyeloablative conditioning. *Hum Gene Ther* 1999;10(11):1783–1790.

77. Kaptein LC, Van Beusechem VW, Riviere I, Mulligan RC, Valerio D. Long-term in vivo expression of the MFG-ADA retroviral vector in rhesus monkeys transplanted with transduced bone marrow cells. *Hum Gene Ther* 1997;8(13):1605–1610.

78. Kiem HP, Heyward S, Winkler A, Potter J, Allen JM, Miller AD, et al. Gene transfer into marrow repopulating cells: comparison between amphotropic and gibbon ape leukemia virus pseudotyped retroviral vectors in a competitive repopulation assay in baboons. *Blood* 1997;90(11):4638–4645.

79. Kiem HP, Andrews RG, Morris J, Peterson L, Heyward S, Allen JM, et al. Improved gene transfer into baboon marrow repopulating cells using recombinant human fibronectin fragment CH-296 in combination with interleukin-6, stem cell factor, FLT-3 ligand, and megakaryocyte growth and development factor. *Blood* 1998;92(6):1878–1886.

80. Lozier JN, Metzger ME, Donahue RE, Morgan RA. The rhesus macaque as an animal model for hemophilia B gene therapy. *Blood* 1999;93(6):1875–1881.

81. Medin JA, Brandt JE, Rozler E, Nelson M, Bartholomew A, Li C, et al. Ex vivo expansion and genetic marking of primitive human and baboon hematopoietic cells. *Ann NY Acad Sci* 1999;872:233–240; discussion 240–242.

82. Morral N, O'Neal W, Rice K, Leland M, Kaplan J, Piedra PA, et al. Administration of helper-dependent adenoviral vectors and sequential delivery of different vector serotype for long-term liver-directed gene transfer in baboons. *Proc Natl Acad Sci USA* 1999;96(22):12,816–12,821.

83. Rossi JJ. Primate in utero gene transfer comes of age. *Mol Ther* 2001;3(2):274,275.

84. Schimmenti S, Boesen J, Claassen EA, Valerio D, Einerhand MP. Long-term genetic modification of rhesus monkey hematopoietic cells following transplantation of adenoassociated virus vector-transduced CD34+ cells. *Hum Gene Ther* 1998;9(18):2727–2734.

85. Sellers SE, Tisdale JF, Agricola BA, Metzger ME, Donahue RE, Dunbar CE, et al. The effect of multidrug-resistance 1 gene versus neo transduction on ex vivo and in vivo expansion of rhesus macaque hematopoietic repopulating cells. *Blood* 2001;97(6):1888–1891.

86. Tarantal AF, O'Rourke JP, Case SS, Newbound GC, Li J, Lee CI, et al. Rhesus monkey model for fetal gene transfer: studies with retroviral- based vector systems. *Mol Ther* 2001;3(2):128–138.

87. Winkler A, Kiem HP, Shields LE, Sun QH, Andrews RG. Gene transfer into fetal baboon hematopoietic progenitor cells. *Hum Gene Ther* 1999;10(4):667–677.

88. Wu T, Kim HJ, Sellers SE, Meade KE, Agricola BA, Metzger ME, et al. Prolonged high-level detection of retrovirally marked hematopoietic cells in nonhuman primates after transduction of CD34+ progenitors using clinically feasible methods. *Mol Ther* 2000;1(3):285–293.

89. Xu LC, Karlsson S, Byrne ER, Kluepfel-Stahl S, Kessler SW, Agricola BA, et al. Long-term in vivo expression of the human glucocerebrosidase gene in nonhuman primates after CD34+ hematopoietic cell transduction with cell-free retroviral vector preparations. *Proc Natl Acad Sci USA* 1995;92(10):4372–4376.

90. Abkowitz JL, Persik MT, Shelton GH, Ott RL, Kiklevich JV, Catlin SN, et al. Behavior of hematopoietic stem cells in a large animal. *Proc Natl Acad Sci USA* 1995;92(6):2031–2035.

91. Kim HJ, Tisdale JF, Wu T, Takatoku M, Sellers SE, Zickler P, et al. Many multipotential gene-marked progenitor or stem cell clones contribute to hematopoiesis in nonhuman primates. *Blood* 2000;96(1):1–8.

92. Mahmud N, Devine SM, Weller KP, Parmar S, Sturgeon C, Nelson MC, et al. The relative quiescence of hematopoietic stem cells in nonhuman primates. *Blood* 2001;97(10):3061–3068.

93. Anderson WF. Human gene therapy. *Nature* 1998;392(6679 Suppl):25–30.

94. Heim DA, Dunbar CE. Hematopoietic stem cell gene therapy: towards clinically significant gene transfer efficiency. *Immunol Rev* 2000;178:29–38.

95. Hoffman R. Progress in the development of systems for in vitro expansion of human hematopoietic stem cells. *Curr Opin Hematol* 1999;6(3):184–191.

96. Novelli EM, Cheng L, Yang Y, Leung W, Ramirez M, Tanavde V, et al. Ex vivo culture of cord blood CD34+ cells expands progenitor cell numbers, preserves engraftment capacity in nonobese diabetic/severe combined immunodeficient mice, and enhances retroviral transduction efficiency. *Hum Gene Ther* 1999;10(18):2927–2940.

97. Piacibello W, Sanavio F, Severino A, Dane A, Gammaitoni L, Fagioli F, et al. Engraftment in nonobese diabetic severe combined immunodeficient mice of human CD34(+) cord blood cells after ex vivo expansion: evidence for the amplification and self-renewal of repopulating stem cells. *Blood* 1999;93(11):3736–3749.

98. Ueda T, Tsuji K, Yoshino H, Ebihara Y, Yagasaki H, Hisakawa H, et al. Expansion of human NOD/SCID-repopulating cells by stem cell factor, Flk2/Flt3 ligand, thrombopoietin, IL-6, and soluble IL-6 receptor. *J Clin Invest* 2000;105(7):1013–1021.

99. Lu L, Xiao M, Shen RN, Grigsby S, Broxmeyer HE. Enrichment, characterization, and responsiveness of single primitive CD34 human umbilical cord blood hematopoietic progenitors with high proliferative and replating potential. *Blood* 1993;81(1):41–48.

100. Peters SO, Kittler EL, Ramshaw HS, Quesenberry PJ. Murine marrow cells expanded in culture with IL-3, IL-6, IL-11, and SCF acquire an engraftment defect in normal hosts. *Exp Hematol* 1995;23(5):461–469.

101. van der Loo JC, Ploemacher RE. Marrow- and spleen-seeding efficiencies of all murine hematopoietic stem cell subsets are decreased by preincubation with hematopoietic growth factors. *Blood* 1995;85(9):2598–2606.

102. Brugger W, Heimfeld S, Berenson RJ, Mertelsmann R, Kanz L. Reconstitution of hematopoiesis after high-dose chemotherapy by autologous progenitor cells generated ex vivo. *N Engl J Med* 1995;333(5):283–287.

103. Williams SF, Lee WJ, Bender JG, Zimmerman T, Swinney P, Blake M, et al. Selection and expansion of peripheral blood CD34+ cells in autologous stem cell transplantation for breast cancer. *Blood* 1996;87(5):1687–1691.

104. Tisdale JF, Hanazono Y, Sellers SE, Agricola BA, Metzger ME, Donahue RE, et al. Ex vivo expansion of genetically marked rhesus peripheral blood progenitor cells results in diminished long-term repopulating ability. *Blood* 1998;92(4):1131–1141.
105. Brandt JE, Bartholomew AM, Fortman JD, Nelson MC, Bruno E, Chen LM, et al. Ex vivo expansion of autologous bone marrow CD34(+) cells with porcine microvascular endothelial cells results in a graft capable of rescuing lethally irradiated baboons. *Blood* 1999;94(1):106–113.
106. Anderson WF. Gene therapy. The best of times, the worst of times. *Science* 2000;288(5466):627–629.
107. Li XC, Strom TB, Turka LA, Wells AD. T cell death and transplantation tolerance. *Immunity* 2001;14(4):407–416.
108. Yu X, Carpenter P, Anasetti C. Advances in transplantation tolerance. *Lancet* 2001;357(9272):1959–1963.
109. Knechtle SJ. Knowledge about transplantation tolerance gained in primates. *Curr Opin Immunol* 2000;12(5):552–556.
110. Fuchimoto Y, Huang CA, Yamada K, Shimizu A, Kitamura H, Colvin RB, et al. Mixed chimerism and tolerance without whole body irradiation in a large animal model. *J Clin Invest* 2000;105(12):1779–1789.
111. Wekerle T, Kurtz J, Ito H, Ronquillo JV, Dong V, Zhao G, et al. Allogeneic bone marrow transplantation with co-stimulatory blockade induces macrochimerism and tolerance without cytoreductive host treatment. *Nat Med* 2000;6(4):464–469.
112. Spitzer TR, Delmonico F, Tolkoff-Rubin N, McAfee S, Sackstein R, Saidman S, et al. Combined histocompatibility leukocyte antigen-matched donor bone marrow and renal transplantation for multiple myeloma with end stage renal disease: the induction of allograft tolerance through mixed lymphohematopoietic chimerism. *Transplantation* 1999;68(4):480–484.
113. Bartholomew AM, Powelson J, Sachs DH, Bailin M, Boskovic S, Colvin R, et al. Tolerance in a concordant nonhuman primate model. *Transplantation* 1999;68(11):1708–1716.
114. Kawai T, Abrahamian G, Sogawa H, Wee S, Boskovic S, Andrew D, et al. Costimulatory blockade for induction of mixed chimerism and renal allograft tolerance in nonhuman primates. *Transplant Proc* 2001;33(1-2):221,222.
115. Pittenger MF, Mackay AM, Beck SC, Jaiswal RK, Douglas R, Mosca JD, et al. Multilineage potential of adult human mesenchymal stem cells. *Science* 1999;284(5411):143–147.
116. Devine SM, Hoffman R. Role of mesenchymal stem cells in hematopoietic stem cell transplantation. *Curr Opin Hematol* 2000;7(6):358–363.
117. Koc ON, Lazarus HM. Mesenchymal stem cells: heading into the clinic. *Bone Marrow Transplant* 2001;27(3):235–239.
118. Devine SM, Bartholomew AM, Mahmud N, Nelson M, Patil S, Hardy W, et al. Mesenchymal stem cells are capable of homing to the bone marrow of non-human primates following systemic infusion. *Exp Hematol* 2001;29(2):244–255.

24 In Vivo Models for the Study of Graft-vs-Host Disease and Graft-vs-Tumor Effects

Kai Sun, MD, PhD, William J. Murphy, PhD, and Lisbeth A. Welniak, PhD

CONTENTS

1. OVERVIEW: NONPRIMATE ANIMAL MODELS

While nonprimate studies of graft-vs-host disease (GVHD) most commonly use rodent models, the field of allogeneic transplantation and treatment of GVHD also owes much to its study in dogs. Donnall Thomas, in collaboration with other investigators at Fred Hutchinson Cancer Center, pioneered the field of allogeneic bone marrow transplantation with his work in beagles. The use of outbred animals requires detailed knowledge of the major histocompatibility complex (MHC) complex for these species and the availability of reagents for tissue typing. More recently, the miniature swine model has been added to the repertoire of models available to investigators. While this model has not gained prominence with investigators of GVHD, it is used to study mechanisms of tolerance in allogeneic and xenogeneic hematopoietic cell and/or organ transplantation. The swine model has advantages for translational work because its body size and composition is comparable to humans. Likewise, the sheep model has been used to study issues of tolerance in xenogeneic hematopoietic cell transplantation.

More commonly, rodent models have been used to study GVHD. These models have the advantage of inbred strains, availability of resources, and the ability of researchers to perform studies with sufficient numbers of animals to give adequate power to survival studies. The mouse model is more common than rats, and the rest of this review will focus on murine models.

This chapter will consider several aspects of mouse models of GHVD. These aspects cover important considerations for the researcher choosing a model, as well as for readers of studies,

From: *Current Clinical Oncology: Allogeneic Stem Cell Transplantation*
Edited by: Mary S. Laughlin and Hillard M. Lazarus © Humana Press Inc., Totowa, NJ

so that they may be more informed about the strengths and limitations of interpreting mouse experimentation in GVHD.

2. MOUSE MODELS: ELEMENTS TO CONSIDER IN A MODEL FOR ALLOGENEIC TRANSPLANT-GVHD

2.1. Basic Considerations in Establishing a Mouse Model of GVHD

It was observed by Billingham *(1)* that the following elements are required for development of GVHD. The graft must contain immunocompetent cells. These cells have since been recognized to be mature T cells *(2)*. The donor T cells must recognize antigenic differences on the host tissues. And finally, the host must be incapable of rejecting the donor cells *(1)*.

The need for mature donor T cells in the development of GVHD has been well-documented and, in general, the severity of disease correlates with the number of donor T cells transfused *(2)*. MHC major and/or minor mismatches, where the host tissue expresses an antigen not present in the donor, are the primary sources of antigenic stimulus for GVHD. However, GVH reactions can be elicited in syngeneic and autologous transplants *(3)*, so that dysregulation and inappropriate recognition of self antigens in the reconstituted immune system may also promote GVHD. The third requirement, the inability of host cells to reject the donor graft, is usually achieved by conditioning the recipient with immunosuppressive chemotherapy and/or radiotherapy. However, in some situations, immunosuppressive conditioning is not required, as when the recipient is immunodeficient or the donor cells do not express MHC antigens differently from the host as occurs in a parent into F1 transplant.

2.2. Mouse Strains

The most common laboratory strains of inbred mice—C57BL/6, BALB/c, and C3H—are also commonly used for GVHD studies, but a broad range of donor–host combinations are available. Selection of mouse strains is dependent upon the degree of MHC major and minor antigen mismatch desired, the availability of reagents, histocompatible tumor lines, specialized mice such as transgenics, or animals with spontaneous or targeted mutations. The phenotype of the different strains may also play a role in model selection.

Cross-breeding of mouse strains has generated a wide selection of possible donor–host mouse combinations based on major and minor MHC mismatches. The use of full MHC disparate mismatched donor-recipient pairs is frequently employed in the laboratory even though the clinical situation usually involves only minor histocompatibility antigen differences. As with the clinical situation where GVHD is usually a consequence of allogeneic hematopoietic cell transplantation, the full MHC disparate murine models of GVHD use high dose radiation with or without concomitant chemotherapy, followed by allogeneic bone marrow transplant to induce immunosuppression of the host and introduce a source of alloreactive T cells along with hematopoietic rescue. Typically, the T cell dose in mouse bone marrow cell preparations is insufficient to induce acute lethal GVHD, and the mouse transplant requires the addition of donor-derived T cells, either purified or as a component of unfractionated splenocytes and/or lymph node cells. Also, mice, as opposed to man, are now specific-pathogen-free which necessitates use of larger numbers of T cells or more extensive conditioning.

BALB/c ($H-2^d$) and C57BL/6 ($H-2^b$) animal strains comprise a common donor–recipient combination that is an example of fully mismatched MHC with multiple minor mismatched histocompatibility antigens. This combination has multiple advantages including availability of the parental strains, as they are two of the most commonly used inbred strains of laboratory mice. Because of the high use of these strains, many of the gene knock-out animals are available on BALB/c or C57BL/6 backgrounds, with sufficient backcrossing to be considered as congenic to the appropriate strain. Well-documented tumor cells lines are available for evaluation of concurrent graft-vs-tumor (GVT) effects. Finally, there is a large body of knowledge regarding strain-specific immunologic function such as dominant Th1 vs Th2 functions and allogeneic-reactive responses.

In some instances, an investigator wishes to examine fully disparate major MHC incompatible responses in the absence of minor histocompatibility differences. Strain combinations such as donor C57BL/6 (H-2^b, T18b) cells into B10.BR (H-2^k, T18a) recipients fulfill this requirement *(4)*. These strains are congenic, differing only at the major histocompatibility locus and the T18 minor histocompatibility thymic antigen, where T18b determines the absence of the antigen (TL$^-$). Many H2 congenic strains are available for study, allowing the investigator to find strain combinations that meet the needs of the study.

There are a few well-studied donor–recipient congenic strain pairs that involve a single antigen mismatch. Several H2 mutants are available on a C57BL/6 background. The most commonly studied of these mutants in the field of GVHD is the class I mutant *bm1*, and the class II mutant *bm12*. These mutants have been used in two different model systems. The first is acute lethal GVHD following lethal radiation and bone marrow transplant (BMT), the second model uses sublethal irradiation and T cell transfer, which results in allogeneic destruction of recipient bone marrow. Both model systems will be reviewed.

The use of single class I or class II mutants are useful in establishing the role of CD4+ and CD8+ subsets in GVHD. Transfer of B6.C-H2^{bm12}/KhEg (*bm12*) bone marrow along with an additional source of T cells following a lethal dose of whole body irradiation can result in acute lethal GVHD, demonstrating in this situation, where only a class II mismatch exists between the graft and host, that CD8+ cells are not required for the disease *(5,6)*. Likewise, although not as effective in the absence of CD4+ cell help, CD8+ cells can induce fatal GVHD following transfer of B6.C-H2^{bm1}/KhEg (*bm1*) bone marrow and T cells after lethal whole body irradiation *(6–8)*. While acute lethal GVHD can occur in mouse models involving a single MHC class I or class II mismatch after lethal total body irradiation (TBI) and BMT, a second model has proven to be independent of subset help, and the extent of disease is proportional to the input of allogeneic-reactive T cells. These models also utilize the *bm1* and *bm12* mutants paired with C57BL/6 mice, but in this model the recipients are conditioned with a sublethal dose of TBI and purified donor T cells. Selection of purified donor CD8+ (for *bm1*/B6 pairs) or CD4+ (for *bm12*/B6 pairs) lymph node T-cells is not required, but does allow enumeration of specific T cell doses *(9,10)*. In the absence of donor-derived hematopoietic stem cells, the donor T cells infusion results in bone marrow failure in the recipient animal. The cell destruction is specific, as donor-derived bone marrow cells will engraft and prevent hematopoietic failure *(9)*.

Cross-breeding of common mouse strains has generated a variety of congenic animals that are matched at the major histocompatibility locus, but are mismatched at a number of minor histocompatibility loci. In four of six tested murine strain combinations, infusion of purified donor-derived CD8+ T cells was sufficient to generate acute lethal GVHD, while infusion of donor CD4+ cells were poor inducers of acute lethal GVHD. However, this finding is not universal, since in the other two strain combinations, purified CD4+ cells were not only sufficient to generate acute lethal GVHD, but were more potent than purified CD8+ cells *(11)*. The opposing outcomes derived from protocols that were similar except for the strain combinations employed point to the multifactorial nature of this disease and the importance of not overinterpreting findings based on a single animal model.

The previous murine models of acute lethal GVHD have focused on strain combinations in which the recipient requires conditioning to induce extensive immunosuppression and render the host unable to effectively reject the donor graft. Another common murine model uses haploidentical transplants (C57BL/6 into B6D2F1 [C57BL/6 × DBA/2]) to avoid the need to overcome host rejection of the graft via T cell-dependent mechanisms. It is necessary to note that in this model, the host natural killer (NK) cells are still capable of graft rejection. This model involves the transfer of parental cells (P) into a F1 hybrid strain recipient. Lethal radiation is not required to suppress host T cell immunity, since the recipient T cells do not recognize the parental cells as foreign although the investigator may chose to set up the model as a BMT. The only barrier to donor T cell engraftment in this model is hybrid resistance by host NK cells (12). However, transfer of sufficient numbers of donor cells (50 million and higher) will overcome recipient NK cell rejection of the graft (13). A unique feature of this model is the ability to select for acute or chronic GVHD based on the source of donor cells. It has been well-documented that infusion of C57BL/6 donor splenocytes into B6D2F1 results in acute lethal GVHD, while infusion of donor DBA/2 splenocytes results in chronic GVHD, although other parental and F1 hybrid strains can be used (14,15). Additional discussion of this model will occur in the section discussing murine models of chronic GVHD.

The wide range of inbred laboratory mouse strains, and the depth of knowledge regarding the differences in disease susceptibility across these strains, permits selection of mouse strain combinations that may enhance the probability of observing a putative activity. The caveat is that results obtained with a single mouse strain combination may fail to realize the specificity of the observation to the genetic background of the test animal. Strikingly different results may occur in different strain combinations, even if the degree of histocompatibility mismatch does not differ. Take for example the various strain combinations of BALB/c, C57BL/6, and C3H. These animals are fully mismatched at the major ($H2^d$, $H2^b$, and $H2^k$, respectively) and minor histocompatibility loci. BALB/c are more radiosensitive than C57BL/6 and C3H mice; they are also poor rejectors of MHC-mismatched grafts (16). This finding may or may not be related to the bias in BALB/c mice toward a Th2 phenotype. In contrast, the C57BL/6 and C3H mice respond to immunological challenge with a strong Th1 response and are also more radioresistant. Investigations into the role of cytokines that influence Th subset development may have different results depending on the choice of donor and host strains. An occurrence of different outcomes would be difficult to interpret as the result of skewing of the T helper subset phenotype, due to the other parameters that may influence outcome in these animals, such as difference in the strain response to the conditioning regimen.

Another challenge to the interpretation of animal models of GVHD is the use of mice with targeted deficiencies, or less commonly, overexpression of a particular gene product. The loss or overexpression of a protein during the development of the animal can often result in obvious and/or subtle differences. In more obvious examples, examination of the role of lymphotoxin-α (LT-α) in the recipient mouse through the use of an LT-α deficient animal is complicated by the lack of normal lymphoid architecture in the host animal (17). It is, therefore, impossible to distinguish between the role of LT-α and normal lymphoid tissue in GVHD. The more subtle example is demonstrated by considering the use of donor cells from LT-α deficient animals. Does the development of T cells, NK cells and possibly hematopoietic cells in the absence of LT-α result in an increased or decreased susceptibility to morbidity and mortality after allogeneic BMT, independent of the inability of the grafted cells to produce LT-α during the test period (18)? The use of knock-out and transgenic animals are a powerful tool for the researcher, but appropriate controls must be run to rule out these possibilities. Neutralizing antibodies that target protein can confirm the observations made in the experiments involving knock-out animals (19). The power of the knock-out animal is the completeness of the blockade and the selectivity of the blockade to inhibit production in only the donor graft or the recipient animal.

2.3. Conditioning

Conditioning is another pivotal element closely associated with the type and the severity of murine GVHD models, in addition to the other elements of strain combinations, histoincompatibility, donor T lymphocytes subset, and cell dose infused. In murine GVHD/graft-vs-leukemia (GVL) models, in order to facilitate engraftment of donor cells as well as reduce tumor burden, the host mice often receive cytoreductive conditioning consisting of TBI and/or chemotherapeutic agents before donor T lymphocyte infusion with or without bone marrow cell transplantation. The need for BMT is dependent on the severity of cytoreduction. TBI is the most common form of conditioning performed on recipient mice. As discussed above, the mice from different strains may have distinct radiosensitivity, so the TBI dose necessary to achieve myeloablation may be different between strains; for example, the lethal dose for C57BL/6 mice is 900–1000 cGy, but 800–900cGy for BALB/c mice, and 350–400cGy for C.B17 severe combined immunodeficiency (SCID) mice. However, the cleaniness of the animal facility plays an important role in the amount of TBI needed to produce 100% lethality without hematopoietic stem cell rescue. In the murine models of allogeneic BMT/GVHD, there are two categories of conditioning regimens that are frequently used, conventional myeloablative and reduced toxicity (20,21), and the former can be further divided into high and low dose myeloablative regimens (22). The incidence and severity of acute GVHD are closely associated with the intensity and toxicity of conditioning regimens. This was extensively studied by Hill and Ferrara, who showed that increased acute GVHD mortality and morbidity was associated with increases in the dose of TBI from 900 to 1300 cGy in several murine donor–recipient strain combination models (22). The study supports the hypothesis that high dose myeloablative conditioning of host mice contributes to the development of acute GVHD because it results in more severe tissue damage and a breakdown of normal barriers which leads to amplification of cytokine release (22,23). In recent years, reduced toxicity regimens with partial conditioning have been used in the study of murine GVHD/GVL. This approach can set up durable donor chimerism and seems to have a lower rate of GVHD in murine GVHD models (24); this is partly because in mixed chimerism, the residual host T cells can resist GVHD by a veto-like effect (25). However, GVL activity may be compromised in mixed chimeras (26).

Partial conditioning of host mice also affects the type of GVHD. Claman et al. (27) developed a GVHD model by injecting the B10.D2 bone marrow cells and lymphocytes into irradiated BALB/c mice. Preparation of the mice with lethal irradiation resulted in acute GVHD, but mice that received sublethal irradiation developed chronic GVHD skin damage (27). Similarly, the kind of conditioning regimen can also affect the type of GVHD. The study by Xun and Widmer found that conditioning with TBI, followed by allogeneic incompatible splenocyte infusion, induced acute GVHD in C.B-17 SCID mice, whereas animals conditioned with the chemotherapeutic agents cyclophosphamide or a combination of busulfan and cyclophosphamide developed chronic GVHD (28). Moreover, the timing of conditioning also affected the induction and development of acute GVHD. The severity of acute GVHD in either immunocompetent recipient mice or the recipient mice with SCID decreased when cell infusion was delayed after TBI (28,29). Likewise, delaying injection of allogeneic (parental) lymphoid cells to F1 hybrid host mice after the host mice were conditioned with cyclophosphamide also reduced the severity of acute GVHD (30).

2.4. Microflora

The data showing that the incidence and severity of acute GVHD in germ-free mice or conventional mice treated with gastrointestinal decontamination are decreased compared to conventional mice indicate that the microflora of host mice, including housing and normal and pathogenic flora, have an influence on the development of GVHD (31). The bacterial flora in the gut is an especially important factor for the induction of intestinal lesions of acute GVHD in mice, since bacterial flora may up-regulate minor histocompatiblity antigens (mHAg) in host mice, leading to cross-reactivity with the recipient's epithelial tissue antigens and promotion of host-reactive donor type T cells activation, with subsequent increases in bacterial lipopolysaccharide (LPS) translocation and finally, enhanced acute GVHD *(22,32)*. Some studies have shown a critical role for LPS in the induction of cytokine dysregulation, which contributes to GVHD *(33,34)*. Use of LPS antagonists can prevent GVHD while preserving T cell responses to host antigens and GVL activity in an experimental mouse model *(34)*.

3. ACUTE GVHD MODELS

Studying acute GVHD in mice allows the investigator to obtain detailed knowledge of acute GVHD pathophysiology, which cannot be studied in humans. The shortcoming is that the present GVHD murine models do not always exactly parallel or reflect clinical human GVHD conditions. There are three major murine acute GVHD models. The most common acute GVHD model analogous to the clinical acute GVHD in humans involves lethal or sublethal conditioning of recipient mice with TBI and/or myeloablative drugs, such as busulfan and cyclophosphamide, followed by transfer of allogeneic bone marrow cells (BMC) and calculated T cells from donor mice whose MHC (H-2 system) loci and/or multiple minor antigens are different from the host mice. The second model consists of induction of acute GVHD in immune competent adult mice that is not preceded by a conditioning regimen, where the donor T cells are from a parental strain (P_1) and the recipient is a haploidentical hybrid $[(P_1 \times P_2)F_1]$. Conditioning is not required because recipient mice lack donor-reactive T cells. Host NK cells' rejection of donor cells can be overcome by sufficient cell doses. Therefore, adoptive transfer of T cells from one of two homozygous parental (P) donors into $(P_1 \times P_2)$ F_1 host mice can engraft and result in the alloreaction of donor T cells to the antigens derived from the other parental strain *(35)*. The addition of conditioning can permit engraftment of donor bone marrow cells if a haploidentical hematopoietic transplant model is desired. A third model utilizes SCID mice, which lack both functional T and B lymphoid cells and, therefore, cannot reject foreign donor cells, except by NK mediated rejection *(36)*. Lower numbers of allogeneic H-2 incompatible donor splenocyte with or without bone marrow cells, even xenografts of human T lymphocytes *(37)*, can readily engraft these mice, and acute GVHD can be induced in these mice *(38)* with or without preparative conditioning.

3.1. Timing

As noted above, the timing of preparative regimens and adoptive cell transfer can influence the induction of acute GVHD. Administration of cytoreductive chemotherapeutic agents or TBI immediately preceding infusion of allogeneic donor T cell results in high mortality, but delaying infusion of donor T cells for 1–3 wk after a BMT with the same conditioning regimen markedly decreased the mortality associated with acute GVHD *(39,40)*. Delaying the BMT by as little as 4 d after TBI may result in the prevention of acute GVHD *(29)*. Thus, the severity of acute GVHD is closely associated with not only the mouse strain combination chosen, the degree of histocompatibility between donor and host, the donor T lymphocytes subset and number to be transplanted, and the dose of conditioning applied, but also the timing of the conditioning regimen.

3.2. T Cell Sources

Unlike clinical allogeneic BMT, infusion of donor BMC alone does not usually result in lethal acute GVHD in murine allogeneic BMT. In order to devise a vigorous lethal acute GVHD model, it is often necessary to infuse allogeneic donor T cells along with BMC. Purified T cells from the lymph node or unfractionated spleen cells can serve as a T cell source, and the incidence and severity of GVHD are closely associated with the numbers of donor mature T cells infused *(2)*.

It is worth noting that the severity and type of GVHD is strain-dependent. For example, transfer of spleen cells from C57BL/6 ($H2^b$) mice into the BALB/c ($H2^d$) host mice after lethal TBI will result in strong lethal GVHD, while transfer of spleen cells from BALB/c mice to the B6 host mice after lethal TBI results in only a comparatively weak GVH response *(41)*. Likewise, transfer of spleen cells from C57BL/6 ($H2^b$) mice to the C57BL/6 × DBA/2F$_1$ (B6D2F$_1$; $H2^{b/d}$) host mice results in acute GVHD, while transfer of the spleen cells from DBA/2 ($H2^d$) mice to the B6D2F1 host mice can result in chronic GVHD *(42)*. Animal models for chronic GVHD have not been extensively studied, and have usually been used for examination of autoimmune responses *(43)* since host autoreactive B cell expansion plays a critical role in these P → F$_1$ models.

3.3. T1 and T2 Subsets and GVHD

Acute GVHD has been postulated to be a disease associated with a Th$_1$/Tc$_1$ response. Several lines of evidence support this hypothesis. Interleukin (IL)-12 is an important cytokine in the differentiation and function of Th$_1$ cells. Administration of antibodies to IL-12 in some models of murine acute GVHD polarized the allogeneic response toward Th2 cytokine production and decreased the incidence and severity of disease *(44,45)*. Infusion of T cells polarized by ex vivo culture to secrete Th$_2$ associated cytokines diminished but did not eliminate acute GVHD *(46)*. Mobilization of peripheral blood cells is associated with polarization of T cells to a Th2 phenotype, and this shift in cytokine response is postulated to be the cause of decreased incidence and severity of acute GVHD in mice *(47,48)*. However, the paradigm of Th$_1$ and Th$_2$ may not hold. Cytokines associated with a Th1 response may play a role in both immunostimulation and immunosuppression. Loss of interferon (IFN)-γ, a classic Th1 cytokine, is associated with accelerated acute GVHD *(19)* in mouse BMT models of the disease.

3.4. Assessment of Acute Murine GVHD

During acute GVHD, an early period of lymphoid hyperplasia is followed by immunosuppression, weight loss, and mortality *(14,42,49)*. The various criteria for the assessment of acute GVHD in mice are described here.

3.4.1. SURVIVAL

Mortality is a primary parameter used to assess murine acute GVHD. Depending on the model, the first death due to GVHD can be seen on or after the first week following allogeneic-BMT *(2)*. The percent of mice surviving and the average onset of death is representative of the severity of lethal acute GVHD.

3.4.2. CLINICAL PARAMETERS OF MURINE ACUTE GVHD

The degree and severity of systemic acute GVHD can be assessed by clinical parameters that have been considered reliable indicators of acute GVHD in murine models *(22)*. These clinical parameters consist of weight loss, posture, activity, fur texture and skin integrity, diarrhea, facial edema (squinty eyes) and weight loss, which is the most critical parameter associated with acute GVHD. A scoring system was set up by Hill and colleagues that depends on these clinical parameters and can be used in the evaluation of acute GVHD. Mice can be evaluated and graded with a semiquantitative score for each criterion, so a clinical index that reflects the degree and severity of systemic acute GVHD can be generated by the summation of the individual criteria scores *(33,50,51)*.

3.4.3. HISTOPATHOLOGY

While the degree and severity of systemic acute GVHD in mice can be diagnosed based on overall survival and a clinical scoring system, histopathologic criteria can support the evaluation of systemic acute GVHD *(10,22)*. Histopathologic evaluation can demonstrate organ-specific differences in acute GVHD that may occur during the examination of the importance of various factors that influence the disease *(52)*. In addition to the determination of qualitative difference in histology, some investigators have used semiquantitative systems to compare the degree of specific organ damage in target tissues (i.e., gut and lung) *(10,33)*.

3.4.4. CYTOKINE DETERMINATION

Study of acute GVHD in recent years has focused on the pivotal role of inflammatory cytokines in acute GVHD pathophysiology *(53)*. There are considerable data available to demonstrate that serum level of tumor necrosis factor (TNF)-α and IL-1β are closely associated with the development and severity of acute GVHD in mice *(54)*. The production of IFN-γ from spleen cells increases in mice with acute GVHD *(45)*, so the measurement of some cytokines may also help to assess the severity of acute GVHD in mice *(55)*.

4. CHRONIC GVHD MODELS

Chronic GVHD is a syndrome of disordered immune regulation with features of autoimmunity and immunodeficiency *(56–58)*. Murine chronic GVHD models are characterized by formation of autoantibodies *(59,60)* and an increase in collagen deposition *(58)*. Murine chronic GVHD shows clinical phenomena that are similar to those seen in patients with autoimmune diseases, such as scleroderma *(57)* and Sjogren's disease, as well as the syndrome that closely resembles systemic lupus erythematosus (SLE) *(61)*. In mice, chronic GVHD can develop as a long-term gradually evolving disease following the resolution of acute GVHD or through the induction of the disease in selected P → F_1 cGVHD models *(61–64)*. Induction and maintenance of chronic GVHD in mice is dependent on the persistence of host–reactive donor T cells, which cannot be deleted or tolerized to host antigens in vivo *(65)*. In contrast to acute GVHD, chronic GVHD is considered a classic Th2-type response *(66,67)*, and administration of a Th_1 cytokine can convert chronic GVHD to acute disease *(68)*, although neutralization of the same cytokine diminished acute GVHD without development of chronic GVHD *(45)*. Although Th2 cytokines are produced from donor-derived CD4+ T cells in chronic GVHD, IFN-γ is also produced *(69)*.

4.1. Analysis of Chronic GVHD in Mice

4.1.1. HISTOPATHOLOGY, CYTOKINE DETERMINATION, AND MEASUREMENT OF AUTOANTIBADY

Due to the slow development nature of the disease, analysis of murine chronic GVHD is often performed more than 60 d after transplantation. Analysis may include identification and measurement of autoantibodies and immune complexes, use of histological and immunopathological techniques, measurement of serum cytokines associated with inflammation, and scoring evidence of clinical disease.

4.1.2. DETECTION OF AUTOANTIBODIES

The expression of several autoantibodies can be assessed by enzyme-linked immunosorbent assay (ELISA). Autoantibodies associated with chronic GVHD include antibodies to nuclear antigens *(62,70)* and renal antigens *(71,72)*. A direct Crithidia assay can be used to detect serum anti-double-stranded (ds) DNA Ab *(73)*.

4.1.3. HISTOLOGICAL CHANGES CHARACTERISTIC OF CHRONIC GVHD

Murine chronic GVHD can be manifested by extensive scleroderma-like skin lesions, and serial skin biopsies need to be taken to assess disease *(27)*. In addition to histologic examination, skin collagen content can be assessed by histochemical methods.

In the murine chronic GVHD with SLE-like disease, the presence of glomerular lesions can be assessed by morphologic examination of kidney tissue sections taken 3 or 5 mo after induction of disease for overall severity, and immunofluorescence microscopy can be used to detect specific components of immune complexes in the glomerular lesions.

The degree of inflammation in the liver and small bowel can be graded semiquantitatively for evidence of pathological changes consistent with chronic GVHD. In the liver, scoring criteria may include portal infiltration by inflammatory cells and abnormal bile duct epithelial morphology *(74)*.

4.1.4. MEASUREMENT OF SERUM CYTOKINES

The proinflammatory and anti-inflammatory cytokines, TNF-α, IFN-γ, and IL-10 serum level can be measured by highly sensitive radio-immunoassay or ELISA to help assess murine chronic GVHD *(66)*.

4.2. Correlation of Murine Chronic GVHD with Human Disease

Although the currently available chronic GVHD murine models are unable to exactly parallel or reflect clinical chronic GVHD conditions, they are believed to be unique experimental models correlated with several human disease.

SLE is an autoimmune disease that is characterized by the formation of autoantibodies. Although almost any organ of the body can be involved, lupus nephritis is a major symptom and the main cause of death. Chronic GVHD induced in C57BL/10 × DBA/2 F_1 mice following adoptive transfer of parental DBA/2 spleen cells has been proposed as an adequate experimental model for studying severe immune complex glomerulonephritis associated with SLE because all of the histologic patterns occurring in human lupus nephritis can also be seen in these mice. Interaction between donor T cells and recipient B cells results in polyclonal B cell activation followed by production of a range of autoantibodies, including anti-ds and -ssDNA, anti-red blood cell, and anti-T cell anticytoskeletal autoantibodies are associated with this model *(62)*. Severe glomerulonephritis results from the deposition of immune complexes in the glomeruli of these mice. In addition to human SLE, models of chronic GVHD in mice can be used to study human scleroderma, which is a chronic and progressive disease characterized mainly by increasing collagen deposition in many organs. Adoptive transfer of splenocytes from B10.D2 mice into sublethally-irradiated minor histocompatibility antigen-mismatched, BALB/c mice results in a disease that resembles many features of the scleroderma in humans, including cutaneous fibrosis, loss of dermal fat, atrophy of dermal appendages, mast cell depletion, and a mononuclear cell infiltration *(57)*. In this model, liver and gastrointestinal tract injuries include inflammatory destruction of the intrahepatic bile ducts and the bowel mucosa.

5. GVL MODELS

Murine models play an indispensable role in the study of GVHD/GVL. The finding of GVL/GVT phenomenon and the concept of GVL/GVT were attributed not only to observations in clinical allogeneic-BMT but also to the study of experimental allogeneic-BMT in mice *(75–77)*. Tumor-bearing mouse models have been widely used in the research field of GVL/GVT. Induction of leukemia can be accomplished by the intravenous injection of an appropriate dose of cells from a leukemia cell line or fresh tumor cells into the lateral tail vein of immunocompetent syngeneic mice. The mice are then monitored for development of physical symptoms of disease, and survival time is determined *(78)*. The reproducible death from leukemia in tumor-bearing mice usually varies in a dose-dependent fashion *(79–81)*. The modulation of GVHD can change the outcome of survival. The goal of many animal studies of GVHD is to minimize the disease without concurrent loss of the GVL effect. In clinical allogeneic-BMT, the GVL effect is most evident in patients with chronic myelogenous leukemia (CML) compared to patients with other forms of leukemia or lymphoma *(82)*, however, the field of study lacks a good murine CML model. There are some commonly studied tumor cells lines used for development and analysis of GVL in mice.

- The C1498 (H-2^b) leukemia cell line was originally derived as a spontaneous myeloid tumor line from a C57BL/6 female mouse *(80,81,83,84)*.
- The EL4 (H-2^b) lymphoma cell line was originally derived as a T cell leukemia/lymphoma tumor line from a C57BL/6 mouse *(83–87)*.
- The P815 (H-2^d, CD45.2+) is a mastocytoma derived from a DBA/2 mouse *(88)*. P815 tumor cells injected intravenously metastasize into the spleen and liver of host mice *(89,90)*.
- A-20 (H-2^d) is derived from a spontaneous B cell leukemia/lymphoma from a BALB/c mouse *(91)*.

The mouse can also serve as a vessel to study human GVL or graft versus tumor (GVT) effects. SCID or non-obese diabetic (NOD)/SCID mice can be injected with human tumor cells followed by adoptive transfer of human immune cells to evaluate the GVL effect in this human–mouse chimera model *(92–94)*.

Recently, the use of mice with specific defects in cytotoxic function has demonstrated the differential role of these specialized cellular mechanisms in GVHD and GVL *(95–97)*. Both CD4+ cells and CD8+ cells can mediate GVHD-associated cytotoxic activity through perforin or Fas pathways *(98)*. In a similar manner, the use of neutralizing antibodies demonstrates the differential outcomes when pro-inflammatory cytokines are depleted in the GHVD/GVL mouse models *(32)*.

6. CONCLUDING REMARKS

Murine models provide a unique experimental approach for the study into the pathophysiology of GVHD and GVL. A broad range of donor–host strain combinations are available to compare MHC disparities on a variety of distinctive genetic backgrounds. Murine models have multiple advantages in that they offer consistent inbred populations for comparison of different treatment groups and provide specific deficiency mutations and transgenic and knock-out strains for further study of GVHD. Hence, new insights from murine models of GVHD/GVL may provide great contributions toward the advancement of clinical therapeutic strategies for the prevention of GVHD and the enhancement of GVL.

ACKNOWLEDGMENTS

The content of this publication does not necessarily reflect the views or policies of the Department of Health and Health Services, nor does mention of trade names, commercial products, or organizations imply endorsement by the U.S. Government. This project has been funded in whole or in part with Federal funds from the National Cancer Institute, National Institutes of Health, under Contract No. NO1-CO-56000.

REFERENCES

1. Billingham RE, Brent L. A simple method for inducing tolerance of skin homografts in mice. *Transplant Bull.*1957;4:67–71.
2. Korngold B, Sprent J. Lethal graft-versus-host disease after bone marrow transplantation across minor histocompatibility barriers in mice. Prevention by removing mature T cells from marrow. *J Exp Med* 1978;148:1687–1698.
3. Hess AD, Horwitz L, Beschorner WE, Santos GW. Development of graft-vs.-host disease-like syndrome in cyclosporine-treated rats after syngeneic bone marrow transplantation. I. Development of cytotoxic T lymphocytes with apparent polyclonal anti-Ia specificity, including autoreactivity. *J Exp Med* 1985;161:718–730.

4. Vallera DA, Carroll SF, Snover DC, Carlson GJ, Blazar BR. Toxicity and efficacy of anti-T-cell ricin toxin A chain immunotoxins in a murine model of established graft-versus-host disease induced across the major histocompatibility barrier. *Blood* 1991;77:182–194.

5. Sprent J, Schaefer M, Korngold R. Role of T cell subsets in lethal graft-versus-host disease (GVHD) directed to class I versus class II H-2 differences. II. Protective effects of L3T4+ cells in anti-class II GVHD. *J Immunol* 1990;144:2946–2954.

6. Mowat AM, Sprent J. Induction of intestinal graft-versus-host reactions across mutant major histocompatibility antigens by T lymphocyte subsets in mice. *Transplantation* 1989;47:857–863.

7. Sprent J, Schaefer M, Gao EK, Korngold R. Role of T cell subsets in lethal graft-versus-host disease (GVHD) directed to class I versus class II H-2 differences. I. L3T4+ cells can either augment or retard GVHD elicited by Lyt-2+ cells in class I different hosts. *J Exp Med* 1988;167:556–569.

8. Williams FH, Thiele DL. The role of major histocompatibility complex and non-major histocompatibility complex encoded antigens in generation of bile duct lesions during hepatic graft-vs.-host responses mediated by helper or cytotoxic T cells. *Hepatology* 1994;19:980–988.

9. Sprent J, Surh CD, Agus D, Hurd M, Sutton S, Heath WR. Profound atrophy of the bone marrow reflecting major histocompatibility complex class II-restricted destruction of stem cells by CD4+ cells. *J Exp Med* 1994;180:307–317.

10. Blazar BR, Taylor PA, Sehgal SN, Vallera DA. Rapamycin, a potent inhibitor of T-cell function, prevents graft rejection in murine recipients of allogeneic T-cell-depleted donor marrow. *Blood* 1994;83:600–609.

11. Korngold R, Sprent J. Variable capacity of L3T4+ T cells to cause lethal graft-versus-host disease across minor histocompatibility barriers in mice. *J Exp Med* 1987;165:1552–1564.

12. Cudkowicz G, Bennett M. Peculiar immunobiology of bone marrow allografts. II. Rejection of parental grafts by resistant F 1 hybrid mice. *J Exp Med* 1971;134:1513–1528.

13. Knobloch C, Dennert G. Loss of F1 hybrid resistance to bone marrow grafts after injection of parental lymphocytes. Demonstration of parental anti-F1 T killer cells and general immunosuppression in the host. *Transplantation* 1988;45:175–183.

14. Pals ST, Radaszkiewicz T, Gleichmann E. Allosuppressor- and allohelper-T cells in acute and chronic graft-vs- host disease. IV. Activation of donor allosuppressor cells is confined to acute GVHD. *J Immunol* 1984;132:1669–1678.

15. Tschetter JR, Mozes E, Shearer GM. Progression from acute to chronic disease in a murine parent-into-F(1) model of graft-versus-host disease. *J Immunol* 2000;165:5987–5994.

16. Bennett M, Yu YY, Stoneman E, et al. Hybrid resistance: 'negative' and 'positive' signaling of murine natural killer cells. *Semin Immunol* 1995;7:121–127.

17. De Togni P, Goellner J, Ruddle NH, et al. Abnormal development of peripheral lymphoid organs in mice deficient in lymphotoxin. *Science* 1994;264:703–707.

18. Iizuka K, Chaplin DD, Wang Y, et al. Requirement for membrane lymphotoxin in natural killer cell development. *Proc Natl Acad Sci USA* 1999;96:6336–6340.

19. Murphy WJ, Welniak LA, Taub DD, et al. Differential effects of the absence of interferon-gamma and IL-4 in acute graft-versus-host disease after allogeneic bone marrow transplantation in mice. *J Clin Invest* 1998;102:1742–1748.

20. Quesenberry PJ, Stewart FM, Becker P, et al. Stem cell engraftment strategies. *Ann NY Acad Sci* 2001;938:54–61.

21. Ballen KK, Becker PS, Stewart FM, Quesenberry PJ. Manipulation of the stem cell as a target for hematologic malignancies. *Semin Oncol* 2000;27:512–523.

22. Hill GR, Crawford JM, Cooke KR, Brinson YS, Pan L, Ferrara JL. Total body irradiation and acute graft-versus-host disease: the role of gastrointestinal damage and inflammatory cytokines. *Blood* 1997;90:3204–3213.

23. Murphy WJ, Blazar BR. New strategies for preventing graft-versus-host disease. *Curr Opin Immunol* 1999;11:509–515.

24. Sykes M, Szot GL, Swenson KA, Pearson DA. Induction of high levels of allogeneic hematopoietic reconstitution and donor-specific tolerance without myelosuppressive conditioning. *Nat Med* 1997;3:783–787.

25. Weiss L, Slavin S. Prevention and treatment of graft-versus-host disease by down- regulation of anti-host reactivity with veto cells of host origin. *Bone Marrow Transplant* 1999;23:1139–1143.

26. Truitt RL, Atasoylu AA. Impact of pretransplant conditioning and donor T cells on chimerism, graft-versus-host disease, graft-versus-leukemia reactivity, and tolerance after bone marrow transplantation. *Blood* 1991;77:2515–2523.

27. Claman HN, Jaffee BD, Huff JC, Clark RA. Chronic graft-versus-host disease as a model for scleroderma. II. Mast cell depletion with deposition of immunoglobulins in the skin and fibrosis. *Cell Immunol* 1985;94:73–84.

28. Xun CQ, Thompson JS, Jennings CD, Brown SA, Widmer MB. Effect of total body irradiation, busulfan-cyclophosphamide, or cyclophosphamide conditioning on inflammatory cytokine release and development of acute and chronic graft-versus-host disease in H-2- incompatible transplanted SCID mice. *Blood* 1994;83:2360–2367.

29. Xun CQ, Tsuchida M, Thompson JS. Delaying transplantation after total body irradiation is a simple and effective way to reduce acute graft-versus-host disease mortality after major H2 incompatible transplantation. *Transplantation* 1997;64:297–302.
30. Lehnert S, Rybka WB. Amplification of the graft-versus-host reaction by cyclophosphamide: dependence on timing of drug administration. *Bone Marrow Transplant* 1994;13:473–477.
31. Heidt PJ, Vossen JM. Experimental and clinical gnotobiotics: influence of the microflora on graft-versus-host disease after allogeneic bone marrow transplantation. *J Med* 1992;23:161–173.
32. Hill GR, Teshima T, Gerbitz A, et al. Differential roles of IL-1 and TNF-alpha on graft-versus-host disease and graft versus leukemia. *J Clin Invest* 1999;104:459–467.
33. Cooke KR, Kobzik L, Martin TR, et al. An experimental model of idiopathic pneumonia syndrome after bone marrow transplantation: I. The roles of minor H antigens and endotoxin. *Blood* 1996;88:3230–3239.
34. Cooke KR, Gerbitz A, Crawford JM, et al. LPS antagonism reduces graft-versus-host disease and preserves graft-versus-leukemia activity after experimental bone marrow transplantation. *J Clin Invest* 2001;107:1581–1589.
35. Hakim FT, Sharrow SO, Payne S, Shearer GM. Repopulation of host lymphohematopoietic systems by donor cells during graft-versus-host reaction in unirradiated adult F1 mice injected with parental lymphocytes. *J Immunol* 1991;146:2108–115.
36. Murphy WJ, Kumar V, Bennett M. Acute rejection of murine bone marrow allografts by natural killer cells and T cells. Differences in kinetics and target antigens recognized. *J Exp Med* 1987;166:1499–1509.
37. Mosier DE, Gulizia RJ, Baird SM, Wilson DB. Transfer of a functional human immune system to mice with severe combined immunodeficiency. *Nature* 1988;335:256–259.
38. Purtilo DT, Falk K, Pirruccello SJ, et al. SCID mouse model of Epstein-Barr virus-induced lymphomagenesis of immunodeficient humans. *Int J Cancer* 1991;47:510–517.
39. Johnson BD, Drobyski WR, Truitt RL. Delayed infusion of normal donor cells after MHC-matched bone marrow transplantation provides an antileukemia reaction without graft-versus- host disease. *Bone Marrow Transplant* 1993;11:329–336.
40. Johnson BD, Truitt RL. Delayed infusion of immunocompetent donor cells after bone marrow transplantation breaks graft-host tolerance allows for persistent antileukemic reactivity without severe graft-versus-host disease. *Blood* 1995;85:3302–3312.
41. Speiser DE, Bachmann MF, Shahinian A, Mak TW, Ohashi PS. Acute graft-versus-host disease without costimulation via CD28. *Transplantation* 1997;63:1042–1044.
42. Williamson E, Garside P, Bradley JA, Mowat AM. IL-12 is a central mediator of acute graft-versus-host disease in mice. *J Immunol* 1996;157:689–699.
43. Via CS, Shearer GM. Murine graft-versus-host disease as a model for the development of autoimmunity. Relevance of cytotoxic T lymphocytes. *Ann NY Acad Sci* 1988;532:44–50.
44. Welniak LA, Blazar BR, Wiltrout RH, Anver MR, Murphy WJ. Role of interleukin-12 in acute graft-versus-host disease(1). *Transplant Proc* 2001;33:1752,1753.
45. Williamson E, Garside P, Bradley JA, More IA, Mowat AM. Neutralizing IL-12 during induction of murine acute graft-versus-host disease polarizes the cytokine profile toward a Th2-type alloimmune response and confers long term protection from disease. *J Immunol* 1997;159:1208–1215.
46. Krenger W, Cooke KR, Crawford JM, et al. Transplantation of polarized type 2 donor T cells reduces mortality caused by experimental graft-versus-host disease. *Transplantation* 1996;62:1278–1285.
47. Pan L, Delmonte J, Jr., Jalonen CK, Ferrara JL. Pretreatment of donor mice with granulocyte colony-stimulating factor polarizes donor T lymphocytes toward type-2 cytokine production and reduces severity of experimental graft-versus-host disease. *Blood* 1995;86:4422–4429.
48. Pan L, Bressler S, Cooke KR, Krenger W, Karandikar M, Ferrara JL. Long-term engraftment, graft-vs.-host disease, and immunologic reconstitution after experimental transplantation of allogeneic peripheral blood cells from G-CSF-treated donors. *Biol Blood Marrow Transplant* 1996;2:126–1133.
49. Gorczynski RM, Kennedy M, Robillard M. Graft-versus-host disease in murine bone marrow transplantation. I. Modification of GVHD by preimmunization of recipients with spleen cells of primary recipients undergoing GVHD. *Immunol Lett* 1985;11:281–291.
50. Blazar BR, Taylor PA, Panoskaltsis-Mortari A, Gray GS, Vallera DA. Coblockade of the LFA1:ICAM and CD28/CTLA4:B7 pathways is a highly effective means of preventing acute lethal graft-versus-host disease induced by fully major histocompatibility complex-disparate donor grafts. *Blood* 1995;85:2607–2618.
51. Blazar BR, Taylor PA, Snover DC, Sehgal SN, Vallera DA. Murine recipients of fully mismatched donor marrow are protected from lethal graft-versus-host disease by the in vivo administration of rapamycin but develop an autoimmune-like syndrome. *J Immunol* 1993;151:5726–5741.
52. Nikolic B, Lee S, Bronson RT, Grusby MJ, Sykes M. Th1 and Th2 mediate acute graft-versus-host disease, each with distinct end-organ targets. *J Clin Invest* 2000;105:1289–1298.
53. Baker KS, Allen RD, Roths JB, Sidman CL. Kinetic and organ-specific patterns of cytokine expression in acute graft-versus-host disease. *Bone Marrow Transplant* 1995;15:595–603.

54. Krenger W, Hill GR, Ferrara JL. Cytokine cascades in acute graft-versus-host disease. *Transplantation* 1997;64:553–558.

55. Fujimori Y, Takatsuka H, Takemoto Y, et al. Elevated interleukin (IL)-18 levels during acute graft-versus-host disease after allogeneic bone marrow transplantation. *Br J Haematol* 2000;109:652–657.

56. Fialkow PJ, Gilchrist C, Allison AC. Autoimmunity in chronic graft-versus-host disease. *Clin Exp Immunol* 1973;13:479–486.

57. Jaffee BD, Claman HN. Chronic graft-versus-host disease (GVHD) as a model for scleroderma. I. Description of model systems. *Cell Immunol* 1983;77:1–12.

58. Mekori YA, Claman HN. Is graft-versus-host disease a reliable model for scleroderma? *Ric Clin Lab* 1986;16:509–513.

59. Rolink AG, Radaszkiewicz T, Melchers F. The autoantigen-binding B cell repertoires of normal and of chronically graft-versus-host-diseased mice. *J Exp Med* 1987;165:1675–1687.

60. van Rappard-Van der Veen FM, Kiesel U, Poels L, et al. Further evidence against random polyclonal antibody formation in mice with lupus-like graft-vs-host disease. *J Immunol* 1984;132:1814–1820.

61. Rolink AG, Pals ST, Gleichmann E. Allosuppressor and allohelper T cells in acute and chronic graft-vs.-host disease. II. F1 recipients carrying mutations at H-2K and/or I-A. *J Exp Med* 1983;157:755–771.

62. Gleichmann E, Van Elven EH, Van der Veen JP. A systemic lupus erythematosus (SLE)-like disease in mice induced by abnormal T-B cell cooperation. Preferential formation of autoantibodies characteristic of SLE. *Eur J Immunol* 1982;12:152–159.

63. Rolink AG, Gleichmann E. Allosuppressor- and allohelper-T cells in acute and chronic graft-vs.-host (GVH) disease. III. Different Lyt subsets of donor T cells induce different pathological syndromes. *J Exp Med* 1983;158:546–558.

64. Gelpi C, Martinez MA, Vidal S, et al. Different strains of donor parental lymphoid cells induce different models of chronic graft-versus-host disease in murine (Balb/c x A/J)F1 hybrid hosts. *Clin Immunol Immunopathol* 1990;56:298–310.

65. Shustov A, Luzina I, Nguyen P, et al. Role of perforin in controlling B-cell hyperactivity and humoral autoimmunity. *J Clin Invest* 2000;106:R39–47.

66. Allen RD, Staley TA, Sidman CL. Differential cytokine expression in acute and chronic murine graft-versus-host-disease. *Eur J Immunol* 1993;23:333–337.

67. Meyers CM, Tomaszewski JE, Glass JD, Chen CW. The nephritogenic T cell response in murine chronic graft-versus-host disease. *J Immunol* 1998;161:5321–5330.

68. Via CS, Rus V, Gately MK, Finkelman FD. IL-12 stimulates the development of acute graft-versus-host disease in mice that normally would develop chronic, autoimmune graft-versus-host disease. *J Immunol* 1994;153:4040–4047.

69. Parkman R. Clonal analysis of murine graft-vs-host disease. I. Phenotypic and functional analysis of T lymphocyte clones. *J Immunol* 1986;136:3543–3548.

70. Portanova JP, Claman HN, Kotzin BL. Autoimmunization in murine graft-vs-host disease. I. Selective production of antibodies to histones and DNA. *J Immunol* 1985;135:3850–3856.

71. Bruijn JA, van Leer EH, Baelde HJ, Corver WE, Hogendoorn PC, Fleuren GJ. Characterization and in vivo transfer of nephritogenic autoantibodies directed against dipeptidyl peptidase IV and laminin in experimental lupus nephritis. *Lab Invest* 1990;63:350–359.

72. Bruijn JA, Hogendoorn PC, Corver WE, van den Broek LJ, Hoedemaeker PJ, Fleuren GJ. Pathogenesis of experimental lupus nephritis: a role for anti-basement membrane and anti-tubular brush border antibodies in murine chronic graft-versus-host disease. *Clin Exp Immunol* 1990;79:115–1122.

73. Brinkman K, van Dam A, van den Brink H, Termaat RM, Berden J, Smeenk R. Murine monoclonal antibodies to DNA. A comparison of MRL/lpr NZB/W and chronically graft-versus-host-diseased mice. *Clin Exp Immunol* 1990;80:274–280.

74. Nonomura A, Koizumi H, Yoshida K, Ohta G. Histological changes of bile duct in experimental graft-versus-host disease across minor histocompatibility barriers. I. Light microscopic and immunocytochemical observations. *Acta Pathol Jpn* 1987;37:763–773.

75. Glass B, Uharek L, Zeis M, et al. Allogeneic peripheral blood progenitor cell transplantation in a murine model: evidence for an improved graft-versus-leukemia effect. *Blood* 1997;90:1694–1700.

76. Weiss L, Nusair S, Reich S, Sidi H, Slavin S. Induction of graft versus leukemia effects by cell-mediated lymphokine-activated immunotherapy after syngeneic bone marrow transplantation in murine B cell leukemia. *Cancer Immunol Immunother* 1996;43:103–108.

77. Morecki S, Moshel Y, Gelfend Y, Pugatsch T, Slavin S. Induction of graft vs. tumor effect in a murine model of mammary adenocarcinoma. *Int J Cancer* 1997;71:59–63.

78. Asai O, Longo DL, Tian ZG, et al. Suppression of graft-versus-host disease and amplification of graft-versus-tumor effects by activated natural killer cells after allogeneic bone marrow transplantation. *J Clin Invest* 1998;101:1835–1842.

79. Blazar BR, Taylor PA, Boyer MW, Panoskaltsis-Mortari A, Allison JP, Vallera DA. CD28/B7 interactions are required for sustaining the graft-versus- leukemia effect of delayed post-bone marrow transplantation spleno-cyte infusion in murine recipients of myeloid or lymphoid leukemia cells. *J Immunol* 1997;159:3460–3473.

80. Boyer MW, Vallera DA, Taylor PA, et al. The role of B7 costimulation by murine acute myeloid leukemia in the generation and function of a CD8+ T-cell line with potent in vivo graft- versus-leukemia properties. *Blood* 1997;89:3477–3485.

81. Boyer MW, Orchard PJ, Gorden KB, Anderson PM, McLvor RS, Blazar BR. Dependency on intercellular adhesion molecule recognition and local interleukin-2 provision in generation of an in vivo CD8+ T-cell immune response to murine myeloid leukemia. *Blood* 1995;85:2498–2506.

82. Porter DL, Collins RH, Jr., Shpilberg O, et al. Long-term follow-up of patients who achieved complete remission after donor leukocyte infusions. *Biol Blood Marrow Transplant* 1999;5:253–261.

83. Tanaka KK, Roberts E. Biological Studies of E.L.4 Lymphoma and C1498 Leukemia in Susceptible (C56BL) and Resistant (B10.D2) mice. *Cancer Res* 1964;24:1785–1797.

84. Blazar BR, Taylor PA, Panoskaltsis-Mortari A, et al. Blockade of CD40 ligand-CD40 interaction impairs CD4+ T cell-mediated alloreactivity by inhibiting mature donor T cell expansion and function after bone marrow transplantation. *J Immunol* 1997;158:29–39.

85. Yang YG, Sergio JJ, Pearson DA, Szot GL, Shimizu A, Sykes M. Interleukin-12 preserves the graft-versus-leukemia effect of allogeneic CD8 T cells while inhibiting CD4-dependent graft-versus-host disease in mice. *Blood* 1997;90:4651–4660.

86. Sykes M, Abraham VS, Harty MW, Pearson DA. IL-2 reduces graft-versus-host disease and preserves a graft-versus-leukemia effect by selectively inhibiting CD4+ T cell activity. *J Immunol* 1993;150:197–205.

87. Sykes M, Harty MW, Pearson DA. Strain dependence of interleukin-2-induced graft-versus-host disease protection: evidence that interleukin-2 inhibits selected CD4 functions. *J Immunother* 1994;15:11–21.

88. Dunn YB, Potter M. A transplantable mast-cell neoplasm in the mouse. *J Natl Cancer Inst* 1957;18:587.

89. Teshima T, Hill GR, Pan L, et al. IL-11 separates graft-versus-leukemia effects from graft-versus-host disease after bone marrow transplantation. *J Clin Invest* 1999;104:317–325.

90. de La Selle V, Riche N, Dorothe G, Bruley-Rosset M. CD8+ cytotoxic T cell repertoire implicated in grafts-versus-leukemia effect in a murine bone marrow transplantation model. *Bone Marrow Transplant* 1999,23.951–958.

91. Kim KJ, Kanellopoulos-Langevin C, Merwin RM, Sachs DH, Asofsky R. Establishment and characterization of BALB/c lymphoma lines with B cell properties. *J Immunol* 1979;122:549–554.

92. Borgmann A, Baldy C, von Stackelberg A, et al. Childhood all blasts retain phenotypic and genotypic char-acteristics upon long-term serial passage in NOD/SCID mice. *Pediatr Hematol Oncol* 2000;17:635–650.

93. Xun CQ, Thompson JS, Jennings CD, Brown SA. The effect of human IL-2-activated natural killer and T cells on graft- versus-host disease and graft-versus-leukemia in SCID mice bearing human leukemic cells. *Trans-plantation* 1995;60:821–827.

94. Harris DT. In vitro and in vivo assessment of the graft-versus-leukemia activity of cord blood. *Bone Marrow Transplant* 1995;15:17–23.

95. Hsieh MH, Korngold R. Differential use of FasL- and perforin-mediated cytolytic mechanisms by T-cell subsets involved in graft-versus-myeloid leukemia responses. *Blood* 2000;96:1047–1055.

96. Schmaltz C, Alpdogan O, Horndasch KJ, et al. Differential use of Fas ligand and perforin cytotoxic pathways by donor T cells in graft-versus-host disease and graft-versus-leukemia effect. *Blood* 2001;97:2886–2895.

97. Tsukada N, Kobata T, Aizawa Y, Yagita H, Okumura K. Graft-versus-leukemia effect and graft-versus-host disease can be differentiated by cytotoxic mechanisms in a murine model of allogeneic bone marrow transplan-tation. *Blood* 1999;93:2738–2747.

98. Jiang Z, Podack E, Levy RB. Major histocompatibility complex-mismatched allogeneic bone marrow trans-plantation using perforin and/or Fas ligand double-defective CD4(+) donor T cells: involvement of cytotoxic function by donor lymphocytes prior to graft-versus-host disease pathogenesis. *Blood* 2001;98:390–397

25

Allogeneic Effector Cell Populations
Separating GVL from GVHD

Michael R. Verneris, MD and Robert S. Negrin, MD

1. INTRODUCTION

The success of allogeneic transplantation in the treatment of malignant hematopoietic disorders is due to a combination of both the chemo-irradiation based conditioning regiment as well as a potent graft-vs-leukemia (GVL) effect imparted by the allogeneic hematopoietic cell graft. Although the exact contributions of either the conditioning regimen or allogeneic antileukemia effects are difficult to directly evaluate and are likely related to the disease and remission status, it is evident that GVL mechanisms are critically important. Some inference of the relative importance of either the conditioning regimen or GVL effects can be gained by examining the situations of identical twin and nonmyelablative bone marrow transplantation (BMT). The higher rate of disease recurrence following identical twin (as compared to matched sibling) BMT, is likely due to a reduced (or lack of) GVL response *(1–6)*. Despite this, there is improved survival following identical twin transplantation (as compared to standard chemotherapy) and thus an effect of high dose, cytotoxic chemotherapy *(7)*. In nonmyeloablative BMT, recipients receive relatively low dose conditioning agents and immunosuppressive drugs. This type of conditioning regiment allows for the engraftment of the allogeneic hematopoietic graft, yet has modest effects on the residual malignant cells. Early data show a substantial proportion of patients achieving complete remissions mainly due to GVL imparted by the allogeneic hematopoietic cells *(8–14)*.

The inverse correlation between leukemia recurrence and the development of graft-vs-host disease (GVHD) further supports the role of the immune system in the eradication of residual malignant cells, since relationships exist between leukemia free survival and the presence of

From: *Current Clinical Oncology: Allogeneic Stem Cell Transplantation*
Edited by: Mary S. Laughlin and Hillard M. Lazarus © Humana Press Inc., Totowa, NJ

acute *(6,15)* and especially chronic GVHD *(6,15,16)*. Additionally, donor leukocyte infusion (DLI) is now an established treatment for relapse of some diseases post-BMT (i.e., chronic myeloid leukemia [CML]) *(17)*. DLI is associated with both GVL and GVHD in a significant proportion of patients. Conversely, GVHD and GVL do not necessarily occur together, since some patients develop GVHD without benefiting from GVL. Such observations have led investigators to speculate whether GVL exists in the absence of GVHD. In support of the separability of GVHD from GVL, Ringden and coworkers observed that patients without GVHD during allogeneic BMT were statistically more likely to experience leukemia-free survival than those receiving an autograft *(18)*. While improved survival in the allogeneic group is suggestive of a GVL effect (without GVHD), there may be other explanations, such as contamination of autologous marrow with clonogenic malignant cells, for this result. A more convincing study supporting GVL without GVHD was performed using CD8+ T cell-depleted DLI for the treatment of relapsed CML. A significant number (43%) of patients entered either hematological or cytogenetic remissions without overt signs of GVHD *(19)*. Similarly, in a dose escalation study of DLI for the treatment of relapsed CML, Mackinnon and coworkers found that a dose of 1×10^7 lymphocytes/body weight was sufficient to induce remissions in at least 8 out of 21 patients, but only 1 out of 21 patients developed GVHD, again showing that GVL is separable from GVHD *(20)*.

Given that the practice of BMT or DLI involves the transfer of heterogeneous populations of fully differentiated lymphocytes, the occurrence of GVL and GVHD is not surprising. Contained within these unseparated preparations are likely to be cell populations with a higher propensity for GVHD than GVL or vice versa. Identification of lymphocyte subsets with a reduced capacity for GVHD is desirable since it would lead to the transfer of defined highly purified cellular products. Whether or not such an approach is ultimately successful remains to be determined, but for the first time, it is clinically tenable given: (i) the improved understanding of lymphocyte subset classification and function; (ii) an increased interest in immune based therapies at a clinical level; and (iii) technological enhancements in cell separation techniques (magnetic bead sorting, antibody based columns, high speed sorting). This chapter will therefore focus on preclinical studies and whenever available, clinical studies of various lymphocyte populations that may mediate GVL with the possibility of attenuated GVHD when adoptively transferred in the post-BMT period.

2. MECHANISMS OF TUMOR CELL KILLING

Regardless of the GVL conferring cell type, the general mechanics of tumor cell killing are typically shared. First, adhesion of the effector cell to a potential target occurs, allowing for more definitive identification. This initial contact occurs through a variety of receptor/ligand pairs mainly involved in cell adhesion (ICAM/LFA-1, CD2/LFA-3, etc.) (reviewed in ref. *21*). Next, target specificity takes place using specific receptor–ligand pairs (T cell receptor [TCR]/ major histocompatibility complex [MHC], TCR/CD1, natural killer [NK] cell receptor/MHC class I, etc.). If productive, effector cell activation occurs and results in target cell killing through three broad cellular pathways: (i) granzymes/perforin; (ii) tumor necrosis factor (TNF) superfamily molecules; and (iii) soluble mediators (Fig. 1).

As the effector cell contacts the target cell, a synapse-like junction is formed, which allows for localized release of granule contents. When the effector cell is triggered to kill the target, intracellular granules fuse with the cell membrane, and granule exocytosis occurs (Fig. 1A). Contained within the granules of effector cells are a variety of molecules that induce target cell apoptosis. The best characterized of these molecules are perforin and granzymes. Once released into the extracellular space, perforin inserts into the cell membrane and polymerizes in a Ca^{++}-

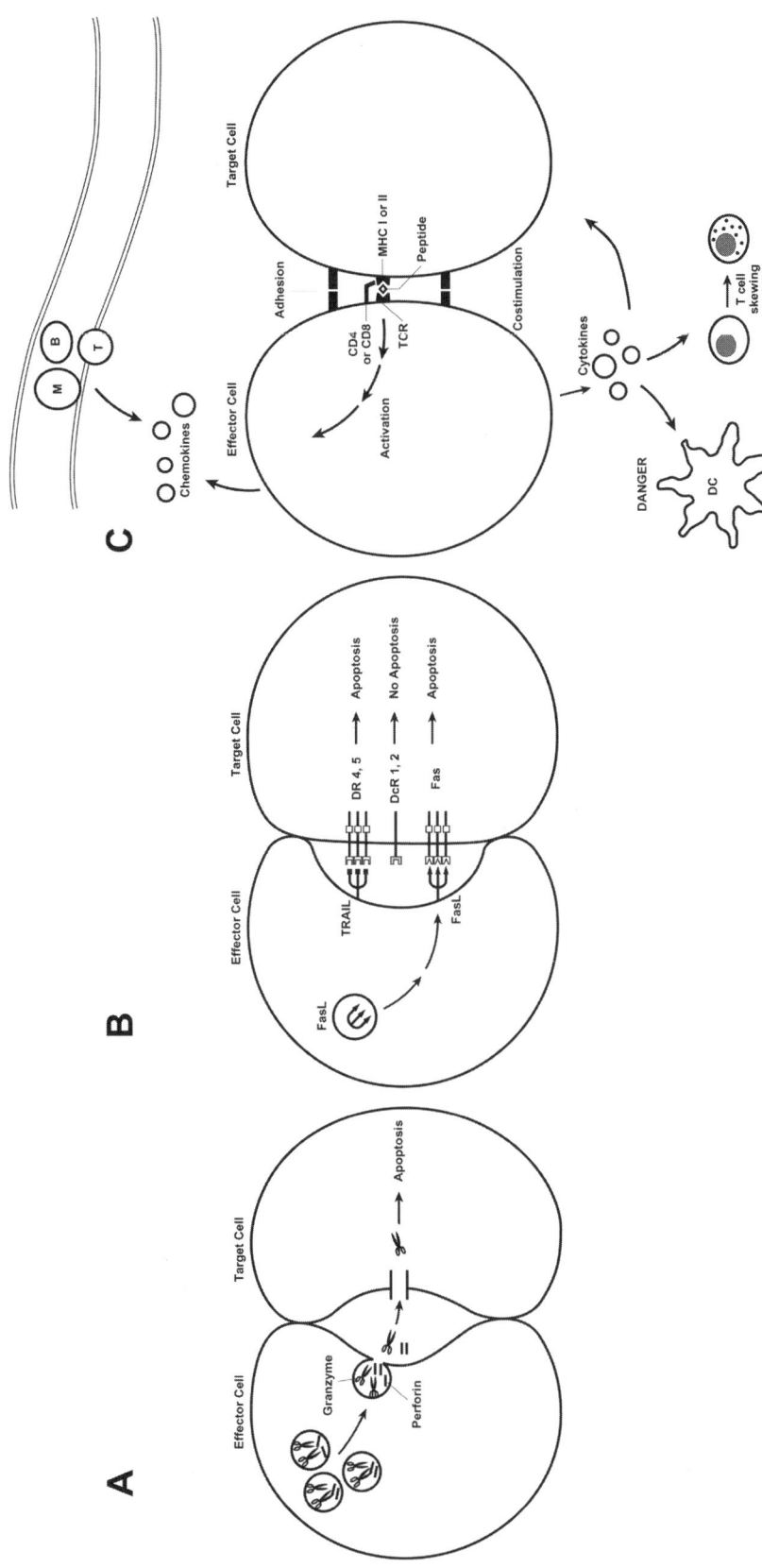

Fig. 1. Mechanisms of effector cell killing. There are three pathways that are used either separately or in combination in target cell killing. These include: **(A)** the release of preformed granule contents. Perforin (lines) and granzyme (scissors) are stored in granules, which are released into a synapse-like space between the effector and target. Perforin then inserts into the target cell membrane, allowing granzyme access to the cytoplasm where it mediates proteolysis and inducing apoptosis. **(B)** Also stored in preformed vesicles is FasL which binds to it's receptor, Fas (CD95). TRAIL is shown on the cell surface and can bind to a variety of receptors; some capable of transmitting an intracellular apoptotic signal (DR 4 and 5) and others that are not able to induce target cell apoptosis (DR 1 and 2). **(C)** The secretion of soluble mediators by the effector cell influences antitumor immunity through the chemo-attraction of other cell types (chemokines) and by the activating APCs, thereby skewing T cell responses and direct sensitization of the target cell for apoptosis (cytokines).

dependent manner to create membrane pores 100–200 Å in diameter *(22,23)*. While perforin induces target cell necrosis, more recent studies show that its true function may be to facilitate entry of other granule contents into the target cell cytoplasm *(24)*. Such molecules include a family of serine proteases called granzymes. Upon entry into the target cell cytosol, these molecules activate the proteolytic machinery within the target itself, inducing apoptosis *(25)*. The substrates for granzymes include those used by the TNF superfamily members as well as other cell death pathways *(26)*. To date, 11 different granzyme molecules have been identified, but the functional significance of this diversity is unknown *(27)*. A variety of other molecules are also found within the effector cell which are likely to induce target cytolysis. One such molecule is granulysin, which has been shown to induce tumor cytolysis in vitro, but their exact role in cytotoxic T lymphocyte (CTL) effector function is less well characterized *(28)*.

As another class of effector molecules, the TNF superfamily has generated considerable interest over the past 10 yr since members of this family play an essential role in both cellular activation and proliferation (CD30L, CD40L), as well as cell death (TNF-α, Fas ligand [FasL], and TNF-related apoptosis-inducing ligand [TRAIL]) *(29–31)*. For the purpose of this discussion, we will only address FasL and TRAIL, both of which are expressed by NK and T cells and participate in antitumor responses *(32,33)*. FasL and TRAIL have specific counter receptors present on a variety of both malignant and nonmalignant cells. For FasL, there is a single receptor, CD95 or Fas *(34)*. There are a total of five receptors to which TRAIL can bind to, and two are capable of inducing apoptosis (TRAIL-R1 [DR4] and TRAIL-R2 [DR5]). Two nonsignaling receptors (TRAIL-R3 [DcR1] and TRAIL-R4 [D$_c$R2]) and a soluble receptor (OPG, osteoprotegerin) do not cause apoptosis in target cells (reviewed in refs. *35* and *36*).

Both FasL and TRAIL induce trimerization of their cognate receptors on the target cells. This in turn activates a cascade of enzymes (*cysteine asp*artate-specific prote*ases* [caspases]), which induce to target cell apoptosis. Initial investigations suggested that FasL was present on the cell surface, but recent studies have refined this notion. Using confocal immunofluorescence, Bossi and Griffiths have elegantly determined that FasL is contained within cytoplasmic granules and is brought to the effector cell surface upon activation, thereby maintaining target specificity and minimizing injury to surrounding tissues *(37)* (Fig. 1B). Once on the cell surface, FasL is rapidly cleaved to a soluble form by matrix metalloproteases *(38)*. Most studies suggest that soluble FasL is either inactive or a weak inducer of apoptosis, thus cleavage from the cell surface may be a form of regulation of FasL-mediated immune responses. The cellular location of TRAIL may be different since it has been found on the surface of liver NK cells *(33)*. Whether TRAIL is regulated in the same manner as FasL (via cleavage from the cell surface) has not yet been definitively determined. Unlike FasL, TRAIL does not induce apoptosis in normal tissues *(39–42)*; thus this level of regulation may not be necessary. However, recent studies have questioned whether normal tissue is truly resistant to the apoptosis inducing effects of TRAIL *(43)*.

Activated T cells and NK cells produce a variety of soluble mediators that have both local and systemic effects. Such mediators include cytokines and chemokines that can affect the immune system and/or tumor targets in a variety of ways, including skewing of the immune response toward a Th1 or Th2 pattern, the chemoattracting of other cell types to tumor sites, activating of "bystander" cells, influencing antigen presentation, and directly sensitizing tumor cells to apoptosis (Fig. 1C).

3. ANTIGEN SPECIFIC CYTOTOXIC T CELLS

After release from the bone marrow, the majority of T cell precursors migrate to the thymus where they are positively and negatively selected based on the appropriate interactions with self-MHC molecules. After successful positive and negative selection, they are released into the peripheral circulation *(44)*. The majority of peripheral blood T cells express the α/β T cell receptor/CD3 complex and either the CD4 or CD8 co-receptors. T cells become activated upon TCR recognition of peptide antigens presented by antigen-presenting cells (APCs), such as B cells and dendritic cells (DCs). Antigens recognized by CD8$^+$ T cells are small peptide fragments (8–10 amino acids in length) complexed with MHC class I, while CD4$^+$ T cells recognize slightly larger peptide fragments (14–18 amino acids, sometimes up to 28 amino acids) presented by MHC class II *(45,46)*. In addition to presenting peptide antigens to T cells, DCs also provide essential co-stimulatory signals (CD80/CD86) and cytokines (interleukin [IL]-12, TNF-α, and interferon [IFN]) which enhance their own antigen presentation capacity and T cell activation *(47,48)*. After encounter with APCs, T cells expand clonally, develop cytolytic effector function and differentiate into long-lived memory cells.

A prerequisite for applying antigen-specific T cell immune responses to cancer therapy requires that: (i) unique and identifiable antigens are presented by tumor cells; and (ii) T cells can recognize these antigens. Since many of the tumor-specific antigens are essentially self-antigens (see below), it is questionable whether such self-reactive T cells actually exist. In fact, tolerance toward a variety of self-antigens has not been established or at least can be overcome *(49)*, and tumor reactive T cells have been identified in both experimental models and humans (see below). Tumor-specific antigens can be classified into four broad groups: (i) unique fusion proteins created by chromosomal translocations (e.g., 9;22, 15;17, etc); (ii) antigens whose overexpression contributes to oncogenesis (N-myc, Her2/neu); (iii) antigens whose expression is tissue restricted to the malignant tissue (protease 3 in myeloid cells, minor histocomapability antigens HA-1 and -2 on hematopoietic tissue and tyrosinase, MART-1/melan, in melanoma); and (iv) potentially universal tumor antigens, such as telomerase *(50–52)*.

Approaches to induce either primary or secondary T cell responses against malignancies have varied in both technique and success. In high-risk melanoma patients, intramuscular injection of adjuvant with peptides derived from the MART-1 protein resulted in both the induction of T cell immunity and demonstrable clinical responses in a number of patients. T cell interferon-γ secretion (postvaccination) correlated strongly with relapse free survival, suggesting that antigen-specific T cells contributed to survival *(53)*. In this study, the adjuvant presumably induced APC activation and peptide uptake followed by presentation to T cells. Instead of using adjuvant, investigators have also isolated and pulsed APCs ex vivo with either tumor-specific peptides or whole protein. Using this technique, Hsu and coworkers *(54)* used peripheral blood DCs and purified idiotype Ig protein for the treatment of patients with follicular lymphoma. They demonstrated antitumor responses in vitro and significant clinical responses in three out of four patients treated *(54)*. Since isolation of peripheral blood DCs is difficult, similar approaches have used peripheral blood monocytes in combination with cytokines to generate DCs in vitro. These cells were pulsed with tumor associated peptides as described above and reinfused. Like the above study, some patients showed both immunological and clinical response *(55)*. Rather than directly transfer APCs, some investigators have used APCs to prime T cells ex vivo. Rooney et al. have used this approach to generate Epstein-Barr virus (EBV)-specific T cells and have shown that they are highly effective in preventing (and treating) EBV lymphoproliferative disease occurring after T cell-depleted BMT *(56)*. Similar results were obtained for cytomegalovirus *(CMV) (57)*. Whether such vigorous immunity toward nonviral tumor antigens can be induced remains to be determined.

Another approach to generate antigen-specific T cell tumor immunity is to modify tumor cells to express immunostimulatory molecules, thereby enhancing their immunogenicity. In animal models and pre-clinical human studies such approaches have proven productive. Choudhury and coworkers cultured CML cells in IL-4, granulocyt-macrophage colony-stimulating factor (GM-CSF), and TNF-α to generate tumor cells with properties of DCs (expression of co-stimulatory molecules) which were then able to stimulate autologous antigen-specific T cells, while uncultured CML blasts could not induce such a response *(58)*. Malignant cells driven to become APCs were also generated from pre-B acute lymphocytic leukemia (ALL) samples after CD40 cross-linking. ALL blasts up-regulated co-stimulatory molecules and were then able to prime a cytolytic CTL response in vitro *(59)*. Gene transfer techniques have also been used to induce the expression of co-stimulatory molecules to generate tumor immunity. Both ALL and acute myelogenous leukemia (AML) cells transduced with the co-stimulatory molecule CD80 led to the generation of allogeneic CTLs *(60,61)*. Other modifications of tumor cells have included the transfer of cytokine genes. Vaccination with IL-12 secreting AML cells mediated elimination of residual AML and protected animals from future AML challenge *(62)*.

Another area of research focuses on enhancing T cell trafficking to sites of malignant disease. In recent years, there has been a rapid characterization of molecules that influence cellular migration. Chemokines are a large family of proteins that have potent chemoattractant properties, inducing T cell migration to sites of antigen presentation, inflammation, and tumor sites. Preclinical studies using tumor cells modified to secrete chemokines have proven to be effective. Murine tumor cells modified with both the IL-2 and lymphotactin genes induced infiltration of T cell and tumor elimination *(63)*.

A major advance for the characterization of antigen-specific T cells has been the development of MHC-tetramers. MHC-tetramers are soluble MHC molecules assembled with defined peptides that specifically bind to the T cell receptor of antigen-specific T cells. MHC-tetramers can be conjugated with a fluorogenic dye and used as reagents to identify, enumerate, and isolate antigen specific T cells by fluorescence-activated cell sorting (FACS) analysis *(64)*. MHC-tetramers have been used to identify antigen-specific T cells in patients with melanoma, cervical carcinoma, and CML *(55,65–67)*. In some patients, tumor-specific T cells account for 2% of all CD8+ T cells *(67)*. Isolation of tetramer staining CD8+ T cells in melanoma patients revealed that these cells had been previously activated, but do not proliferate, produce cytokines or mediate cytotoxicity against peptide-pulsed targets. While the above defect was observed in tumor specific T cells, CMV-specific T cells from the same individuals were normal, suggesting that although the immune system can recognize tumors, there is a selective dysfunction in tumor-specific T cells *(67)*. Conversely, in some diseases, the presence of tumor-reactive CTLs appears to be functional, since T cells reactive against a peptide derived from proteinase-3 (PR-1) predicted responses to either IFN-α treatment or allogeneic BMT in patients with CML *(68)*. Tetramer staining has also been used to monitor responses to immunotherapeutic interventions. In some studies, an increase in tetramer staining cells correlated with responses *(55)*, while in other cases it did not *(66)*, again confirming the complex interactions of the endogenous T cell response in cancer patients.

Tumor-specific immunity is the goal of immunotherapy. Indeed, if the antigen is chosen correctly, CTLs can provide specificity and memory with, theoretically, little risk for GVHD. Studies of antigen-specific CTLs adoptively transferred following transplantation in both murine and human studies have confirmed this concept *(56,69)*. But such an approach to cancer therapy is technically challenging, since the identification of tumor-associated antigens is complex and labor-intensive. Given the heterogeneity of the human MHC and that the peptide/MHC interaction is highly specific, a large number of peptides would be necessary to treat all individuals with a single disease. Thus the development of antigen-specific T cells either with peptide-pulsed DCs or by ex vivo generation, will likely require individualized therapies. The use of tumor modified vaccines circumvents such problems, since malignant tissue from each individual could be cryopreserved and used in the future, but there are practical concerns with using a whole tumor vaccine. One cannot control which antigens are being presented, and there is at least the theoretical risk of inducing autoimmunity. In fact, using a murine model of BMT, Anderson has shown that modified malignant cells induced both GVHD and GVL *(70)*. Therefore, while antigen-specific T cells have promise, there are many practical concerns that must be overcome before their widespread use and promise is achieved.

4. NK CELLS

NK cells make up approx 10% of circulating peripheral blood lymphocytes and are defined phenotypically by the lack of CD3 and by the presence of Fcγ III receptor (CD16) and neural cell adhesion molecule (N-CAM) (CD56) (in humans) or by the expression of NK1.1 and DX5 (in rodents). NK cells are functionally characterized by their ability to mediate MHC-unrestricted cytolysis of either virally infected or malignant transformed targets. Accordingly, patients with selective deficiencies of NK cells are at higher risk for the development of uncontrolled viral infections *(71,72)*, and NK cells from these patients have markedly reduced cytolysis against the NK sensitive erythroleukemia target cell line K562 *(73–75)*.

The adoptive transfer of NK cells following allogeneic transplantation holds promise since a large body of evidence supports their potent antitumor activity. Freshly isolated NK cells recognize and lyse some cultured malignant cell lines and autologous tumor targets *(76)*. IL-2-activated NK cells, referred to as lymphokine-induced killer (LAK) cells, have a broader spectrum of tumor killing and are capable of killing a wide range of cultured tumor cells *(76,77)*. One of the largest in vitro studies of LAK cells was performed by Teichmann and coworkers who examined the sensitivity of >250 patient-derived leukemia samples and found that the same leukemia specimen was either susceptible or nonsusceptible to LAK-mediated lysis from multiple donors. The majority of samples (62%) were susceptible to lysis by multiple donors. Greater than 60% of acute leukemias (AML or ALL) and most CML blast crisis samples were sensitive to lysis (92%), while only 39% of chronic phase CML samples were killed. Patient-derived LAK cells were also evaluated in this study, and in 63% of samples, there was autologous anti-leukemia activity *(77)*. Similarly, many in vivo animal experiments have demonstrated an important role of either endogenous *(78)* or adoptively transferred NK cells in the control of a variety of tumors *(79)*. While the original description of the clinical application of LAK cells was encouraging, with nearly half of chemotherapy refractory patients showing some response to LAK therapy *(80)*, subsequent studies have yielded less impressive results *(81–86)*. Further, such therapy is associated with considerable toxicity due to the requirement for exogenous IL-2 administration *(87)*.

How NK cells recognize targets was unknown until the recent cloning and characterization of a rapidly expanding family of cell surface receptors. The unifying theme is that these receptors detect the presence or absence of classical or nonclassical MHC class I molecules on target cells *(88,89)*. Depending upon the receptor, engagement leads to either NK cell inhibition or activation.

The majority of NK cell receptors identified thus far fall into the inhibitory category. Engagement of these receptors (with class I MHC molecules) leads to an inhibition of NK cell-mediated responses (Fig. 2A). Conversely, when NK cells encounter a potential target and the inhibitory receptor is not engaged, the NK cell is triggered to induce target cytolysis (Fig. 2B). Such functions were initially predicted by Ljunggren and Karre and coined the "missing self hypothesis" *(90)*. The commonality between these inhibitory NK cell receptors is that the cytoplasmic tail contains immunoreceptor tyrosine-based inhibition motif (ITIM) residues. Receptor cross-linking recruits Src homology 2 domain-containing phosphatase (SHP)-1 and SH-2-containing inositol polyposphate 5-phosphatase (SHIP), which in turn inhibits NK cell-mediated cytotoxicity *(91,92)*.

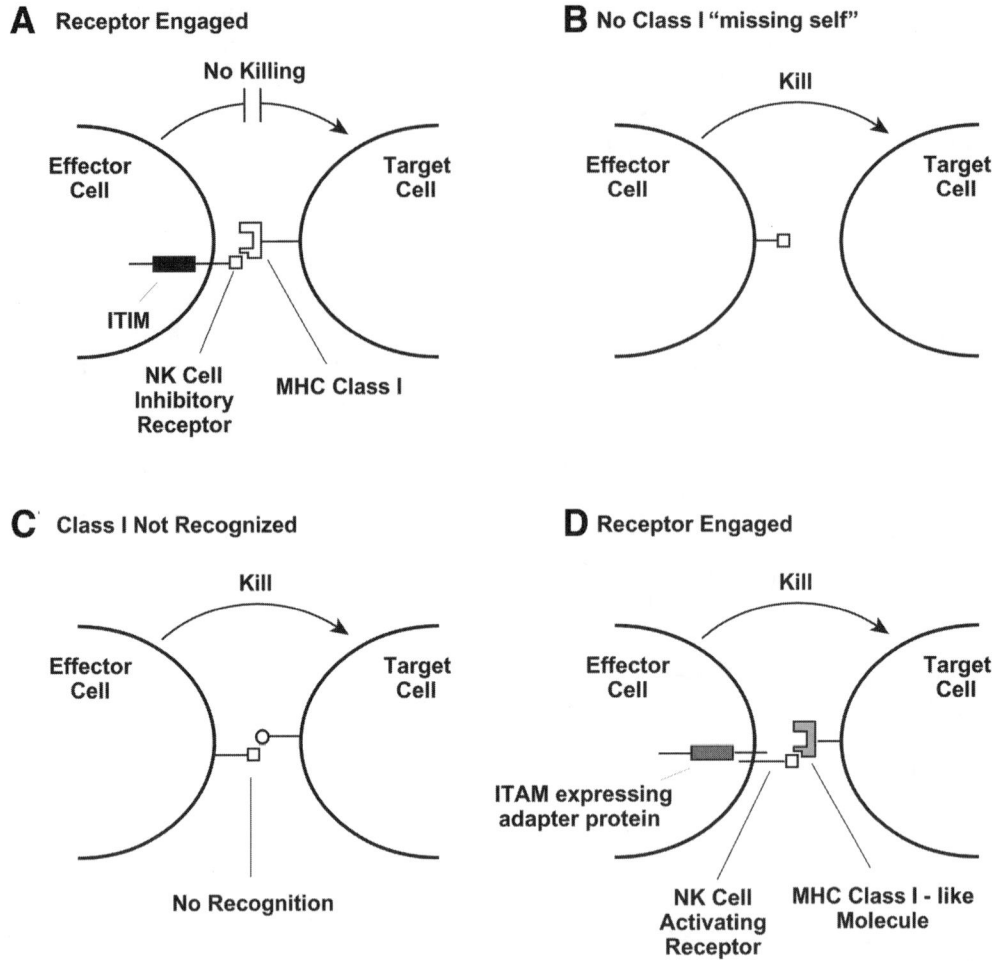

Fig. 2. Missing self hypothesis and NK cell activating receptors. NK cells recognize the presence or absence of target cell MHC class I (or class I-like) molecules. When NK cell inhibitory receptors are engaged (**A**) killing is inhibited. Conversely, when NK cell-inhibitory receptors are not engaged, either due to the lack of MHC class I (**B**) or due to MHC mismatch (**C**), killing occurs. When NK cell-activating receptors are engaged, killing is triggered (**D**).

Activating NK cell-associated molecules have also recently been identified, which trigger cytotoxicity. This rapidly expanding group of proteins is less well-characterized, yet the unifying theme is that they lack cytoplasmic ITIM motifs necessary for inhibitory signaling. For transmission of activating signals, most of these receptors require interactions with the adapter proteins CD3ζ, FceRIg, and DAP 12, all of which express cytoplasmic immunoreceptor tyrosine-based activating (ITAM) motifs. Phosphorylation of these motifs in turn recruits ZAP70 and Syk, resulting in NK cell cytokine synthesis and cytotoxicity *(88,93)*. Other activating adapter proteins use DAP 10, which lacks ITAM motifs and, instead, signals through phoshatidylinositol 3-kinase *(94)*. Additional activating receptors, such as 2B4, use no adapter molecules or ITAM signaling motifs *(95)*.

NK cell cytotoxicity must be a tightly regulated process, integrating both positive and negative signals from both activating and inhibitory receptors, respectively. Understanding such regulation may be essential for clinical applicability. In fact, both the inhibitory and the activating receptors can be expressed by the same NK cell *(96)*. In vitro studies suggest that

NK cell triggering occurs after an integration of many cell surface signals from such receptors *(96)*. Given the current understanding of this system, it appears that inhibitory signals dominate over activating signals. This is supported by the relatively larger numbers of inhibitory receptors relative to activating receptors, as well as the direct experimental evidence showing NK cell inhibition when both inhibitory and activating receptors are simultaneously engaged *(96)*.

NK receptors have been divided into the C-type lectin receptors and the immunoglobulin superfamily inhibitory receptors. Within each of these families there exist both activating and inhibitory receptors. The C-type lectin receptors are further subdivided into the Ly49 molecules and the CD94/NKG2 heterodimers. The Ly49 receptors are present only on murine NK cells, and while a human homologue has been identified, it appears to be a pseudogene *(97)*. To date, at least nine different Ly49 (Ly49 *A, C, D, E, F, G, H I, K*) molecules have been identified *(98)*. Most have been shown to bind class I molecules and, thus, directly interrogate a potential target for the presence or absence of cell surface MHC class I. While the majority of the receptors in this family appear to be inhibitory, the Ly49D and Ly49H receptors have activating function *(99)*.

The other member of C type lectin receptors is the disulfide-linked heterodimer between the invariant CD94 chain and various members of the NKG2 complex (NKG2A, NKG2C, and NKG2E). Unlike Ly49, both CD94 and NKG2 molecules have been identified in both primates and rodents *(100,101)*. Instead of directly detecting the expression of class I on the cell surface, the CD94/NKG2A/C/E heterodimer detects the *level* of MHC class I expression. This is because the counter receptor on the target cell (either HLA-E, human or Qa-1, mouse) is stable only when a leader sequence (AMAPRTLLL) of classical MHC class I is presented in the peptide-binding groove *(102–104)*.

A distantly related member of the NKG2 family is NKG2D, sharing only partial sequence homology with the other members *(105)*. NKG2D does not heterodimerize with CD94, but rather forms a homodimer and signals through the adapter molecule DAP-10 *(94)*. NKG2D has NK cell-activating function and recognizes the MHC class I-related chain A (MICA) and B (MICB) in humans *(94,106)*. MICA/B are stress-induced and have been found mainly on epithelial-derived tumors *(107,108)*. Recent studies suggest that cell lines derived from other malignancies and leukemia also express these ligands *(96)*. Experimintal data show that some NK cells recognize tumor targets that do not express MICA and MICB, suggesting that there are other ligands for NKG2D *(96)*. Murine NKG2D has also been characterized. The ligands for murine NKG2D—H60 and Rae-1—have a strikingly low level of homology to one another and to MICA/B *(109)*. Soluble NKG2D binds to a variety of NK-sensitive tumor cell lines, suggesting that NKG2D ligands are expressed on murine malignant tissue *(109)*. Interestingly, the promoter elements for Rae-1 contains a retinoic acid responsive element *(110)*, possibly ascribing a novel antitumor activity of this drug.

The other large group of NK cell inhibitory receptors are the killer inhibitory receptors (KIRs). KIRs have only been identified in humans, and based on cDNA data it is estimated that there are approx 12 individual genes *(89)*. Classification is based on both the number of extracellular Ig domains (either 2 or 3, designated KIR2D or KIR3D) and the length of the intracellular signaling domain (either long or short, designated either KIR2DL or KIR2DS) (Table 1). In general, receptors bearing the long intracellular domains contain an ITIM region necessary for the inhibition of cytotoxicity, while receptors with short intracellular domain lack such regions and are activating.

Lastly, a group of Ig family member receptors, which lack ITIM motifs, have recently been described and are referred to as the natural cytotoxicity receptors (NCRs) *(111)*. NCRs have been identified by generating antibodies to NK cells and using them in a redirected killing assay. In this assay, an anti-NK cell antibody is combined with a Fc-bearing target, and the

Table 1
KIR Designation and Epitope Recognition

Name	Alternate name	Recognition	Inhibitory (ITIM)
KIR2DL1	p58.1 (CD158a-long form)	HLA-Cw 2, 4, 5, 6	Yes
KIR2DL2/3	p58.2 (CD158b-long form)	HLA-Cw 1,3,7, 8	Yes
KIR2DL4	p49	HLA-G	Yes
KIR3DL1	p70	HLA-Bw4	Yes
KIR3DL2	p140	HLA-A3, A11	Yes
KIR2DS1	p50.1 (CD158a-short form)	HLA-Cw4	No
KIR2DS2	p50.2 (CD158b-short form)	?HLA-C	No
KIR2DS3	—	?	No
KIR2DS4	p50.3	?HLA-C	No
KIR2DS5	—	?	No
KIR3DS1	—	?HLA-B	No

Adapted with permission from refs. 203–205.

ability of the NK cell to kill the target is measured and compared to an irrelevant antibody. If the antibody recognizes and induces cross-linking of activating receptors, cytolysis is triggered. Four NCR family members termed NKp46, NKp44, NKp30, and NKp80 have recently been identified using this method. NKp46 is found on all NK cells, and in some individuals there is bimodal expression of NKp46, with some NK clones being NKp46[bright] and others being NKp46[dull]. High receptor density of NKp46 on NK cells strongly correlates with tumor cytotoxicity and appears to identify subsets of NK cells with high antitumor activity (112–114). Like NKp46, NKp30 has been identified on NK clones and cooperates with NKp46 in target recognition (115). NKp44 is an activating ligand only found on activated NK cells (116,117). The expression of NKp44 on activated NK cells only may help explain the increased spectrum of tumor recognition of LAK cells compared to NK cells (109). NKp80 is also found on NK cells and a small subset of freshly isolated CD3+CD56+ T cells. This receptor appears to cooperate with the other NCRs in the recognition of phytohemagglutinin antigen (PHA)-activated T cells (118). The exact ligands for the above receptors have not been identified.

Characterizing the cell surface receptors involved in target recognition may be the first step to improved clinical application of NK cells, but an essential question surrounds their capacity to induce GVHD if they are to be used in the post-transplant setting. Murine studies show that full MHC-mismatched IL-2-expanded NK cells do not cause GVHD while retaining their capacity to mediate GVL (119). As well in this model, IL-2-activated NK cells secreted transforming growth factor (TGF)-β, which prevented the induction of lethal T cell-mediated GVHD. Human studies have supported such findings since patients undergoing haploidentical stem cell transplantation have a very early recovery of donor-derived NK cells without any associated GVHD despite the lack of immunosuppressive drugs (120). Since the KIR molecules are not genetically linked to MHC loci, it is possible to select a donor based on NK cell receptors that do not recognize host MHC class I antigens (Fig. 2C). Such a situation would be analogous to the lack of MHC class I (Fig. 2B) and should trigger cytotoxicity. In fact, donor-derived NK clones isolated following transplantation have significant activity against recipient leukemia targets, and this cytotoxicity can be predicted based on the HLA/KIR mismatch. This type of mismatch predicted cytotoxicity against recipient AML and CML cells, but not for ALL, possibly due to the lack of CD54 (ICAM) on ALL blasts (121). Clinical studies support these in vitro observations, since patients with AML and CML undergoing haploidentical BMT with a HLA/KIR mismatch were significantly less likely to relapse (1 out of 28) as compared to those without mismatch (14 out of 47) (122).

Table 2
Properties of Various Subpopulations of NKT Cells

	$CD4^-CD8^-, CD4^+$	$CD8^+$
Thymic-dependent	Yes	No
IL-4 secretion	Yes	BM-Yes; Spleen-No
IFN-γ secretion	Yes	BM-Yes; Spleen-No
TCR receptor	Biased	Nonbiased
CD1-dependent	Yes	No

5. NKT CELLS

Natural killer T cells (NKT cells) are a subset of T cells that have been described in both mouse and man with immune regulatory and tumor surveillance functions. NKT cells express both the TCR/CD3 complex and typical NK cell molecules, NK1.1 (or NKR-P1C, CD161) [123]. NKT cells also express molecules associated with a memory T cell phenotype including CD44[high], CD69[high], CD62L[low], IL-2Rβ (CD122)[high], [123,124]. There is variable expression of other NK-associated markers, including DX-5, Ly49 in rodents [125,126] and NKR-P1A (CD161), CD56 in humans [127].

Three subsets of NKT cells are further defined based on the expression of the co-receptors CD4 and CD8 and include: (i) double negative (DN, CD4-CD8-); (ii) CD4[+]; and (iii) CD8[+]. There are considerable differences between these subsets with respect to TCR expression, CD1 recognition, tissue distribution, thymic dependence, and cytokine production (summarized in Table 2). In mice, the CD4 and the DN subsets are derived from the same (or a similar) lineage, since most express a single invariant TCR α chain (Vα14Jα281) paired with a limited number of Vβ receptors (Vβ8.2 being the most common) [123,128]. In contrast to classical T cells, which recognize peptide in the context of MHC class I or II, the CD4 and many of the DN NKT cells recognize glycolipid in the context of the nonclassical MHC molecule CD1 [129]. Synthetic ligands that bind in the groove of CD1 have been identified and include α-galactosylceramide (α-GalCer) [129,130] (see below). NKT cells can be found in most lymphoid tissues, with CD4[+] NKT cells predominately found in the liver and thymus and DN NKT cells found in the spleen and bone marrow [125]. Most studies suggest that these NKT cells are dependent upon the thymus for development since they are markedly reduced in thymectomized mice, nude mice and arise in Rag[-/-]β2M[-/-] mice after thymus transplantation [131,132]. Upon activation, CD4[+] and DN NKT cells promptly secrete large amounts of IFN-γ, IL-10, and IL-4 which may contribute to their immunoregulatory functions [133,134].

In contrast to CD1-restricted NKT cells, murine CD8[+] NKT and some DN NKT cells are found in CD1[-/-] mice and are thus not dependent on CD1 for their development (125). Moreover, CD8[+]NKT cells express a heterogeneous TCR repertoire and do not express the canonical TCR (Vα14Jα281) expressed on many CD1-restricted NKT cells [125,135]. Thymectomy at d 3 of life leads to a significant reduction in CD4[+] and DN NKT cells in the spleen and thymus, but splenic CD8[+]NKT cells are relatively unchanged in numbers, suggesting that they are either thymus-independent or leave the thymus very early in life [131,133]. With regard to cytokine production, activated splenic CD8[+]NKT cells produce little IFN-γ and IL-4 [133]. In contrast, bone marrow-derived CD8[+]NKT cells produce substantial quantities of IFN-γ and IL-4 [134], thus suggesting significant heterogeneity between CD8[+]NKT cells from different tissues.

In humans, NKT cells have also been identified in the peripheral blood and liver [137,138]. These cells express the Vα24JQ receptor associated with Vβ11 (homologues for the murine receptors Vα14Jα281 and Vβ8.2, respectively) [138]. Like murine NKT cells, three subsets can be identified based on CD4 and CD8 expression, but in contrast to the mouse, there is a larger percentage of CD1-restricted CD8$^+$ NKT cells in humans *(138,139)*. Human Vα24JQ/Vβ11 cells secrete both IL-4 and INF-γ *(138)*. Takahashi and coworkers *(140)* compared the cytokine secretion of CD4$^+$ NKT cells with DN NKT cells. They demonstrated that while there was no difference in INF-γ secretion, CD4$^+$ NKT cells secrete more IL-4 than do DN NKT cells *(140)*.

Since small numbers of NKT cells are found in human peripheral blood, methodologies are being developed to expand such cells ex vivo. Culturing NKT cells with α-GalCer and IL-12 activates NKT cells (increased intracellular granzyme B), but has little effect on cell expansion *(139)*. Expansion of human NKT cells has recently been achieved after culture of peripheral blood T cells with α-GalCer-pulsed DCs and stimulation with IL-7 and/or IL-15 *(141)*. As mentioned above, α-GalCer is a synthetic ligand for CD1 and, thus far, has not been identified in mammalian tissues *(130)*. The identity of the exact natural ligands that are presented to NKT cells have not been precisely determined, but phospholipid extracts from tumor cell lines do bind to CD1 and induce NKT cell activation *(142)*. Thus, NKT cells may be able to respond to endogenous antigens presented by tumor cells.

There is considerable experimental evidence suggesting that NKT cells play a role in tumor surveillance, but the exact nature of this antitumor activity is debated. Treatment of tumor bearing mice with either IL-12, α-GalCer, or α-GalCer pulsed DCs induces NKT cell dependent antitumor activity *(143–145)*. Whether or not this is directly due to NKT cell-mediated cytotoxicity has not been established, since in the above models splenocytes and not purified populations of NKT cells were used to demonstrate antitumor cytotoxicity. NKT cells may mediate tumor clearance indirectly, since their activation induces NK cell proliferation and cytotoxicity, which is, in part, dependent upon their prompt IFN-γ production after activation *(146,147)*. In humans, there is evidence for direct antitumor activity since either α-GalCer-stimulated CD3$^+$ cells or NKT cell clones mediate perforin-dependent tumor cytolysis in vitro *(140,148,149)*.

It should be noted that NKT cells have also been implicated in tumor progression and recurrence. Tamada and coworkers *(150)* isolated tumor-infiltrating NKT cells from B16 melanoma injected mice. These cultured NKT cells could inhibit antitumor CTL generation both through the elaboration of TGF-β and cytolysis of cells expressing co-stimulatory molecules *(150)*. There may be differences between these cultured NKT cells and freshly isolated NKT cells, since the DN cells in this study did not produce IL-4 upon stimulation, as do freshly isolated NKT cells. In another study using a model of tumor growth, followed by regression, and finally recurrence, it was shown that CD4$^+$ NKT cells play an essential role in tumor recurrence phase due to the secretion of IL-13 *(151)*. Thus, the secretion of counterregulatory cytokines in some systems may inhibit antitumor activity.

Few studies have addressed whether or not NKT cells induce GVHD. Zeng and coworkers have found that bone marrow NKT cells transplanted across major histocomaptability barriers did not induce GVHD and are capable of suppressing GVHD induced by peripheral blood CD4$^+$ and CD8$^+$ cells *(152)*. Protection from GVHD was lost if BM NKT cells were used from IL-4$^{-/-}$ mice, suggesting that in this model, IL-4 plays an essential role in GVHD protection. Some caution is warranted, since other investigators have shown that host-derived NKT cells can be demonstrated in the thymus during acute GVHD *(153)*. Whether these cells actually contribute to GVHD (or arise in response to GVHD) was not determined, but it was shown that the host NKT cells contributed to the cytotoxicity of the thymus-containing cells.

6. CIK CELLS

For some time, it has been known that small numbers of human peripheral blood T cells express the NK cell marker CD56 and that these freshly isolated cells have NK like cytotoxicity

(MHC-unrestricted) against tumor targets *(154)*. Culture conditions have been developed that allow for the expansion of T cells with similar attributes, i.e., expression of CD56 and broad MHC-unrestricted cytotoxicity against a variety of tumor targets without prior exposure *(155–157)*. Subsequent studies showed that these ex vivo expanded cells, termed cytokine-induced killer cells (CIK cells), were in fact not derived from either NK cells or CD3+CD56+ precursor cells, but rather from either CD3+CD4-CD8-, CD3+CD8+, or even CD3+CD4+CD8+ cells *(158)*.

The culture conditions used to generate CIK cells include the prestimulation of cells with IFN-γ, followed by a cross-linking CD3 antibody and intermediate dose IL-2 (300 U/mL). Cells are fed with fresh media every 3 to 4 d and after 14–21 d there is an approx 100- to 500-fold expansion of CD3+CD56+ cells *(158)*. Using these conditions, we have generated CIK cells from peripheral blood, bone marrow, cord blood (in humans) and spleen, thymus and liver (in mice). Prestimulation of cells with IFN-γ leads to monocyte activation, which enhances CD3+CD56+ expansion through both the secretion of IL-12 and CD58/LFA3 co-stimulation *(159)*. Other studies support these findings, since cultures of lymphocytes under identical conditions and IL-12 (as compared to IL-2) lead to higher numbers of CD3+CD56+ cells *(160)*.

We have previously shown that these ex vivo-activated and -expanded cells have significant antitumor activity. Using a severe combined immunodeficiency disease (SCID)/Hu model of lymphoma, CIK cells were more effective than LAK cells in curing animals *(158)*. Autologous CIK cells can be generated from patients with chronic phase CML, and the majority of samples (12 out of 13) were Philadelphia (Ph) chromosome negative by cytogenetic analysis *(161)*. When CML was engrafted into SCID mice, a significant proportion of the animals could be rescued by administration of autologous CIK cells *(161)*. Similarly, we have expanded CIK cells from patients with AML and found them to have activity against autologous AML blasts *(162)*. CIK cells are more effective in mediating cytotoxicity against cell lines derived from hematopoeitic malignancies than solid tumors. To augment the antitumor activity against solid tumor targets, we have used bispecific antibodies to redirect CIK cells to target cells. CD3xHer2/neu bispecific antibody (bsAb)-redirected CIK cells are significantly more effective in mediating in vitro tumor cytolysis when compared to CIK cells or CIK cells and a control bsAb. Similarly, bsAb-redirected CIK cells are more effective in eradicating residual breast, ovarian, and primitive neural ectodermal tumor (PNET) cell lines engrafted into SCID mice (unpublished results).

The cell surface structures involved in CIK cell recognition of tumor targets is not well understood. To date, there is no evidence supporting a T cell receptor-based identification of targets, since antibodies against CD3, CD4, CD8, TCR α/β, MHC I and II are unable to block cytotoxicity *(156)*. ICAM and LFA-1 are the only molecules known to be involved in cytotoxicity, since antibodies against these molecules attenuates cytotoxicity *(156)*. Blocking cytoplasmic granule release inhibits cytotoxicity, suggesting a perforin based mechanism *(163)*. We have recently generated a homologous population of activated T cells from murine splenocytes, with the cell surface phenotype of CD8+ NKT cells *(164)*. These cells have many of the same attributes as human CIK cells, namely expression of NK cell markers (NK1.1 and DX5) and MHC-unrestricted cytotoxicity against a variety of targets without prior exposure. To address the mechanism of cytotoxicity, cells were expanded from either FasL deficient (gld) or perforin gene knock-out (pfp) mice. Cytotoxicity assays demonstrate that the FasL deficient mice have cytotoxicity identical to wild-type mice, yet cells derived from the pfp animals were devoid of any cytolytic activity both in vitro and in vivo *(165)*.

Using murine-expanded CD8+ NKT cells we investigated their propensity to induce GVHD when transplanted across major histocompatability barriers. Transplantation experiments were performed using purified allogeneic hematopoietic stem cells (HSCs) alone or with adoptively transferred splenocytes or expanded CD8+ NKT cells. Mice that received unactivated splenocytes (1×10^6) all died of acute lethal GVHD. Conversely, mice that received 10× the number of expanded CD8[+] NKT cells had mild weight loss, but were otherwise without evidence of GVHD (ruffled fur, diarrhea). To test whether expanded CD8[+] NKT cells mediated GVL effects, a murine model of persistent lymphoma after HSC transplantation was utilized. Mice transplanted with FACS-purified HSCs alone all died of lymphoma while approx 50% of the animals that received HSCs and expanded CD8[+] NKT cells were rescued from lymphoma and did not have GVHD *(165)*. There are multiple possible explanations as for why the ex vivo-expanded CD8[+] NKT cells cause less GVHD than unexpanded cells. Expanded CD8[+] NKT cells have undergone multiple rounds of expansion, and the same cellular events that occur in GVHD are not likely to occur (i.e., T cell activation and cytokine storm). Expanded CD8[+] NKT cells express both TGF-β and low levels of IL-10, a combination of cytokines that have been shown by others to prevent alloreactivity *(166)*. Lastly, expanded CD8[+] NKT cells constitutively secrete IFN-γ, which can be protective in murine GVHD *(167)*. In contrast to wild-type expanded CD8[+] NKT cells, those expanded from IFN-γ[-/-] mice induce rapid lethal GVHD *(164)*.

Given the above encouraging preclinical results, we have recently performed a phase I, dose escalation trial using autologous CIK cells in patients with relapsed–refractory lymphoma (Hodgkin's and non-Hodgkin's). The goals of this study were to: (i) determine whether sufficient numbers of cells could be generated in a clinical laboratory setting; and (ii) to determine the safety of administration of ex vivo-expanded and -activated cells. The target doses were 1×10^9–1×10^{10} cells. Sufficient quantities of cells could be generated from patients with relapsed malignancies. The total cellular expansion and the numbers of CD3[+]CD56[+] cells varied amongst donors. The infusion of cells was well-tolerated. Given these results, phase II studies are now underway in autologous and allogeneic settings. A similar strategy was utilized to treat patients with hepatoma following surgical resection in a prospective randomized trial. The patients who received ex vivo-activated T cells had a statically significant reduction in disease recurrence and prolonged survival *(168)*.

7. γ/δ T CELLS

The majority of peripheral blood T cells express the αβ TCR, but a small percentage of cells (approx 5–10%) express the γδ TCR. γδ T cells are a unique subset of T cells, since they differ from the αβ T cells in the type of antigens recognized and in the ability to identify stressed or transformed cells. While α/β T cells are primed by APCs to recognize peptide fragments complexed with MHC molecules, the same is not true for γδ T cells. Some lines of evidence suggest that γδ T cells recognize protein without the need for antigen presentation *(169)*. Evaluating the CDR3 length of αβ, γδ, and immunoglobulin receptors, Rock and coworkers determined that γδ T cell receptors may be more like immunoglobulin than αβ TCRs *(170)*. The types of antigens that γδ T cells recognize seem to be completely different from αβ T cells. Using γδ T cell clones, it has been determined that at least one type of antigen recognized by γδ T cells is nonclassical MHC class I molecules (T10 and T22). Interestingly, although these molecules do not bind peptide, they are still able to stimulate these clones, even when expressed in *Drosophila* or recombinantly in bacteria or when immobilized on solid phase *(169)*.

A variety of substances have been identified which lead to γδ T cell activation and proliferation. These include mycobacterial extracts (PPD), random copolymer of glutamic acid and tyrosine (poly GT), tetanus toxoid, heat-shock proteins, and phosphate containing nonpeptide molecules *(171)*. Recently, it has been shown that bisphosphonates induce activation and proliferation of a specific subset of human peripheral blood γδ T cells (Vγ9/Vδ2) *(172)*. While bisphosphonates have been used clinically to prevent bone readsorption, some studies have shown that bisphoshonates may have a direct antimyeloma effect *(173)*. Based on this, Kunzmann and coworkers *(174)* expanded γδ T cells from patients with myeloma and determined that expanded γδ T cells mediated cytolysis against myeloma cell lines. Furthermore, cultures of patient-derived bone marrow cells in the presence of bisphosphonates showed a reduction in plasma cells, which was γδ T cell-dependent *(174)*.

Multiple studies have evaluated the role of γδ T cells in both infections and immunosurveillance against malignancies. These studies have implicated γδ T cells in the protection against mycobacteria, listeria, salmonella, mycoplasma, and viruses including CMV and herpes simplex virus (HSV) *(171)*. Interestingly, all of these pathogens have intracellular phases, leading to the hypothesis that γδ T cells may not be directly responding to microbial antigens, but rather to "cellular stress" induced by such pathogens. Other forms of cellular stress include malignant transformation, and γδ T cells have been postulated to provide immunosurveillance against malignancies. Recently, some γδ T cells expressing the $V_\delta 1$ receptor have been shown to recognize the stress-induced MHC class I-related molecules MICA and MICB *(108,175)*. Further, autologous leukemia cells may stimulate the expansion of γδ T cells *(176)*. In vitro studies show that either freshly isolated or in vitro-activated γδ T cells mediate cytotoxicity against a variety of tumor targets including lymphoma *(177)*, myeloma *(174)*, glioblastoma multiforme *(178)*, and oral malignancies *(179)*. Indeed, tumor-infiltrating γδ T cells have been found in many human malignancies *(180–187)*. In one animal model, the accumulation of γδ T cells in tumor tissue was detrimental to antitumor activity, since they were found to secrete TGF-β and IL-10, which suppressed αβ T cells and NK cells. Removal of γδ T cells or antibody blockade of TGF-β and IL-10 improved antitumor CTL development and NK activity *(188)*.

Whether or not γδ T cells induce GVHD is not well established, since some clinical studies have found that γδ T cells are correlated with the onset of GVHD *(189)*, while others show that the loss of γδ T cells is associated with chronic GVHD *(190)*. Still others have found no significant correlation between GVHD and the numbers of γδ T cells in the infused stem cell graft *(191)*, during immune reconstitution *(192)*, or in GVHD lesions themselves *(193,194)*. Animal studies have been equally confusing since some implicate γδ T cells in the pathology of GVHD *(195–197)*, while others have shown that γδ T cells can be safely transplanted without GVHD *(198,199)*. In vitro studies have demonstrated that γδ T cells suppress alloreactivity through a veto mechanism *(200)*, suggesting that under some circumstances γδ T cells may be able to suppress active GVHD.

Very few studies have addressed the potential of γδ T cells to mediate GVL. Lamb and coworkers found that elevations in peripheral blood γδ T cells after T cell-depleted BMTs were associated with a significantly improved disease-free survival (88 vs 31%) at 30 mo posttransplant *(201)*. The antibody used to T cell deplete the BM in this study (T10B9) selectively depletes α/β T cells, suggesting that the γδ T cells in the infused marrow may be beneficial. Lastly, γδ T cells may play an important role in stem cell engraftment, since one group has shown a potential role in the facilitation of BM engraftment *(198,199)* and in the recovery of neutrophils after transplantation *(190)*.

8. CONCLUSION

Disease recurrence is the most common cause of treatment failure in BMT, and strategies aimed at reducing (or treating) relapse will have a significant impact on improving overall survival. It is clear that donor-derived lymphocytes play a crucial role in both the eradication of residual malignant cells and the induction of GVHD. Studies suggest that GVHD and GVL can be separable. Strategies aimed at preserving GVL activity and reducing GVHD are highly desirable. Here, we have tried to outline the preclinical data on various cell populations that

Table 3
Properties of the Various Cell Populations[a]

Cell type	Phenotype	% of PBLs	Expandability	Structures used for target recognition (on effector cells)	Counter receptors (on target cells)
Cytotoxic T cells	CD3$^+$CD8$^+$CD56$^-$TCRα/β$^+$	0.1–10%	Moderate	α/β TCR	MHC I
NK cells	CD3$^-$CD16$^+$CD56$^+$ TCR$^-$	5–10%	Poor	KIR, Ly49, NKG2, NCRs	MHC I and MHC I-like molecules
NK-T cells	CD3$^+$CD4$^{-/+}$CD8$^-$TCRα/β$^+$	~1%	Poor—moderate	α/β TCR	CD1
CIK cells	CD3$^+$CD8$^+$CD56$^+$ TCRα/β$^+$	n/a	Moderate—excellent	adhesion molecules, ? NKG2, ? other	?
γ/δ T cells	CD3$^+$CD4$^-$CD8$^-$TCRγ/δ$^+$	1–5%	Moderate—excellent	γ/δ TCR, ? NKG2D, ? other	Stress-related molecules, ? MICA and MICB, ? other

[a]Based on the predominate surface phenotype and approximate percentages of cells derived from either in murine or human studies.

may retain antitumor activities but have a reduced propensity for the induction of GVHD (Table 3). It is hoped that if purified populations of cells are adminstered to patients, this second generation of DLI will allow us to more accurately treat minimal residual disease with greater efficacy and reduced risk.

REFERENCES

1. Fefer A, Sullivan KM, Weiden P, et al. Graft versus leukemia effect in man: the relapse rate of acute leukemia is lower after allogeneic than after syngeneic marrow transplantation. *Prog Clin Biol Res* 1987;244:401–408.
2. Fefer A, Cheever MA, Greenberg PD. Identical-twin (syngeneic) marrow transplantation for hematologic cancers. *J Natl Cancer Inst* 1986;76:1269–1273.
3. Weiden PL, Flournoy N, Thomas ED, et al. Antileukemic effect of graft-versus-host disease in human recipients of allogeneic-marrow grafts. *N Engl J Med* 1979;300:1068–1073.
4. Gale RP, Horowitz MM, Ash RC, et al. Identical-twin bone marrow transplants for leukemia. *Ann Intern Med* 1994;120:646–652.
5. Fefer A, Buckner CD, Thomas ED, et al. Cure of hematologic neoplasia with transplantation of marrow from identical twins. *N Engl J Med* 1977;297:146–148.
6. Horowitz MM, Gale RP, Sondel PM, et al. Graft-versus-leukemia reactions after bone marrow transplantation. *Blood* 1990;75:555–562.
7. Appelbaum FR, Fefer A, Cheever MA, et al. Treatment of non-Hodgkin's lymphoma with marrow transplantation in identical twins. *Blood* 1981;58:509–513.
8. Sykes M, Preffer F, McAfee S, et al. Mixed lymphohaemopoietic chimerism and graft-versus-lymphoma effects after non-myeloablative therapy and HLA-mismatched bone-marrow transplantation. *Lancet* 1999;353:1755–1759.
9. Childs R, Epperson D, Bahceci E, Clave E, Barrett J. Molecular remission of chronic myeloid leukaemia following a non-myeloablative allogeneic peripheral blood stem cell transplant: in vivo and in vitro evidence for a graft-versus-leukaemia effect. *Br J Haematol* 1999;107:396–400.
10. Slavin S, Nagler A, Naparstek E, et al. Nonmyeloablative stem cell transplantation and cell therapy as an alternative to conventional bone marrow transplantation with lethal cytoreduction for the treatment of malignant and nonmalignant hematologic diseases. *Blood* 1998;91:756–763.
11. Champlin R, Khouri I, Giralt S. Graft-vs.-malignancy with allogeneic blood stem cell transplantation: a potential primary treatment modality. *Pediatr Transplant* 1999;3(Suppl 1):52–58.
12. Giralt S, Khouri I, Champlin R. Non myeloablative "mini transplants." *Cancer Treat Res* 1999;101:97–108.
13. Slavin S, Or R, Prighozina T, et al. Immunotherapy of hematologic malignancies and metastatic solid tumors in experimental animals and man. *Bone Marrow Transplant* 2000;25(Suppl 2):S54–57.
14. Champlin R, Khouri I, Shimoni A, et al. Harnessing graft-versus-malignancy: non-myeloablative preparative regimens for allogeneic haematopoietic transplantation, an evolving strategy for adoptive immunotherapy. *Br J Haematol* 2000;111:18–29.
15. Sullivan KM, Weiden PL, Storb R, et al. Influence of acute and chronic graft-versus-host disease on relapse and survival after bone marrow transplantation from HLA-identical siblings as treatment of acute and chronic leukemia. *Blood* 1989;73:1720–1728.
16. Ringden O, Labopin M, Gluckman E, et al. Graft-versus-leukemia effect in allogeneic marrow transplant recipients with acute leukemia is maintained using cyclosporin A combined with methotrexate as prophylaxis. Acute Leukemia Working Party of the European Group for Blood and Marrow Transplantation. *Bone Marrow Transplant* 1996;18:921–929.
17. Kolb HJ, Mittermuller J, Clemm C, et al. Donor leukocyte transfusions for treatment of recurrent chronic myelogenous leukemia in marrow transplant patients. *Blood* 1990;76:2462–2465.
18. Ringden O, Labopin M, Gorin NC, et al. Is there a graft-versus-leukaemia effect in the absence of graft-versus-host disease in patients undergoing bone marrow transplantation for acute leukaemia? *Br J Haematol* 2000;111:1130–1137.
19. Alyea EP, Soiffer RJ, Canning C, et al. Toxicity and efficacy of defined doses of CD4(+) donor lymphocytes for treatment of relapse after allogeneic bone marrow transplant. *Blood* 1998;91:3671–3680.
20. Mackinnon S, Papadopoulos EB, Carabasi MH, et al. Adoptive immunotherapy evaluating escalating doses of donor leukocytes for relapse of chronic myeloid leukemia after bone marrow transplantation: separation of graft-versus-leukemia responses from graft-versus-host disease. *Blood* 1995;86:1261–1268.
21. Patarroyo M, Prieto J, Rincon J, et al. Leukocyte-cell adhesion: a molecular process fundamental in leukocyte physiology. *Immunol Rev* 1990;114:67–108.
22. Young JD, Hengartner H, Podack ER, Cohn ZA. Purification and characterization of a cytolytic pore-forming protein from granules of cloned lymphocytes with natural killer activity. *Cell* 1986;44:849–859.

23. Young JD, Podack ER, Cohn ZA. Properties of a purified pore-forming protein (perforin 1) isolated from H-2-restricted cytotoxic T cell granules. *J Exp Med* 1986;164:144–155.

24. Trapani JA, Davis J, Sutton VR, Smyth MJ. Proapoptotic functions of cytotoxic lymphocyte granule constituents in vitro and in vivo. *Curr Opin Immunol* 2000;12:323–329.

25. Talanian RV, Yang X, Turbov J, et al. Granule-mediated killing: pathways for granzyme B-initiated apoptosis. *J Exp Med* 1997;186:1323–1331.

26. Sarin A, Haddad EK, Henkart PA. Caspase dependence of target cell damage induced by cytotoxic lymphocytes. *J Immunol* 1998;161:2810–2816.

27. Kam CM, Hudig D, Powers JC. Granzymes (lymphocyte serine proteases): characterization with natural and synthetic substrates and inhibitors. *Biochim Biophys Acta* 2000;1477:307–323.

28. Pena SV, Krensky AM. Granulysin, a new human cytolytic granule-associated protein with possible involvement in cell-mediated cytotoxicity. *Semin Immunol* 1997;9:117–125.

29. Gruss HJ, Boiani N, Williams DE, Armitage RJ, Smith CA, Goodwin RG. Pleiotropic effects of the CD30 ligand on CD30-expressing cells and lymphoma cell lines. *Blood* 1994;83:2045–2056.

30. Jumper MD, Nishioka Y, Davis LS, Lipsky PE, Meek K. Regulation of human B cell function by recombinant CD40 ligand and other TNF-related ligands. *J Immunol* 1995;155:2369–2378.

31. Ashkenazi A, Dixit VM. Apoptosis control by death and decoy receptors. *Curr Opin Cell Biol* 1999;11:255–260.

32. Smyth MJ, Cretney E, Takeda K, et al. Tumor necrosis factor-related apoptosis-inducing ligand (TRAIL) Contributes to interferon gamma-dependent natural killer cell protection from tumor metastasis. *J Exp Med* 2001;193:661–670.

33. Takeda K, Hayakawa Y, Smyth MJ, et al. Involvement of tumor necrosis factor-related apoptosis-inducing ligand in surveillance of tumor metastasis by liver natural killer cells. *Nat Med* 2001;7:94–100.

34. Takahashi T, Tanaka M, Brannan CI, et al. Generalized lymphoproliferative disease in mice, caused by a point mutation in the Fas ligand. *Cell* 1994;76:969–976.

35. Walczak H, Krammer PH. The CD95 (APO-1/Fas) and the TRAIL (APO-2L) apoptosis systems. *Exp Cell Res* 2000;256:58–66.

36. Abe K, Kurakin A, Mohseni-Maybodi M, Kay B, Khosravi-Far R. The complexity of TNF-related apoptosis-inducing ligand. *Ann NY Acad Sci* 2000;926:52–63.

37. Bossi G, Griffiths GM. Degranulation plays an essential part in regulating cell surface expression of Fas ligand in T cells and natural killer cells. *Nat Med* 1999;5:90–96.

38. Kayagaki N, Kawasaki A, Ebata T, et al. Metalloproteinase-mediated release of human Fas ligand. *J Exp Med* 1995;182:1777–17783.

39. Ashkenazi A, Pai RC, Fong S, et al. Safety and antitumor activity of recombinant soluble Apo2 ligand. *J Clin Invest* 1999;104:155–162.

40. Walczak H, Miller RE, Ariail K, et al. Tumoricidal activity of tumor necrosis factor-related apoptosis-inducing ligand in vivo. *Nat Med* 1999;5:157–63.

41. Wiley SR, Schooley K, Smolak PJ, et al. Identification and characterization of a new member of the TNF family that induces apoptosis. *Immunity* 1995;3:673–682.

42. Pitti RM, Marsters SA, Ruppert S, Donahue CJ, Moore A, Ashkenazi A. Induction of apoptosis by Apo-2 ligand, a new member of the tumor necrosis factor cytokine family. *J Biol Chem* 1996;271:12,687–12,690.

43. Jo M, Kim TH, Seol DW, et al. Apoptosis induced in normal human hepatocytes by tumor necrosis factor-related apoptosis-inducing ligand. *Nat Med* 2000;6:564–567.

44. Sebzda E, Mariathasan S, Ohteki T, Jones R, Bachmann MF, Ohashi PS. Selection of the T cell repertoire. *Annu Rev Immunol* 1999;17:829–874.

45. Engelhard VH. Structure of peptides associated with MHC class I molecules. *Curr Opin Immunol* 1994;6:13–23.

46. Rotzschke O, Falk K. Origin, structure and motifs of naturally processed MHC class II ligands. *Curr Opin Immunol* 1994;6:45–51.

47. Lanzavecchia A, Sallusto F. Dynamics of T lymphocyte responses: intermediates, effectors, and memory cells. *Science* 2000;290:92–97.

48. Moser M, Murphy KM. Dendritic cell regulation of TH1-TH2 development. *Nat Immunol* 2000;1:199–205.

49. Lanzavecchia A. How can cryptic epitopes trigger autoimmunity? *J Exp Med* 1995;181:1945–1948.

50. Robbins PF, Kawakami Y. Human tumor antigens recognized by T cells. *Curr Opin Immunol* 1996;8:628–636.

51. Disis ML, Cheever MA. Oncogenic proteins as tumor antigens. *Curr Opin Immunol* 1996;8:637–642.

52. Vonderheide RH, Hahn WC, Schultze JL, Nadler LM. The telomerase catalytic subunit is a widely expressed tumor-associated antigen recognized by cytotoxic T lymphocytes. *Immunity* 1999;10:673–679.

53. Wang F, Bade E, Kuniyoshi C, et al. Phase I trial of a MART-1 peptide vaccine with incomplete Freund's adjuvant for resected high-risk melanoma. *Clin Cancer Res* 1999;5:2756–2765.

54. Hsu FJ, Benike C, Fagnoni F, et al. Vaccination of patients with B-cell lymphoma using autologous antigen-pulsed dendritic cells. *Nat Med* 1996;2:52–58.

55. Lau R, Wang F, Jeffery G, et al. Phase I trial of intravenous peptide-pulsed dendritic cells in patients with metastatic melanoma. *J Immunother* 2001;24:66–78.

56. Rooney CM, Smith CA, Ng CY, et al. Infusion of cytotoxic T cells for the prevention and treatment of Epstein-Barr virus-induced lymphoma in allogeneic transplant recipients. *Blood* 1998;92:1549–1555.

57. Walter EA, Greenberg PD, Gilbert MJ, et al. Reconstitution of cellular immunity against cytomegalovirus in recipients of allogeneic bone marrow by transfer of T-cell clones from the donor. *N Engl J Med* 1995;333:1038–1044.

58. Choudhury A, Gajewski JL, Liang JC, et al. Use of leukemic dendritic cells for the generation of antileukemic cellular cytotoxicity against Philadelphia chromosome-positive chronic myelogenous leukemia. *Blood* 1997;89:1133–1142.

59. Cardoso AA, Seamon MJ, Afonso HM, et al. Ex vivo generation of human anti-pre-B leukemia-specific autologous cytolytic T cells. *Blood* 1997;90:549–561.

60. Mutis T, Schrama E, Melief CJ, Goulmy E. CD80-Transfected acute myeloid leukemia cells induce primary allogeneic T-cell responses directed at patient specific minor histocompatibility antigens and leukemia-associated antigens. *Blood* 1998;92:1677–1684.

61. Stripecke R, Cardoso AA, Pepper KA, et al. Lentiviral vectors for efficient delivery of CD80 and granulocyte-macrophage- colony-stimulating factor in human acute lymphoblastic leukemia and acute myeloid leukemia cells to induce antileukemic immune responses. *Blood* 2000;96:1317–1326.

62. Dunussi-Joannopoulos K, Runyon K, Erickson J, Schaub RG, Hawley RG, Leonard JP. Vaccines with interleukin-12-transduced acute myeloid leukemia cells elicit very potent therapeutic and long-lasting protective immunity. *Blood* 1999;94:4263–4273.

63. Dilloo D, Bacon K, Holden W, et al. Combined chemokine and cytokine gene transfer enhances antitumor immunity. *Nat Med* 1996;2:1090–1095.

64. Altman JD, Moss PA, Goulder PJ, et al. Phenotypic analysis of antigen-specific T lymphocytes. *Science* 1996;274:94–96.

65. Youde SJ, Dunbar PR, Evans EM, et al. Use of fluorogenic histocompatibility leukocyte antigen-A*0201/HPV 16 E7 peptide complexes to isolate rare human cytotoxic T-lymphocyte- recognizing endogenous human papillomavirus antigens. *Cancer Res* 2000;60:365–371.

66. Lee KH, Wang E, Nielsen MB, et al. Increased vaccine-specific T cell frequency after peptide-based vaccination correlates with increased susceptibility to in vitro stimulation but does not lead to tumor regression. *J Immunol* 1999;163:6292–6300.

67. Lee PP, Yee C, Savage PA, et al. Characterization of circulating T cells specific for tumor-associated antigens in melanoma patients. *Nat Med* 1999;5:677–685.

68. Molldrem JJ, Lee PP, Wang C, et al. Evidence that specific T lymphocytes may participate in the elimination of chronic myelogenous leukemia. *Nat Med* 2000;6:1018–1023.

69. Gao L, Yang TH, Tourdot S, Sadovnikova E, Hasserjian R, Stauss HJ. Allo-major histocompatibility complex-restricted cytotoxic T lymphocytes engraft in bone marrow transplant recipients without causing graft-versus-host disease. *Blood* 1999;94:2999–3006.

70. Anderson LD, Jr., Petropoulos D, Everse LA, Mullen CA. Enhancement of graft-versus-tumor activity and graft-versus-host disease by pretransplant immunization of allogeneic bone marrow donors with a recipient-derived tumor cell vaccine. *Cancer Res* 1999;59:1525–1530.

71. Sullivan JL, Byron KS, Brewster FE, Purtilo DT. Deficient natural killer cell activity in x-linked lymphoproliferative syndrome. *Science* 1980;210:543–545.

72. Merino F, Henle W, Ramirez-Duque P. Chronic active Epstein-Barr virus infection in patients with Chediak-Higashi syndrome. *J Clin Immunol* 1986;6:299–305.

73. Roder JC, Haliotis T, Klein M, et al. A new immunodeficiency disorder in humans involving NK cells. *Nature* 1980;284:553–555.

74. Roder JC, Haliotis T, Laing L, et al. Further studies of natural killer cell function in Chediak-Higashi patients. *Immunology* 1982;46:555–560.

75. Benoit L, Wang X, Pabst HF, Dutz J, Tan R. Defective NK cell activation in X-linked lymphoproliferative disease. *J Immunol* 2000;165:3549–3553.

76. Grimm EA, Mazumder A, Zhang HZ, Rosenberg SA. Lymphokine-activated killer cell phenomenon. Lysis of natural killer-resistant fresh solid tumor cells by interleukin 2-activated autologous human peripheral blood lymphocytes. *J Exp Med* 1982;155:1823–1841.

77. Teichmann JV, Ludwig WD, Thiel E. Cytotoxicity of interleukin 2-induced lymphokine-activated killer (LAK) cells against human leukemia and augmentation of killing by interferons and tumor necrosis factor. *Leuk Res* 1992;16:287–298.

78. Talmadge JE, Meyers KM, Prieur DJ, Starkey JR. Role of NK cells in tumour growth and metastasis in beige mice. *Nature* 1980;284:622–624.

79. Uharek L, Glass B, Gaska T, et al. Natural killer cells as effector cells of graft-versus-leukemia activity in a murine transplantation model. *Bone Marrow Transplant* 1993;12(Suppl 3):S57–60.

80. Rosenberg SA, Lotze MT, Muul LM, et al. Observations on the systemic administration of autologous lymphokine-activated killer cells and recombinant interleukin-2 to patients with metastatic cancer. *N Engl J Med* 1985;313:1485–1492.

81. Dillman RO, Oldham RK, Tauer KW, et al. Continuous interleukin-2 and lymphokine-activated killer cells for advanced cancer: a National Biotherapy Study Group trial. *J Clin Oncol* 1991;9:1233–1240.

82. Foon KA, Walther PJ, Bernstein ZP, et al. Renal cell carcinoma treated with continuous-infusion interleukin-2 with ex vivo-activated killer cells. *J Immunother* 1992;11:184–190.

83. Haruta I, Yamauchi K, Aruga A, et al. Analytical study of the clinical response to two distinct adoptive immunotherapies for advanced hepatocellular carcinoma: comparison between LAK cell and CTL therapy. *J Immunother Emphasis Tumor Immunol* 1996;19:218–223.

84. Sankhla SK, Nadkarni JS, Bhagwati SN. Adoptive immunotherapy using lymphokine-activated killer (LAK) cells and interleukin-2 for recurrent malignant primary brain tumors. *J Neurooncol* 1996;27:133–140.

85. Rosenberg SA, Lotze MT, Yang JC, et al. Prospective randomized trial of high-dose interleukin-2 alone or in conjunction with lymphokine-activated killer cells for the treatment of patients with advanced cancer. *J Natl Cancer* Inst 1993;85:622–632.

86. Yano T, Sugio K, Yamazaki K, et al. Postoperative adjuvant adoptive immunotherapy with lymph node-LAK cells and IL-2 for pathologic stage I non-small cell lung cancer. *Lung Cancer* 1999;26:143–148.

87. Siegel JP, Puri RK. Interleukin-2 toxicity. *J Clin Oncol* 1991;9:694–704.

88. Long EO. Regulation of immune responses through inhibitory receptors. *Annu Rev Immunol* 1999;17:875–904.

89. Lanier LL. NK cell receptors. *Annu Rev Immunol* 1998;16:359–393.

90. Ljunggren HG, Karre K. Host resistance directed selectively against H-2-deficient lymphoma variants. Analysis of the mechanism. *J Exp Med* 1985;162:1745–1759.

91. Tamir I, Dal Porto JM, Cambier JC. Cytoplasmic protein tyrosine phosphatases SHP-1 and SHP-2: regulators of B cell signal transduction. *Curr Opin Immunol* 2000;12:307–315.

92. Rohrschneider LR, Fuller JF, Wolf I, Liu Y, Lucas DM. Structure, function, and biology of SHIP proteins. *Genes Dev* 2000;14:505–520.

93. Lanier LL. Turning on natural killer cells. *J Exp Med* 2000;191:1259–1262.

94. Wu J, Song Y, Bakker AB, et al. An activating immunoreceptor complex formed by NKG2D and DAP10. *Science* 1999;285:730–732.

95. Nakajima H, Colonna M. 2B4: an NK cell activating receptor with unique specificity and signal transduction mechanism. *Hum Immunol* 2000;61:39–43.

96. Pende D, Cantoni C, Rivera P, et al. Role of NKG2D in tumor cell lysis mediated by human NK cells: cooperation with natural cytotoxicity receptors and capability of recognizing tumors of nonepithelial origin. *Eur J Immunol* 2001;31:1076–1086.

97. Westgaard IH, Berg SF, Orstavik S, Fossum S, Dissen E. Identification of a human member of the Ly-49 multigene family. *Eur J Immunol* 1998;28:1839–1846.

98. McQueen KL, Freeman JD, Takei F, Mager DL. Localization of five new Ly49 genes, including three closely related to Ly49c. *Immunogenetics* 1998;48:174–183.

99. Gosselin P, Mason LH, Willette-Brown J, Ortaldo JR, McVicar DW, Anderson SK. Induction of DAP12 phosphorylation, calcium mobilization, and cytokine secretion by Ly49H. *J Leukoc Biol* 1999;66:165–171.

100. Chang C, Rodriguez A, Carretero M, Lopez-Botet M, Phillips JH, Lanier LL. Molecular characterization of human CD94: a type II membrane glycoprotein related to the C-type lectin superfamily. *Eur J Immunol* 1995;25:2433–2437.

101. Vance RE, Tanamachi DM, Hanke T, Raulet DH. Cloning of a mouse homolog of CD94 extends the family of C-type lectins on murine natural killer cells. *Eur J Immunol* 1997;27:3236–3241.

102. Kurepa Z, Hasemann CA, Forman J. Qa-1b binds conserved class I leader peptides derived from several mammalian species. *J Exp Med* 1998;188:973–978.

103. Vance RE, Kraft JR, Altman JD, Jensen PE, Raulet DH. Mouse CD94/NKG2A is a natural killer cell receptor for the nonclassical major histocompatibility complex (MHC) class I molecule Qa-1(b). *J Exp Med* 1998;188:1841–1848.

104. Braud VM, Allan DS, O'Callaghan CA, et al. HLA-E binds to natural killer cell receptors CD94/NKG2A, B and C. *Nature* 1998;391:795–799.

105. Glienke J, Sobanov Y, Brostjan C, et al. The genomic organization of NKG2C, E, F, and D receptor genes in the human natural killer gene complex. *Immunogenetics* 1998;48:163–173.

106. Bauer S, Groh V, Wu J, et al. Activation of NK cells and T cells by NKG2D, a receptor for stress-inducible MICA. *Science* 1999;285:727–729.

107. Groh V, Bahram S, Bauer S, Herman A, Beauchamp M, Spies T. Cell stress-regulated human major histocompatibility complex class I gene expressed in gastrointestinal epithelium. *Proc Natl Acad Sci USA* 1996;93:12,445–12,450.

108. Groh V, Rhinehart R, Secrist H, Bauer S, Grabstein KH, Spies T. Broad tumor-associated expression and recognition by tumor-derived gamma delta T cells of MICA and MICB. *Proc Natl Acad Sci USA* 1999;96:6879–6884.

109. Diefenbach A, Jamieson AM, Liu SD, Shastri N, Raulet DH. Ligands for the murine NKG2D receptor: expression by tumor cells and activation of NK cells and macrophages. *Nat Immunol* 2000;1:119–126.

110. Cerwenka A, Bakker AB, McClanahan T, et al. Retinoic acid early inducible genes define a ligand family for the activating NKG2D receptor in mice. *Immunity* 2000;12:721–727.

111. Moretta A, Bottino C, Vitale M, et al. Activating receptors and coreceptors involved in human natural killer cell-mediated cytolysis. *Annu Rev Immunol* 2001;19:197–223.

112. Sivori S, Pende D, Bottino C, et al. NKp46 is the major triggering receptor involved in the natural cytotoxicity of fresh or cultured human NK cells. Correlation between surface density of NKp46 and natural cytotoxicity against autologous, allogeneic or xenogeneic target cells. *Eur J Immunol* 1999;29:1656–1666.

113. Sivori S, Vitale M, Morelli L, et al. p46, a novel natural killer cell-specific surface molecule that mediates cell activation. *J Exp Med* 1997;186:1129–1136.

114. Pessino A, Sivori S, Bottino C, et al. Molecular cloning of NKp46: a novel member of the immunoglobulin superfamily involved in triggering of natural cytotoxicity. *J Exp Med* 1998;188:953–960.

115. Pende D, Parolini S, Pessino A, et al. Identification and molecular characterization of NKp30, a novel triggering receptor involved in natural cytotoxicity mediated by human natural killer cells. *J Exp Med* 1999;190:1505–1516.

116. Cantoni C, Bottino C, Vitale M, et al. NKp44, a triggering receptor involved in tumor cell lysis by activated human natural killer cells, is a novel member of the immunoglobulin superfamily. *J Exp Med* 1999;189:787–796.

117. Vitale M, Bottino C, Sivori S, et al. NKp44, a novel triggering surface molecule specifically expressed by activated natural killer cells, is involved in non-major histocompatibility complex-restricted tumor cell lysis. *J Exp Med* 1998;187:2065–2072.

118. Vitale M, Falco M, Castriconi R, et al. Identification of NKp80, a novel triggering molecule expressed by human NK cells. *Eur J Immunol* 2001;31:233–242.

119. , Asai O, Longo DL, Tian ZG, et al. Suppression of graft-versus-host disease and amplification of graft-versus-tumor effects by activated natural killer cells after allogeneic bone marrow transplantation. *J Clin Invest* 1998;101:1835–1842.

120. Aversa F, Tabilio A, Velardi A, et al. Treatment of high-risk acute leukemia with T-cell-depleted stem cells from related donors with one fully mismatched HLA haplotype. *N Engl J Med* 1998;339:1186–1193.

121. Ruggeri L, Capanni M, Casucci M, et al. Role of natural killer cell alloreactivity in HLA-mismatched hematopoietic stem cell transplantation. *Blood* 1999;94:333–339.

122. Ruggeri L, Capanni M, Urbani E, et al. KIR epitope incompatibility in the GvH direction predicts control of leukemia relapse after mismatched hematopoietic transplantation. *Blood* 2000;96:479a.

123. Bendelac A, Rivera MN, Park SH, Roark JH. Mouse CD1-specific NK1 T cells: development, specificity, and function. *Annu Rev Immunol* 1997;15:535–562.

124. Watanabe H, Iiai T, Kimura M, et al. Characterization of intermediate TCR cells in the liver of mice with respect to their unique IL-2R expression. *Cell Immunol* 1993;149:331–342.

125. Eberl G, Lees R, Smiley ST, Taniguchi M, Grusby MJ, MacDonald HR. Tissue-specific segregation of CD1d-dependent and CD1d-independent NK T cells. *J Immunol* 1999;162:6410–641.

126. Ortaldo JR, Winkler-Pickett R, Mason AT, Mason LH. The Ly-49 family: regulation of cytotoxicity and cytokine production in murine CD3+ cells. *J Immunol* 1998;160:1158–1165.

127. Sakamoto A, Oishi Y, Kurasawa K, Kita Y, Saito Y, Iwamoto I. Characteristics of T-cell receptor Valpha24JalphaQ T cells, a human counterpart of murine NK1 T cells, from normal subjects. *J Allergy Clin Immunol* 1999;103:S445–451.

128. Godfrey DI, Hammond KJ, Poulton LD, Smyth MJ, Baxter AG. NKT cells: facts, functions and fallacies. *Immunol Today* 2000;21:573–583.

129. Benlagha K, Weiss A, Beavis A, Teyton L, Bendelac A. In vivo identification of glycolipid antigen-specific T cells using fluorescent CD1d tetramers. *J Exp Med* 2000;191:1895–1903.

130. Kawano T, Cui J, Koezuka Y, et al. CD1d-restricted and TCR-mediated activation of valpha14 NKT cells by glycosylceramides. *Science* 1997;278:1626–1629.

131. Hammond K, Cain W, van Driel I, Godfrey D. Three day neonatal thymectomy selectively depletes NK1.1+ T cells. *Int Immunol* 1998;10:1491–1499.

132. Coles MC, Raulet DH. NK1.1+ T cells in the liver arise in the thymus and are selected by interactions with class I molecules on CD4+CD8+ cells. *J Immunol* 2000;164:2412–2418.

133. Hammond KJ, Pelikan SB, Crowe NY, et al. NKT cells are phenotypically and functionally diverse. *Eur J Immunol* 1999;29:3768–3781.

134. Zeng D, Gazit G, Dejbakhsh-Jones S, et al. Heterogeneity of NK1.1+ T cells in the bone marrow: divergence from the thymus. *J Immunol* 1999;163:5338–5345.

135. Emoto M, Zerrahn J, Miyamoto M, Perarnau B, Kaufmann SH. Phenotypic characterization of CD8(+)NKT cells. *Eur J Immunol* 2000;30:2300–2311.

136. Dellabona P, Casorati G, Friedli B, et al. In vivo persistence of expanded clones specific for bacterial antigens within the human T cell receptor alpha/beta CD4-8- subset. *J Exp Med* 1993;177:1763–1771.

137. Ishihara S, Nieda M, Kitayama J, et al. Alpha-glycosylceramides enhance the antitumor cytotoxicity of hepatic lymphocytes obtained from cancer patients by activating CD3-CD56+ NK cells in vitro. *J Immunol* 2000;165:1659–1664.

138. Prussin C, Foster B. TCR V alpha 24 and V beta 11 coexpression defines a human NK1 T cell analog containing a unique Th0 subpopulation. *J Immunol* 1997;159:5862–5870.

139. Van Der Vliet HJ, Nishi N, Koezuka Y, et al. Effects of alpha-galactosylceramide (KRN7000), interleukin-12 and interleukin-7 on phenotype and cytokine profile of human Valpha24+ Vbeta11+ T cells. *Immunology* 1999;98:557–563.

140. Takahashi T, Nieda M, Koezuka Y, et al. Analysis of human V alpha 24+ CD4+ NKT cells activated by alpha-glycosylceramide-pulsed monocyte-derived dendritic cells. *J Immunol* 2000;164:4458–4464.

141. van der Vliet HJ, Nishi N, Koezuka Y, et al. Potent expansion of human natural killer T cells using alpha-galactosylceramide (KRN7000)-loaded monocyte-derived dendritic cells, cultured in the presence of IL-7 and IL-15. *J Immunol Methods* 2001;247:61–72.

142. Gumperz JE, Roy C, Makowska A, et al. Murine CD1d-restricted T cell recognition of cellular lipids. *Immunity* 2000;12:211–221.

143. Eberl G, Lowin-Kropf B, MacDonald HR. Cutting edge: NKT cell development is selectively impaired in Fyn- deficient mice. *J Immunol* 1999;163:4091–4094.

144. Toura I, Kawano T, Akutsu Y, Nakayama T, Ochiai T, Taniguchi M. Cutting edge: inhibition of experimental tumor metastasis by dendritic cells pulsed with alpha-galactosylceramide. *J Immunol* 1999;163:2387–2391.

145. Cui J, Shin T, Kawano T, et al. Requirement for Valpha14 NKT cells in IL-12-mediated rejection of tumors. *Science* 1997;278:1623–1626.

146. Eberl G, MacDonald HR. Selective induction of NK cell proliferation and cytotoxicity by activated NKT cells. *Eur J Immunol* 2000;30:985–992.

147. Carnaud C, Lee D, Donnars O, et al. Cutting edge: cross-talk between cells of the innate immune system: NKT cells rapidly activate NK cells. *J Immunol* 1999;163:4647–4650.

148. Exley M, Porcelli S, Furman M, Garcia J, Balk S. CD161 (NKR-P1A) costimulation of CD1d-dependent activation of human T cells expressing invariant V alpha 24 J alpha Q T cell receptor alpha chains. *J Exp Med* 1998;188:867–876.

149. Nicol A, Nieda M, Koezuka Y, et al. Human invariant valpha24+ natural killer T cells activated by alpha-galactosylceramide (KRN7000) have cytotoxic anti-tumour activity through mechanisms distinct from T cells and natural killer cells. *Immunology* 2000;99:229–234.

150. Tamada K, Harada M, Abe K, et al. Immunosuppressive activity of cloned natural killer (NK1.1+) T cells established from murine tumor-infiltrating lymphocytes. *J Immunol* 1997;158:4846–4854.

151. Terabe M, Matsui S, Noben-Trauth N, et al. NKT cell-mediated repression of tumor immunosurveillance by IL-13 and the IL-4R-STAT6 pathway. *Nat Immunol* 2000;1:515–520.

152. Zeng D, Lewis D, Dejbakhsh-Jones S, et al. Bone marrow NK1.1(-) and NK1.1(+) T cells reciprocally regulate acute graft versus host disease. *J Exp Med* 1999;189:1073–1081.

153. Onoe Y, Harada M, Tamada K, et al. Involvement of both donor cytotoxic T lymphocytes and host NK1.1+ T cells in the thymic atrophy of mice suffering from acute graft-versus- host disease. *Immunology* 1998;95:248–256.

154. Baume DM, Caligiuri MA, Manley TJ, Daley JF, Ritz J. Differential expression of CD8 alpha and CD8 beta associated with MHC-restricted and non-MHC-restricted cytolytic effector cells. *Cell Immunol* 1990;131:352–365.

155. Schmidt-Wolf I, Lefterova P, Johnston V, Jihn D, Blume K, Negrin R. Propagation of large number of T cells with natural killer cell markers. *Br J Haematol* 1994;87:453–458.

156. Schmidt-Wolf IG, Lefterova P, Mehta BA, et al. Phenotypic characterization and identification of effector cells involved in tumor cell recognition of cytokine-induced killer cells. *Exp Hematol* 1993;21:1673–1679.

157. Schmidt-Wolf IGH, Negrin RS, Kiem HP, Blume KG, Weissman IL. Use of a SCID mouse/human lymphoma model to evaluate cytokine-induced killer cells with potent anti-tumor activity. *J Exp Med* 1991;139–149.

158. Lu PH, Negrin RS. A novel population of expanded human CD3+CD56+ cells derived from T cells with potent in vivo antitumor activity in mice with severe combined immunodeficiency. *J Immunol* 1994;153:1687–1696.

159. Lopez RD, Waller EK, Lu PH, Negrin RS. CD58/LFA-3 and IL-12 provided by activated monocytes are critical in the in vitro expansion of CD56+ T cells. *Cancer Immunol Immunother* 2001;49:629–640.

160. Zoll B, Lefterova P, Ebert O, Huhn D, Von Ruecker A, Schmidt-Wolf IG. Modulation of cell surface markers on NK-like T lymphocytes by using IL- 2, IL-7 or IL-12 in vitro stimulation. *Cytokine* 2000;12:1385–1390.

161. Hoyle C, Bangs CD, Chang P, Janek O, Mehta B, Negrin RS. Expansion of philadelphia chromosome-negative CD3+CD56+ cytotoxic cells from chronic myeloid leukemia patients: *in vitro* an *in vivo* efficacy in severe combined immunodeficiency disease mice. *Blood* 1998;92:3318–3327.

162. Alvarnas JC, Linn YC, Hope EG, Negrin RS. Expansion of cytotoxic CD3+ CD56+ cells from peripheral blood progenitor cells of patients undergoing autologous hematopoietic cell transplantation. *Biol Blood Marrow* Transplant 2001;7:216–222.

163. Mehta BA, Schmidt-Wolf IG, Weissman IL, Negrin RS. Two pathways of exocytosis of cytoplasmic granule contents and target cell killing by cytokine-induced CD3+ CD56+ killer cells. *Blood* 1995;86:3493–3499.

164. Baker J, Verneris MR, Ito M, Shizuru JA, Negrin RS. Expansion of cytolytic CD8(+) natural killer T cells with limited capacity for graft-versus-host disease induction due to interferon gamma production. *Blood* 2001;97:2923–2931.

165. Verneris MR, Ito M, Baker J, Arshi A, Negrin RS. Engineering hematopoietic grafts: purified allogeneic hematopoietic stem cells plus expanded CD8+NK-T cells in the treatment of lymphoma. *Biol Blood Marrow Transplant* 2001;10:532–542.

166. Zeller JC, Panoskaltsis-Mortari A, Murphy WJ, et al. Induction of CD4+ T cell alloantigen-specific hyporesponsiveness by IL- 10 and TGF-beta. *J Immunol* 1999;163:3684–3691.

167. Yang YG, Dey BR, Sergio JJ, Pearson DA, Sykes M. Donor-derived interferon gamma is required for inhibition of acute graft-versus-host disease by interleukin 12. *J Clin Invest* 1998;102:2126–2135.

168. Takayama T, Sekine T, Makuuchi M, et al. Adoptive immunotherapy to lower postsurgical recurrence rates of hepatocellular carcinoma: a randomised trial. *Lancet* 2000;356:802–807.

169. Chien YH, Jores R, Crowley MP. Recognition by gamma/delta T cells. *Ann Rev Immunol* 1996;14:511–532.

170. Rock EP, Sibbald PR, Davis MM, Chien YH. CDR3 length in antigen-specific immune receptors. *J Exp Med* 1994;179:323–328.

171. Born W, Cady C, Jones-Carson J, Mukasa A, Lahn M, O'Brien R. Immunoregulatory functions of gamma delta T cells. *Adv Immunol* 1999;71:77–144.

172. Kunzmann V, Bauer E, Wilhelm M. Gamma/delta T-cell stimulation by pamidronate. *N Engl J Med* 1999;340:737,738.

173. Dhodapkar MV, Singh J, Mehta J, et al. Anti-myeloma activity of pamidronate in vivo. *Br J Haematol* 1998;103:530–532.

174. Kunzmann V, Bauer E, Feurle J, Weissinger F, Tony HP, Wilhelm M. Stimulation of gammadelta T cells by aminobisphosphonates and induction of antiplasma cell activity in multiple myeloma. *Blood* 2000;96:384–392.

175. Groh V, Steinle A, Bauer S, Spies T. Recognition of stress-induced MHC molecules by intestinal epithelial gammadelta T cells. *Science* 1998;279:1737–1740.

176. Duval M, Yotnda P, Bensussan A, et al. Potential antileukemic effect of gamma delta T cells in acute lymphoblastic leukemia. *Leukemia* 1995;9:863–868.

177. Fisch P, Meuer E, Pende D, et al. Control of B cell lymphoma recognition via natural killer inhibitory receptors implies a role for human Vgamma9/Vdelta2 T cells in tumor immunity. *Eur J Immunol* 1997;27:3368–3379.

178. Fujimiya Y, Suzuki Y, Katakura R, et al. In vitro interleukin 12 activation of peripheral blood CD3(+)CD56(+) and CD3(+)CD56(-) gammadelta T cells from glioblastoma patients. *Clin Cancer Res* 1997;3:633–643.

179. Laad AD, Thomas ML, Fakih AR, Chiplunkar SV. Human gamma delta T cells recognize heat shock protein-60 on oral tumor cells. *Int J Cancer* 1999;80:709–714.

180. Bachelez H, Flageul B, Degos L, Boumsell L, Bensussan A. TCR gamma delta bearing T lymphocytes infiltrating human primary cutaneous melanomas. *J Invest Dermatol* 1992;98:369–374.

181. Honda S, Sakamoto Y, Fujime M, Kitagawa R. Immunohistochemical study of tumor-infiltrating lympho-cytes before and after intravesical bacillus Calmette-Guérin treatment for superficial bladder cancer. *Int J Urol* 1997;4:68-73.

182. Kitayama J, Atomi Y, Nagawa H, et al. Functional analysis of TCR gamma delta+ T cells in tumour-infiltrating lymphocytes (TIL) of human pancreatic cancer. *Clin Exp Immunol* 1993;93:442–447.

183. Kowalczyk D, Skorupski W, Kwias Z, Nowak J. Flow cytometric analysis of tumour-infiltrating lymphocytes in patients with renal cell carcinoma. *Br J Urol* 1997;80:543–547.

184. Knowles G, O'Neil BW, Campo MS. Phenotypical characterization of lymphocytes infiltrating regressing papillomas. *J Virol* 1996;70:8451–8458.

185. Kluin-Nelemans JC, Kester MG, Oving I, Cluitmans FH, Willemze R, Falkenburg JH. Abnormally activated T lymphocytes in the spleen of patients with hairy-cell leukemia. *Leukemia* 1994;8:2095–2101.

186. Watanabe N, Hizuta A, Tanaka N, Orita K. Localization of T cell receptor (TCR)-gamma delta + T cells into human colorectal cancer: flow cytometric analysis of TCR-gamma delta expression in tumour-infiltrating lymphocytes. *Clin Exp Immunol* 1995;102:167–173.

187. Zhao X, Wei YQ, Kariya Y, Teshigawara K, Uchida A. Accumulation of gamma/delta T cells in human dysgerminoma and seminoma: roles in autologous tumor killing and granuloma formation. *Immunol Invest* 1995;24:607–618.

188. Seo N, Tokura Y, Takigawa M, Egawa K. Depletion of IL-10- and TGF-beta-producing regulatory gamma delta T cells by administering a daunomycin-conjugated specific monoclonal antibody in early tumor lesions augments the activity of CTLs and NK cells. *J Immunol* 1999;163:242–249.

189. Viale M, Ferrini S, Bacigalupo A. TCR gamma/delta positive lymphocytes after allogeneic bone marrow transplantation. *Bone Marrow Transplant* 1992;10:249–253.
190. Yabe M, Yabe H, Hattori K, et al. Transition of T cell receptor gamma/delta expressing double negative (CD4-/CD8-) lymphocytes after allogeneic bone marrow transplantation. *Bone Marrow Transplant* 1994;14:741–746.
191. Cela ME, Holladay MS, Rooney CM, et al. Gamma delta T lymphocyte regeneration after T lymphocyte-depleted bone marrow transplantation from mismatched family members or matched unrelated donors. *Bone Marrow Transplant* 1996;17:243–247.
192. Kawanishi Y, Passweg J, Drobyski WR, et al. Effect of T cell subset dose on outcome of T cell-depleted bone marrow transplantation. *Bone Marrow Transplant* 1997;19:1069–1077.
193. Norton J, al-Saffar N, Sloane JP. An immunohistological study of gamma/delta lymphocytes in human cutaneous graft-versus-host disease. *Bone Marrow Transplant* 1991;7:205–208.
194. Norton J, al-Saffar N, Sloane JP. Immunohistological study of distribution of gamma/delta lymphocytes after allogeneic bone marrow transplantation. *J Clin Pathol* 1992;45:1027,1028.
195. Blazar BR, Taylor PA, Panoskaltsis-Mortari A, Barrett TA, Bluestone JA, Vallera DA. Lethal murine graft-versus-host disease induced by donor gamma/delta expressing T cells with specificity for host nonclassical major histocompatibility complex class Ib antigens. *Blood* 1996;87:827–837.
196. Ellison CA, MacDonald GC, Rector ES, Gartner JG. Gamma delta T cells in the pathobiology of murine acute graft-versus-host disease. Evidence that gamma delta T cells mediate natural killer-like cytotoxicity in the host and that elimination of these cells from donors significantly reduces mortality. *J Immunol* 1995;155:4189–4198.
197. Sakai T, Ohara-Inagaki K, Tsuzuki T, Yoshikai Y. Host intestinal intraepithelial gamma delta T lymphocytes present during acute graft-versus-host disease in mice may contribute to the development of enteropathy. *Eur J Immunol* 1995;25:87–91.
198. Drobyski WR, Majewski D. Donor gamma delta T lymphocytes promote allogeneic engraftment across the major histocompatibility barrier in mice. *Blood* 1997;89:1100–1109.
199. Drobyski WR, Majewski D, Hanson G. Graft-facilitating doses of ex vivo activated gammadelta T cells do not cause lethal murine graft-vs.-host disease. *Biol Blood Marrow Transplant* 1999;5:222–230.
200. Nagai M, Azuma E, Qi J, et al. Suppression of alloreactivity with gamma delta T-cells: relevance to increased gamma delta T-cells following bone marrow transplantation. *Biomed Pharmacother* 1998;52:137–142.
201. Lamb LS, Jr., Henslee-Downey PJ, Parrish RS, et al. Increased frequency of TCR gamma delta + T cells in disease-free survivors following T cell-depleted, partially mismatched, related donor bone marrow transplantation for leukemia. *J Hematother* 1996;5:503–509.
202. Moretta L, Biassoni R, Bottino C, Mingari MC, Moretta A. Human NK-cell receptors. *Immunol Today* 2000;21:420–422.
203. Young NT. Kir genes, killer cells and clinical transplantation. *Transplantation* 1999;68:1626–1628.
204. Long E, Colonna M, Lanier L. Protein Reviews On The Web (PROW). KIR. [National Cancer Institute and National Center for Biotechnology Information]. Available at: (http://www.ncbi.nlm.nih.gov/prow/guide/679664748_g.htm). Accessed June 2, 2001.

26 Dendritic Cells

Immunobiology and Potential Use for Cancer Immunotherapy

David Avigan, MD

CONTENTS

1. INTRODUCTION

Dendritic cells (DCs) represent a complex network of antigen-presenting cells that play a crucial role in the initiation of primary immunity as well as maintaining the balance between immune tolerance and reactivity *(1)*. Skin DCs were first described by Langerhans in 1868, but their function remained a mystery for the next 100 yr. The modern field of DC biology was initiated in 1973 by Steinman and Cohn, who identified a subpopulation of murine splenocytes that had distinctive morphologic and phenotypic characteristics and powerfully stimulated T cell responses *(2)*. DCs have subsequently been described as the most potent antigen-presenting cell which demonstrate the unique capacity to induce primary immune responses. Antigen-presenting cells process protein into peptide epitopes which are subsequently presented in the context of MHC molecules *(3)*. Endogenous proteins undergo processing in the cell cytoplasm and are typically presented in the context of MHC class I molecules resulting in the stimulation of cytotoxic T lymphocyte (CTL) responses. In contrast, exogenous antigens are internalized, processed in MHC class II compartments, and subsequently presented to CD4 (helper) T cells.

From: *Current Clinical Oncology: Allogeneic Stem Cell Transplantation*
Edited by: Mary S. Laughlin and Hillard M. Lazarus © Humana Press Inc., Totowa, NJ

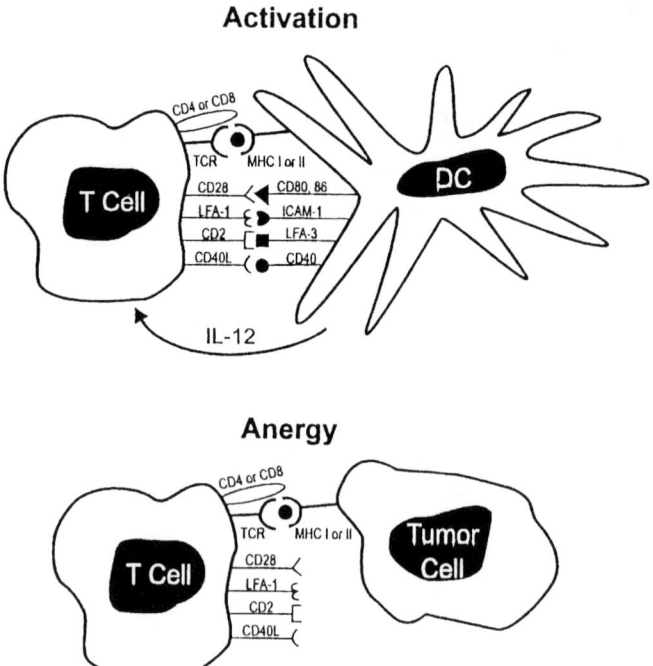

Fig. 1. DCs: immunobiology and potential use of cancer immunotherapy.

In specific settings, cross priming occurs in which antigens from donor cells are captured by antigen-presenting cells and presented in the context of MHC class I molecules *(4)*. Stimulation of naïve T cells requires antigen presentation in the context of co-stimulatory and adhesion molecules, which serve as secondary signals needed for the activation of primary immunity. Antigen-presenting cells, such as B cells and macrophages, are effective in maintaining immune responses, but are incapable of initiating primary responses to novel antigens. In contrast, DC richly express MHC class I, II, co-stimulatory and adhesion molecules and are uniquely potent in initiating cellular immunity (Fig. 1) *(5–7)*.

DCs have emerged as an area of intense interest in the fields of tumor immunotherapy and transplant biology. Tumor cells have been shown to express unique antigens not found in normal adult tissue, allowing for their recognition by host immunity *(8)*. T cells with the capacity to recognize tumor antigens have been identified in the repertoire of patients with malignancy *(9–11)*. However, productive responses are generally not seen, because tumor cells present antigen in the absence of secondary signals necessary for the initiation of primary immunity (Fig. 1) *(12)*. A major focus of tumor immunotherapy has been the use of DCs to reverse tumor-induced anergy by the presentation of antigen in the context of co-stimulatory molecules. DCs manipulated to express tumor antigens have been shown to induce tumor-specific immunity in preclinical animal and human studies, and are now being studied in clinical trials *(13–20)*. Although DCs represent only a small fraction of circulating mononuclear cells, large numbers of DCs can been generated from precursor populations derived from blood, marrow, and cord blood, allowing for the potential clinical use for immunotherapy *(21–24)*.

DCs are essential in the development of tolerance toward self antigens as well as the rejection of allogeneic tissue *(25,26)*. Dendritic cell subpopulations are thought to regulate the presentation of allo-antigens following transplant as well as mediate the deletion of auto-reactive T cell clones through negative selection. As such, the role of DC in modulating

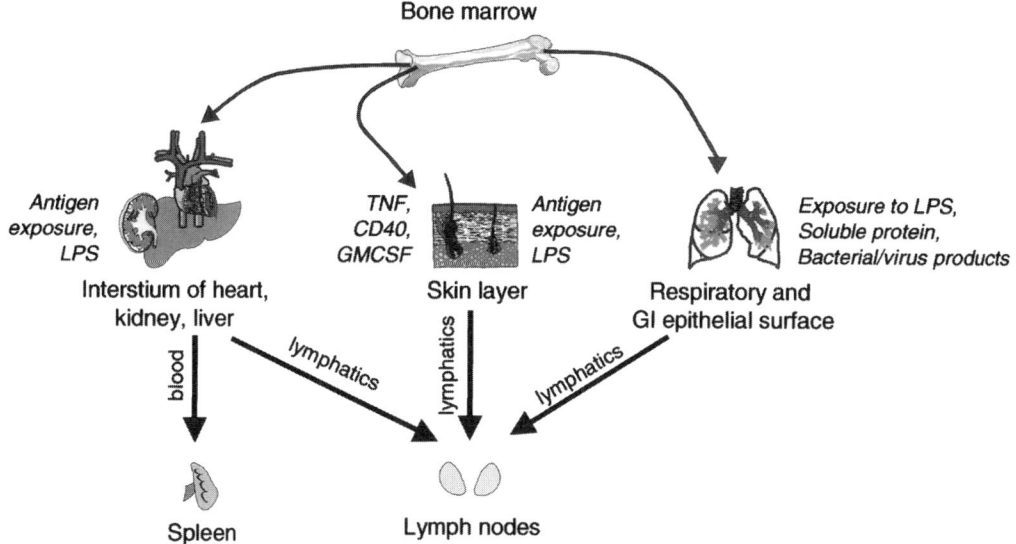

Fig. 2. DCs: immunobiology and potential use of cancer immunotherapy.

rejection and graft-vs-host disease following allogeneic hematopoietic stem cells transplantation has recently been the subject of intense study. In addition, the recovery of DC function following hematopoietic stem cell transplantation and the implications for immune reconstitution are being explored.

This review will focus on hematopoieitic development of myeloid DCs and its intimate link with antigen processing and presentation. Strategies to generate DC populations from precursor populations in vitro and their use in generating tumor vaccines in animal and human models will be analyzed. Preliminary efforts to translate DC-based immunotherapy into the clinical setting will be reviewed. Studies of DC immunobiology in the setting of hematopoietic stem cell transplantation will be reviewed.

2. PHENOTYPIC CHARACTERISTICS OF IMMATURE DCS: TISSUE LOCALIZATION, MIGRATORY PATTERNS, AND FUNCTIONAL PROPERTIES

DCs pass through a complex life cycle, in which their phenotypic characteristics evolve with maturation (Fig. 2) *(27)*. DCs originate from marrow progenitors and subsequently migrate to sites of exposure to foreign antigens. Upon antigen capture, DCs undergo maturation and concurrently migrate to areas of lymphocyte traffic. DCs initiate primary immunity through the selection and stimulation of antigen-specific CTL and activation of CD4+ helper cells that further modulate cellular and humoral immune responses. DCs educate lymphocytes to home towards sites of tissue injury and may subsequently undergo apoptosis following completion of this interaction.

Chimeric murine transplant models have confirmed that DCs develop from bone marrow progenitors *(28)*. In murine studies, DCs have been shown to differentiate from myeloid and lymphoid precursor populations. Lymphoid-derived DCs express $CD8_a$ and share a common precursor with T cells, B cells, and natural killer (NK) cells *(29–31,32)*. Myeloid DC progenitors are defined by the absence of $CD8_a$ expression and exquisite sensitivity to granulocyte-macrophage colony-stimulating factor (GM-CSF).

In humans, DCs differentiate from marrow-derived CD34+ precursors and migrate to sites of antigen uptake *(6)*. DC are found in the epithelial surface of the skin, gastrointestinal tract, and lung, as well as the interstium of all organs with the exception of the immunopriveleged sites of the brain, testis, and eye *(1,33)*. The precise mechanisms that are responsible for the recruitment and localization of DCs in tissue has not been fully elucidated, but appears to be related to intrinsic features of the progenitor cells, as well as the release of cytokine and inflammatory signals. The presence of a "skin homing receptor" on a subset of CD34+ cells is associated with their subsequent migration to the epidermis and their acquisition of phenotype of a Langerhans cell (LC) *(34)*. Expression of E-cadherin by LCs facilitates the binding of these cells into the epidermal layer *(35)*. Intradermal injection of GM-CSF also results in the increased numbers of immature DCs in the skin *(36)*. The migration of DCs into the brochoepithelium is induced by the presence of aerosolized lipopolysaccharide (LPS), soluble protein, bacterial or viral products, or the release of GM-CSF secondary to local inflammation or by pulmonary tumors. Systemic administration of LPS results in the localization of DCs to the interstitium of the heart and kidney. The migration of DCs to the liver is induced by the release of cytokines following the ingestion of colloidal carbon by hepatic kupfer cells. In mouse models, accumulation of immature DCs in the liver and dermis has been demonstrated following exposure to Flt3 ligand (Flt3L) *(37,38)*. Animals treated with daily injections of Flt3L had a dramatic increase in cells expressing class II, CD11c, DEC205, and CD86. DCs were numerically increased in the bone marrow, gastrointestinal lymphoid tissue, peripheral blood, peritoneal cavity, liver, lymph nodes, lung, spleen and thymus.

Migration of DCs precursors is partially mediated through a complex pattern of chemokine signaling. CD34+ derived immature DC express the chemokine receptor, CCR6 *(27,39,40)*. Its associated ligand, MIP-3_a, is released at sites of inflammation in the epithelium of the organs, gut, and skin, and is thought to be the primary mediator responsible for the localization of immature DCs at sites of antigen exposure. Expression of MIP-3_a by malignant cells is associated with the accumulation of immature DCs in the tumor bed *(41)*. Migration of DCs is also facilitated by the expression of proteins with elastase properties allowing for their penetration through basement membranes *(42)*.

LCs represent a well-characterized immature DC population found in the skin, which express CD1_a, Lag antigen, E-cadherin, and contains cytoplasmic inclusion bodies known as Birbeck granules (Fig. 3) *(6,13)*. DCs residing in other tissues do not share all of these morphologic characteristics, but demonstrate similar properties with regard to antigen processing and presentation. The morphology of immature DCs is characterized by a highly organized cytoskelatin, slow motility, and the absence of prominent dendrites. They express low levels of co-stimulatory molecules and are poor stimulators of allogeneic T cell proliferation. Immature DCs demonstrate potent capacity to internalize exogenous antigens. Studies of freshly isolated LCs and bone marrow-derived immature DCs demonstrate the ability to internalize protein latex microspheres, bacille Calmette-Guerin (BCG), colloidal gold, apoptotic and necrotic cell fragments, heat-shock proteins, viral and bacterial products as well as whole bacteria *(43–48)*.

Phagocytic properties of DCs are distinct from that seen with macrophages *(43,49,50)*. Macrophages are responsible for the scavenging and clearance of foreign material, which are transferred to cytoplasmic lysosomal compartments for degradation. DCs are more selective, demonstrating the uptake of smaller quantities of antigen, which are incorporated into MHC class II compartments for subsequent antigen presentation. DC-mediated antigen uptake occurs via both receptor mediated endocytosis as well as macropinocytosis. Immature DCs express Fc$_\gamma$, Fc$_\epsilon$, complement, and mannose receptors thought to mediate internalization of exogenous proteins *(6)*. In contrast to macrophages, DCs express the $\alpha v \beta 5$ integrin, which is crucial for

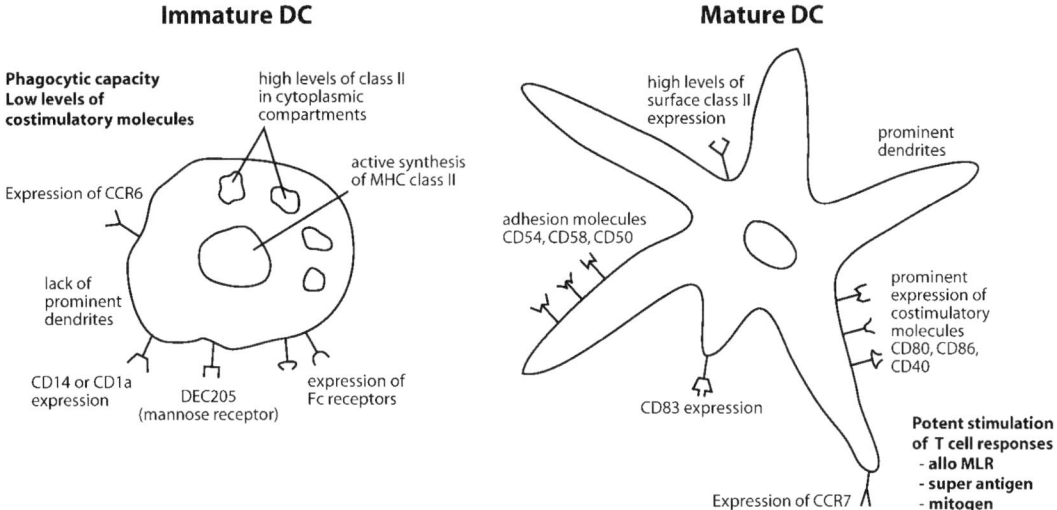

Fig. 3. DCs: immunobiology and potential use of cancer immunotherapy.

the uptake of apoptotic bodies and the subsequent presentation of antigen along the class I pathway *(45)*. An essential component facilitating endocytosis is the presence of the DEC205, a receptor homologous to the macrophage mannose receptor *(51)*. Antigen bound to DEC 205 is transferred via coated pits into endosomal compartments for subsequent processing and presentation in the context of MHC class II molecules. Endocytosis mediated by this pathway has been demonstrated to be 100-fold more effective than bulk macropinocytosis *(52)*. Mannosylation of the ingested antigen markedly increases in immunogenicity with an increase in levels of T cell responsiveness by 200- to 10,000-fold. Human LCs lack mannose receptors and demonstrate poorer phagocytic capacity as compared to interstitial DC *(53)*.

Immature DCs actively synthesize MHC class II molecules which are subsequently bound to the invariant chain in the endoplasmic reticulum and transferred to specialized compartments adjacent to the cell surface (Fig. 4) *(50)*. Exogenous proteins are transferred to these compartments following endocytosis and are separated from their plasma membrane receptor. They subsequently undergo digestion into peptide components, and are bound to MHC class II molecules that have been released from the invariant chain. Cytatstatin C inhibits degradation of the invariant chain and the associated integration of peptide antigens into class II molecules *(54)*. In the absence of maturation signals, undigested proteins may remain in perinuclear lysosomal structures distinguished by the presence of lysosomal membrane proteins *(55)*. In the immature state, expression of MHC class II on the cell surface is limited and is unstable in nature.

Endogenous proteins are degraded and loaded as peptides onto newly synthesized class I molecules in the endoplasmic reticulum. DCs express ubiquitin and TAP proteins necessary for the proteolytic digestion of proteins and transfer of peptides into the endoplasmic reticulum, respectively *(56)*. Alternatively, antigen derived from the uptake of whole cells, apoptotic bodies, and viral infection may be presented along the class I pathway potentially directed by CD1 molecules independent of TAP-mediated processing *(57–59)*.

3. PHENOTYPIC CHARACTERISTICS OF MATURE DC

Upon maturation, DCs migrate as veiled cells via the afferent lymphatics to regional lymph nodes, which serve as the site of antigen recognition and T cell activation *(27)*. During this

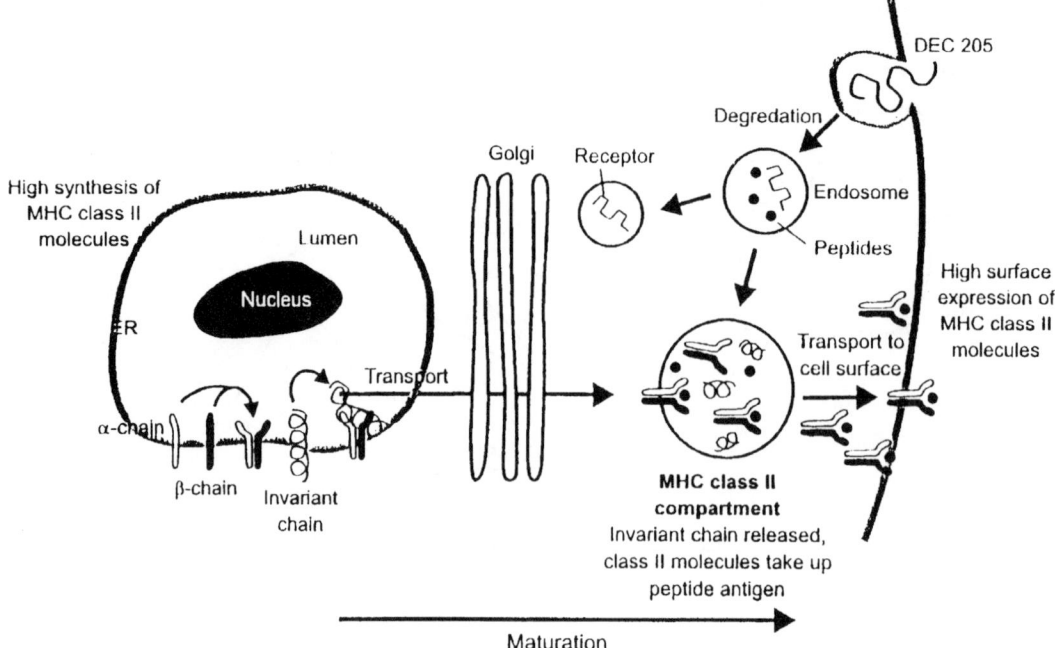

Fig. 4. DCs: immunobiology and potential use of cancer immunotherapy.

process, DCs undergo fundamental changes in their phenotypic and functional characteristics. DCs injected into mouse footpads are subsequently found in the draining popliteal lymph nodes. DCs derived from skin explants in animal and human models migrate through the dermal lymphatics into regional lymph nodes *(60)*. In contrast, DCs found in the interstitium of the solid organs travel through the peripheral blood to designated areas of the spleen. Animal models demonstrate that migration of DCs is dependent on the presence of intact immunity. DCs do not recirculate in the efferent lymphatics, and it is thought that those cells that do not present antigen undergo T cell-mediated apoptosis.

A variety of factors have been demonstrated to induce the maturation and migration of DCs. Loss of E-cadherin and release of type IV collagenase by LCs is associated with their capacity to migrate from skin epithelium and travel toward lymphocyte-rich areas *(61)*. In contrast, ligation of E-cadherin is associated with inhibition of DC maturation *(62)*. Keratinocytes secrete GM-CSF, which induces LC maturation *(63)*. Receptors for GM-CSF are prominently expressed by immature DCs and GM-CSF has been shown to support the differentiation, viability, and long-term survival of DC *(6,64)*. DC maturation is also mediated by inflammatory stimuli, such as whole bacteria, LPS, interleukin (IL)-1, and tumor necrosis factor (TNF)α *(65)*. Ligation of CD40, a member of the TNF receptor family, also induces terminal differentiation of DCs *(66)*. Exposure to LPS results in increased levels of circulating TNFα, which has been shown to upregulate expression of GM-CSF receptors on immature DCs. Exposure to oligodeoxynucleotides containing CpG motifs augments DCs maturation as manifested by a transient increase in antigen processing followed by loss of capacity to internalize and process exogenous protein antigens *(67)*. In contrast, IL-10 has been demonstrated to inhibit the differentiation of DCs, limiting the capacity to stimulate T cell responses *(68)*.

Upon antigen uptake or exposure to inflammatory signals, DCs downregulate CCR6 and lose sensitivity toward macrophage inhibiting protein (MIP)-3α *(27,39,69)*. Conversely, maturing DCs upregulate expression of CCR7 and demonstrate increased sensitivity towards chemokines MIP-3β and 6Ckine *(70)*. Expression of these chemokines is found in lymphatic vessels and the T-cell rich paracortical areas of the draining lymph nodes and mediates migration of DCs through the afferent lymphatics *(71–73)*. Mature DCs release MIP-3β and 6Ckine, further amplifying the effect, as well as attracting naïve T cells to the site of antigen presentation *(74)*. Absence of MIP-3β and 6Ckine expression is associated with deficient homing of DCs and T cells to lymphatic tissue *(75,76)*. Adenoviral transfection of tumor cells with MIP-3α resulted in the migration of DCs into the tumor bed and inhibition of tumor growth *(77)*.

With the onset of maturation, there is a transient increase in the production of cytoplasmic class II molecules and antigen loaded during this period is particularly immunogenic *(50)*. Cytostatin C is downregulated and cathepsin S is increased favoring the removal of the invariant chain and the incorporation of peptide to the MHC class II complex *(54,78,79)*. In addition, human leukocyte antigen (HLA)-DM contained in these compartments promotes binding of peptide with MHC class II molecules. Following exposure to an agent inducing differentiation, such as LPS, peptide-MHC complexes segregate from lysosomal compartments and appear in peripheral vesicles, known as CIIV *(55)*. Terminal maturation is associated with a decrease in the synthesis of MHC molecules, and MHC class II are thrust onto the cell surface resulting in stable presentation of the incorporated antigen. Localization of co-stimulatory molecules and peptide-MHC complexes in the CIIV compartments is subsequently translated to clustering of these molecules on the membrane surface for antigen presentation. Exposure to IL-10 inhibits the translocation of antigen expressing class II molecules onto the plasma membrane *(80)*.

Mature DCs are distinguished morphologically by the presence of prominent dendrites that facilitate motility and provide a large surface area for the simultaneous interaction with multiple T cells *(1,13)*. Morphologic changes are mediated by the actin-bundling protein p55 fascin *(81)*. Fascin expression is augmented by cytokines that induce DC maturation and has been associated with increased capacity to stimulate T cell proliferation *(82)*. Mature DCs are distinguished by low buoyant density, lack of adherant properties, absence of expression of lineage specific surface markers characteristic of T, B, and NK cells, macrophages, and the presence of CD83 in some populations *(6,83)*. Expression of Fc receptors and nonspecific esterase is downregulated and Birbeck granules are no longer detected.

Mature DCs lack phagocytic capacity and are incapable of processing and presenting exogenous protein. Mature cells are far more effective than macrophages and B cells in stimulating mitogen or allogeneic T cell proliferation and induce significantly higher levels of IL-2 secretion *(84–87)*. A single DC is capable of maximally stimulating 100–3000 T cells, and DCs pulsed with only minute concentrations of superantigen can generate significant lymphocyte responses *(88)*. Unlike other antigen-presenting cells, DCs are uniquely capable of inducing CD8 proliferative and CTL responses in the absence of CD4 helper cells *(89)*. DCs manipulated to present antigen through loading with peptide, protein or RNA, transfection with DNA, or viral infection results in the stimulation of powerful CD4 and CD8 responses *(18,19,90–92)*. CD83+ mature DCs induce TH1 responses following repetitive stimulation of T cells. In contrast, co-culture of T cells with immature DCs resulted in upregulation of the inhibitory molecule CTLA-4, lack of proliferation, and an inability for the T cells to subsequently respond to stimulation with mature DCs *(93)*.

DCs derive their potency as antigen-presenting cells from the prominent expression of MHC class I, II, adhesion and co-stimulatory molecules including CD58 (lymphocyte function-related antigen [LFA]-3), CD54 (intercellular adhesion molecule [ICAM]-1), CD50 (ICAM-3), CD40, CD80 (B7-1), and CD86 (B7-2) *(5,7,94)*. Ligation of corresponding molecules on T cells, most notably CD28, provides the essential secondary signals for the initiation of primary immune responses. Interference with this crucial dialogue through antibody blockade abrogates DC- mediated T cell stimulation. Although signaling occurs via the entire network of adhesion and co-stimulatory molecules, disruption of CD86 binding appears paramount, which results in a 70% reduction in T cell stimulation.

DCs also impact on B cell development and function. DCs support the differentiation of naïve and memory B cells toward antibody-secreting plasma cells, and promote class switching necessary for IgA secretion. DCs are thought to play a role in mediating the interaction between CD4 helper cells and B cells (95,96).

4. DC–T CELL INTERACTIONS

DCs initially aggregate with T cells in an antigen-independent manner in an effort to survey the repertoire for T cells with the capacity recognize the presented antigen (97). IL-15 induces the release of chemokines which mediate the migration of T cells to the site of antigen presentation, while IL-1α facilitates T cell clustering around the DC (98,99). Adhesion molecules such as CD11a, CD54, and CD58 are responsible for DC–T cell binding, which is strengthened by the presence of antigen recognition (100). T cell activation is significantly impaired by antibody blockade of these interactions or genetic defects in which animals lack the full complement of adhesion molecules. Presentation of immunodominant epitopes and binding of T cells results in competitive inhibition which suppresses recognition of subdominant epitopes (101).

The activation of T cells is mediated through the ligation of co-stimulatory molecules and the subsequent release of a complex network of cytokines (Fig. 5). CD40L and IL-12 play an important role in DC mediated stimulation of T cells. Upon binding to DCs, T cell expression of CD40L is upregulated. This results in increased expression of MHC class II adhesion and costimulatory molecules prolonged DC survival, and IL-12 secretion (102–105). Ligation of the RANK, a member of the TNF receptor family, and release of IFNα in response to DC-T cell binding also results in the secretion of IL-12 (106–108). IL-12 release is also stimulated by the antigen-specific activation of T cells and exposure of the antigen-presenting cells to inflammatory factors, such as, TNF, segmental allergen challenge (SAC), and LPS (109). IL-12 augments T and NK cell cytotoxicity and biases T cell development towards the TH1 phenotype that is associated with the release of IFNγ (110). IL-12 has been shown to be far more potent than IL-2 in amplifying antigen-specific responses mediated by DCs activation of T cells (111,112). Exogenous IL-12 has been demonstrated to replace the need for helper T cells in generating effective immune responses directed against tumor lines of poor immunogenicity (113). IL-12 enhances T cell proliferation following stimulation with DCs pulsed with tumor peptide, and transfection of murine DCs with with IL-12 gene markedly upregulates their capacity to induce tumor-specific CTL responses.

Mature DCs are immune to Fas-mediated apoptosis while immature DCs are partially sensitive and may undergo apoptosis following interaction with T cells (114,115). Ligation of Fas receptor may paradoxically induce differentiation in immature DCs, leading to upregulation of co-stimulatory molecules (116).

A variety of factors inhibit DC maturation and blunt the capacity of DCs to generate T cell responses. Tumor cells, TH2 clones, B cells, macrophages, and mast cells produce the TH2 cytokines, IL-10, and IL-4 that inhibit antigen-presentation through the downregulation of co-stimulatory molecule expression, and the suppression of the release of inflammatory cytokines such as IL-1, IL-6, IL-8, TNF, and GM-CSF (117,118). Immature DCs release IL-10 following exposure to CD40L (119). IL-10 blunts the capacity of DC to stimulate allogeneic T cell proliferation as well as the release of IL-2 by activated T cells.68 Culture of DC precursor populations in the presence of IL-10 results in a bias toward differentiation along the monocyte lineage. DCs generated in this setting demonstrate impaired capacity to secrete IL-12 and stimulate TH1 responses. DCs generated in the presence of IL-10 induce anergy in potentially

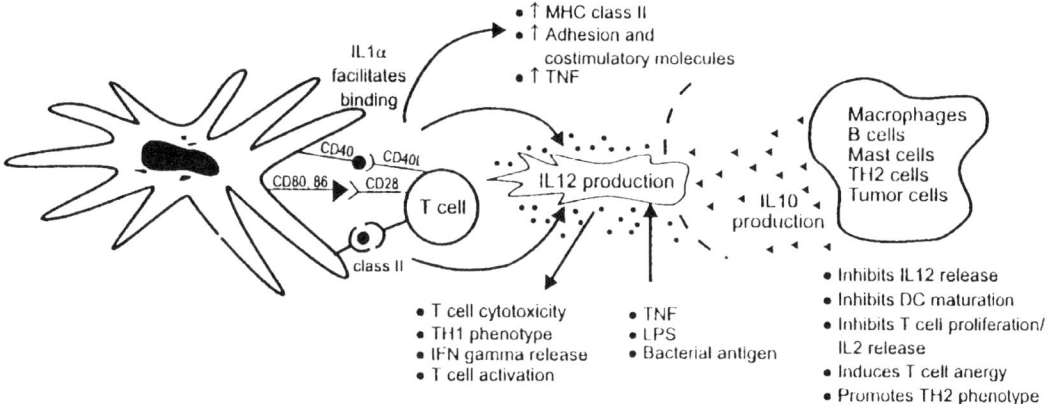

Fig. 5. DCs: immunobiology and potential use of cancer immunotherapy.

reactive T cell populations that is not reversed upon exposure to IL-10 naive DCs. In contrast, DCs that mature in the absence of IL-10 are subsequently resistant to its inhibitory effects. IL-10 secretion has been demonstrated by a variety of malignancies including melanoma, renal cell, and colon cancer, and may play an important role in the tumor evasion of host immunity *(120)*. Tumor cells transfected with IL-10 inhibit migration of DCs to the site of implantation and therefore are rendered less immunogenic to the host. Conversely, expression of IL-4 by TH2 cells induces IL-12 activity as part of a negative feedback loop *(121)*.

Subsets of DC populations demonstrate distinct profiles of cytokine secretion and T cell stimulation *(27)*. Myeloid DCs have been described as DC1, characteristically inducing a TH1-type T cell response. In contrast, CD8α+ lymphoid-derived DCs (DC2) are characterized by the expression of CD123 and favor the secretion of IL-4 and IL-10 by stimulated lymphocytes. CD8α+ DCs were shown to inhibit the capacity of CD8α– DCs to induce responses directed against the tumor/self peptide, P815AB *(122)*. Priming of the CD8α– DCs with IL-12 or CD40L reverses the inhibition while IFNγ enhances it.

5. DC HEMATOPOIESIS

In vitro studies demonstrate that differentiation of DCs may occur along several distinct hematopoieitic pathways. Murine studies have shown that bone marrow progenitors cultured with GM-CSF for 4 to 5 d generate a subpopulation of loosely adherent cells that richly express co-stimulatory and adhesion molecules and potently stimulate allogeneic T cell proliferation *(123)*. Once fully mature, their phenotype is not reversible by the withdrawal of cytokine or exposure to M-CSF. Clonogenic studies in semisolid media demonstrate that myeloid progenitors cultured with GM-CSF generated mixed colonies containing granulocytes, macrophages, and DCs, with the latter comprising approx 1% of the final population. DCs are not found in colonies grown in the presence of G-CSF, IL-3 or M-CSF. Flt3L stimulates the expansion and maturation of early DC progenitors in the bone marrow and results in the increased presence in vivo and in vitro of lymphoid and myeloid DC subsets.124,125

Studies of DC hematopoiesis in humans suggest that DCs and monocytes share a common early lineage but subsequently differentiate from distinct colony-forming units. CD34+ progenitors cultured with GM-CSF alone give rise to mixed myeloid colonies of DCs and macrophages *(126)*. Stem cell factor (SCF) and FLt3L induces the recruitment and proliferation of early progenitors, and their addition to the culture media does not alter the cell populations but results in an increase in the number and size of the colonies *(127,128)*. FLt3L also induces both myeloid and lymphoid DC development.38 TNFα acts in concert with GM-CSF in promoting the differentiation of DCs through its inhibition of granulocyte colony formation and its upregulation of GM-CSF receptor expression on the maturing cells. CD34+ progentors cultured with TNFα and GM-CSF give rise to pure DCs as well as mixed myeloid colonies.

Large yields of DCs may be generated from CD34+ cells isolated from cord blood, bone marrow, and mobilized peripheral blood stem cells that are cultured in the presence of GM-CSF and TNFα *(21,22,129)*. IL-4 suppresses monocyte maturation and improves the purity of DCs in the resultant population. IL-3 and CD40L were found to enhance DCs maturation in suspension cultures. The addition of SCF and Flt3L to suspension cultures results in the expansion of early myeloid progenitors, increasing the total yield of DCs. Flt3L also promotes the generation of CD1a+ and CD1a- immature DC from CD34+ progenitors *(130,131)*. Cell populations generated from CD34+ precursors may pass through distinct intermediate stages of differentiation. In one study, CD34+ cells isolated from cord blood samples and cultured in GM-CSF and TNFα generated two alternative populations of immature DC *(22)*. CD1a+/CD14- cells demonstrated characteristic LC phenotype with the presence of Birbeck granules, lag antigen, and E-cadherin, and a lack of potential to mature toward the monocytic lineage. A second population of CD1a-/CD14+ cells demonstrated greater phagocytic capacity, lack of LC phenotype, and differentiated into monocytes when exposed to M-CSF. However, both immature DC populations differentiated into DCs with a characteristic mature phenotype following culture with GM-CSF and TNFα. These results suggest that DCs may evolve from a unique precursor population or from a progenitor that is shared between the DCs and monocyte lineages. Another study also demonstrated that intermediate DC precursors may mature into DCs or macrophages dependent on the nature of cytokine exposure *(132)*. CD34+ cells cultured for 1 wk with SCF, GM-CSF, and IL-4 generated a small population of DR[bright]/CD14- cells that richly expressed co-stimulatory molecules and were extremely potent stimulators of allogeneic T cell proliferation. A larger number of CD14+ intermediate cells were also isolated that irreversibly differentiated into mature DCs or monocytes when cultured with GM-CSF and TNFα or M-CSF, respectively. In another study, CD34+ cells that had been cultured with SCF, GM-CSF, and TNFα generated two populations of intermediate progeny that were distinguished by levels of expression of the panmyeloid marker, CD13 *(133)*. Upon further culture, the CD13[hi] intermediates progressively expressed CD1a and subsequently adopted a mature DC phenotype. In contrast, CD13[lo] populations matured more slowly, transiently demonstrated a DC phenotype associated with potent allostimulatory activity and increased levels of CD13 expression, but subsequently contained increasing numbers of macrophages with poor antigen-presenting capacity.

DCs may also be generated in significant numbers in vitro from partially differentiated precursors in peripheral blood *(134)*. In one study, two precursor populations were identified as defined by the expression of the integrin, CD11c *(135)*. CD11c+ cells demonstrated greater allostimulatory activity. When placed in culture, both populations developed a phenotype consistent with a mature DC phenotype as defined by the expression of costimulatory molecules and function in assays of antigen presentation. Another study found the presence of CD33[bright] and CD33[dim] populations in peripheral blood mononuclear cells (PBMC) from which monocytes, NK, B, and T cells had been removed *(136)*. CD33[bright] cells manifested aspects of partially mature DC in that they expressed adhesion molecules, stimulated alloge-neic T cell proliferation, and were capable of processing and presenting tetanus protein to autologous T cells. In contrast, CD33[dim] cells initially functioned poorly as antigen-presenting cells, but gradually evolved towards the phenotype of the CD33[bright] cells once in culture. Both populations upregulated expression of co-stimulatory molecules after in vitro culture adopting the phenotype of more mature DCs.

Several investigators have demonstrated that DCs may be derived from more mature monocyte populations *(24)*. Plastic adherent CD14+ PBMC cultured with GM-CSF, TNFα, and IL-4 generate cell populations that are potent in allogeneic mixed leukocyte reaction (MLR) and express CD83 and CD1a *(83)*. Adherent PBMC cultured with GM-CSF and IL-4 yield DCs at an intermediate level of differentiation, with the capacity to stimulate T cell responses. Exposure to IL-4 results in maintaining the capacity of DCs to internalize and present exogenous protein *(137)*. In contrast, the presence of TNFα is associated with the loss of phagocytosis and a more mature phenotype. Blood precursor populations may also evolve toward an LC phenotype under the influence of TGFβ *(138)*.

A variety of agents have been shown to induce terminal differentiation in DCs generated from peripheral blood precursors. Adherent PBMC sthat were first cultured in GM-CSF and subsequently exposed to monocyte-conditioned medium generated large numbers of cells that upregulated CD80, CD86, and CD83, and were particularly effective in stimulating allogeneic T cell proliferation *(139)*. Similarly, the addition of CD40L, TNFα, and LPS results in the terminal differentiation that is not reversed upon removal of cytokines *(27)*. In one study, pulsing of monocyte-derived DCs with keyhole limpet hemocyanin (KLH) or human immunodeficiency virus (HIV)1p24 gag and culture of the cells with TNFα resulted in the adoption of a mature phenotype and the loss of phagocytic capacity *(140)*.

6. DC-MEDIATED CTL RESPONSES

DCs expressing foreign antigens potently induce primary CTL responses. DCs loaded with protein and injected into mouse footpads subsequently appear in draining popliteal lymph nodes, where they activate antigen-specific T cell responses *(60)*. DCs pulsed with the HIV gag or envelope proteins induce primary T cell immunity that demonstrates lysis of peptide-pulsed or virally infected targets *(141)*. In a murine model, mice immunized with DCs loaded with ovalbumin (OVA) peptide demonstrate OVA-specific primary immunity *(90)*. DCs infected in vivo or in vitro with the influenza virus generate potent immunity directed against flu-infected targets *(92)*. DCs infected with wild-type or heat-inactivated influenza virus stimulate CD8+ responses that are effective in lysing flu targets in the absence of T helper cells. Responses are considerably more potent than that generated by DCs pulsed with influenza-derived nucleoprotein or that induced by virally infected monocytes or bulk splenocytes.

A variety of other strategies have been developed to introduce foreign antigens into DCs.

The use of viral vectors have been pursued in an effort to induce expression of gene products that are subsequently processed by endogenous mechanisms and presented along the class I pathway. Adenoviral vectors have demonstrated remarkable efficiency in the transference of genes into DCs, but antigen specific responses may be limited by background reactions directed against viral proteins *(91)*. Retroviral vectors do not induce prominent anti-viral responses but require the presence of dividing cells *(142,143)*. CD34+ cells that have undergone retroviral transfection have been subsequently cultured in vitro with cytokines and differentiated into DCs. Using this strategy, effective transfer of the marker gene, β-galactosidase, has been seen in 35–67% of the target population with preservation of the retroviral DNA in the cellular genome for up to 20 d. Introduction of foreign antigens into DCs has also been accomplished by the use of liposomal RNA or DNA, although subsequent surface expression was weak and less effective than adenoviral transfer *(144)*. Another strategy has been the in vivo loading of DCs following the inoculation with naked DNA *(145)*. Protein is expressed by cells at the site of injection, and antigen is then taken up by DCs recruited to the site of inflammation.

7. DC-BASED IMMUNOTHERAPY FOR CANCER

Strategies to introduce tumor antigens into DCs have been pursued in an effort to induce tumor-specific CTL responses. One approach has been the in vivo loading of tumor antigens by DCs recruited to the site of malignancy. The presence of DCs in the tumor bed has been shown to directly inhibit tumor growth *(146)*. Tumor cells genetically engineered to express GM-CSF or co-administered with GM-CSF-secreting cells induce tumor-specific immunity through the recruitment of DCs to the site of inoculation with subsequent internalization and presentation of tumor antigens *(147)*. Inoculation of animals with C-26 colon carcinoma cells that were transduced with GM-CSF and CD40L resulted in the heavy infiltration of DC at the tumor site and spontaneous regressions of disease *(148)*. Infiltrating DCs expressed the murine leukemia virus antigen that was taken up in vivo from the C-26 cells. In another study, DCs genetically engineered to express IL-12 inhibited growth of established tumors through the presentation of in vivo-acquired tumor antigens and the resultant infiltration of tumor-specific CD4 and CD8 T cells *(149)*.

Systemic administration of Flt3L results in the tissue accumulation of DCs and the potential internalization, processing, and presentation of tumor antigens at the site of malignant disease. Therapy with Flt3L has been shown to induce tumor regression in animal models. A significant proportion of mice challenged with a syngeneic methylchlorine-induced fibrosarcoma were rendered disease-free following treatment with Flt3L *(150)*. Tumor-specific immunity was transferred to irradiated naïve animals by the transfer of CD8+ splenocytes. In another study, animals treated with Flt3L were protected from challenge with a murine mammary carcinoma line. Eighty percent of animals treated for 10 d were protected from tumor challenge at d 1 or 4 of therapy *(151)*. However, the protection was transient and all animals that were subsequently re-challenged developed tumors. Transfection of the tumor cells with a gene expressing human or murine Flt3L resulted in more durable protection against challenge with wild-type tumor. Flt3L has also been shown to induce regression of liver metastases in a murine model *(152)*. In another study, animals treated with the combination of radiation and Flt3L experienced a decrease in pulmonary metastases and improved survival as compared to those treated with FLt3L alone *(153)*. The investigators postulated that radiation facilitated the loading of tumor antigens onto infiltrating DCs.

A variety of in vitro strategies to introduce tumor antigens into DCs have also been examined in animal models. (Fig. 6). Exogenous loading of DCs with tumor peptides bearing the appropriate HLA restriction results in their incorporation into empty MHC complexes located on the cell surface. This approach allows for the use of DCs with a mature phenotype, which lack the capacity for phagocytosis but are potent stimulators of T cell proliferation. Response to individual peptides is governed by their affinity to MHC binding and their capacity to induce responses against variant epitopes *(154)*. In one study, vaccination with DCs loaded with OVA peptide generated CTL responses that demonstrated in vitro lysis of syngeneic tumor cells pulsed with OVA peptide or transfected with the OVA gene *(90)*. In another model, animals vaccinated with DC pulsed with an immunogenic OVA peptide were subsequently protected from an otherwise lethal challenge with tumor cells manipulated to express the OVA gene *(15)*. More significantly, animals were subsequently resistant to challenge with the wild-type parent tumor line. These results suggest that the recognition of OVA peptide on the tumor cells following DCs vaccination secondarily resulted in heightened recognition of other tumor antigens.

In another study, animals were immunized with DCs loaded with one of three tumor-associated peptides, mut1 (lewis lung carcinoma), human papillomavirus (HPV) peptide (virally induced sarcoma line), or OVA peptide (melanoma cell line transfected with the OVA gene) *(155)*. Vaccination with peptide-pulsed DCs resulted in protection from subsequent

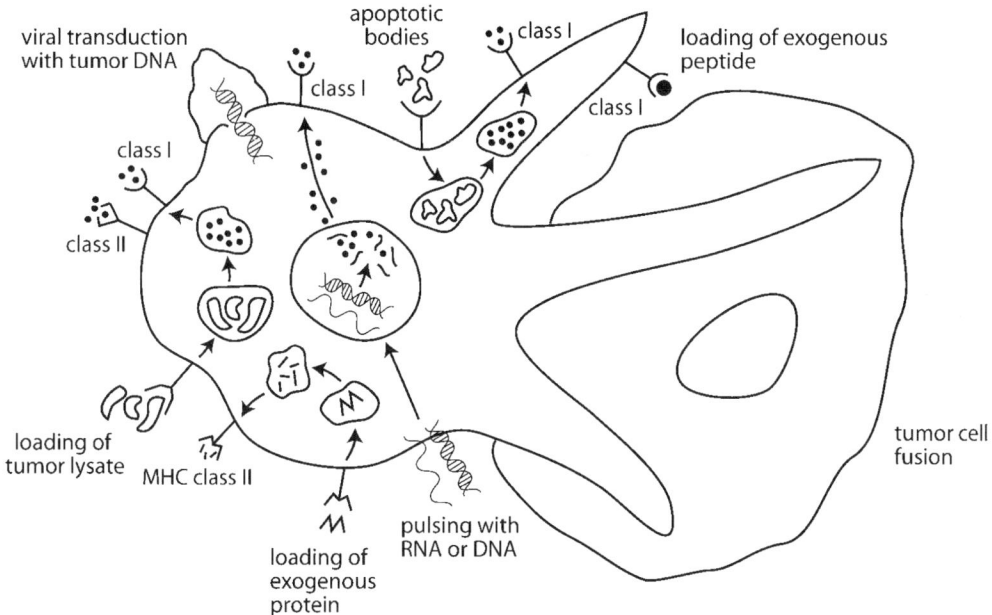

Fig. 6. DCs: immunobiology and potential use of cancer immunotherapy.

challenge with the antigen-expressing tumor line. DCs generated from precursor populations cultured with GM-CSF and IL-4 were more effective in generating tumor specific immunity than those cultured with GM-CSF and TNFα or GM-CSF alone. In a treatment model, animals were rendered disease free when inoculated with tumor and subsequently immunized with peptide-pulsed DCs within 7–14 d. The therapeutic efficacy was lost if the tumor cells were given more time to establish themselves, suggesting that DC-based immunotherapy is most potent in the absence of bulky disease. Another study demonstrated that tumor immunity generated by vaccination with DCs pulsed with HPV peptide was abrogated by treatment of animals with antibody directed against CD8+ cells *(156)*. A murine model examined the immunogenicity of DCs pulsed with a peptide generated from a mutant p53 gene product that was derived from a sarcoma cell line *(157)*. Immunized animals were protected from tumor challenge and inhibition of tumor growth was seen in animals treated within 7 d following tumor inoculation. DCs genetically manipulated to express B7-1, intercellular adhesion molecule-1, and LFA-3 demonstrated heightened capacity to present peptide antigens to autologous T cells *(158)*.

The capacity of peptide-pulsed DCs to generate effective immunity directed against human tumors has also been examined. DCs loaded with the melanoma-associated antigens tyrosinase, gp100, and Melan A were capable of inducing CTL responses in vitro following the repetitive stimulation of naïve T cell populations *(159)*. Lysis was demonstrated of peptide-loaded targets as well as HLA-matched melanoma cell lines expressing the appropriate antigens. Similarly, DCs loaded with a carcinoembryonic antigen (CEA) peptide potently stimulated mediated lysis of antigen-expressing tumor cell lines in an HLA-restricted fashion *(160)*. Peptides derived from the BCR/ABL fusion region have also been shown to be immunogenic when presented by antigen-loaded DCs. CD4-mediated responses were generated that lysed CML cells containing the associated breakpoint region *(161)*. T cells stimulated with DCs pulsed with a bcr-abl peptide lyse patient-derived chronic myeloid leukemia (CML) cells containing the same breakpoint, but not autologous monocytes *(162,163)*. In one study, pulsing of DCs with a Her2neu peptide, which was altered to augment binding to the MHC complex resulted in higher levels of CTL activity *(164)*. Of note, weekly immunization resulted in decreased levels of response, while animals vaccinated every 3 wk did not experience diminution in CTL immunity.

Although effective in animal models, the efficacy of peptide-pulsed DCs in generating tumor specific immunity is limited. The immunogenecity of identified antigens is variable, the stability of antigen presentation following exogenous pulsing is uncertain, and the clinical efficacy of an immune response directed against a single epitope may be muted. Of note, patient-derived CTL induced by DCs pulsed with p53-derived peptides were unable to lyse autologous squamous cell carcinoma cells due to the downregulation of expression of this epitope.165 In addition, there is a lack of defined tumor-specific peptides in many malignancies, and treatment is limited to patients of a particular HLA genotype.

Another approach to designing DC-based tumor vaccines is through the exogenous loading of whole proteins. In this way, multiple epitopes may be presented in the appropriate HLA context. In one study, DCs pulsed with the β-galactosidase protein stimulated CTL-mediated lysis of tumor cells manipulated to present this antigen (19). In an animal model, vaccination with DCs pulsed with lymphoma-derived idiotype protein, resulted in protection from challenge with tumor cells and the generation of an anti-idiotype response (166). CD14+ moncytes cultured with GM-CSF and IL-4 internalized and processed patient-derived idiotype protein, and effectively stimulated T cell responses following exposure to TNFα, LPS, or CD40L as a maturational signal (167,168). In another study, idiotype protein was shown to be transferred to DCs located at the tumor site, which subsequently presented the antigen to CD4+ T cells (169). DCs presenting idiotype antigen declined in number with tumor progression. The efficacy of protein loading may also be limited in that it is dependent on the use of DCs with the capacity to internalize and process antigen, and the ability of T cell repertoire to recognize presented epitopes is less easily defined. The processing of exogenous proteins also results in their presentation along a class II pathway, producing a primary helper as compared to cytotoxic T cell response.

Another approach to introducing tumor antigens into DCs has been the use of viral vectors to insert genes encoding for tumor-specific proteins. In this way, tumor antigens are processed through endogenous mechanisms and presented along a class I pathway, resulting in a cytotoxic T cell response. Vaccination with DCs that had undergone transduction with an adenoviral vector expressing the MART1 gene resulted in protective immunity against a MART1-expressing fibrosarcoma cell line (170). In another study, animals were vaccinated with DCs that had been infected with a replication-deficient adenoviral vector expressing the β-galactosidase gene (171). Immunized animals demonstrated resistance to challenge with a β-galactosidase-expressing colon cancer line, and those with established disease experienced inhibition of tumor growth. DCs transduced with adenovirus expressing gp100 induced CD4-mediated CTL responses resulting in tumor rejection (172). In this model, tumor protection was independent of CD8 T cells and did not require the presence of IL-12.

DCs infected with recombinant fowlpox virus bearing the OVA gene successfully stimulated antigen-specific T cell responses (173). DCs infected with vaccinia virus bearing melanoma-derived gp100 stimulated CTL responses that lysed HLA-matched targets that had been pulsed with a variety of gp100-derived peptides (174). A potential concern regarding the use of viral vectors is their generation of potent immunologic responses directed against viral proteins. These antigens are potentially far more immunogenic and may overwhelm the response against the designated tumor antigens and prevent repetitive dosing from being effective. Another potential limitation of this approach is the demonstration that viral infection may be associated with decreased DC function (175).

Another strategy for the introduction of tumor-specific genes into DCs has been through the use of retroviral vectors (142,143). Investigators have explored the feasibility of the retroviral insertion of tumor genes into CD34+ cells that are subsequently differentiated into DCs in the presence of cytokines. Using this approach, stable expression of the MUC-1 tumor antigen was generated in DCs derived from retrovirally transfected precursor cells *(176)*. Similarly, the MART1 gene was expressed in approx 25% of DC following its retroviral insertion into CD34+ cells that were then cultured with SCF, TNFα, and GM-CSF *(177)*. In another study, retroviral transduction of DC with the β-galactosidase gene resulted in signficant CTL responses against a β-galactosidase-expressing tumor in excess of that seen with DC-pulsed with peptide *(178)*. Vaccination of animals resulted in regression of established pulmonary metastases. Vaccination with DCs transduced with an adenoviral vector bearing the MAGE-1 gene resulted in suppression of tumor growth in a subcutaneous melanoma model, with 10% of animals experiencing long-term survival. In contrast, vaccination with tumor cells expressing IL-12, GM-CSF, or CD40L were unable to contain tumor progression *(179)*. Paradoxically, levels of MAGE-1 expression were significantly higher in tumor cells as compared to DCs.

Transfer of tumor-specific genes into DCs has also been accomplished through the use of tumor-derived RNA. This strategy is facilitated by established methods to isolate and amplify RNA from biopsy specimens, allowing for its potential general applicability in the clinical setting. DCs pulsed with RNA encoding OVA protein or with whole RNA from OVA expressing tumor cells stimulated OVA-specific CTL *(180)*. Mice vaccinated with RNA-loaded DCs were protected from challenge with OVA-expressing tumors, and resulted in the reduction in lung metastases when used therapeutically. DCs transfected with RNA encoding for HPV E6 and E7 oncoproteins stimulate CTL responses that recognize antigen expressing human cervical carcinoma cells *(181)*. DCs pulsed with CEA-mRNA stimulate tumor specific CD8+ CTL *(18)*. Similarly, DCs pulsed with RNA encoding for prostate-specific antigen (PSA) induced CTL responses against cells expressing PSA but not kallikrein, a self antigen that shares homology with PSA *(182)*. In another study, DCs pulsed with either B16 cell extract or whole tumor RNA were able to protect animals from challenge with tumor in the central nervous system (CNS) and led to improved survival in animals with established disease *(14)*. DCs transfected with RNA encoding for the MUC-1 tumor antigen induced tumor-specific responses in immunized animals resulting in protection from tumor challenge and regression of established disease *(183)*. Vaccination with DCs cotransfected with MUC-1 RNA and IL-12 resulted in MUC-1-specific responses in a transgenic murine model.

All of the above mentioned strategies involve the targeting of known tumor associated antigens. The use of single gene products for DC-based immune strategies limits one to a small group of potential antigens of uncertain immunogenicity. Immunotherapeutic approaches that rely on induction of immunity against a particular antigen are also potentially subject to tumor cell resistance mediated by the downregulation of expression of that single gene product. One approach to circumvent this limitation is the pulsing of DCs with antigens extracted from whole tumor cells. Mice vaccinated with DCs pulsed with acid-eluted peptides from tumor cells were protected from challenge with immunogenic tumors *(184)*. Of note, this strategy was less efficacious in setting poorly immunogenic tumors with immunized animals experiencing only a delay in tumor growth. Similarly, in a melanoma and fibrosarcoma model, immunization of animals with DCs pulsed with tumor lysate resulted in regression of established disease *(185)*. DCs loaded with lysate generated by freeze-thawing of an Epstein-Barr virus (EBV) transformed lymphoblastoid cell lines (LCL) line stimulated tumor-specific CD4+ and CD8+ responses with a TH1 phenotype *(186)*. Lysates generated by membrane extraction affinity-purified MHC class I and II peptides and acid-eluted peptides were less immunogenic and did not generate significant responses. Loading of DCs with lysate prior to terminal maturation with TNFα, IL-1β, and prstaglandin E (PGE)$_2$ was the most effective approach in generating tumor immunity. Another study examined the capacity of monocyte-derived immature DCs to process and present tumor antigens from tumor cells that had undergone lethal γ irradiation or exposure to anti-Fas antibody *(187)*.

Another strategy for generating tumor immunity involves the use of apoptotic bodies as a means of introducing tumor antigens into DCs with subsequent cross-presentation along the class I pathway *(188,189)*. DCs were found to express a unique receptor αvβ5 integrin which facilitates phagocytosis of apoptotic bodies and is downregulated upon maturation *(45)*. Macrophages ingest apoptotic bodies more readily, but do not express this receptor and lack the capacity to cross present antigenic material from the apoptotic bodies. In one study, DCs demonstrated the capacity to internalize necrotic as well as apoptotic tumor bodies, but only the latter induced DCs maturation and resulted in potent CD8+ tumor-specific responses *(190)*. In another study, DCs internalized apoptotic bodies generated by the irradiation of vector-producing cell lines expressing the MAGE-3. DCs stimulated autologous T cells with resultant lysis of MAGE-3-expressing tumor cells. In another study, DCs pulsed with melanoma cells that underwent apoptosis were more effective in generating tumor responses than those loaded with live or necrotic cells *(191)*.

One strategy that is currently being explored for the generation of DC-based immunotherapy for leukemia has been the differentiation in vitro of leukemic clones into DCs. In this manner, tumor antigens retained from the malignant clone can be endogenously processed and presented by a functionally active antigen-presenting cell. CML cells cultured with GM-CSF and IL-4 developed phenotypic characterisitics of DCs that contained the bcr-abl translocation *(192,193)*. Stimulation of autologous T cells resulted in cytotoxic activity against CML cells and bcr-abl-expressing targets as well as the inhibition of growth in CML clonogenic precursors in colony forming assays in vitro. Retroviral transduction with the gene encoding for IL-7 further increased the potency of bcr-abl-expressing DCs generated from CML patients *(194)*. Investigators have also demonstrated that functionally active DCs can be generated from acute myeloid and leukemia cells *(195,196)*. Leukemic blasts were cultured in cytokines and subsequently found to express co-stimulatory molecules such as CD80, CD86, and CD40, DC-specific markers such as CD83, and retained the chromosomal abnormalities of the original leukemic clone. DCs stimulated autologous T cell-lysed leukemic targets. Of note, immature CD34+/CD38- leukemia progenitors are resistant to differentiating toward DCs *(197)*.

A potent strategy for designing DC-based tumor vaccines involves the fusion of DCs with tumor cells. In this approach, multiple tumor antigens, including those yet unidentified, are presented in the context of DC-mediated co-stimulation. The potential simultaneous presentation of endogenously synthesized and internalized antigens along the class I and II pathways, respectively, results in a highly potent immune response. In an animal model, murine MC38 adenocarcinoma cells were fused to syngeneic bone marrow-derived DC *(16)*. The MC38 line was transfected with the human mucin glycoprotein (MUC-1) gene to serve as a tumor-specific marker. Fusion cells expressed MUC-1 , MHC class I, II, and the co-stimulatory molecules B7-1 and B7-2. Animals vaccinated with fusion cells were protected from an otherwise lethal challenge of MC38 cells but not a bladder carcinoma line. In a treatment model, animals vaccinated with fusion cells up to 18 d following the infusion of MC38/MUC-1 cells were rendered disease-free. In contrast, control animals were found to have widespread pulmonary metastases. DC/tumor fusions were also found to break immunologic tolerance toward the MUC1 tumor antigen in transgenic mouse models *(198)*. In another study, vaccination with fusion cells resulted in protection from tumor challenge as well as efficacy as therapy for metastatic disease in melanoma and lung carcinoma models *(199)*. Another investigator reported that 50% of animals with disseminated plasmacytoma were rendered disease-free after inoculation with DC/tumor fusions *(200)*. Similar findings were observed in animals vaccinated with B16 melanoma cells fused to syngeneic DCs genetically engineered to express GM-CSF. Animals with pulmonary metastases experienced regression of disease with prolonged survival *(201)*.

Subsequent studies have demonstrated that DC/tumor fusions are potent stimulators of tumor-specific immunity in preclinical human studies in breast and ovarian cancer *(17,202)*. Fusion cells were generated from patient-derived tumor cells and autologous DCs, and were found to co-express tumor antigens and DC-derived co-stimulatory molecules. Fusion cells induced prominent tumor-specific CTL responses in vitro following a single stimulation. CTLs did not lyse autologous monocytes and were inhibited by incubation with anti-class I antibody. T cells stimulated by DCs, tumor cells, or DCs and tumor cells that had been co-cultured but not fused, demonstrated minimal lysis of autologous tumor cells.

8. DC-BASED IMMUNOTHERAPY: CLINICAL STUDIES

DC-based tumor immunotherapy is now being pursued in the clinical setting. One strategy involves the attempt to mobilize DCs in vivo in an effort to augment presentation of tumor antigens. In one study, patients with colon cancer were treated with Flt3L prior to resection of metastatic lesions in the lung or liver *(203)*. Increased numbers of CD11c/CD14- DC were noted in the peripheral blood as well as at the tumor margins of Flt3L treated patients. Clinical responses have also been demonstrated in patients with melanoma and breast cancer undergoing injection with autologous DCs directly into the tumor bed *(204)*.

Vaccination of patients with DCs pulsed with tumor peptides has been studied in clinical trials. Sixteen patients with melanoma were treated with DCs pulsed with melanoma peptides or lysate as well as KLH to induce helper responses *(20)*. Following vaccination, 11 out of 16 patients developed DTH responses to DCs pulsed with melanoma peptides, and associated tumor-specific CTL responses were noted. Six out of 16 patients showed evidence of clinical response. In another study, 14 melanoma patients were treated with DCs pulsed with several melanoma peptides *(205)*. Peptide-specific DTH responses were seen in four patients, and two patients showed evidence of clinical regression. No significant toxicities were noted. In another study, 17 previously untreated patients with prostate cancer underwent monthly intravenous infusions with DCs pulsed with prostate-specific membrane antigen (PSMA) peptides *(206)*. Three partial responders and one complete response was noted. No significant treatment related toxicity was reported. Immunological assessment revealed that clinical response was associated with skin test response to recall antigens, T cell responsiveness to cytokines, and, in some patients, cytotoxicity against the immunizing peptides *(207)*. A phase I trial was conducted in which 10 patients with breast and ovarian cancer underwent vaccination with DCs pulsed with Her2neu- or MUC1-derived peptides *(208)*. In five out of 10 patients, peptide-specific CTL responses were noted with immunodominance of two particular epitopes. Patients undergoing vaccination with DC pulsed with peptides eluted from CNS tumors demonstrated cellular immune responses and intratumoral T cell infiltration *(209)*. In another study, 18 patients with metastatic melanoma underwent vaccination with CD34+-derived DCs pulsed with several melanoma peptides *(210)*. Sixteen out of 18 patients demonstrated evidence of T cell response to the control antigens, influenza, and KLH, and at least one of the melanoma peptides. Of note, clinical response was associated with response to at least two melanoma peptides. Vaccination of 21 prostate cancer patients with DCs pulsed with a xenogeneic PAP peptide resulted in antigen-specific T cell responses and disease stabilization in 11 and six patients, respectively *(211)*.

Another strategy that is examined in the clinical setting has been the vaccination of patients with DCs pulsed with tumor-associated proteins. In one study, patients with low grade lymphoma underwent vaccination with DCs pulsed with idiotype protein. In an initial report, all patients showed evidence of idiotype-specific cellular immunity, while humoral responses were absent *(212)*. In a follow-up report, eight out of 10 patients demonstrated idiotype-specific cellular immunity. Disease response was seen in four patients, including two patients who experienced a complete response. Of a cohort of lymphoma patients undergoing vaccination following completion of chemotherapy, 70% remain without evidence of progression with a median follow up of 43 mo *(213)*. Titzer et al. reported on 11 patients with multiple myeloma who were treated with CD34-derived DCs pulsed with idiotype protein *(214)*. Four out of 10 patients developed evidence of increase idiotype-specific cellular immunity as determined by ELIspot analysis, and three patients showed evidence of anti-idiotype humoral response. One patient demonstrated evidence of marrow regression of plasma cells. Another study examined the impact of the infusion of DCs pulsed with idiotype protein following high0dose chemotherapy with stem cell rescue in patients with multiple myeloma *(215)*. Four out of 26 patients demonstrated evidence of idiotype-specific T cell proliferative responses in the post-transplant period.

Prominent clinical responses were reported in patients with metastatic renal cancer who were treated with fusions generated from patient-derived tumor cells and allogeneic DCs *(216)*. Seven out of 17 patients experienced at least 50% regression of disease, with four patients entering a complete remission. Disease response was noted in bone, soft tissue, and visceral sites with little associated toxicity.

9. DC IMMUNOTHERAPY: POTENTIAL LIMITING FACTORS

One concern regarding DC immunotherapy is the potential induction of T cell responses directed against self antigens. In a transgenic mouse model, animals vaccinated with DCs pulsed with tumor peptides demonstrated regression of established disease *(217)*. However, when the antigen was co-expressed in pancreatic β islet cells, arterial smooth muscle cells, and myocardial tissue, vaccination was associated with the development of diabetes, severe arteritis, and myocarditis, respectively. Another potential limiting factor in developing DCs immunotherapy is that cancer patients demonstrate deficiencies in cellular immunity. Patient-derived dendritic cells exhibit diminished functional capacity that potentially allows for the escape of tumor cells from immunosurveillance *(13,218)*. DCs isolated from tumor tissue are typically poor stimulators of T cell proliferation. Tumor cells may secrete IL-6, IL-10, and M-CSF which inhibit DC maturation. Tumor cells secrete high levels of MIP-3α, resulting in the migration of immature DCs into the tumor bed. In contrast, the more functionally active mature DCs are characteristically found in the peritumoral areas *(41)*. Fewer DCs have been found in primary sites of disease in patients with metastatic disease *(219)*. The tumor-associated antigens, MUC-1 and HER-2/neu, are internalized by DCs, but are not consistently transported to late MHC class II endosomes thus abrogating their ability to undergo appropriate processing and presentation *(220)*. DCs isolated from peripheral blood and tumor-draining lymph nodes were studied in 93 patients with breast, head and neck, and lung cancer *(221)*. Decreased numbers of circulating mature DCs was noted and impaired function was seen in DCs derived from both lymph nodes and blood, suggesting a systemic effect of the tumor. Partial reversal of these findings was noted after tumor resection. In contrast, functionally active DCs derived from patients with malignancy can be generated from precursor populations cultured in vitro with cytokines. DCs generated from patients with multiple myeloma, breast cancer, lymphoma, and renal cancer have been shown to prominently express co-stimulatory molecules and stimulate autologous and allogeneic T cell responses *(222–224)*.

10. CHARACTERIZATION OF DCS FOLLOWING AUTOLOGOUS AND ALLOGENEIC HEMATOPOIETIC CELL TRANSPLANTATION

The role of dendritic cells in the recovery of cellular immunity following autologous stem cell transplantation has been investigated. The nature of cytokine mobilization determines the character of DCs precursors in the graft and may have an impact on posttransplant immune reconstitution *(225)*. DCs generated in vitro from precursor populations isolated following autologous transplantation demonstrate normal phenotypical and functional characteristics *(223,226)*.

The nature of DCs reconstitution following allogeneic transplantation is likely to have profound implications for the development of donor/host tolerance with clinical implications for the incidence of rejection, graft-vs-host disease (GVHD), infection, and disease relapse. Levels of circulating DCs are suppressed following allogeneic transplant and in patients who develop GVHD *(227)*. In one study, DCs were found to be predominantly of donor origin in the early post-transplant period *(228)*. In a murine model, residual host DCs were uniquely responsible for the induction of GVHD *(229)*.

The nature of the recovering DCs subpopulations and their functional characteristics is strongly associated with levels of alloreactivity and tolerance. In animal models of solid organ transplants, treatment with immature DCs, lymphoid derived DCs, or DCs following blockade of the CD40 pathway resulted in prolonged survival of the allograft tissue *(230–232)*. Manipulation of DC populations by extracorporeal photochemotherapy resulted in improvement in chronic GVHD *(233)*. DCs generated from patients treated with FK506 following allogeneic transplantation demonstrate decreased functional capacity. Exposure to corticosteroids results in inhibited maturation and the expression of costimulatory molecules *(234,235)*. In animal model, G-CSF mobilized stem cell donors demonstrate decreased production of TNFα and IL-12 by DCs following exposure to LPS *(236)*. Following G-CSF mobilization of allogeneic donors, increased numbers of circulating lymphoid DCs (DC2) are found that are poor stimulators of T cell proliferation and may mediate tolerance *(237)*. This finding was thought to potentially explain the lack of increase in acute GVHD associated with allogeneic peripheral blood stem cell grafts, despite the increased numbers of T cells as compared to bone marrow. In patients undergoing allogeneic peripheral blood stem cell transplantation, increased numbers of DC2 in the stem cell graft was associated with decreased incidence of GVHD and increased risk of relapse *(238)*.

The use of DC posttransplant to boost cellular immunity directed against infectious pathogens and tumor cells is now being explored. Preclinical transplant models have demonstrated DC-mediated induction of T cell responses to cytomegalovirus (CMV), aspergillus, and candida *(239–241)*. In one report, a posttransplant patient demonstrated clinical response following treatment with donor-derived DCs that had been pulsed with irradiated autologous leukemia cells, as well as T cells that had been primed in vitro *(242)*.

11. CONCLUSION

DCs are potent antigen-presenting cells that play a crucial role in the initiation of cellular immunity and the maintenance of the delicate balance between tolerance and immune recognition. DC function is intimately linked to hematopoietic development. The use of DC-based immunotherapy has emerged as a major field of investigation and has yielded promising preliminary findings. Its integration into hematopoietic stem cell transplantation offers a potential avenue to modulate tumor-specific immunity and improve outcomes. Ongoing efforts in this arena will hopefully bear fruit in the struggle to generate an effective means to generating clinically meaningful immunotherapeutic strategies.

ACKNOWLEDGMENTS

Baldev Vasir, Ph.D., Zachary Avigan, and Jean-Claude Tetreault.

REFERENCES

1. Steinman RM. The dendritic cell system and its role in immunogenicity. *Annu Rev Immunol* 1991;9:271–296.

2. Steinman RM, Cohn ZA. Identification of a novel cell type in peripheral lymphoid organs of mice. I. Morphology, quantitation, tissue distribution. *J Exp Med* 1973;137:1142–1162.

3. Germain RN. The biochemistry and cell biology of antigen presentation by MHC class I and class II molecules. Implications for development of combination vaccines. *Ann NY Acad Sci* 1995;754:114–125.

4. Harding FA, McArthur JG, Gross JA, et al. CD28-mediated signalling co-stimulates murine T cells and prevents induction of anergy in T-cell clones. *Nature* 1992;356:607–609.

5. Young JW, et al. The B7/BB1 antigen provides one of several costimulatory signals for the activation of CD4+ T lymphocytes by human blood dendritic cells in vitro. *J Clin Invest* 1992;90:229–237.

6. Young JW, Steinman RM. The hematopoietic development of dendritic cells: a distinct pathway for myeloid differentiation. *Stem Cells* 1996;14:376–387.

7. Inaba K, et al. The tissue distribution of the B7-2 costimulator in mice: abundant expression on dendritic cells in situ and during maturation in vitro. *J Exp Med* 1994;180:1849–1860.

8. Boon T, van der Bruggen P. Human tumor antigens recognized by T lymphocytes. *J Exp Med* 1996;183:725–729.

9. Carrel S, Johnson JP. Immunologic recognition of malignant melanoma by autologous T lymphocytes. *Curr Opin Oncol* 1993;5:383–389.

10. Cox AL, et al. Identification of a peptide recognized by five melanoma-specific human cytotoxic T cell lines. *Science* 1994;264:716–719.

11. Kawakami Y, et al. Identification of a human melanoma antigen recognized by tumor- infiltrating lymphocytes associated with in vivo tumor rejection. *Proc Natl Acad Sci USA* 1994;91:6458–6462.

12. Speiser DE, et al. Self antigens expressed by solid tumors Do not efficiently stimulate naive or activated T cells: implications for immunotherapy. *J Exp Med* 1997;186:645–653.

13. Avigan D. Dendritic cells: development, function and potential use for cancer immunotherapy. *Blood Rev* 11999;3:51–64.

14. Ashley DM, et al. Bone marrow-generated dendritic cells pulsed with tumor extracts or tumor RNA induce antitumor immunity against central nervous system tumors. *J Exp Med* 1997;186:1177–1182.

15. Celluzzi CM, Mayordomo JI, Storkus WJ, et al. Peptide-pulsed dendritic cells induce antigen-specific CTL-mediated protective tumor immunity. *J Exp Med* 1996;183:283–287.

16. Gong J, Chen D, Kashiwaba M, et al. Induction of antitumor activity by immunization with fusions of dendritic and carcinoma cells. *Nat Med* 1997;3:558–561.

17. Gong J, et al. Activation of antitumor cytotoxic T lymphocytes by fusions of human dendritic cells and breast carcinoma cells. *Proc Natl Acad Sci USA* 2000;97:2715–2718.

18. Nair SK, et al. Induction of primary carcinoembryonic antigen (CEA)-specific cytotoxic T lymphocytes in vitro using human dendritic cells transfected with RNA. *Nat Biotechnol* 1998;16:364–369.

19. Paglia P, Chiodoni C, Rodolfo M, et al. Murine dendritic cells loaded in vitro with soluble protein prime cytotoxic T lymphocytes against tumor antigen in vivo. *J Exp Med* 1996;183:317–322.

20. Nestle FO, et al. Vaccination of melanoma patients with peptide- or tumor lysate-pulsed dendritic cells. *Nat Med* 1998;4:328–332.

21. Bernhard H, et al. Generation of immunostimulatory dendritic cells from human CD34+ hematopoietic progenitor cells of the bone marrow and peripheral blood. *Cancer Res* 1995;55:1099–1104.

22. Caux C, et al. CD34+ hematopoietic progenitors from human cord blood differentiate along two independent dendritic cell pathways in response to GM-CSF+TNF alpha. *J Exp Med* 1996;184:695–706.

23. Szabolcs P, Feller ED, Moore MA, et al. Progenitor recruitment and in vitro expansion of immunostimulatory dendritic cells from human CD34+ bone marrow cells by c-kit-ligand, GM- CSF, and TNF alpha. *Adv Exp Med Biol* 1995;378:17–20

24. Romani N, et al. Proliferating dendritic cell progenitors in human blood. *J Exp Med* 1994;180:83–93.

25. Russo V, et al. Acquisition of intact allogeneic human leukocyte antigen molecules by human dendritic cells. *Blood* 2000;95:3473–3477.

26. Hirano A, et al. Graft hyporeactivity induced by donor-derived dendritic cell progenitors. *Transplant Proc* 2000;32:260–264.

27. Banchereau J, et al. Immunobiology of dendritic cells. *Annu Rev Immunol* 2000;18:767–811.

28. Katz SI, Tamaki K, Sachs DH. Epidermal Langerhans cells are derived from cells originating in bone marrow. *Nature* 1979;282:324–326.

29. Wu L, Li CL, Shortman K. Thymic dendritic cell precursors: relationship to the T lymphocyte lineage and phenotype of the dendritic cell progeny. *J Exp Med* 1996;184:903–911.

30. Shortman K, et al. The linkage between T-cell and dendritic cell development in the mouse thymus. *Immunol Rev* 1998;165:39–46.

31. Vremec D, Shortman K. Dendritic cell subtypes in mouse lymphoid organs: cross-correlation of surface markers, changes with incubation, and differences among thymus, spleen, and lymph nodes. *J Immunol* 1997;159:565–573.

32. Traver D, et al. Development of CD8alpha-positive dendritic cells from a common myeloid progenitor. *Science* 2000;290:2152–2154. (2000).

33. Sertl K, et al. Dendritic cells with antigen-presenting capability reside in airway epithelium, lung parenchyma, and visceral pleura. *J Exp Med* 1986;163:436–451.

34. Strunk D, Egger C, Leitner G, et al. A skin homing molecule defines the langerhans cell progenitor in human peripheral blood. *J Exp Med* 1997;185:1131–1136.

35. Jakob T, Udey MC. Regulation of E-cadherin-mediated adhesion in Langerhans cell-like dendritic cells by inflammatory mediators that mobilize Langerhans cells in vivo. *J Immunol* 1998;160:4067–4073.

36. Austyn JM. New insights into the mobilization and phagocytic activity of dendritic cells. *J Exp Med* 1996;183:1287–1292.

37. Drakes ML, Lu L, Subbotin VM, et al. In vivo administration of flt3 ligand markedly stimulates generation of dendritic cell progenitors from mouse liver. *J Immunol* 1997;159:4268–4278.

38. Esche C, et al. Interleukin-12 and Flt3 ligand differentially promote dendropoiesis in vivo. *Eur J Immunol* 2000;30:2565–2575.

39. Dieu MC, et al. Selective recruitment of immature and mature dendritic cells by distinct chemokines expressed in different anatomic sites. *J Exp Med* 1998;188:373–386.

40. Power CA, et al. Cloning and characterization of a specific receptor for the novel CC chemokine MIP-3alpha from lung dendritic cells. *J Exp Med* 1997;186:825–835.

41. Bell D, et al. In breast carcinoma tissue, immature dendritic cells reside within the tumor, whereas mature dendritic cells are located in peritumoral areas. *J Exp Med* 1999;190:1417–1426.

42. Kobayashi Y. Langerhans' cells produce type IV collagenase (MMP-9) following epicutaneous stimulation with haptens. *Immunology* 1997;90:496–501.

43. Steinman RM, Swanson J. The endocytic activity of dendritic cells. *J Exp Med* 1995;182:283–288.

44. Rubartelli A, Poggi A, Zocchi MR. The selective engulfment of apoptotic bodies by dendritic cells is mediated by the alpha(v)beta3 integrin and requires intracellular and extracellular calcium. *Eur J Immunol* 1997;27:1893–900.

45. Albert ML, et al. Immature dendritic cells phagocytose apoptotic cells via alphavbeta5 and CD36, and cross-present antigens to cytotoxic T lymphocytes. *J Exp Med* 1998;188:1359–1368.

46. Arnold-Schild D, et al. Cutting edge: receptor-mediated endocytosis of heat shock proteins by professional antigen-presenting cells. *J Immunol* 1999;162:3757–3760.

47. Todryk S, et al. Heat shock protein 70 induced during tumor cell killing induces Th1 cytokines and targets immature dendritic cell precursors to enhance antigen uptake. *J Immunol* 1999;163, 1398-408. (1999).

48. Inaba K, Inaba M, Naito M, et al. Dendritic cell progenitors phagocytose particulates, including bacillus Calmette-Guerin organisms, and sensitize mice to mycobacterial antigens in vivo. *J Exp Med* 1993;178:479–488.

49. Kampgen E, et al. Class II major histocompatibility complex molecules of murine dendritic cells: synthesis, sialylation of invariant chain, and antigen processing capacity are down-regulated upon culture. *Proc Natl Acad Sci USA* 1991;88:3014–3018.

50. Watts C. Immunology. Inside the gearbox of the dendritic cell. *Nature* 1997;388:724,725.

51. Jiang W, et al. The receptor DEC-205 expressed by dendritic cells and thymic epithelial cells is involved in antigen processing. *Nature* 1995;375:151–155.

52. Tan MC, et al. Mannose receptor-mediated uptake of antigens strongly enhances HLA class II-restricted antigen presentation by cultured dendritic cells. *Eur J Immunol* 1997;27:2426–2435.

53. Mommaas AM, et al. Human epidermal Langerhans cells lack functional mannose receptors and a fully developed endosomal/lysosomal compartment for loading of HLA class II molecules. *Eur J Immunol* 1999;29:571–580.

54. Pierre P, Mellman I. Developmental regulation of invariant chain proteolysis controls MHC class II trafficking in mouse dendritic cells. *Cell* 1998;93:1135–1145.

55. Turley SJ, et al. Transport of peptide-MHC class II complexes in developing dendritic cells. *Science* 2000;288:522–527.

56. Bates EE, et al. Identification and analysis of a novel member of the ubiquitin family expressed in dendritic cells and mature B cells. *Eur J Immunol* 1997;27:2471–2477.

57. Pfeifer JD, et al. Phagocytic processing of bacterial antigens for class I MHC presentation to T cells. *Nature* 1993;361:359–362.

58. Kovacsovics-Bankowski M, Clark K, Benacerraf B, et al. Efficient major histocompatibility complex class I presentation of exogenous antigen upon phagocytosis by macrophages. *Proc Natl Acad Sci USA* 1993;90:4942–4946.

59. Kovacsovics-Bankowski M, Rock KL. A phagosome-to-cytosol pathway for exogenous antigens presented on MHC class I molecules. *Science* 1995;267:243–246.

60. Inaba K, Metlay JP, Crowley MT, et al. Dendritic cells pulsed with protein antigens in vitro can prime antigen-specific, MHC-restricted T cells in situ. *J Exp Med* 1990;172:631–640.

61. Tang A, Amagai M, Granger LG, et al. Adhesion of epidermal Langerhans cells to keratinocytes mediated by E- cadherin. *Nature* 1993;361:82–85.

62. Riedl E, et al. Ligation of E-cadherin on in vitro-generated immature Langerhans-type dendritic cells inhibits their maturation. *Blood* 2000;96:4276–4284.

63. Witmer-Pack MD, Olivier W, Valinsky J, et al. Granulocyte/macrophage colony-stimulating factor is essential for the viability and function of cultured murine epidermal Langerhans cells. *J Exp Med* 1987;166:1484–1498.

64. Kampgen E, et al. Understanding the dendritic cell lineage through a study of cytokine receptors. *J Exp Med* 1994;179:1767–1776.

65. Santiago-Schwarz F, Divaris N, Kay C, et al. Mechanisms of tumor necrosis factor-granulocyte-macrophage colony- stimulating factor-induced dendritic cell development. *Blood* 1993;82:3019–3028.

66. Flores-Romo L, et al. CD40 ligation on human cord blood CD34+ hematopoietic progenitors induces their proliferation and differentiation into functional dendritic cells. *J Exp Med* 1997;185:341–349.

67. Askew D, Chu RS, Krieg AM, et al. CpG DNA induces maturation of dendritic cells with distinct effects on nascent and recycling MHC-II antigen-processing mechanisms. *J Immunol* 2000;165:6889–6895.

68. Morel AS, Quaratino S, Douek DC, et al. Split activity of interleukin-10 on antigen capture and antigen presentation by human dendritic cells: definition of a maturative step. *Eur J Immunol* 1997;27:26–34.

69. Sallusto F, et al. Rapid and coordinated switch in chemokine receptor expression during dendritic cell maturation. *Eur J Immunol* 1998;28:2760–2769.

70. Chan VW, et al. Secondary lymphoid-tissue chemokine (SLC) is chemotactic for mature dendritic cells. *Blood* 1999;93:3610–3616.

71. Gunn MD, et al. A chemokine expressed in lymphoid high endothelial venules promotes the adhesion and chemotaxis of naive T lymphocytes. *Proc Natl Acad Sci USA* 1998;95:258–263.

72. Saeki H, Moore AM, Brown MJ, et al. Cutting edge: secondary lymphoid-tissue chemokine (SLC) and CC chemokine receptor 7 (CCR7) participate in the emigration pathway of mature dendritic cells from the skin to regional lymph nodes. *J Immunol* 1999;162:2472–2475.

73. Ngo VN, Tang HL, Cyster JG. Epstein-Barr virus-induced molecule 1 ligand chemokine is expressed by dendritic cells in lymphoid tissues and strongly attracts naive T cells and activated B cells. *J Exp Med* 1998;188:181–191.

74. Campbell JJ, et al. Chemokines and the arrest of lymphocytes rolling under flow conditions. *Science* 1998;279:381–384.

75. Gunn MD, et al. Mice lacking expression of secondary lymphoid organ chemokine have defects in lymphocyte homing and dendritic cell localization. *J Exp Med* 1999;189:451–460.

76. Nakano H, et al. A novel mutant gene involved in T-lymphocyte-specific homing into peripheral lymphoid organs on mouse chromosome 4. *Blood* 1998;91:2886–2895.

77. Fushimi T, Kojima A, Moore MA, et al. Macrophage inflammatory protein 3alpha transgene attracts dendritic cells to established murine tumors and suppresses tumor growth. *J Clin Invest* 2000;105:1383–1393.

78. Cresswell P. Invariant chain structure and MHC class II function. *Cell* 1996;84:505–507.

79. Castellino F, Zhong G, Germain RN. Antigen presentation by MHC class II molecules: invariant chain function, protein trafficking, and the molecular basis of diverse determinant capture. *Hum Immunol* 1997;54:159–169.

80. Koppelman B, Neefjes JJ, de Vries JE, et al. Interleukin-10 down-regulates MHC class II alphabeta peptide complexes at the plasma membrane of monocytes by affecting arrival and recycling. *Immunity* 1997;7:861–871.

81. Mosialos G, et al. Circulating human dendritic cells differentially express high levels of a 55-kd actin-bundling protein. *Am J Pathol* 1996;148:593–600.

82. Al-Alwan MM, Rowden G, Lee TD, et al. Fascin is involved in the antigen presentation activity of mature dendritic cells. *J Immunol* 2001;166:338–345.

83. Zhou LJ, Tedder TF. Human blood dendritic cells selectively express CD83, a member of the immunoglobulin superfamily. *J Immunol* 1995;154:3821–3835.

84. Steinman RM, Witmer MD. Lymphoid dendritic cells are potent stimulators of the primary mixed leukocyte reaction in mice. *Proc Natl Acad Sci USA* 1978;75:5132–5236.

85. Van Voorhis WC, et al. Relative efficacy of human monocytes and dendritic cells as accessory cells for T cell replication. *J Exp Med* 1983;158:174–191.

86. Cassell DJ, Schwartz RH. A quantitative analysis of antigen-presenting cell function: activated B cells stimulate naive CD4 T cells but are inferior to dendritic cells in providing costimulation. *J Exp Med* 1994;180:1829–1840.

87. Ellis J, et al. Antigen presentation by dendritic cells provides optimal stimulation for the production of interleukin (IL) 2, IL 4 and interferon-gamma by allogeneic T cells. *Eur J Immunol* 1991;21:2803–2809.

88. Bhardwaj N, Friedman SM, Cole BC, et al. Dendritic cells are potent antigen-presenting cells for microbial superantigens. *J Exp Med* 1992;175:267–273.

89. Inaba K, Young JW, Steinman RM. Direct activation of CD8+ cytotoxic T lymphocytes by dendritic cells. *J Exp Med* 1987;166:182–194.

90. Porgador A, Gilboa E. Bone marrow-generated dendritic cells pulsed with a class I-restricted peptide are potent inducers of cytotoxic T lymphocytes. *J Exp Med* 1995;182:255–260.

91. Arthur JF, et al. A comparison of gene transfer methods in human dendritic cells. *Cancer Gene Ther* 1997;4:17–25.

92. Bhardwaj N, et al. Influenza virus-infected dendritic cells stimulate strong proliferative and cytolytic responses from human CD8+ T cells. *J Clin Invest* 1994;94:797–807.

93. Jonuleit H, Schmitt E, Schuler G, et al. Induction of interleukin 10-producing, nonproliferating CD4(+) T cells with regulatory properties by repetitive stimulation with allogeneic immature human dendritic cells. *J Exp Med* 2000;192:1213–1222.

94. Caux C, et al. B70/B7-2 is identical to CD86 and is the major functional ligand for CD28 expressed on human dendritic cells. *J Exp Med* 1994;180:1841–1847.

95. Dubois B, et al. Critical role of IL-12 in dendritic cell-induced differentiation of naive B lymphocytes. *J Immunol* 1998;161:2223–2231.

96. Dubois B, et al. Dendritic cells enhance growth and differentiation of CD40-activated B lymphocytes. *J Exp Med* 1997;185:941–951.

97. Steinman RM, Inaba K. The binding of antigen presenting cells to T lymphocytes. *Adv Exp Med Biol* 1988;237:31–41.

98. Jonuleit H, et al. Induction of IL-15 messenger RNA and protein in human blood-derived dendritic cells: a role for IL-15 in attraction of T cells. *J Immunol* 1997;158:2610–2615.

99. Koide SL, Inaba K, Steinman RM. Interleukin 1 enhances T-dependent immune responses by amplifying the function of dendritic cells. *J Exp Med* 1987;165:515–530.

100. Hauss P, Selz F, Cavazzana-Calvo M, et al. Characteristics of antigen-independent and antigen-dependent interaction of dendritic cells with CD4+ T cells. *Eur J Immunol* 1995;25:2285–2294. (1995).

101. Kedl RM, et al. T cells compete for access to antigen-bearing antigen-presenting cells. *J Exp Med* 2000;192:1105–1113.

102. Caux C, et al. Activation of human dendritic cells through CD40 cross-linking. *J Exp Med* 1994;180:1263–1272.

103. McLellan AD, Sorg RV, Williams LA, et al. Human dendritic cells activate T lymphocytes via a CD40: CD40 ligand- dependent pathway. *Eur J Immunol* 1996;26:1204–1210.

104. Kelsall BL, Stuber E, Neurath M, et al. Interleukin-12 production by dendritic cells. The role of CD40-CD40L interactions in Th1 T-cell responses. *Ann NY Acad Sci* 1996;795:116–126.

105. Cella M, et al. Ligation of CD40 on dendritic cells triggers production of high levels of interleukin-12 and enhances T cell stimulatory capacity: T-T help via APC activation. *J Exp Med* 1996;184:747–752.

106. Anderson DM, et al. A homologue of the TNF receptor and its ligand enhance T-cell growth and dendritic-cell function. *Nature* 1997;390:175–179.

107. Wong BR, et al. TRANCE (tumor necrosis factor [TNF]-related activation-induced cytokine), a new TNF family member predominantly expressed in T cells, is a dendritic cell-specific survival factor. *J Exp Med* 1997;186:2075–2080.

108. Foster GR, Germain C, Jones M, et al. Human T cells elicit IFN-alpha secretion from dendritic cells following cell to cell interactions. *Eur J Immunol* 2000;30:3228–3235.

109. Verhasselt V, et al. Bacterial lipopolysaccharide stimulates the production of cytokines and the expression of costimulatory molecules by human peripheral blood dendritic cells: evidence for a soluble CD14-dependent pathway. *J Immunol* 1997;158:2919–2925.

110. Macatonia SE, et al. Dendritic cells produce IL-12 and direct the development of Th1 cells from naive CD4+ T cells. *J Immunol* 1995;154:5071–5079.

111. Bhardwaj N, Seder RA, Reddy A, et al. IL-12 in conjunction with dendritic cells enhances antiviral CD8+ CTL responses in vitro. *J Clin Invest* 1996;98:715–722.

112. Koch F, et al. High level IL-12 production by murine dendritic cells: upregulation via MHC class II and CD40 molecules and downregulation by IL-4 and IL-10. *J Exp Med* 1996;184:741–746.

113. Zitvogel L, et al. IL-12-engineered dendritic cells serve as effective tumor vaccine adjuvants in vivo. *Ann NY Acad Sci* 1996;795:284–293.

114. Leverkus M, et al. Maturation of dendritic cells leads to up-regulation of cellular FLICE- inhibitory protein and concomitant down-regulation of death ligand- mediated apoptosis. *Blood* 2000;96:2628–2631.

115. Lu L, et al. Fas ligand (CD95L) and B7 expression on dendritic cells provide counter- regulatory signals for T cell survival and proliferation. *J Immunol* 1997;158:5676–5684.

116. Rescigno M, et al. Fas engagement induces the maturation of dendritic cells (DCs), the release of interleukin (IL)-1beta, and the production of interferon gamma in the absence of IL-12 during DC-T cell cognate interaction: a new role for Fas ligand in inflammatory responses. *J Exp Med* 2000;192:1661–1668.

117. Steinbrink K, Wolfl M, Jonuleit H, et al. Induction of tolerance by IL-10-treated dendritic cells. *J Immunol* 1997;159:4772–4780.

118. Allavena P, et al. IL-10 prevents the differentiation of monocytes to dendritic cells but promotes their maturation to macrophages. *Eur J Immunol* 1998;28:359–369.

119. de Saint-Vis B, et al. The cytokine profile expressed by human dendritic cells is dependent on cell subtype and mode of activation. *J Immunol* 1998;160:1666–1676.

120. Qin Z, Noffz G, Mohaupt M, et al. Interleukin-10 prevents dendritic cell accumulation and vaccination with granulocyte-macrophage colony-stimulating factor gene-modified tumor cells. *J Immunol* 1997;159:770–776.

121. Hochrein H, et al. Interleukin (IL)-4 is a major regulatory cytokine governing bioactive IL-12 production by mouse and human dendritic cells. *J Exp Med* 2000;192:823–833.

122. Grohmann U, et al. A tumor-associated and self antigen peptide presented by dendritic cells may induce T cell anergy in vivo, but IL-12 can prevent or revert the anergic state. *J Immunol* 1997;158:3593–3602.

123. Inaba K, et al. Generation of large numbers of dendritic cells from mouse bone marrow cultures supplemented with granulocyte/macrophage colony-stimulating factor. *J Exp Med* 1992;176:1693–1702.

124. Maraskovsky E, et al. Dramatic increase in the numbers of functionally mature dendritic cells in Flt3 ligand-treated mice: multiple dendritic cell subpopulations identified. *J Exp Med* 1996;184:1953–1962.

125. Pulendran B, et al. Developmental pathways of dendritic cells in vivo: distinct function, phenotype, and localization of dendritic cell subsets in FLT3 ligand- treated mice. *J Immunol* 1997;159:2222–2231.

126. Young JW, Szabolcs P, Moore MA. Identification of dendritic cell colony-forming units among normal human CD34+ bone marrow progenitors that are expanded by c-kit-ligand and yield pure dendritic cell colonies in the presence of granulocyte/macrophage colony-stimulating factor and tumor necrosis factor alpha. *J Exp Med* 1995;182:1111–1119.

127. Saraya K, Reid CD. Stem cell factor and the regulation of dendritic cell production from CD34+ progenitors in bone marrow and cord blood. *Br J Haematol* 1996;93:258–264.

128. Curti A, Fogli M, Ratta M, et al. Stem cell factor and FLT3-ligand are strictly required to sustain the long-term expansion of primitive CD34+DR- dendritic cell precursors. *J Immunol* 2001;166:848–854. (2001).

129. Szabolcs P. Moore MA, Young JW. Expansion of immunostimulatory dendritic cells among the myeloid progeny of human CD34+ bone marrow precursors cultured with c-kit ligand, granulocyte-macrophage colony-stimulating factor, and TNF-alpha. *J Immunol* 1995;154:5851–5861.

130. Strobl H, et al. flt3 ligand in cooperation with transforming growth factor-beta1 potentiates in vitro development of Langerhans-type dendritic cells and allows single-cell dendritic cell cluster formation under serum-free conditions. *Blood* 1997;90:1425–1434.

131. Arrighi JF, Hauser C, Chapuis B, et al. Long-term culture of human CD34(+) progenitors with FLT3-ligand, thrombopoietin, and stem cell factor induces extensive amplification of a CD34(-)CD14(-) and a CD34(-)CD14(+) dendritic cell precursor. *Blood* 1999;93:2244–2252.

132. Szabolcs P, et al. Dendritic cells and macrophages can mature independently from a human bone marrow-derived, post-colony-forming unit intermediate. *Blood* 1996;87;4520–4530.

133. Rosenzwajg M, Canque B, Gluckman JC. Human dendritic cell differentiation pathway from CD34+ hemato-poietic precursor cells. *Blood* 1996;87:535–544.

134. O'Doherty U, et al. Dendritic cells freshly isolated from human blood express CD4 and mature into typical immunostimulatory dendritic cells after culture in monocyte-conditioned medium. *J Exp Med* 1993;178:1067–1076.

135. O'Doherty U, et al. Human blood contains two subsets of dendritic cells, one immunologically mature and the other immature. *Immunology* 1994;82:487–493.

136. Thomas R, Lipsky PE. Human peripheral blood dendritic cell subsets. Isolation and characterization of precursor and mature antigen-presenting cells. *J Immunol* 1994;153:4016–4028.

137. Sallusto F, Lanzavecchia A. Efficient presentation of soluble antigen by cultured human dendritic cells is maintained by granulocyte/macrophage colony-stimulating factor plus interleukin 4 and downregulated by tumor necrosis factor alpha. *J Exp Med* 1994;179:1109–1118.

138. Ito T, et al. A CD1a+/CD11c+ subset of human blood dendritic cells is a direct precursor of Langerhans cells. *J Immunol* 1999;163:1409–1419.

139. Bender A, Sapp M, Schuler G, et al.. Improved methods for the generation of dendritic cells from nonproliferating progenitors in human blood. *J Immunol Methods* 1996;196:121–135.

140. Schlienger K, Craighead N, Lee KP, et al. Efficient priming of protein antigen-specific human CD4(+) T cells by monocyte-derived dendritic cells. *Blood* 2000;96:3490–3498.

141. Mehta-Damani A, Markowicz S, Engleman EG. Generation of antigen-specific CD8+ CTLs from naive precursors. *J Immunol* 1994;153:996–1003.

142. Song ES, et al. Antigen presentation in retroviral vector-mediated gene transfer in vivo. *Proc Natl Acad Sci USA* 1997;94:1943–1948.

143. Aicher A, et al. Successful retroviral mediated transduction of a reporter gene in human dendritic cells: feasibility of therapy with gene-modified antigen presenting cells. *Exp Hematol* 1997;25:39–44.

144. Alijagic S, et al. Dendritic cells generated from peripheral blood transfected with human tyrosinase induce specific T cell activation. *Eur J Immunol* 1995;25:3100–3107.

145. Casares S, Inaba K, Brumeanu TD, et al. Antigen presentation by dendritic cells after immunization with DNA encoding a major histocompatibility complex class II-restricted viral epitope. *J Exp Med* 1997;186:1481–1486.

146. Chapoval AI, Tamada K, Chen L. In vitro growth inhibition of a broad spectrum of tumor cell lines by activated human dendritic cells. *Blood* 2000;95:2346–2351.

147. Shen Z, Reznikoff G, Dranoff G, et al. Cloned dendritic cells can present exogenous antigens on both MHC class I and class II molecules. *J Immunol* 1997;158:2723–2730.

148. Chiodoni C, et al. Dendritic cells infiltrating tumors cotransduced with granulocyte/macrophage colony-stimulating factor (GM-CSF) and CD40 ligand genes take up and present endogenous tumor-associated antigens, and prime naive mice for a cytotoxic T lymphocyte response. *J Exp Med* 1999;190:125–133.

149. Furumoto K, et al. Spleen-derived dendritic cells engineered to enhance interleukin-12 production elicit therapeutic antitumor immune responses. *Int J Cancer* 2000;87:665–672.

150. Lynch DH, et al. Flt3 ligand induces tumor regression and antitumor immune responses in vivo. *Nat Med* 1997;3:625–631.

151. Chen K, et al. Antitumor activity and immunotherapeutic properties of Flt3-ligand in a murine breast cancer model. *Cancer Res* 1997;57:3511–3516.

152. Peron JM, et al. FLT3-ligand administration inhibits liver metastases: role of NK cells. *J Immunol* 1998;161:6164–6170.

153. Chakravarty PK, et al. Flt3-ligand administration after radiation therapy prolongs survival in a murine model of metastatic lung cancer. *Cancer Res* 1999;59:6028–6032.

154. Bullock TN, Colella TA, Engelhard VH. The density of peptides displayed by dendritic cells affects immune responses to human tyrosinase and gp100 in HLA-A2 transgenic mice. *J Immunol* 2000;164:2354–2361.

155. Mayordomo JI, et al. Bone marrow-derived dendritic cells pulsed with synthetic tumour peptides elicit protective and therapeutic antitumour immunity. *Nat Med* 1995;1:1297–1302.

156. De Bruijn ML, et al. Immunization with human papillomavirus type 16 (HPV16) oncoprotein-loaded dendritic cells as well as protein in adjuvant induces MHC class I-restricted protection to HPV16-induced tumor cells. *Cancer Res* 1998;58:724–731.

157. Mayordomo JI, et al. Therapy of murine tumors with p53 wild-type and mutant sequence peptide-based vaccines. *J Exp Med* 1996;183:1357–1365.

158. Hodge JW, et al. Enhanced activation of T cells by dendritic cells engineered to hyperexpress a triad of costimulatory molecules. *J Natl Cancer Inst* 2000;92:1228–1239.

159. Bakker AB, et al. Generation of antimelanoma cytotoxic T lymphocytes from healthy donors after presentation of melanoma-associated antigen-derived epitopes by dendritic cells in vitro. *Cancer Res* 1995;55:5330–5334.

160. Alters SE, et al. Dendritic cells pulsed with CEA peptide induce CEA-specific CTL with restricted TCR repertoire. *J Immunother* 1998;21:17–26.

161. Mannering SI, McKenzie JL, Fearnley DB, et al. HLA-DR1-restricted bcr-abl (b3a2)-specific CD4+ T lymphocytes respond to dendritic cells pulsed with b3a2 peptide and antigen-presenting cells exposed to b3a2 containing cell lysates. *Blood* 1997;90:290–297.

162. Nieda M, et al. Dendritic cells stimulate the expansion of bcr-abl specific CD8+ T cells with cytotoxic activity against leukemic cells from patients with chronic myeloid leukemia. *Blood* 1998;91:977–983.

163. Osman Y, et al. Generation of bcr-abl specific cytotoxic T-lymphocytes by using dendritic cells pulsed with bcr-abl (b3a2) peptide: its applicability for donor leukocyte transfusions in marrow grafted CML patients. *Leukemia* 1999;13:166–174.

164. Serody JS, Collins EJ, Tisch RM, et al. T cell activity after dendritic cell vaccination is dependent on both the type of antigen and the mode of delivery. *J Immunol* 2000;164:4961–4967.

165. Hoffmann TK, et al. Generation of T cells specific for the wild-type sequence p53(264-272) peptide in cancer patients: implications for immunoselection of epitope loss variants. *J Immunol* 2000;165:5938–5944.

166. Flamand V, et al. Murine dendritic cells pulsed in vitro with tumor antigen induce tumor resistance in vivo. *Eur J Immunol* 1994;24:605–610.

167. Ratta M, et al. Efficient presentation of tumor idiotype to autologous T cells by CD83(+) dendritic cells derived from highly purified circulating CD14(+) monocytes in multiple myeloma patients. *Exp Hematol* 2000;28:931–940.

168. Osterroth F, Garbe A, Fisch P, et al. Stimulation of cytotoxic T cells against idiotype immunoglobulin of malignant lymphoma with protein-pulsed or idiotype-transduced dendritic cells. *Blood* 2000;95:1342–1349.

169. Dembic Z, Schenck K, Bogen B. Dendritic cells purified from myeloma are primed with tumor-specific antigen (idiotype) and activate CD4+ T cells. *Proc Natl Acad Sci USA* 2000;97:2697–2702.

170. Ribas A, et al. Genetic immunization for the melanoma antigen MART-1/Melan-A using recombinant adenovirus-transduced murine dendritic cells. *Cancer Res* 1997;57:2865–2869.

171. Song W, et al. Dendritic cells genetically modified with an adenovirus vector encoding the cDNA for a model antigen induce protective and therapeutic antitumor immunity. *J Exp Med* 1997;186:1247–1256.

172. Wan Y, Bramson J, Pilon A, et al. Genetically modified dendritic cells prime autoreactive T cells through a pathway independent of CD40L and interleukin 12: implications for cancer vaccines. *Cancer Res* 2000;60:3247–3253.

173. Brown M, et al. Dendritic cells infected with recombinant fowlpox virus vectors are potent and long-acting stimulators of transgene-specific class I restricted T lymphocyte activity. *Gene Ther* 2000;7:1680–1689.

174. Yang S, et al. Dendritic cells infected with a vaccinia vector carrying the human gp100 gene simultaneously present multiple specificities and elicit high-affinity T cells reactive to multiple epitopes and restricted by HLA-A2 and -A3. *J Immunol* 2000;164:4204–4211.

175. Jenne L, Hauser C, Arrighi JF, et al. Poxvirus as a vector to transduce human dendritic cells for immunotherapy: abortive infection but reduced APC function. *Gene Ther* 2000;7:1575–1583.

176. Henderson RA, et al. Human dendritic cells genetically engineered to express high levels of the human epithelial tumor antigen mucin (MUC-1). *Cancer Res* 1996;56:3763–3770.

177. Reeves ME, Royal RE, Lam JS, et al. Retroviral transduction of human dendritic cells with a tumor-associated antigen gene. *Cancer Res* 1996;56:5672–5677.

178. Specht JM, et al. Dendritic cells retrovirally transduced with a model antigen gene are therapeutically effective against established pulmonary metastases. *J Exp Med* 1997;186:1213–1221.

179. Klein C, Bueler H, Mulligan RC. Comparative analysis of genetically modified dendritic cells and tumor cells as therapeutic cancer vaccines. *J Exp Med* 2000;191:1699–1708.

180. Boczkowski D, Nair SK, Snyder D, et al. Dendritic cells pulsed with RNA are potent antigen-presenting cells in vitro and in vivo. *J Exp Med* 1996;184:465–472.

181. Thornburg C, Boczkowski D, Gilboa E, et al. Induction of cytotoxic T lymphocytes with dendritic cells transfected with human papillomavirus E6 and E7 RNA: implications for cervical cancer immunotherapy. *J Immunother* 2000;23:412–418.

182. Heiser A, et al. Human dendritic cells transfected with RNA encoding prostate-specific antigen stimulate prostate-specific CTL responses in vitro. *J Immunol* 2000;164:5508–5514.

183. Koido S, et al. Induction of antitumor immunity by vaccination of dendritic cells transfected with MUC1 RNA. *J Immunol* 2000;165:5713–5719.

184. Zitvogel L, et al. Therapy of murine tumors with tumor peptide-pulsed dendritic cells: dependence on T cells, B7 costimulation, and T helper cell 1-associated cytokines. *J Exp Med* 1996;183:87–97.

185. DeMatos P, Abdel-Wahab Z, Vervaert C, et al. Pulsing of dendritic cells with cell lysates from either B16 melanoma or MCA-106 fibrosarcoma yields equally effective vaccines against B16 tumors in mice. *J Surg Oncol* 1998;68:79–91.

186. Herr W, et al. Mature dendritic cells pulsed with freeze-thaw cell lysates define an effective in vitro vaccine designed to elicit EBV-specific CD4(+) and CD8(+) T lymphocyte responses. *Blood* 2000;96:1857–1864.

187. Nouri-Shirazi M, et al. Dendritic cells capture killed tumor cells and present their antigens to elicit tumor-specific immune responses. *J Immunol* 2000;165:3797–3803.

188. Russo V, et al. Dendritic cells acquire the MAGE-3 human tumor antigen from apoptotic cells and induce a class I-restricted T cell response. *Proc Natl Acad Sci USA* 2000;97:2185–2190.

189. Albert ML, Sauter B, Bhardwaj N. Dendritic cells acquire antigen from apoptotic cells and induce class I-restricted CTLs. *Nature* 1998;392:86–89.

190. Sauter B, et al. Consequences of cell death: exposure to necrotic tumor cells, but not primary tissue cells or apoptotic cells, induces the maturation of immunostimulatory dendritic cells. *J Exp Med* 2000;191:423–434.

191. Shaif-Muthana M, McIntyre C, Sisley K, et al. Dead or alive: immunogenicity of human melanoma cells when presented by dendritic cells. *Cancer Res* 2000;60:6441–6447.

192. Choudhury A, et al. Use of leukemic dendritic cells for the generation of antileukemic cellular cytotoxicity against Philadelphia chromosome-positive chronic myelogenous leukemia. *Blood* 1997;89:1133–1142.

193. Chen X, Regn S, Raffegerst S, et al. Interferon alpha in combination with GM-CSF induces the differentiation of leukaemic antigen-presenting cells that have the capacity to stimulate a specific anti-leukaemic cytotoxic T-cell response from patients with chronic myeloid leukaemia. *Br J Haematol* 2000;111:596–5607.

194. Westermann J, et al. Bcr/abl+ autologous dendritic cells for vaccination in chronic myeloid leukemia. *Bone Marrow Transplant* 2000;26(Suppl 2):S46–49.

195. Cignetti A, et al. CD34(+) acute myeloid and lymphoid leukemic blasts can be induced to differentiate into dendritic cells. *Blood* 1999;94:2048–2055.

196. Choudhury BA, et al. Dendritic cells derived in vitro from acute myelogenous leukemia cells stimulate autologous, antileukemic T-cell responses. *Blood* 1999;93:780–786.

197. Costello RT, et al. Human acute myeloid leukemia CD34+/CD38- progenitor cells have decreased sensitivity to chemotherapy and Fas-induced apoptosis, reduced immunogenicity, and impaired dendritic cell transformation capacities. *Cancer Res* 2000;60:4403–4411.

198. Gong J, et al. Reversal of tolerance to human MUC1 antigen in MUC1 transgenic mice immunized with fusions of dendritic and carcinoma cells. *Proc Natl Acad Sci USA* 1998;95:6279–6283. (1998).

199. Celluzzi CM, Falo LD. Physical interaction between dendritic cells and tumor cells results in an immunogen that induces protective and therapeutic tumor rejection. *J Immunol* 1998;160:3081–3085.

200. Lespagnard L, et al. Dendritic cells fused with mastocytoma cells elicit therapeutic antitumor immunity. *Int J Cancer* 1998;76:250–258.

201. Cao X, et al. Therapy of established tumour with a hybrid cellular vaccine generated by using granulocyte-macrophage colony-stimulating factor genetically modified dendritic cells. *Immunology* 1999;97:616–625.

202. Gong J, et al. Fusions of human ovarian carcinoma cells with autologous or allogeneic dendritic cells induce antitumor immunity. *J Immunol* 2000;165:1705–1711.

203. Morse MA, et al. Preoperative mobilization of circulating dendritic cells by Flt3 ligand administration to patients with metastatic colon cancer. *J Clin Oncol* 2000;18:3883–3893.

204. Triozzi PL, et al. Intratumoral injection of dendritic cells derived in vitro in patients with metastatic cancer. *Cancer* 2000;89:2646–2654.

205. Mackensen A, et al. Phase I study in melanoma patients of a vaccine with peptide-pulsed dendritic cells generated in vitro from CD34(+) hematopoietic progenitor cells. *Int J Cancer* 2000;86:385–392.

206. Murphy GP, et al. Higher-dose and less frequent dendritic cell infusions with PSMA peptides in hormone-refractory metastatic prostate cancer patients. *Prostate* 2000;43:59–62.

207. Lodge PA, Jones LA, Bader RA, et al. Dendritic cell-based immunotherapy of prostate cancer: immune monitoring of a phase II clinical trial. *Cancer Res* 2000;60:829–833.

208. Brossart P, et al. Induction of cytotoxic T-lymphocyte responses in vivo after vaccinations with peptide-pulsed dendritic cells. *Blood* 2000;96:3102–3108.

209. Yu JS, Wheeler CJ, Zeltzer PM, et al. Vaccination of malignant glioma patients with peptide-pulsed dendritic cells elicits systemic cytotoxicity and intracranial T cell infiltration. *Cancer Res* 2001;61:842–847.

210. Banchereau J, Plauka AK, Dhodapkar M, et al. Immune and clinical responses in patients with metastatic melanoma to CD34+ progenitor-derived dendritic cell-vaccine. *Cancer Res* 2001;61:6451–6458.

212. Hsu FJ, et al. Vaccination of patients with B-cell lymphoma using autologous antigen- pulsed dendritic cells. *Nat Med* 1996;2:52–58.

211. Fong L, Brockstedt D, Benike C, et al. Dendritic cell-based xenoantigen vaccination for prostate cancer immunotherapy. *J Immunol* 2001;167:7150–7156.

213. Timmerman JM, Czerwinski DK, Davis TA, et al. Idiotype-pulsed dendritic cell vaccination for B-cell lymphoma: clinical and immune responses in 35 patients. *Blood* 2002;99:1517–1526.

214. Titzer S, et al. Vaccination of multiple myeloma patients with idiotype-pulsed dendritic cells: immunological and clinical aspects. *Br J Haematol* 2000;108:805–816.

215. Liso A, et al. Idiotype vaccination using dendritic cells after autologous peripheral blood progenitor cell transplantation for multiple myeloma. *Biol Blood Marrow Transplant* 2000;6:621–627.

216. Kugler A, et al. Regression of human metastatic renal cell carcinoma after vaccination with tumor cell-dendritic cell hybrids. *Nat Med* 2000;6:332–336.

217. Ludewig B, et al. Immunotherapy with dendritic cells directed against tumor antigens shared with normal host cells results in severe autoimmune disease. *J Exp Med* 2000;191:795–804.

218. Gabrilovich DI, et al. Production of vascular endothelial growth factor by human tumors inhibits the functional maturation of dendritic cells. *Nat Med* 1996;2:1096–1103.

219. Tsuge T, Yamakawa M, Tsukamoto M. Infiltrating dendritic/Langerhans cells in primary breast cancer. *Breast Cancer Res Treat* 2000;59:141–152.

220. Hiltbold EM, Vlad AM, Ciborowski P, et al. The mechanism of unresponsiveness to circulating tumor antigen MUC1 is a block in intracellular sorting and processing by dendritic cells. *J Immunol* 2000;165:3730–3741.

221. Almand B, et al. Clinical significance of defective dendritic cell differentiation in cancer. *Clin Cancer Res* 2000;6:1755–1766.

222. Raje N, et al. Bone marrow and peripheral blood dendritic cells from patients with multiple myeloma are phenotypically and functionally normal despite the detection of Kaposi's sarcoma herpesvirus gene sequences. *Blood* 1999;93:1487–1495.

223. Avigan D, et al. Immune reconstitution following high-dose chemotherapy with stem cell rescue in patients with advanced breast cancer. *Bone Marrow Transplant* 2000;26:169–176.

224. Chaperot L, et al. Differentiation of antigen-presenting cells (dendritic cells and macrophages) for therapeutic application in patients with lymphoma. *Leukemia* 2000;14:1667–1677.

225. Avigan D, et al. Selective in vivo mobilization with granulocyte macrophage colony- stimulating factor (GM-CSF)/granulocyte-CSF as compared to G-CSF alone of dendritic cell progenitors from peripheral blood progenitor cells in patients with advanced breast cancer undergoing autologous transplantation. *Clin Cancer Res* 1999;5:2735–2741.

226. Galy A, Rudraraju S, Baynes R, et al. Recovery of lymphocyte and dendritic cell subsets after autologous CD34+ cell transplantation. *Bone Marrow Transplant* 2000;25:1249–1255.

227. Fearnley DB, Whyte LF, Carnoutsos SA, Cook AH, Hart DN. Monitoring human blood dendritic cell numbers in normal individuals and in stem cell transplantation. *Blood* 1999;93:728.

228. Auffermann-Gretzinger S, Lossos IS, Vayntrub TA, Leong W, Grumet FC, Blume KG, et al. Rapid establishment of dendritic cell chimerism in allogeneic hematopoietic cell transplant recipients. *Blood* 2002;99:1442.

229. Shlomchik WD, Couzens MS, Tang CB, McNiff J, Robert ME, Liu J, et al. Prevention of graft versus host disease by inactivation of host antigen-presenting cells. *Science*1999; 285:412.
230. O'Connell PJ, Li W, Wang Z, Specht SM, Logar AJ, Thomson AW. Immature and mature CD8alpha+ dendritic cells prolong the survival of vascularized heart allografts. *J Immunol* 2002;168:143.
231. Niimi M, Shirasugi N, Ikeda Y, Kan S, Takami H, Hamano K. Operational tolerance induced by pretreatment with donor dendritic cells under blockade of CD40 pathway. *Transplantation* 2001;72:1556.
232. Lutz MB, Suri RM, Niimi M, Ogilvie AL, Kukutsch NA, Rossner S, et al. Immature dendritic cells generated with low doses of GM-CSF in the absence of IL-4 are maturation resistant and prolong allograft survival in vivo. *Eur J Immunol* 2000;30:1813.
233. Alcindor T, Gorgun G, Miller KB, Roberts TF, Sprague K, Schenkein DP, et al. Immunomodulatory effects of extracorporeal photochemotherapy in patients with extensive chronic graft-versus-host disease. *Blood* 2001;98:1622.
234. Rea D, et al. Glucocorticoids transform CD40-triggering of dendritic cells into an alternative activation pathway resulting in antigen-presenting cells that secrete IL-10. *Blood* 2000;95:3162–3127.
235. Matyszak MK, Citterio S, Rescigno M, et al. Differential effects of corticosteroids during different stages of dendritic cell maturation. *Eur J Immunol* 2000;30:1233–1242.
236. Reddy V, et al. G-CSF modulates cytokine profile of dendritic cells and decreases acute graft-versus-host disease through effects on the donor rather than the recipient. *Transplantation* 2000;69:691–693.
237. Arpinati M, Green CL, Heimfeld S, et al. Granulocyte-colony stimulating factor mobilizes T helper 2-inducing dendritic cells. *Blood* 2000;95:2484–2490.
238. Waller EK, Rosenthal H, Jones TW, Peel J, Lonial S, Langston A, Redei I, et al. Larger numbers of CD4(bright) dendritic cells in donor bone marrow are associated with increased relapse after allogeneic bone marrow transplantation. *Blood* 2001;97:2948.
239. Vannucchi AM, Glinz S, Bosi A, Caporale R, Rossi-Ferrini P. Selective ex vivo expansion of cytomegalovirus-specific CD4+ and CD8+ T lymphocytes using dendritic cells pulsed with a human leucocyte antigen A*0201-restricted peptide. *Br J Haematol* 2001;113:479.
240. Grazziutti M, Przepiorka D, Rex JH, Braunschweig I, Vadhan-Raj S, Savary CA. Dendritic cell-mediated stimulation of the in vitro lymphocyte response to Aspergillus. *Bone Marrow Transplant* 2001;27:647.
241 Bacci A, Montagnoli C, Perruccio K, Bozza S, Gaziano R, Pitzurra L, et al. Dendritic cells pulsed with fungal RNA induce protective immunity to Candida albicans in hematopoietic transplantation. *J Immunol* 2002;168:2904.
242. Fujii S, Shimizu K, Fujimoto K, Kiyokawa T, Tsukamoto A, Sanada I, et al. Treatment of post-transplanted, relapsed patients with hematological malignancies by infusion of HLA-matched, allogeneic-dendritic cells (DCs) pulsed with irradiated tumor cells and primed T cells. *Leuk Lymphoma* 2001;42:357.

VII EPILOGUE

27 Epilogue

James R. Mason and Ernest Beutler

1. INTRODUCTION

Allogeneic stem cell transplantation is without doubt a work in progress. As this text so well illustrates, the field of allogeneic stem cell transplantation has evolved from a halting beginning, poorly accepted by the medical profession a mere 35 yr ago, to an established therapy in the management of a variety of malignant and non-malignant conditions. Indeed, in the process of this evolution traditional, allogeneic bone marrow transplantation has become nearly extinct, replaced by the use of peripheral blood stem cells and submyeloablative conditioning regimens. We can now only speculate about the role of allogeneic stem cell transplantation over the next few decades. It is likely that the diseases we currently treat by stem cell transplantation will continue to be targets for this type of therapy and that more than incremental advances will be made in their curability. Yet, it is likely that truly exciting advances in stem cell transplantation will be in some totally new directions.

2. THE FUTURE OF HEMATOPOIETIC STEM CELL THERAPY

2.1. Submyeloablative Allogeneic Transplantation

Submyeloablative allogeneic transplantation provides us with one window of what the future may hold. We now recognize, of course, that ablative doses of chemotherapy are not necessary for hematopoietic stem cell engraftment. Indeed, recent trials have suggested that extraordinarily low doses of chemotherapy or radiation therapy are sufficient to allow the engraftment of hematopoietic cells from the donor. These cells then interact with the host to produce a variety of effects, including reconstitution of the immune system and, most importantly, a graft-vs-malignancy effect. Currently the use of submyeloablative allogeneic transplantation is primitive at best. Multiple centers throughout the world are attempting to optimize the conditioning regimen, emphasizing ever less intense conditioning regimens, and making the procedure safer and more tolerable for the elderly and for those with organ toxicities from prior therapies or disease. At the same time ways to enhance the graft-vs-malignancy phenomenon are being explored.

From: *Current Clinical Oncology: Allogeneic Stem Cell Transplantation*
Edited by: Mary S. Laughlin and Hillard M. Lazarus © Humana Press Inc., Totowa, NJ

2.2. Donor Cells for Patients without HLA-Matched Family Donors

Despite these encouraging advances in hematopoietic and nonhematopoietic stem cell therapy, one major obstacle remains: the availability of healthy donor stem cells. This is a particularly acute problem for hematopoietic cell grafting, but perhaps for nonhematopoietic grafting as well. Many of the patients who most need healthy donor mesenchymal or stem cells cannot serve as the autologous hematopoietic donor because of their own inherent disease. Several possible solutions may be considered. One is to rely on the traditional approach of haploidentical transplantation but not limit donors to family members. With the expansion and use of modern databases, potential donors exist for up to 90% of patients. To date, however, results of transplantation from unrelated haploidentical donors have been disappointing; significant rates of graft-vs-host disease occur and the need for very intensive chemotherapy regimens results in significant patient morbidity. Another approach is the more effective treatment of graft-vs-host disease. Although improvements have been made, the human leukocyte antigen (HLA) barrier remains very much just that: a barrier. The use of other sources of stem cells has been considered. It has been widely known for many years that there are sufficient stem cells in umbilical cord blood to perform an allogeneic transplant. There are some limitations in cell number related to the size of the recipient, but here again, the main problem is the HLA barrier. Although lower in this case due to the inherent phenotype of the cord blood cells, it still remains in place, and graft-vs-host disease, graft rejection, and other issues are still germane to this field. Vigorous attempts have been made to set up national umbilical cord blood banks. However, these banks are very still much in their infancy, and umbilical cord blood is seldom used for adult transplantation in the United States. Fetal stem cells are another exciting potential source of primitive pluri-potential cells. The ethical and social debate that is engendered by their use continues, however, and has effectively hampered the development of this field.

2.3. The Universal Stem Cell

The holy grail of allogeneic stem cell research is the universal donor stem cell and development of the bioreactor in which to produce it. Clearly, producing such cells should be one of our major goals, for not until we are able to generate large numbers of HLA-compatible allogeneic cells (whether they be hematopoietic or nonhematopoietic) will it be possible to employ genetically engineered grafts for the benefit of all patients. This goal has not eluded us for the want of trying. A great deal of effort has been expended to devise various "cocktails" of cytokines known or hoped to stimulate the proliferation of the normally indolent stem cell. While it has been possible to goad this cell into some proliferation (usually at the expense of also causing maturation), we are far from being able to produce the very large numbers of stem cells that are needed. Science moves forward through both empiricism and rational inquiry. In our attempts to amplify stem cells, empiricism has failed us, and rational inquiry has not carried us far enough to be able to apply our knowledge of the regulation of hematopoietic stem cells to their culture in the laboratory. What we need to understand is how the division of stem cells is regulated in nature. What triggers the division of a multipotential stem cell into two multipotential stem cells? One can presume that it must be the proper balance between the various transcriptional factors that activate the mechanism of cell division while, at the same time, the factors that restrain the differentiation of the stem cell into a more mature differentiated hematopoietic cell are inhibited. Unless some lucky break suddenly sheds light on this mysterious mechanism, the answer will probably come only gradually through meticulous investigation of the cellular biology of stem cells. Such an understanding may well come about within the next few years. This optimistic assessment is based on nothing more or less than that the development of technologies for studying gene expression in cells is moving ahead very rapidly.

Even when we are able to amplify stem cells by many-fold, creating cells that can be given to any recipient seems an even more difficult challenge: how are we to persuade the HLA-incompatible host to accept them and, conversely, to persuade grafted cells to accept the host? Better understanding of the mechanism by which the immune system distinguishes between self and non-self could bring us the key for avoiding rejection of universal stem cells and avoiding their rejection of the host. Many negative regulators of the immune response exist and are being better understood. It is becoming increasingly apparent that the activation of T lymphocytes is a complex phenomenon that requires numerous intercellular interactions. Modulation of some of these interactions is being explored in an effort to selectively blunt the immune response.

2.4. Regulating the Direction of Differentiation of Hematopoietic Stem Cells

With better understanding of regulatory mechanisms, it may be possible to direct their differentiation by the administration of small molecules to the patient. This approach was pioneered using the bacterial Tet promoter, which is the promoter that is regulated by tetracycline (1). Genetic engineering allows it to be extended to other effectors. Cells can be engineered to respond positively or negatively to a molecule such as tetracyline, thus turning on or off the targeted gene. It is quite conceivable that a stem cell can be altered so that if drug A is given it is driven to differentiate into platelet, while drug B will promote differentiation into a granulocyte.

2.5. The Use of Autologous Nonhematopoietic Stem Cells

A major problem intrinsic to autologous transplantation is that the disease being treated is usually the result of a somatic mutation in the hematopoietic lineage, and that harvesting the abnormal cells from the patient and returning them to the marrow is not likely to effect a cure. Surprisingly, some success has been achieved in acute leukemia and chronic granulocytic leukemia by infusing remission marrow that may be sufficiently free of mutant cells so as to make possible a cure. In reality, the results of this now-standard approach are far from satisfactory.

It had long been conventional wisdom that each tissue contains stem cells that will repopulate the cells of that lineage but not of other lineages. However, the seminal observations of Friedenstein some 30 yr ago (2) had shown that this was not necessarily the case; fibroblastic adherent cells that had been isolated from bone marrow could be induced to differentiate into bone. We are only now seeing the possibilities for harvesting, growing, and differentiating mesenchymal stem cells and other nonhematopoietic stem cells. Preliminary experiments (3) suggest the ability to produce an ex vivo expansion of mesenchymal progenitor cells of up to 16,000-fold, and these are as yet the crudest of experiments at a time of only minimal understanding of the potential of the nonhematopoietic stem cell. Muscle and neural cells have been shown in recent years to serve as hematopoietic precursors in mice, and if this proves to be the case in man, it could solve this problem. One can envision that a muscle biopsy, for example, could be a source of myoblasts that would be free of the disease-producing mutation of a patient with acute leukemia and repopulate the marrow of the patient.

The concept that stem cells may have the capacity to replace tissues other than those of the organ in which they originated can, of course, be carried far beyond the hematopoietic system. One can easily imagine a time in the near future when nonhematopoietic or mesenchymal cells extracted from peripheral blood by leukopheresis, or perhaps better yet, standard phlebotomy, are expanded ex vivo many thousand-fold and genetically engineered to differentiate into tissues needed for the ailing patient. Cells may be engineered to home to and target those tissues in need of repair and then differentiate into their appropriate cellular structure.

Better understanding of stem cells, their regulation, and their potential for forming or repopulating many different tissues heralds a different type of future: a future in which surgery, chemotherapy, and radiation therapy, currently the stalwarts of medical treatment, are viewed as antiquated, and have instead been replaced by cellular therapy using genetically engineered cells designed to repair tissues and organs to their original state.

ACKNOWLEDGMENT

This is manuscript number 14063-MEM from The Scripps Research Institute. Supported by the Stein Endowment Fund.

REFERENCES

1. Gossen M, Bujard H. Tight control of gene expression in mammalian cells by tetracycline-responsive promoters. *Proc Natl Acad Sci USA* 1992;89:5547–5551.
2. Friedenstein AJ, Piatetzky-Shapiro II, Petrakova KV. Osteogenesis in transplants of bone marrow cells. *J Embryol Exp Morphol* 1966;16:381–390.
3. Lazarus HM, Haynesworth SE, Gerson SL, et al. Ex vivo expansion and subsequent infusion of human bone marrow-derived stromal progenitor cells (mesenchymal progenitor cells): implications for therapeutic use. *Bone Marrow Transplant* 1995;16:557–564.

INDEX